INFERTILITY
COUNSELING
A COMPREHENSIVE HANDBOOK
FOR CLINICIANS

For our husbands, Sheldon Robert Burns, MD and Barry Truitt
Covington, and our children, Alicen Christina Burns and Evan
Robert Burns, Michelle Skiff Covington, Brendan Truitt
Covington, and Laura Stratford Covington. You are the wind
beneath our wings.

INFERTILITY COUNSELING

A COMPREHENSIVE HANDBOOK
FOR CLINICIANS

Edited by

Linda Hammer Burns, PhD
Department of Obstetrics and Gynecology,
University of Minnesota Medical School,
Minneapolis, Minnesota, USA

Sharon N. Covington, MSW
Department of Obstetrics and Gynecology,
Georgetown University School of Medicine,
Washington, DC, USA

Foreword by

Roger D. Kempers, MD
Medical Director, American Society for Reproductive Medicine
Editor Emeritus, *Fertility and Sterility*

The Parthenon Publishing Group
International Publishers in Medicine, Science & Technology

NEW YORK   LONDON

Published in the USA by
The Parthenon Publishing Group Inc.
One Blue Hill Plaza
PO Box 1564, Pearl River
New York 10965, USA

Published in the UK and Europe by
The Parthenon Publishing Group Limited
Casterton Hall, Carnforth
Lancs. LA6 2LA, UK

First published 1999 in hardback

This edition published 2000 in paperback

Library of Congress Cataloging-in-Publication Data
Data available on request

British Library Cataloguing in Publication Data
Data available on request

ISBN 1-84214-065-5

Typeset by Martin Lister Publishing Services, Carnforth, UK

Printed and bound in the USA

Contents

List of Contributors

Linda Hammer Burns, PhD
Assistant Professor
Department of Obstetrics and Gynecology
University of Minnesota Medical School
Minneapolis, Minnesota

Director, Psychological Services
Reproductive Health Associates
St Paul, Maryland
(Chapters 1, 8, 9, 11, 25)

Sharon N. Covington, MSW
Director, Psychological Support Services
Shady Grove Fertility Centers
Rockville, Maryland

Clinical Assistant Professor
Department of Obstetrics and Gynecology
Georgetown University School of Medicine
Washington DC
(Chapters 1, 12, 16, 18, 26)

G. David Adamson, MD
Director, Fertility and Reproductive Health
Institute of Northern California
Palo Alto and San Jose, California

Clinical Professor
Department of Obstetrics and Gynecology
Stanford University School of Medicine
Stanford, California

Assistant Clinical Professor
University of California, San Francisco
(Chapter 28)

Linda D. Applegarth, EdD
Clinical Assistant Professor of Psychology
Departments of Psychiatry and Obstetrics
and Gynecology
Cornell University Medical College
New York, New York

Director, Psychological Services
The Center for Reproductive Medicine and
Infertility
The New York Hospital—Cornell Medical
Center
New York, New York
(Chapters 5, 20)

Randi G. Barrow, JD, Esq.
Attorney, Private Practice
Santa Monica, California
(Chapter 27)

Diane N. Clapp, BSN, RN
Medical Information Director
National RESOLVE, Inc.
Boston, Massachusetts

Private Practice
Lexington, Massachusetts
(Chapter 28)

Dorothy A. Greenfeld, MSW
Clinical Social Worker
Yale Center for Reproductive Medicine
New Haven, Connecticut

Assistant Clinical Professor
Department of Obstetrics and Gynecology
Yale University School of Medicine
New Haven, Connecticut
(Chapter 19)

Elaine R. Gordon, PhD
Psychologist, Private Practice
Santa Monica, California
(Chapter 27)

Nancy Hafkin, PhD
Psychologist, Private Practice
Bethesda, Maryland
(Chapter 16)

Hilary Hanafin, PhD
Psychologist, Private Practice
Los Angeles, California

Coordinator, Psychological Services
The Center for Surrogate Parenting and
Egg Donation
Beverly Hills, California
(Chapter 21)

Mary Casey Jacob, PhD
Associate Professor
Departments of Psychiatry and Obstetrics
and Gynecology
University of Connecticut School of
Medicine
Farmington, Connecticut
(Chapter 14)

William R. Keye, Jr., MD
Director, Division of Reproductive
Endocrinology
Department of Obstetrics and Gynecology
William Beaumont Hospital
Royal Oak, Michigan

Clinical Associate Professor
Department of Obstetrics and Gynecology
University of Michigan School of Medicine
Ann Arbor, Michigan
(Chapter 2)

Sheryl A. Kingsberg, PhD
Assistant Professor of Reproductive Biology
and Psychiatry
Case Western Reserve University School of
Medicine
University Hospitals of Cleveland
Cleveland, Ohio
(Chapters 15,20)

Susan Caruso Klock, PhD
Assistant Professor
Departments of Obstetrics, Gynecology,
and Psychiatry
Northwestern University School of
Medicine
Chicago, Illinois
(Chapter 3)

Bonnie S. LeRoy, MS
Director, Graduate Program in Genetic
Counseling
Institute of Human Genetics
University of Minnesota
Minneapolis, Minnesota
(Chapter 11)

Donald B. Maier, MD
Director, Division of Reproductive
Endocrinology and Infertility
Associate Professor
Department of Obstetrics and Gynecology
University of Connecticut Health Center
Farmington, Connecticut

Director, Division of Reproductive
Endocrinology and Infertility
St. Francis Hospital and Medical Center
Hartford, Connecticut
(Chapter 10)

Louise U. Maier, PhD
Psychologist, Private Practice
Avon Psychological Associates
Avon, Connecticut
(Chapter 10)

Sherry D. Molock, PhD
Associate Professor of Psychology
Director, Clinical Psychology Program
Department of Psychology
Howard University
Washington, DC
(Chapter 13)

Christopher R. Newton, PhD
Psychologist
London Health Sciences Centre

Assistant Professor
Department of Obstetrics and Gynecology
University of Western Ontario
London, Ontario, Canada
(Chapter 6)

Miriam B. Rosenthal, MD
Associate Professor of Psychiatry and
Reproductive Biology
Case Western Reserve School of Medicine

Director, Division of Behavioral Medicine
in Obstetrics and Gynecology
University MacDonald Women's Hospital
Cleveland, Ohio
(Chapter 15)

Linda P. Salzer, MSS
Social Worker, Private Practice
Englewood, New Jersey
(Chapter 22)

Gretchen Sewall, RN, MSW
Fertility and Endocrine Center
Department of Obstetrics and Gynecology
University of Washington
Seattle, Washington
(Chapter 23)

Harriet Fishman Simons, PhD
Social Worker, Private Practice

Adjunct Assistant Professor of Research
Smith College School of Social Work
Wellesley, Massachusetts
(Chapter 17)

Constance Hoenk Shapiro, PhD
Department Head and Professor
Department of Human and Community
Development
University of Illinois at Urbana–
Champaign
Urbana, Illinois
(Chapter 7)

Annette L. Stanton, PhD
Associate Professor of Psychology
Director, Graduate Specialty in Clinical
Health Psychology
University of Kansas
Lawrence, Kansas
(Chapter 8)

Katherine E. Williams, MD
Women's Wellness Clinic
Stanford University Medical Center
Stanford, California
(Chapter 4)

Aline P. Zoldbrod, PhD
Psychologist, Private Practice
Lexington, Massachusetts
(Chapter 18)

Foreword

Over the past two decades, our knowledge and understanding of reproductive medicine have been substantially expanded through extraordinary theoretical, investigative and clinical research. This has led to many remarkable advances in the reproductive medicine technologies designed for the treatment of infertility. Newly created frontiers have been continuous. The advent of these wonders has simultaneously brought enormous challenges to other disciplines. Among these, bioethics has been challenged to provide thoughtful recommendations for a wide array of new ethical issues. Another field, reproductive health psychology, has been propelled into an important role in reproductive medicine. The resulting discipline is that of Infertility Counseling, vital to excellence in the diagnosis and treatment of infertility. Infertility Counseling as a specialty combines mental health professionals with careers as social workers, psychologists, psychiatrists, marriage and family therapists and psychiatric nurses. These dedicated practitioners provide invaluable support through patient education and emotional and therapeutic counseling.

During the past two decades, as Editor-in-Chief of *Fertility and Sterility*, I was privileged to review and publish many important juried papers on investigative and clinical advances in reproductive medicine. During that time, mental health professionals took their proper place among the teams that managed the care of infertile couples. It was with great pride that *Fertility and Sterility* published many excellent contributions to the scientific literature these professionals generated. These articles, as cited in the bibliographies of the chapters of this book, included studies of psychosocial issues, psychological evaluations and counseling strategies. A number of these exceptional reports, including editorials, came from the two co-authors of this book, Sharon N. Covington, MSW, and Linda Hammer Burns, PhD, and their leadership skills, as evidenced by their clinical research published in *Fertility and Sterility*, as well as other journals; their roles as founding members and chairs of the Mental Health Professional Group of the American Society for Reproductive Medicine, and their devoted membership on committees that developed documents such as Qualification Guidelines for Infertility Counselors are all a matter of record. Their efforts helped to establish Infertility Counseling as an integral professional service in the care of infertile couples.

With the maturation of this specialty has come the urgent need for a comprehensive, integrated ready source of information. The authors once again have taken a leadership position by crafting this exhaustive state-of-the-art textbook. Drawing from their extensive backgrounds in education, research and clinical practice, they have carefully organized a selection of chapters covering the full range of topics on infertility counseling. A valuable inclusion in the book is the section of appendices. This contains a collection of the guideline documents developed by committees from the Mental Health Professional Group as well as sample consent forms for a variety of clinical situations. The book's chapters were carefully edited for consistency and balance.

The authors direct the readers' attention to historical perspectives, theoretical consideration and currently recommended therapeutic interventions. While they have contributed many of the chapters themselves, a number of critical sections have been provided by distinguished colleagues based on their special knowledge and experience in specific areas.

This important book is designed for serious students and practitioners of infertility counseling. It will be a valuable resource text for medical libraries and will grace the personal libraries of mental health professionals, students of reproductive medicine, clinicians and educators alike.

Roger D. Kempers, MD
Medical Director
American Society for Reproductive Medicine
Birmingham, AL

Editor Emeritus
Fertility and Sterility

Preface

Writers are really people who write books not because they are poor, but because they are dissatisfied with the books which they could buy but do not like.

Walter Benjamin

There are any number of reasons why people write (or edit) books, although it is difficult to say that actually editing a book was our initial motivation when we started this project. Furthermore, it is difficult to say *when* this project began. One view is that it began when Sharon was one of the instrumental founding members of the Mental Health Professional Group—a group of motivated and inspired mental health professionals who had the idea that infertility counseling was an important and integral specialty in its own right. Another view is that it began at the American Society for Reproductive Medicine in Seattle in 1996, when we realized at the same time that there was no book on infertility counseling and that perhaps there might be an interest in one. What surprised us most when we began to float this idea was how many people agreed it was a good idea.

Over the years we each have worked with the American Society of Reproductive Medicine, which we remember as the American Fertility Society, in a variety of capacities including as chairs of the Mental Health Professional Group and on various ASRM committees. And although this work helped us meld special relationships with the society's directors and staff, we were overwhelmed with their enthusiasm and encouragement about this project. Every time (and it was many) we needed help they responded promptly and usually in spades!

Each and every one deserves a special thank you, but most especially Dr Roger Kempers, Dr Ben Younger, Nancy Hayley, Kathy Fleck, Michelle Parker, and Jennifer Kelly who, in their best southern hospitality, made us feel that our requests warranted special attention.

Most importantly we wish to thank our contributors, all of whom are highly respected professionals in their own right. For the majority, their contributions have not simply been their chapters, but their professional encouragement, expertise, and/or suggestions. We appreciate their effort, time, and investment in this field which many have seen develop into a respected professional specialty due to their own efforts. Finally, we wish to express our appreciation for their willingness to contribute their expertise and knowledge to this volume and for their patience and tolerance of our suggestions, critiques, and 'improvements'. We hope (and think) that, despite our sometimes exacting demands, we have kept their friendships and they are well aware of our gratitude.

We must also thank our respective practices and colleagues with whom we work each day. For Linda, this has been at the University of Minnesota Medical School, Department of Obstetrics and Gynecology, as well as Reproductive Health Associates. First, a special thanks must go to Dr George Tagatz, who, so many years ago, said in such a casual and disarming way, 'Linda, how would you like to work here?' and then let me design and implement a program of infertility counseling which grew into a program of women's health psychology. His confidence, and that of Department Chair, Dr Leo Twiggs, have been instrumental, and I wish to thank them for 'letting me do my thing' with their blessings. A special thanks must go to the secretarial staff, who were wonderful in compensating for me when I had too many balls in the air. At Reproductive Health Associates I owe a special debt to all my colleagues, but especially the physicians and nurses for being exceedingly helpful, often by providing curbside consultation or late night conferencing. These include Drs Theodore Nagel, Jasques Stassart, Jack Malo, John Pryor, and Hugh Hensleigh, and nurses Deb Pearo, Selina Blatz, and Neda Tasson. They have all tolerated my big ideas (even when a bit wary) and supported my various other commitments and interests without complaint. In addition, I owe a special debt of gratitude to psychologists Sue V. Petzel, PhD and Barbara Senneseth, MA, who provided encouragement and ideas as well as a willingness to pick up the slack when I was preoccupied or overwhelmed. A simple thank you is not enough and I hope they know how much I appreciate them and their friendship. I feel especially privileged and blessed to have worked with colleagues who have provided not only support but camaraderie.

For Sharon, this has been the entire staff of the Shady Grove Fertility Centers who have given their expertise, enthusiasm, and support whenever necessary: specifically my colleagues on the counseling staff. Katherine Hirsch, LCSW-C, Patricia Sachs, LCSW-C, Carol Toll, LCSW-C, and Catherine Tuck, MA deserve special thanks for having tolerated my stress level, assisting with helpful feedback on some of my chapters, and picking up on additional responsibilities when necessary. A special appreciation is extended to Dr Arthur Sagoskin, who has always shared my vision of the need for infertility counseling, and whose good nature and genuine concern have continually been a source of strength to me. In addition, Drs Denise Murray, Eric Weidra, Michael Levy, Robert Stillman, and Gil Mottla have generously shared their expertise and have never seemed to have minded being cornered at the office for a quick consult on this book. Undoubtedly, I have always felt a tremendous and unwavering support from our outstanding nursing staff at Shady Grove, with special recognition to Karen Moore, Kathy Bugga, and Susan Knox, who believed in this project from the beginning, Deep appreciation is extended to dear friends and colleagues Linda Applegarth, EdD and Nancy Hafkin, PhD, who helped (or put up with) me from beginning to end, with guidance, direction, humor, and loving support, and to Dr Paul Feldman, whose vision and support started me on my path to infertility counseling.

Of course, we realize that a book such as this could not have been written without a fair bit of clinical expertise, and for that we owe a special debt of gratitude to our patients. In their suffering and resilience they taught us, and from their pain and transcendence we learned. We feel honored and privileged to have been included in their journeys through infertility. We are who we are today because of these special clients, and this project could not have been possible without them.

Without a doubt, we owe a special debt to our families, who kept our equilibrium through personal and family crises, developmental transitions, and daily hassles. Our children pitched in as teenage computer experts, research assistants, receptionists, secretarial staff, and *aides-de-camp*, with only minimal good-natured grumbling. Our husbands, who from ground zero thought this was a good idea, provided more encouragement and support than can be described. They never wavered in their affection and comfort, lifting our lagging spirits, tolerating our self-imposed work schedules, and filling in on our family and social obligations when we could not. We feel especially blessed to have such special husbands and families and, obviously, could not have completed this book without them.

Finally, we would be remiss without thanking our publishers at Parthenon, and especially Nat Russo and Roseann Caserio, who were enthusiastic from the start and let us develop this book with our own vision. A special thanks to Paul Smith, our editor in London, who provided excellent editorial assistance, while also exhibiting impressive patience and tolerance with two inexperienced Yankees. We would also be remiss without thanking each other. We are not quite certain what the dynamics were that made it so amazingly easy and smooth to work together, but it was. While the trials and tribulations of our professional and personal lives pressed on, we somehow were able to keep a forward motion with patience, understanding, and a good sense of humor. In the process, we mastered every form of modern-day communication, across continents and through all forms of weather—not to mention living together for extended periods. Our amicable and enjoyable partnership has probably been due in large measure to our shared vision of this book, so that whenever trouble arose we returned to focus on that shared vision. Our agreeable partnership may also have been the result of our own personal characteristics which we have come to value and appreciate in each other: communication, compromise, intelligence, good-humor, and work ethic.

Linda Hammer Burns
Sharon N. Covington

I. OVERVIEW

1

Psychology of Infertility

Linda Hammer Burns, PhD, and Sharon N. Covington, MSW

A child within my mind. I see
the eye, the hands. I see you also there.
I see you waiting with an honest care,
Within my mind, within my body
And birth and death close to us constantly.

Elizabeth Jennings

Yearning for children and the heartbreak of barrenness have been a part of life since the beginning of mankind, chronicled throughout history by religious accounts, myths, legends, art, and literature. Whether driven by biological drive, social necessity, or psychological longing, the pursuit of a child or children has compelled men and women to seek a variety of remedies, sometimes even extreme measures. In fact, in all cultures involuntary childlessness is recognized as a crisis that has the potential to threaten the stability of individuals, relationships, and communities. Every society has culturally approved 'solutions' to infertility involving, either alone or together, alterations of social relationships (e.g., divorce, adoption), spiritual intercession (e.g., prayer, pilgrimage to spiritually powerful site,) or medical interventions (e.g., taking of herbs, consultation with 'medicine man')[1].

While spiritual and medical remedies for infertility are common and often employed early on by infertile couples, social solutions demanding the alteration of relationships have been shown to be the last alternative individuals or couples usually consider[1]. Typically, infertile couples are reluctant to jeopardize or disturb close relationships, perhaps because social changes are usually permanent or because they hope or believe infertility will be a temporary problem. By the same token, reluctance to consider social solutions may be due to the hope and promise often attributed to medical and/or spiritual interventions. Nonetheless, infertile couples employ all three measures— social, spiritual, and medical—as remedies for their involuntary childlessness; numerous examples of these remedies exist throughout history and across all cultures[1].

One of the most renowned social solutions to involuntary childlessness is King Henry VIII of England, who changed the religion and laws of a country to accommodate the need for a child (albeit a male child). Divorce, polygamy, and extramarital affairs remain, as they have long been, social solutions to infertility, as do various forms of adoption and fostering. Examples of other social solutions include the continuing practice in some African and middle Eastern cultures of multiple wives in response to infertility (or lack of a son) or the traditional East Asian custom requiring an eldest brother to provide one of his own sons to a childless younger brother. Community involvement in the realignment of social relationships is exemplified by the native peoples of two small islands off the coast of South America in which infertility was addressed by raiding the neighboring island to steal small children for childless women. Demonstrable in each of these examples is the social and emotional distress and expense of solutions involving the alteration of social relationships. This explains, in part, the reluctance of individuals to pursue these alternatives until other remedies have been exhausted.

Since antiquity, the appeal of religious faith and the power of belief in spirits and gods as a remedy for infertility can be found in nearly all cultures. Fertility symbols, special gods, and fertility rites and customs are apparent from the highly erotic art of India, to the Celtic goddess of fertility carved into stoned walls of ancient Irish castles, to specially shaped and painted Navajo pottery. In addition, the special spiritual power of certain places to enhance fertility can be seen in a phallic-shaped rock on the island of Maui in Hawaii, as well as in the pilgrimages made by infertile women of the Carib tribe in Mexico to Isla de las Mujeres (Island of Women) and by many infertile Roman Catholic women to Medjugorje in Yugoslavia. Nevertheless, the importance of faith either as a means of solving infertility or as a source of comfort cannot be minimized, and religious faith remains a powerful resource for many infertile individuals even today.

Medical solutions to infertility are the most common and, it may be argued, most acceptable solutions to infertility in 20th-century America. In the past, medical treatments for infertility often focused on eating special foods, vaginal treatments, or medicines enhancing male sexual potency. For example, there is a custom in Africa of applying a special powder made from the crushed roots of nine trees to the penis to enable a man to have sexual intercourse three times a night[2]. Other examples of medical treatments include the eating of spiders by Siberian women, the use by African women of vaginal pessaries made of wool dipped in peanut oil and wrapped in two cloves of garlic, and 19th-century Western physicians' recommendations of bleeding with leeches or carrying St John's Wort[2]. Whether the 'primitive' medical treatments of the past or the sophisticated assisted reproductive technologies commonplace today, medical treatments for infertility have particular power and influence for infertile couples.

Finally, infertility as a recognizable crisis across all cultures and throughout history represents the fundamental importance of children and parenting to men and women, their families, and societies. While infertility typically triggers remedy-seeking behaviors, the nature of acceptable remedies is influenced by a variety of factors, such as individual preferences, culture, religion, place, or point in history.

The focus of this book is the complex psychological aspects of infertility and the provision of infertility counseling. As such, this chapter will serve both as an overview of the psychology of infertility and an introduction to the content of the book. It will outline the scope and depth of issues involved in:

- infertility counseling, assessment, and treatment

- medical diagnosis of infertility and its treatment, including atypical medical conditions and special populations

- alternative family building, involving adoption and third-party reproduction

- post-infertility issues such as pregnancy and parenting

- infertility counseling clinical practice issues.

HISTORICAL OVERVIEW

In colonial America, children were necessary for propagation of the colonies and, most important, for economic survival. Further, childlessness was thought to be the result of a woman's sinful ways, and the very idea of attempting to alleviate infertility was viewed as defiance of the will of God[3,4]. People who were voluntarily childless were called 'shirkers', as they failed to contribute to the economic stability and well-being of the community[3]. However, infertility did not necessarily mean that a couple faced childlessness or exclusion from the community. Most couples took in the children of family members or 'adopted' children from siblings as biological heirs while the biological parents continued to maintain ties with the children[4]. Cultural shifts during the 18th century affected family life and patterns of family formation, moving American families away from a communal society to a society founded on single-family units of married couples and their offspring[4].

Before the industrial revolution of the 19th century, children were valued primarily for their economic utility. With the institution of child labor laws, a monumental social change occurred: Children were displaced from the work force and came to be valued for their affectional ties, companionship, and stimulation. Thus, children became *functionally worthless* but *emotionally priceless* companions. Griel[5] suggests that this shift in values may explain differences in the meaning of children to men and women. Historically, men invested in having children (especially sons) out of a need to have a material and spiritual heir; children, like wives, were the chattel property of men. With the industrial revolution, children became less valuable as *economic* investments providing economic return and more valuable as *emotional* investments providing emotional warmth and affection, typically the domain of women. It was this value shift that, Griel speculates, accounts for the decline in men's investment in children.

By the beginning of the 20th century, reproduction had become less a matter of having children than of having the *right* children: only worthy parents were fit to bear and rear worthy children. This cultural shift, termed the *privatization of happiness*, represented a shift in American society from the community as a source of emotional investment and reward to a society in which the family is the ideological center of happiness[3]. In this view, the current high value of children— 'a child at any price'—is the result of contemporary American culture in that 'public life appears bankrupt and alienating, [so that] Americans with or without children will continue their pursuit of happiness in the ... private areas of their lives' and children will remain the focus of this private drive[3].

While infertility rates have remained surprisingly the same for a century (10–13%)[6], the use and availability of infertility treatment have dramatically increased, especially over the past 25 years. Furthermore, although men are infertile as often as women, throughout the past three centuries in America, women have disproportionately borne the medical, social, and cultural burden of a couple's failure to conceive[4]. Now, at the end of the 20th century, infertility has been converted from a social state to a medical condition: a process of 'medicalization' of infertility in which there has been a shift in emphasis from 'coping with childlessness through social means (e.g., participating in the rearing of others' children), to a dependence on medical intervention'[4]. While social conditions have limited the availability of children for adoption, assisted reproductive technologies have increased the notion of perfect 'designer' infants available to an increasing array of infertile, childless, and even repeat parents. Now the cultural and social pressures on the infertile couple are not simply the consequences of their childlessness, but pressures to use (or at least consider) assisted reproductive technologies.

REVIEW OF LITERATURE

Original investigations into the psychological aspects of infertility focused on individual psychopathology and were largely based on theoretical speculations or anecdotal information rather than rigorous scientific investigation. Much of the research was exploratory, relied on researcher-designed instruments rather than standard measures, lacked control or comparison groups, and were plagued by small numbers. Although the scientific rigor of psychosocial investigations remains a continuing problem, in actuality, the overall quality and quantity of studies have dramatically improved over the past 20 years, as have the researchers and the availability of research funds.

More recently, the focus of research on the psychological aspects of infertility has shifted from individual psychopathology to more holistic/interactive views of infertility and to the impact of advancing assisted reproductive technologies. Consequently, there has been a shift from a singular focus on the individual to assessments and interventions aimed at groups, such as couples and families. In addition, while research and clinical experience continue to indicate that the vast majority of infertile men and women *do not* experience significant levels of psychological trauma or psychopathology, the use of advanced medical technology and/or third-party reproduction involving a plethora of additional stressors may increase psychological distress during specific periods of the treatment cycle. As such, investigations into responses to assisted reproduction have again involved the interactive aspects of medical technology and individual and couple response, as well as medical outcome.

Each aspect of the psychology of infertility addressed in this volume has involved some measure of psychosocial research and, as such, is included in the chapters addressing the specific topic. The following review of research provides an overview of current research on the psychology of infertility, focusing on four areas: motivations for parenthood in infertile couples, psychological reactions to infertility, psychological responses to infertility in men versus women, and psychological responses to assisted reproductive technologies.

Motivations for Parenthood

Hoffman and Hoffman[7] in a conceptualization of motivations for parenthood in a normal population enumerated eight categories: adult status and social identity, expansion of self, moral values, group ties and affection, stimulation and fun, achievement and creativity, power and influence, social comparison, and economic utility. In a study of motives for having children in involuntarily childless couples, van Balen and Trimbos-Kemper[8] found that the desire for children was very strong, especially among women, even after a lengthy (8.6 years) period of infertility. For both men and women, the primary motive for wanting children was happiness and well-being, while social control and continuity were unimportant to both men and women. Newton and colleagues[9] assessed motives for parenthood of infertile women and men participating in an in vitro fertilization program, reporting that women placed greatest emphasis on fulfilling gender-role requirements, while men were more likely to stress a desire for marital completion as motivation. Although the long period of infertility treatment appears to stimulate the process of thinking and rethinking the reasons for having children, most couples do not abandon the desire for a family. Furthermore, this process may help infertile men and women develop a more realistic perception of the demands and rewards of children.

Psychological Reactions to Infertility

In a comprehensive review of available research on psychological reactions to infertility, Dunkel-Schetter and Lobel[10] investigated both descriptive and empirical research. Their conclusion on descriptive reports was that a greater focus was placed on the emotional effects of infertility than on loss of control, changes in identity or esteem, or social effects. And while the descriptive literature characterized infertile individuals as a group in substantial distress, the authors concluded that research subjects may represent a unique and select sample of individuals who decided to pursue medical treatment or infertility counseling. They further suggested that the psychological effects of infertility represent a web of interrelated reactions rather than distinct or independent responses.

In terms of the empirical research, Dunkel-Schetter and Lobel[10] concluded that the evidence *did not* clearly indicate that negative effects accompany infertility, although there is some evidence of adverse effects in a few studies. They found that 'empirical evidence from scientifically rigorous research on the psychological effects of infertility does not support contentions that specific reactions are common'[10]. While several studies have indicated abnormally high levels of depression or low self-esteem, few have replicated these findings. Furthermore,

methodologically rigorous research suggests that the majority of people with infertility *do not* experience clinically significant emotional reactions, loss of self-esteem, or adverse marital and sexual consequences. However, there were indications that infertility affects individual identity and self-image, especially in terms of present and ideal selves. Dunkel-Schetter and Lobel concluded 'that the average infertile individual does not experience severe or clinically significant distress, marital problems, sexual problems, or other psychological difficulties, or is there evidence for a set sequence of emotional reactions'.

Psychological Responses in Men versus Women

Research on gender differences in psychological responses to infertility indicate that women experience greater levels of psychosocial distress in response to infertility than men[5,11-14]. In a review of empirical research on gender differences, Wright and colleagues[15] concluded that women tended to be more distressed by the infertility experience and its medical treatment than men, even when the infertility diagnosis was not attributable to her[16-18] or when the diagnosis was ambiguous[19,20]. However, women also appear to be more likely to seek information and assistance and may be better able to identify and access other areas of potential social support outside of their marriages[5,11,21]

Infertility diagnosis appears to be a factor in men's psychological adjustment to infertility, in that men with male-factor infertility exhibit more negative emotional response to infertility including more feelings of stigma, loss, and poor self-esteem[16]. In addition, men tend to make more self-denigrating remarks if the infertility diagnosis is male-factor. In coping with emotional responses to infertility, men appear more often to use denial, distancing, avoidance, and withdrawal into themselves and are less likely to seek social support, counseling, or discussions with caregivers[11,15,21]. One longitudinal study of infertile men found that a man's coping strategy with earlier phases of infertility impacted his long-term adjustment: Men who substituted an object (e.g., house, pet, garden) or a child (e.g., leading a church youth group) to nurture during this period were more likely to achieve generativity and parenthood, while those who used self-centered substitutes (e.g., body building) failed to achieve either generativity or fatherhood by midlife[22].

Psychological Responses to Assisted Reproductive Technologies

Over the past 20 years in vitro fertilization (IVF) has moved from an experimental procedure to an accepted medical treatment with over 15,000 IVF babies born worldwide. However, despite these advances, IVF and its variations continue to have only minimal success rates, typically less than 20%; in 1993, for example, 81.2% of attempted IVFs did not result in pregnancy[18]. While as recently as 10 years ago IVF was the last available medical treatment modality available for infertile couples, now variations of IVF, including third-party reproduction (e.g., donated gametes, gestational carrier) and assisted medical technologies (e.g., intracytoplasmic sperm injection), are increasingly available. However, these options also strain traditional meanings of parenthood and have the potential for endangering the fetus, the physical health of the mother, and emotional or marital equilibrium, as well as transmitting unknown genetic disorders. As such, an increasing number of studies have investigated psychological well-being before, during, and after assisted reproduction to assess psychological factors as mediating forces in successful outcomes and psychological response to unsuccessful outcomes.

In an early review of psychological studies of IVF and embryo transfer (IVF/ET) participants, Mazure and Greenfeld[23] investigated (1) psychological profiles of women and their partners requesting IVF/ET, (2) clinical reports describing the psychological experience of IVF/ET and providing recommendations for counseling both before and during IVF/ET, and (3) follow-up studies of IVF/ET participants. They found that IVF/ET participants scored within normal limits on measurements of preexisting psychopathology and that researchers consistently had difficulty documenting reactive anxiety or stress-related emotional difficulties using standardized psychological tests, even though there was clinical evidence of these reactions.

In short, individuals undergoing assisted reproduction appear to be at no greater risk for psychological disturbances, although there may be a greater risk of anxiety, distress, and grief, especially if the procedure is unsuccessful[24-27]. Factors contributing to grief reaction following unsuccessful IVF/ET included a belief that the treatment is the couple's last chance at having a biological child, preexisting psychological illness, and overestimation of personal success[25,26,28-31]. More recent research has shown that mood (anxiety, depression, or distress) probably fluctuates in both men and women over the course of an assisted reproductive treatment cycle: anxiety and depression increasing on oocyte-retrieval day, decreasing on embryo-transfer day, and rising again on pregnancy-testing day. However, severity of response appears to diminish with repeat cycles[26,32,33].

Much of current research on third-party reproduction has been descriptive studies of oocyte donors and gestational carriers: motivation (altruism), socioeconomic status (middle class), age (under 30), education (some college), and marital status (single). Research also has focused on the psychological suitability and/or stability of participants, with the majority of research indicating that *accepted* donors and gestators were at no increased risk of developing psychopathology during or as a result of participation, although there was evidence of history of past traumatic experiences or loss related to reproduction[34-43].

THEORETICAL PERSPECTIVE

Theoretical approaches to infertility have evolved over the years from what Berg and Wilson[44] referred to as the *psychogenic infertility model*, in which demonstrable psychopathology was thought to play an etiological role in infertility, to a *psychological sequelae model*, in which psychological factors were considered the result of infertility. More recently, theoretical approaches have adopted systemic or psychosocial models rather than the individual psychopathology or psychogenic approaches more common in the past. The application of a broader spectrum of theoretical approaches has led to a less individualistic perspective and more holistic approach in which the interactions among individuals, couples, and social and medical factors are considered. These perspectives have also increased understanding of individual and couple differences and resiliency, while providing research foundations and therapeutic interventions.

Psychogenic Infertility Model

The psychogenic infertility model (also referred to as a psychosomatic medicine approach) was introduced in the 1930s and reached its height of popularity during the pronatalist period of the 1950s and 1960s. At a time when up to 50% of infertility problems could not be medically diagnosed or treated, psychological explanations of reproductive problems in terms of causation or treatment were considered helpful and reasonable. However, the vast majority of these theories focused on psychological (and subconscious) disturbances *in women*, contending that neurotic conflicted feelings about motherhood or their own mothers prevented conception and therefore assumption of an adult role. Fischer[45] described two personality styles in women contributing to infertility: the weak, emotionally immature, overprotected type, and the ambitious, masculine, aggressive, and dominating career type. The 'weak' woman was thought to be unable to separate/differentiate from her mother or express her anger in a direct fashion, or she had an abnormal fear of sex, motherhood, pregnancy, and labor that inhibited reproductive ability. 'Ambitious' women were infertile because 'becoming pregnant meant accepting sexual feelings, being comfortable in competing with a stronger maternal figure, giving up the fantasy of remaining a child, and not having to compete with an unborn child'[46].

Typically, 'psychogenically infertile' men were thought to have domineering mothers who overcontrolled their sons by threatening withdrawal of love, expecting conformity to their rigid moral codes, or creating anxiety within their sons as a result of their own sexual inhibitions[47]. Men, too, were thought to have conflicted feelings about parenthood or masculinity causing infertility[48]. This theory was recycled during the sexual revolution of the 1960s in descriptions of the 'new impotence'—men experiencing impotence as a result of performance pressure from 'liberated' women who expected sexual encounters to be mutually rewarding[49].

The psychogenic infertility model fell into disfavor partly as a result of the increased ability of reproductive medicine to diagnose and treat infertility problems. During the past 20 years, infertility of unknown etiology has been 5% or less, eliminating the necessity and/or feasibility of psychological causes of reproductive failure. More importantly, several reviewers of the psychogenic infertility literature concluded that the preponderance of studies revealed no consistent or striking evidence of psychological causes of infertility[50–53].

Psychoanalytic Theory

Psychoanalytic theory, based on Freud's theory of personality, provided the basis for the psychogenic model. It contended that psychological disorders resulted from anxiety produced by unresolved conflicts and forces of which a person may be unaware. Infertility, when not caused by organic pathology, was considered a defense against the dangers inherent in the procreative function[54]. A defense is an unconscious function of the ego to protect the self against the dangers originating within the self, that is, the physiological process of reproductive function. Further, maladjustment occurs when a person relies on too many defense mechanisms (e.g., repression) or when defense mechanisms fail. In short, psychosomatic infertility is caused by unresolved oedipal issues, conflicted sexual identity, and defenses against the conflictual relationship between self and parents (i.e., a woman's hostile identification with her mother)[48].

Psychological Sequelae Model

The psychological sequelae model developed in the late 1970s, facilitated by the work of Menning[55], introduced the concept that infertility was an emotionally difficult experience, impacting all aspects of an individual and couple's life. Hence, infertility was the *consequence* and not the cause of childlessness. The psychological sequelae model encompasses a broad view of the interrelationships of individual, couple, family, society, and reproductive medicine. It integrates different theoretical frameworks to provide an eclectic picture of the psychological aspects of infertility and treatment approaches. The psychological sequelae approach includes the theory of ego and self psychology, developmental and crisis theory, grief and loss theory, cognitive-behavioral theory, family systems theory, and gender-based theories.

Ego and Self Psychology Theory

Psychoanalytic theory has continued to contribute to the understanding of infertility primarily through ego psychology and object relations. Ego psychology or the psychology of self is based on the principles of psychoanalysis in which the ego (an individual's perceived sense of self) is formed early as the central psychic structure. Narcissistic responses, including fantasies of grandiosity and uniqueness, can impair object-relatedness and reality testing. Narcissistic injuries can lead to rage reactions and other regressive responses. According to self psychology, the narcissistic trauma of infertility is experienced as an injury to self-cohesion leading to anxiety, fragmentation, and more archaic forms of self-organization. Hence, a reorganization of the self is necessary to cope with the lost ideal as a biological parent and the loss of one's biological immortality.

Kohut's[56] *psychology of self*, based on psychoanalytic theory, views a stable sense of self as central to happiness and well-being. When a loss is fundamental to an individual's sense of self, there is a perceptible self-deficit with concomitant loss of hopefulness, depression, and feelings of shame. Predictably, altered self-concept and self-image are significant factors for both infertile men and women, although frequently for different reasons: Women often feel inadequate and deficient for failing to fulfill personal and societal roles, while men typically feel inferior, ashamed, and angry.

Internalization of the infertility experienced is instrumental in managing the narcissistic wounds of infertility, according to Olshansky[57]. Thus, to move away from infertility as a central focus in life, infertile individuals must make it a part of their individual identity and self-definition. Sandelowski's[58] research on this perspective indicated that integration of the infertility experience involves defining infertility functionally, behaviorally, empirically, and phenomenologically, giving meaning and purpose to a painful experience resulting in triumph over it. However, this research also found that not all individuals needed to make infertility a part of their personal identity to deal with it appropriately.

The concept of *stigma* in infertile men and women contains a self-perception of loss, role failure, and diminished esteem. Stigma involves the failure to fulfill cultural norms and extends to the social identity of the whole person, polluting his or her other accomplishments[59]. Infertile men and women often express feelings of defectiveness, inadequacy, inferiority, worthlessness, and guilt. Recent research indicates that men and women do not differ in feelings of stigma: Men with male-factor infertility were more stigmatized than men without male-factor infertility, and women were stigmatized by infertility regardless of whether it was attributable to male or female factor[16]. Infertility, as an externally invisible 'defect', increases feelings of inferiority, differentness, and spoiled identity[60,61].

Developmental and Crisis Theory

Erickson[62] proposed a *developmental life stage model* in which eight psychosocial stages of development from infancy to adulthood were outlined along with psychological tasks for completion in each stage. According to Erickson, early adulthood involves the ability to form close and lasting relationships characterized by intimacy (versus isolation), while middle adulthood is concerned with establishing and guiding the next generation, characterized by the psychosocial achievement of generativity (versus self-absorption). Failure to establish intimate relationships or generativity results in isolation and stagnation, during which the individual fails to mature, achieve developmental tasks, or follow societal expectations, causing feelings of despair and abnormality.

Menning[55] applied the developmental stage model to infertility by pointing out that the inability to procreate creates a block to the adult tasks of intimacy and generativity. The block contributes to the infertile couple's experience by emphasizing both psychological tasks and social expectations that are impossible for them to achieve. Having internalized the tasks and expectations of relationships and parenthood (or intimacy and generativity), the infertile man or woman usually feels more pressure than less traditionally socialized or more psychologically egocentric individuals. Furthermore, pressures to perform certain tasks or achieve specific milestones result in feelings of dysynchronization with peers, failure, stigma, and inferiority.

Menning[55] also suggested that this developmental block precipitated a life crisis for the infertile person or couple. *Crisis theory* is based on individual response and adaptation to a crisis in which the individual is thrown into a state of helplessness and coping strategies are no longer successful in mastering the problem. The crisis state cannot continue and is resolved over time, leading to improved adaptation by strengthened coping abilities, to a return to previous equilibrium, or to poor adaptation if coping resources have failed. As a life crisis, infertility is considered an insolvable problem that threatens important life goals, taxes personal resources, and arouses unresolved problems from the past. Menning contended that infertility involved a period of emotional disequilibrium, with the potential for either maladjustment or positive growth, that pushes people toward resolution and homeostasis. The crisis of infertility may reawaken earlier experiences of loss, and the outcome is usually dependent on the quality of available social support during the crisis, the individual's perception of the crisis, internal resources for managing the crisis, and, significantly, the infertile couple's ability to give meaning to the experience and achieve personal growth through it.

Grief and Loss Theory

The *grief and loss model* was initially applied to infertility by Menning[63] to explain the typical feelings and psychological responses to infertility in both men and women. Menning applied the five stages of Kübler-Ross's death and dying model (shock, denial, anger, bargain, acceptance) to describe the typical feelings and the myriad of losses grieved during infertility, including the loss of hopes, dreams, future plans, marital satisfaction, self-esteem, sense of control, belief in the fairness of life, health and well-being, and, most important, the 'dream child'. In addition, Menning contended that infertility losses evoke a predictable pattern of feelings requiring recognition, working through, and overcoming in order to attain effective resolution.

It has been suggested that a *stage model* of bereavement may imply a process that 'fixes' the individual at a particular place

despite intervening variables[64]. For this reason, a *phase model* is recommended that serves as a guide for a free-flowing process in which the individual moves back and forth while grieving. A 'process-directed' approach is Bowlby's[65] grief model, based on attachment and human information-processing theory in which the phases of grief are: (1) numbing, (2) yearning and searching, (3) disorganization and despair, and (4) reorganization[65]. This model or modifications of it (e.g., Sanders[64] and Parkes[66]) provide a dynamic approach that not only acknowledges typical responses to grief but recognizes the necessity for the individual's active participation in the process[64,66]. In addition, the application of grief models helps define (and perhaps predict) a couple's response to the loss of their longed-for child. It also provides a guide for the infertility counselor in terms of therapeutic interventions and facilitation of recovery. Sanders[64], in a model that moves the bereaved gradually from external to internal self-awareness, suggested that psychoanalytic/client-centered therapies are most suited to the initial phase of grief (numbing, shock, and awareness of loss), while humanistic/ existential therapies are most appropriate to phases two and three (yearning, searching, disorganization and despair) and behavioral therapies to phase four (reorganization, healing and renewal). Through the experience and expression of emotions involved in the grieving process, the infertile couple is thought to move toward an acceptance of their infertile state, engage in the exploration of alternative plans, and begin to move forward with their lives[21].

The *keening syndrome* refers to the Irish custom of mourning in which the women, weeping and wailing, prepared the dead body for burial, while the men sat soberly around the edges of the room watching (and often passing a bottle.) The keening syndrome refers to the way in which many couples grieve the losses of infertility: Women weep and men watch, with the result that the husband becomes the 'forgotten mourner' because he is not as verbal and expressive with his grief as she is. Ultimately, failure to acknowledge and appropriately grieve the losses of infertility impacts a couple's long-term adjustment to infertility, as well as prospective decisions regarding treatment and family-building alternatives. In many ways, this approach highlights not only gender differences in grief and mourning but also how women often assume the role of primary mourner, bearing an unequal share of the emotional burden of a couple's grief. Some have suggested that this is because women are proportionately more distressed than men, while others argue that it represents a common marital pattern in which women assume responsibility for the couple's emotional well-being.

Unruh and McGrath[67] objected to the application of the grief model to infertility because it failed to address the ongoing, chronic nature of infertility. They contended that infertility is a *chronic sorrow*, in which the pain of the loss is not forgotten but periodically remembered and mourned, even after infertility is no longer an issue in the couple's or individual's life. By contrast, Stanton and Dunkel-Schetter[21] pointed out that the conceptualization of infertility as a major life crisis involving grief is valuable in that it has helped stimulate the development of support groups, increase awareness among professionals, and legitimize adjustment to infertility as a problem worthy of empirical study.

Cognitive-Behavioral Theory

Cognitive-behavioral theory is based on a unique combination of behaviorism and cognitive psychology: Behaviorism focuses on changing overt behaviors rather than on understanding subjective feelings, unconscious processes, or motivations, while cognitive psychology involves changing thought processes. Cognitive psychology applies social learning principles that are based on three basic propositions: (1) Cognitive activity affects behavior, (2) which can be monitored, and (3) behavioral changes can be affected through cognitive changes. Sometimes referred to as the *biopsychosocial model* when applied to health psychology or behavioral medicine, it is based on the premise that biological, psychological, and social factors are interrelated influences on health and illness. Cognitive-behavioral application to infertility emphasizes current behavior, thoughts, and feelings about the medical situation rather than long-term, in-depth discussions of early childhood experiences, unconscious motivations, or inner psychic conflicts as causal factors of infertility. Taymor was the first to refer to infertility as a *biopsychosocial crisis* because it involves interaction among physical conditions predisposing to infertility, medical interventions addressing infertility, reactions of others, and individual psychological characteristics[68].

The *chronic illness model*, based on cognitive-behavioral theory, is a synergistic model of chronic illness in which there is an ongoing, reciprocal relationship among physical, cognitive, affective, social, and behavioral factors. In short, each individual's perspective (based on idiosyncratic attitudes, beliefs, and unique schema) interacts reciprocally with emotional factors, social influences, behavioral responses, and sensory phenomena[69]. The application of chronic illness theory to infertility highlights how infertility involves chronicity of treatment, physical impairment, separation from support system and/or lack of support, loss of key roles, disruption of future plans, assault on self-image and self-esteem, loss of autonomy and control, uncertain and unpredictable futures, distressing emotions, extensive array of adjustment demands, and disease-related factors such as permanent changes in bodily functions[69]. The aims of this approach are to (1) reduce stress, (2) reduce disability and improve physical functioning, (3) reduce symptoms, and (4) limit inappropriate use of medical care[70]. In short, this approach helps infertile individuals reduce the stress, disability, and symptoms of medical treatment through adaptation and by becoming an active participant in infertility treatment.

The *stress and coping model* is based on the work of Hans Seyle[71], who during the 1930s began a systematic study of stress and its impact on physical health. According to Seyle, people respond to stress in three stages: (1) an initial short-term stage of alarm, (2) a longer period of resistance, and (3) a final stage of exhaustion. *Stress* has also been conceptualized as a stimulus, with stressors from major life events (e.g., illness, divorce) or daily hassles[72]. Lazarus and Folkman[73] used a definition of stress that involved 'a relationship between the person and the environment that is appraised by the person as taxing or exceeding his or her resources and endangering his or her well-being'[73]. *Coping* refers to the process by which a person takes some action to manage external or internal demands that cause stress and tax the individual's inner resources.

Fundamental to stress and coping theory is the individual's perception of the stressor, other stressful life events, coping skills, resilience, and social support. Variables in the response to stress include personality, cognition, social environment, gender, and culture. Stanton and Dunkel-Schetter[21] suggested that infertility is characterized by the dimensions that individuals usually find most stressful: unpredictability, negativity, uncontrollability, and ambiguity. As such, infertility is a stressor that takes place over an extended period of time, is beyond the control of the individuals involved, and entails negative consequences, responses, and outcomes that are unknown and unpredictable. Coping techniques for managing the crisis involve not only assessment of the individual's and couple's resources, personality, perceptions of the stressor, and response to the stress but also how these are applied to the stressor (infertility) to achieve adaptive adjustment.

The stress and coping approach has become instrumental in attempts to determine which behavioral techniques (e.g., relaxation, expression of emotion) may facilitate conception and parenthood, in what some have considered a recycling of the psychogenic infertility model. While cognitive-behavior theory provides conceptualization and therapeutic direction for individuals experiencing infertility, Stanton and Dunkel-Schetter[21] suggest that it provides little direction for furthering our knowledge of systematic variability in adjustment. However, they also suggest that the application of stress and coping theory to infertility provides a greater understanding of (1) the conditions under which infertility is likely to be perceived as stressful, (2) factors most likely to facilitate or impede adjustment in infertile couples or individuals, and (3) guidance in defining what constitutes successful psychological adjustment to infertility.

Family Systems Theory

Family systems theory is based on a systemic approach to disturbed interactions of the individuals in a family, in contrast to traditional psychological approaches focusing on disturbances within individuals. Family systems theory is based on the principles of family systems, structure, and relationship interactions that are the subject of therapeutic assessment and intervention. The application of family systems theory to infertility focuses on the impact of infertility on marriage, the couple, their families of origin, or the individual within the context of these relationship systems.

The *family life stage model* defines the series of life stages and expectable timelines that most people pass through in a predictable manner over the family's life cycle[74]. Parenthood, as a family life stage, represents the establishment of a new family, precipitating structural and relationship changes in the family intergenerationally. Because infertility represents the inability to proceed through family life stages in a predictable and socially conforming fashion, couples stuck in the 'couple stage' of the family life cycle often have difficulty adapting to the ambiguity that infertility or uncertain parenthood entails. Matthews and Matthews[60], using the family life stage model, suggested that the identity confusion and role adjustments of infertility precipitates family stress and crisis. Accordingly, infertility as a 'transition to nonparenthood' represents the infertile couple's inability to make the anticipated transition to parenthood, resulting in confused life tasks, uncertain roles, and blurred boundaries in their own relationship and between their relationship and their families of origin.

Family boundary ambiguity[75] refers to ambiguity in family relationships and roles that impair family functioning. In short, confused or blurred boundaries make family systems and family members uncomfortable. Boundary ambiguity in infertility occurs on three levels: (1) the fantasy child as a psychologically present and physically absent member of the infertile marriage, (2) one or both partners as a 'marginal person', dividing loyalties between his/her family of origin and creating unclear boundaries in both families as a result of the inability to differentiate effectively, and

(3) biological/hereditary ambiguity as a result of adoption and/or third-party reproduction, which obscures family ties or continuity and therefore boundaries[75]. Some infertile couples may respond to infertility with rigid boundaries (particularly regarding medical treatment or considerations of family-building options) in an attempt to protect themselves from invasions of privacy or blurred family boundaries. This action may cause greater isolation when rigid boundaries result in alienation or isolation from family members. By contrast, too permeable boundaries may create unclear relationship definitions and invasions of privacy when the intimate details of the infertile couple's reproductive lives are inappropriately discussed by family members or family-building options are influenced more by family-of-origin opinions than by the couple's own wishes.

Infertility is an *intergenerational family developmental crisis* preventing parents and siblings from proceeding through life cycle stages (e.g., not yet grandparents, inability to share parenthood with siblings). Family pressures to have children may be increased for the infertile individual if she or he is an only child (perhaps signaling unresolved infertility issues in previous generations) or the last family member to carry on the family name, or has siblings who are cut off from the family or are childless by choice[76]. Family history of infertility, pregnancy losses, reproductive failures, and unresolved deaths and losses may precipitate the reemergence of long-buried issues or highlight flawed family coping patterns. In addition, significant other family stressors or crisis such as parental retirement or divorce, sibling marriages or childbirth, family illness or deaths, and/or family patterns of chronic chaos or dysfunction may overshadow the couple's infertility crisis, further isolating them from their families or simply making family members unavailable to provide support even when they may wish to.

Gender-Based Theories

Historically, psychological theory on gender has tended to reinforce traditional and conventional generalizations on the differences between men and women by associating women with 'relatedness' and men with 'autonomy'[77]. This dichotomy is further evidenced in the way infertile women and men typically describe their experiences and responses to infertility: Women emote and need to express their feelings of distress to others, while men repress and isolate themselves in an effort to be 'strong and masculine'. Nevertheless, there is growing evidence in psychology and in the psychology of infertility that men and women differ in terms of psychological perspectives and responses to various experiences including infertility.

The psychology of women, beginning with the work of Horney[78], was originally based on adaptations of male psychological theory and focused on the importance of self-realization for women. Probably, it is fair to say that *all* psychological theories suggest in one way or another that a 'woman's reproductive capacity shapes her mental life'[77]. Motherhood and reproduction, as the foundations of a woman's life and identity, were considered powerful factors in a woman's self-perception, personal fulfillment, and life choices. This theoretical approach became the foundation for psychogenic infertility theories and, perhaps more importantly, enhanced the effect of infertility on women by diminishing the choices of women who could not have children.

More recent feminist theories, based on developmental psychology and the psychology of self, have focused on women's development, self-actualization, and definitions of the central issues in women's lives. Current feminist theory holds that central to a woman's life and sense of self are relationships and her sense of connection to others[79]. According to this approach, the quality of a woman's intimate relationships determines her emotional stability, while psychological disturbance is the result of disconnections and violations in her intimate relationships. In terms of infertility, the importance of relationships for women must be considered an influential factor in her decision-making, adjustment to infertility, consideration of family-building alternatives, and marital satisfaction. Relationship disturbance may be experienced by women in terms of disconnection from her spouse, and the inability to connect with the potential child, extended family, or friends.

Feminists have traditionally been opposed to all uses of reproductive technology because it implies women's surrendering control of their reproductive lives to the primarily white, male medical establishment and being reduced to 'breeder' status (especially regarding surrogacy and gestational carriers). To that end, Unruh and McGrath[67] suggested that infertile women have (1) the right to have control over their bodies, particularly their reproductive capabilities, and to actively participate in their health care, (2) been commonly blamed for the conditions that have caused them personal distress, (3) been socialized to value themselves primarily through their childbearing roles, and (4) more in common with each other than their differences in fertility. 'Infertility treatment thus provides a paradigmatic example of a medical situation in which throughout much of its history the doctors have been men, the patients women, and the focus of attention on the sexual organs'[4].

Traditional definitions of male psychology have often been based on assumptions and expectations of male behavior emphasizing self-reliance, success, and aggression, as exemplified by Staudacher's[80] description of five primary coping styles of men: (1) remaining silent, (2) engaging in solitary mourning or 'secret' grief, (3) taking physical or legal action, (4) becoming immersed in an activity or work, or (5) exhibiting addictive behaviors. With the feminist movement, the psychology of men began to address the hazards of traditional male socialization, especially expectations that men maintain emotional stoicism, deny emotional vulnerability, remain preoccupied with work, achievement, and success, and engage in forceful and interpersonally aggressive behavior[82,83]. Further, it emphasized how the alienation of men from their feelings often lead to emotional isolation, impairment of physical health, and self-destructive behaviors[82]. More recently, the men's movement has encouraged a redefinition of masculinity based on the importance of relationships, comfort with the expression of feelings, and greater self-understanding and self-acceptance.

CLINICAL ISSUES AND THERAPEUTIC INTERVENTIONS

Although an understanding of the psychology of infertility is fundamental to infertility counseling, it is also paramount that the infertility counselor be knowledgeable of reproductive medicine, including medical diagnosis and current treatment options for infertility. As such, an overview of the medical aspects of infertility is provided, as well as a review of medical conditions or circumstances of particular relevance to infertility and its treatment. With this foundation of knowledge of reproductive medicine, the infertility counselor can address the clinical and therapeutic issues important to the psychology of infertility including:

- assessment

- treatment modalities
- medical counseling issues
- special populations
- third-party reproduction and other means of alternative family building
- post-infertility issues
- infertility counseling practice issues.

Assessment

As will be noted, psychological care of the infertile individual or couple including assessment and treatment takes place within a wide array of contexts and circumstances, such as self-referral for psychotherapy or mandatory educational counseling. Psychosocial assessment in infertility is generally for the purposes of information gathering about the individual/couple's personal history, psychiatric history, and current level of functioning, as well as a review of the infertility experience in terms of its impact on family, psychiatric health, relationships, reproductive history, and sexual history (see Comprehensive Psychosocial History of Infertility: Appendix 2). Psychological testing and/or a structured interview are the methods typically used for gathering this information, thereby facilitating assessment and treatment. Like other forms of psychological treatment, infertility counseling involves interventions based on careful psychosocial assessment of the patient/couple for disturbance, psychopathology, and possibly the need for psychotropic medication.

While there is no evidence of increased incidence of psychiatric problems in infertile patients, individuals may develop psychological distress in response to the stresses of medical treatment or experience the reemergence of preexisting psychopathology (e.g., depression, eating disorders). Whether newly emergent or preexisting, emotional distress can impair quality of life, impact medical treatment, and pose challenging management problems for the medical staff. As such, psychological care involves a variety of treatment modalities including *psychiatric or psychopharmacological treatment*. Whether psychiatric care is adjunctive or primary care, the practitioner must be aware of the unique treatment demands and challenges of patients undergoing infertility treatment while also requiring psychiatric care.

Treatment Modalities

Infertility counselors, as mental health professionals, typically employ a variety of treatment modalities, rarely endorsing a single approach. *Individual counseling* is useful for addressing personal distress and dysfunction, whether caused or exacerbated by infertility. It provides a safe and trusting relationship with the therapist, allowing growth and healing from the pain of infertility or past psychological injury or illness. *Couple counseling* is useful in addressing relationship or marital problems, particularly those involving communication, decision-making, and conflict resolution. It is a particularly appropriate approach for infertility that is usually a 'couple problem', involving the grieving of shared losses for both partners, interupted sexual practices, and considerable couple stressors (e.g. financial strain, extended medical treatment). *Group counseling* is helpful to couples and individuals needing validation or personal perspective in promoting psychological growth. Group members aid in normalizing and sharing the infertility experience, as well as ameliorating feelings of isolation and stigma.

Within the context of these three methods of therapy delivery, different counseling approaches may be used. *Behavioral medicine* as a therapeutic approach to infertility is helpful in that it integrates cognitive-behavioral therapy and health psychology, emphasizing the patient's role in medical care. It offers stress management and coping interventions, such as cognitive restructuring, guided imagery, and relaxation techniques. *Sexual counseling* is often both necessary and beneficial for infertile couples who typically encounter problems related to sexual health either as a result of medical treatment or in response to the infertility diagnosis. Whether the infertility counselor provides these counseling services or refers to another professional for adjunctive care, it is evident that diverse treatment modalities are beneficial in assisting infertile patients.

Medical Counseling Issues

Medical conditions affecting fertility include conditions causing infertility (e.g., cancer treatment, genetic disorders), resulting in infertility (e.g., premature ovarian failure), or affecting infertility treatment (e.g., endometriosis). *Medically complicating conditions* or special medical circumstances often involve a variety of psychological issues with the potential for precipitating emotional crisis and understandably impacting reproductive treatment decisions. Diagnosis of a disease or genetic disorder (whether related or unrelated to infertility) during the course of infertility evaluation or treatment can result in a dual crisis of health and fertility in which the patient must deal with illness (even mortality) that amplifies the typical reactions to infertility of loss, defectiveness, and abnormality. Finally, it has become increasingly common for infertile patients to undergo *genetic counseling* or genetic screening for reasons of parental age, reproductive or medical history of genetic disorders, or diagnosis of the reproductive problem. Understandably, the process of genetic counseling and/or the diagnosis of a genetic problem can cause significant distress and complicate adjustment to infertility.

For couples who may have spent years of anticipation, time, energy, and money to conceive a much desired pregnancy, pregnancy loss or the death of a newborn is especially bitter and cruel. *Pregnancy loss* (whether spontaneous or planned) can be an emotionally traumatic experience involving varying degrees of grief, diminished self-esteem, and marital distress. Spontaneous losses—ectopic pregnancy, miscarriage, stillbirth, or infant death—may potentially trigger acute grief responses, clinical depression, and/or the reemergence of unresolved past losses. Planned terminations (e.g., for reasons of multifetal reduction or genetic defects) are often grieved and mourned in the same manner as spontaneous losses, although social stigma associated with abortion may increase isolation and guilt about the 'chosen' loss of a longed-for child.

Special Populations

The psychology of infertility for diverse populations and circumstances (as distinct from white, middle-class, heterosexual, young, first-married couples) involves the recognition of disparate responses and unique social circumstances, typically influencing therapeutic approaches and counseling interventions. Knowledge of cross-cultural factors in infertility can assist the therapist's provision of appropriate support, direction, and intervention, as well as improving establishment of the therapeutic alliance. Issues of *race, culture, and religion* impact each infertile couple's experience of infertility either by influencing their perspective, defining their approach to treatment or family-building options, or impacting their psychological adjustment.

Social changes involving women taking increasing control of their reproductive capabilities have contributed to the dramatic increase in *single women and lesbian couples* seeking infertility services, whether or not they are technically infertile. Other social changes are evident as *older couples* who have delayed childbearing for any number of reasons and *remarried couples* who want a child together present for reproductive services. Furthermore, if there is an infertility diagnosis, the etiology is more likely to be related to age or prior reproductive decisions (e.g., surgical sterilization) resulting in different, and often more complex, psychological issues. Finally, treatment for these patients (lesbian couples, single women, older, and remarried couples) may entail the use of assisted reproduction and/or donated gametes, with concomitant special psychological considerations, issues, and adjustments.

Couples affected by *secondary infertility* are not 'childless' but are unable to expand their families as they wish. Whether or not they have had prior difficulty conceiving, these couples encounter many of the same psychological issues of infertility as other couples and are often equally as distressed and isolated. However, they face the additional challenges of parenting and decision-making about treatment and alternative family building within the context of their present family constellation.

Third-Party Reproduction and Other Means of Alternative Family Building

For some infertile couples, traditional medical treatments will not be successful, and they must reconsider previous decisions about parenthood and decide whether to maintain their family as it is (e.g., couple, single-child family) or pursue other family-building alternatives such as adoption or third-party reproduction. All of these alternatives involve the conscious decision to stop current medical treatment, redefine family, and grieve the experience of pregnancy, birth, and/or their own genetically shared, biological child. For some couples, childlessness may be redefined as *child-free*, and their decision not to continue medical treatment may involve enhancing the benefits of couplehood, redefining the meaning of family, or the pursuit of other life goals. Other couples prefer more traditional family-building alternatives such as *adoption* or foster care and will discover the plethora of rewards not only of parenthood but of sharing their lives with a child needing parents. Finally, the pursuit of parenthood through the various forms of third-party reproduction (donated sperm, eggs, or embryos, surrogacy, and gestational carrier) is another positive means of family building that challenges traditional beliefs or customs.

While considerations of adoption and childlessness seem fairly straightforward to most infertile individuals, third-party reproduction can be daunting in its complexity. To a large extent, current practices in third-party reproduction are based on traditions associated with sperm donation, used therapeutically in the United States for over 100 years and involving donor anonymity and family secrecy. However, the development of assisted reproduction technologies (e.g., IVF) over the last 20 years now enables couples to build their family through the use of donated oocytes and embryos and to utilize the services of surrogates and gestational carriers. The psychological complexities of these forms of family building have precipitated considerations and recommendations for the care of all participants—recipients and donors—involving assessment, preparation, education, and support.

Couples considering the use of donated sperm, egg, or embryos must first address the emotional consequences of reproductive failure as individuals and as couples. Having decided to build their family through the use of donated gametes or embryos, they, as the *recipient couple*, must grieve the biological, genetically-shared child they had hoped for. In addition, they must mutually agree that their best alternative to genetic parenthood is assisted reproduction and the use of donated sperm, egg, or embryo. Further, they must decide on the type of donation with which they are comfortable—anonymous donor or known donor (e.g., family member)—and on their level of openness about the child's conception.

The other patient participants in third-party reproduction are the donors, surrogates, and gestational carriers who facilitate parenthood for infertile couples. Preparation of gamete donors varies. Anonymous *sperm donor* preparation has primarily been restricted to medical screening while *oocyte donors* have received more extensive assessment and preparation because the donation process is medically intrusive and demanding. *Embryo donors* are usually infertile couples who relinquish cryopreserved embryos or extra embryos from a current IVF cycle that they do not plan to use themselves. This option is sometimes referred to as 'preimplantation adoption'. Preparation of embryo donors has involved assessment of couple agreement as well as helping them understand the implications of their donation, socially, legally, and psychologically. Preparation of *surrogates and gestational carriers* has typically involved psychological assessment, education, definition of the reproductive relationship parameters, and ongoing support, sometimes even after the pregnancy and relinquishment of the child as the 'ultimate gift'.

Postinfertility Counseling Issues

Pregnancy after infertility is precious but often fraught with anxiety and worry. Psychological adjustment to this unique pregnancy typically presents a myriad of new issues, including possible multiple gestation, potential serious maternal/fetal health risks, decisions regarding multifetal reduction, complications requiring high-tech intervention and prolonged bed rest, or adjustment to a pregnancy that is not genetically related to or carried by the 'contracting' mother. In short, previously infertile pregnant women and their spouses, expecting a blissful experience, are often surprised by an exceedingly challenging experience that diminishes happiness and expectations.

Parenting and family adjustment after infertility entail all the normal developmental tasks of parenthood and family life, but often with unique demands. The special issues for these parents may involve older parenthood, parenting multiples, parenting an only child after secondary infertility, or the complex dilemmas of parenting after third-party reproduction. Parenthood against a backdrop of reproductive loss and highly technical medical conception requires special psychological preparation, education, and adjustment to its special joys and challenges.

Infertility Counseling Practice Issues

Infertility counseling is a new and emerging field in which mental health professionals (social workers, psychologists, psychiatrists, psychiatric nurses, and marriage and family therapists) have become increasingly important professionals in reproductive medicine, genetics, and perinatalogy. There are positive and negative approaches to the various ways in which infertility counseling services may be provided: independent practitioner working with a medical clinic, independent contractor/consultant, or employee of the clinic. However infertility counseling services are provided, it is important that the infertility counselor be prepared to provide excellent mental health services with a clear understanding of medical issues. Further, the infertility counselor must have a keen awareness of the ethical issues involved in infertility and the legal dimensions of treatment (e.g., third-party reproduction) to advise patients appropriately.

Physicians and nurses in reproductive medicine are closely involved in the care and understanding of their patients, promoting general well-being, assessing and supporting emotional needs, counseling on treatment decisions, and providing support during intrusive medical procedures and treatment failures. Infertility counselors work closely with physicians and nurses as part of the reproductive medicine team providing comprehensive patient care. As such, appropriate referral to the infertility counselor by a physician and/or nurse typically entails patient assessment, education, and communication, emphasizing the opportunity for patient benefit and reward from the counseling experience.

FUTURE IMPLICATIONS

As a new and emerging mental health profession, infertility counseling applies mental health treatment to the fields of reproductive medicine, genetic medicine, and perinatology. Over the past 20 years, it has seen dynamic growth in terms of the number of professionals working in the field, the amount of scientific research, professional development, and increasing presence in a wide variety of infertility clinics and medical treatment facilities. Worldwide mental health professionals working in the field of infertility counseling have provided comprehensive patient care, while establishing programs, standards of professional education, practice guidelines, and more recently professional qualifications and quality assurance for consumers. As such, it is safe to say that infertility counseling may be a new, as well as a dynamically growing, field of mental health marked by a group of multidisciplinary professionals working together with a wide variety of medical professionals to provide comprehensive patient care, increase consumer awareness and education, and improve patient response to medical treatment. Future developments in this field involve its continuing definition as a mental health profession, qualifications for caregivers, and education and training for professionals wishing to enter the field.

SUMMARY

- Although infertility has existed since the beginning of time, the social and historical context of reproductive choice has changed dramatically in the last century and become significantly more complex for couples medically, socially and psychologically.

- While research and clinical experience continue to indicate that the vast majority of infertile men and women do not experience significant levels of psychological trauma, the use of advanced medical technology and/or third-party reproduction may increase psychological distress during specific periods of treatment.

- There has been an evolution in the psychological theoretical view of infertility over the years from a psychogenic model, in which infertility is the result of psychopathology, to a psychological sequelae model, in which psychological difficulties are the consequence of infertility.

- Clinical intervention combines an understanding of the medical and psychological aspects of infertility. Intervention is based on careful assessment, use of appropriate treatment modalities, and an understanding of the complex issues and circumstances involved in infertility counseling practice.

REFERENCES

1. Rosenblatt PC, Peterson P, Portner J, *et al.* A cross-cultural study of responses to childlessness. *Behav Sci Notes* 1973;8:221–31

2. Sha JL. *Mothers of Thyme: Customs and Rituals of Infertility and Miscarriage*. Ann Arbor, MI: Lida Rose Press, 1990

3. May ET. *Barren in the Promised Land: Childless Americans and the Pursuit of Happiness*. New York: Basic Books, 1995

4. Marsh M, Ronner W. *The Empty Cradle: Infertility in America from Colonial Times to the Present*. Baltimore: Johns Hopkins University Press, 1996

5. Griel AL. *Not Yet Pregnant: Infertile Couples in Contemporary America*. New Brunswick, NJ: Rutgers University Press, 1991

6. Mosher WD, Pratt WF. Fertility and infertility in the United States. *Advance Data* 1990;3–5

7. Hoffman LW, Hoffman M. The value of children to parents. In: Fawcett JT, ed. *Psychological Perspectives on Population*. New York: Basic Books, 1973;19–73

8. van Balen F, Trimbos-Kemper TCM. Involuntary childless couples: Their desire to have children and their motives. *J Psychosom Obstet Gynaecol* 1995;16: 137–44

9. Newton CR, Hearn MT, Yuzpe AA, Houle M. Motives for parenthood and response to failed in vitro fertilization: Implications for counseling. *J Assist Reprod Technol Genet* 1992;9:24–31

10. Dunkel-Schetter C, Lobel M. Psychological reactions to infertility. In: Stanton AL, Dunkel-Schetter C, eds. *Infertility: Perspectives from Stress and Coping Research*. New York: Plenum Press, 1991;29–57

11. Abbey A, Andrews FM, Halman LJ.

Gender's role in responses to infertility. *Psychol Women Q* 1991;15:295–316

12. Berg BJ, Wilson JF, Weingartner PJ. Psychological sequelae of infertility treatment: The role of gender and sex-role identification. *Soc Sci Med* 1991;33:1071–80

13. Koropatnick S, Daniluk J, Pattinson HA. Infertility: A non-event transition. *Fertil Steril* 1993;59:163–71

14. Link PW, Darling CA. Couples undergoing treatment for infertility: Dimensions of life satisfaction. *J Sex Marital Ther* 1986;12:46–59

15. Wright J, Duchesne C, Sabourin S, *et al.* Psychosocial distress and infertility: Men and women respond differently. *Fertil Steril* 1991;55:100–8

16. Nachtigall RD, Quiroga SS, Tschann JM, *et. al.* Stigma, disclosure, and family functioning among parents with children conceived through donor insemination. *Fertil Steril* 1997;68:1–7

17. Mason MC. *Male Infertility—Men Talking.* London: Routledge, 1993

18. Daniluk JC. Gender and infertility. In: Leiblum SR, ed. *Infertility: Psychological Issues and Counseling Strategies.* New York: Wiley, 1997; 103–25

19. Daniluk JC. Infertility: Intrapersonal and interpersonal impact. *Fertil Steril* 1988; 49:982–90

20. McEwan KL, Costello CG, Taylor PJ. Adjustment to infertility. *J Abnorm Psychol* 1987; 96:108–16

21. Stanton AL, Dunkel-Schetter C. Psychological adjustment to infertility. In: Stanton AL, Dunkel-Schetter C, eds. *Infertility: Perspectives from Stress and Coping Research.* New York: Plenum Press, 1991;3–16

22. Snarey J, Son L, Kuihne, *et al.* The role of parenting in men's psychosocial development: A longitudinal study of early adulthood infertility and midlife generativity. *Dev Psychol* 1987;23:593–603

23. Mazure CM, Greenfeld DA. Psychological studies of in vitro fertilization/embryo transfer participants. *J In Vitro Fertil Emb Transfer* 1989;6:242–56

24. Downey J, Yingling S, McKinney M. Mood disorders, psychiatric symptoms and distress in women presenting for infertility evaluation. *Fertil Steril* 1989;52:425–32

25. Rosenthal MB. Psychiatric aspects of infertility and assisted reproductive technologies. *Infertil Reprod Med Clin North Am* 1993;4:471–82

26. Boivin J, Takefman JE, Tulandi T, Brender W. Reactions to infertility based on extent of treatment failure. *Fertil Steril* 1995; 63:801–7

27. Leiblum S, Kemmann E, Lane MK. Psychological concomitants of in vitro fertilization. *J Psychosom Obstet Gynaecol* 1987; 6:165–78

28. Baram D, Tourelot E, Muechler E, *et al.* Psychosocial adjustment following unsuccessful in vitro fertilization. *J Psychosom Obstet Gynaecol* 1988;9:181–90

29. Newton CR, Hearn MT, Yuzpe AA. Psychological assessment and follow-up after in vitro fertilization: Assessing the impact of failure. *Fertil Steril* 1990;54:879–86

30. Greenfeld D, Haseltine F. Candidate selection and psychosocial consideration of in vitro fertilization procedures. *Clin Obstet Gynecol* 1986;29:119–26

31. Collins A, Freeman EW, Boxer AS, Tureck R. Perceptions of infertility and treatment stress in females as compared with males entering in vitro fertilization treatment. *Fertil Steril* 1992;57:350–6

32. Merari D, Feldberg D, Elizur A, *et al.* Psychological and hormonal changes in the course of in vitro fertilization. *J Assist Reprod Technol Genet* 1992;9:161–9

33. Beaurepaire J, Jones M, Theiring P, *et al.* Psychosocial adjustment in infertility and its treatment: Male and female responses at different stages of IVF/ET treatment. *J Psychosom Res* 1994;38:229–40

34. Weil E, Cornet D, Sibony C, *et al.* Psychological aspects in anonymous and non-anonymous oocyte donation. *Hum Reprod* 1994; 9:1344–7

35. Braverman AM. Surrogacy and gestational carrier programs: Psychological issues. *Infertil Reprod Med Clin North Am* 1993;4:517–31

36. Braverman AM, Corson SL. Characteristics of participants in a gestational carrier program. *J Assist Reprod Technol Genet* 1992;9:353–7

37. Schover LR. Psychological aspects of oocyte donation. *Infertil Reprod Med Clin North Am* 1993;4:483–515

38. Schover LR, Collins RL, Quigley MM, *et al.*

Psychological follow-up of women evaluated as oocyte donors. *Hum Reprod* 1991;6:1487–91

39. Schover LR, Reis J, Collins RL, *et al*. The psychological evaluation of oocyte donors. *J Psychosom Obstet Gynaecol* 1990;11:583–90

40. Parker PJ. Motivations of surrogate mothers: Initial findings. *Am J Psychiatry* 1983; 140: 117–18

41. Steadman JH, McCloskey GT. The prospect of surrogate mothering: Clinical concerns. *Can J Psychiatry* 1987;32:545

42. Bartlett JA. Psychiatric issues in non-anonymous oocyte donation. *Psychosomatics* 1991;32:433–7

43. Lessor R, Cervantes N, O'Connor N, *et al*. An analysis of social and psychological characteristics of women volunteering to be oocyte donors. *Fertil Steril* 1993;53:65

44. Berg BJ, Wilson JF. Psychiatric morbidity in the infertile population: A reconceptualization. *Fertil Steril* 1990;53:654–61

45. Fischer IC. Psychogenic aspects of infertility. *Fertil Steril* 1953;4:466–71

46. Rothman D, Kaplan AH, Nettles E. Psychosomatic infertility. *Am J Obstet Gynecol* 1962;83:373–81

47. Belonoschkin B. Psychosomatic factors and matrimonial infertility. *Int J Fertil* 1962; 7:29–36

48. Rubenstein BB. An emotional factor in infertility: A psychosomatic approach. *Fertil Steril* 1951;2:80–6

49. de Watteville H. Psychologic factors in the treatment of sterility. *Fertil Steril* 1957;8:12–24

50. Walker HE. Psychiatric aspects of infertility. *Urol Clin North Am* 1978;5:481–8

51. Denber HCB. Psychiatric aspects of infertility. *J Reprod Med* 1978;20:23–9

52. Edelmann RJ, Connolly KJ. Psychological aspects of infertility. *Br J Med Psychol* 1986;59:209–19

53. Noyes RW, Chapnick EM. Literature on psychology and infertility: A critical analysis. *Fertil Steril* 1964;15:543–58

54. Benedek T. Infertility as a psychosomatic defense. *Fertil Steril* 1952;3:527–41

55. Menning BE. The emotional needs of infertile couples. *Fertil Steril* 1980;34:313–19

56. Kohut H. *The Restoration of the Self*. New York: International Universities Press, 1977

57. Olshansky EF. Identity of self as infertile: An example of theory-generating research. *Adv Nurs Sci* 1987;9:54–63

58. Sandelowski M. The color gray: Ambiguity and infertility. *Image J Nurs Sch* 1987; 19:70–4

59. Goffman E. *Stigma: Notes on the Management of Spoiled Identity*. Englewood Cliffs, NJ: Prentice Hall, 1963

60. Matthews R, Matthews AM. Infertility and involuntary childlessness: The transition to nonparenthood. *J Marriage Fam* 1986; 48:641–9

61. Miall CE. Perceptions of informal sanctioning and the stigma of involuntary childlessness. *Deviant Behav* 1985;6:383–403

62. Erickson E. *Childhood and Society*. New York: Norton, 1950

63. Menning BE. *Infertility: A Guide to the Childless Couple*. Englewood Cliff, NJ: Prentice Hall, 1980

64. Sanders CM. *Grief: The Mourning After*. New York: Wiley, 1989

65. Bowlby J. *Attachment and Loss: Loss, Sadness, and Depression*, vol. 3. New York: Basic Books, 1980

66. Parkes CM. *Bereavement: Studies in Grief in Adult Life*. New York: International Universities Press, 1972

67. Unruh AM, McGrath PJ. The psychology of female infertility: Toward a new perspective. *Health Care Women Int* 1985; 6:369–81

68. Cook EP. Characteristics of the biopsychosocial crisis of infertility. *J Couns Dev* 1987;65:465–70

69. Turk DC, Salovey P. Cognitive-behavioral treatment of illness behavior. In: Nicassio PM, Smith TW, eds. *Managing Chronic Illness: A Biopsychosocial Perspective*. Washington, DC: American Psychological Association, 1995;245–84

70. Sharpe M, Peveler R, Mayou R. The psychological treatment of patients with functional somatic symptoms: A practical guide. *J Psychosom Res* 1992;36;515–29

71. Seyle H. *The Stress of Life*. New York: McGraw-Hill, 1956

72. Lazarus RS, Cohen JB. Environmental stress. In: Altman I, Wohlwill JF, eds. *Human Behavior and the Environment: Current Theory and Research*. New York:

Plenum Press, 1977

73. Lazarus RS, Folkman S. *Stress, Appraisal, and Coping*. New York: Springer, 1984

74. Carter E, McGoldrick M. *The Family Life Cycle*. New York: Gardner, 1980

75. Burns LH. Infertility as boundary ambiguity: One theoretical perspective. *Fam Process* 1987;26:359–72

76. Mikesell SG, Stohner M. Infertility and pregnancy loss: The role of the family consultant. In: Mikesell RH, Lusterman D, McDaniel SH, eds. *Integrating Family Therapy: Handbook of Family Psychology and Systems Theory*. Washington, DC: American Psychological Association, 1995;421–36

77. Ireland MS. *Reconceiving Women: Separating Motherhood from Female Identity*. New York: Guilford Press, 1993

78. Horney K. *Feminine Psychology*. New York: Norton, 1967/1973

79. Miller JB. Women's psychological development: Connections, disconnections, and violations. In: Berger MM, ed. *Women Beyond Freud: New Concepts of Feminine Psychology*. New York: Brunner/Mazel, 1994;79–98

80. Staudacher C. *Men & Grief*. Oakland, CA: New Harbinger Publications, 1991

81. Meth RL, Pasick RS. *Men in Therapy: The Challenge of Change*. New York: Guilford Press, 1990

82. Philpot CL, Brooks GR, Luterman D, Nutt RL. *Bridging Separate Gender Worlds*. Washington DC: American Psychological Association, 1997

83. Goldberg H. *The Hazards of Being Male*. In: *Self-Destruction to Self-Care*. New York: New American Library, 1979

2

Medical Aspects of Infertility for the Counselor

William R. Keye, Jr., MD

Fortunately when religion was strong and science weak, men mistook magic for medicine; now, when science is strong and religion weak, men mistake medicine for magic.

Thomas Szasz

The term *infertility* is commonly used to describe the inability to conceive during 1 year of sexual intercourse without contraception. This time interval is chosen because of the observation that approximately 25% of couples will conceive within the first month, 60% within 6 months, and 80% within 12 months of unprotected sexual intercourse[1]. However, many couples consider themselves to be infertile if they conceive but, due to a miscarriage, are unable to deliver a living child. *Primary infertility* is defined as the failure to conceive by a couple who has never conceived (30% of infertile couples), while *secondary infertility* refers to the failure to conceive by a couple who had previously conceived (70% of infertile couples). In general, the evaluation and treatment of couples with primary or secondary infertility, as well as the causes, are the same.

It is estimated that 8–14% of couples experience infertility. While there is an impression that infertility has become more prevalent, recent data suggest this is not true. The proportion of couples experiencing infertility has apparently not changed since 1965[2]. What is increasing is the demand for medical services for infertility and the publicity and public awareness of infertility and new high-tech treatments such as in vitro fertilization (IVF).

Table 1 Causes of infertility

Disorders of ovulation	30%
Abnormality of semen	22%
Abnormal fallopian tubes	17%
Unexplained	14%
Other disorders: cervical and uterine disorders, immunological problems, infection, sexual dysfunction	12%
Endometriosis	5%

(Reproduced from ref. 3, with permission)

The causes of infertility may be categorized as seen in Table 1[3]. The major causes of infertility include (1) failure to ovulate, (2) failure to deliver adequate numbers of healthy sperm to the fallopian tubes, (3) blockage or obstruction of the fallopian tubes, (4) endometriosis or adhesions in the pelvis of the woman that interfere with capture of the egg by the fallopian tube, (5) poor timing or technique of intercourse, (6) infections of the reproductive tract or immunological barriers to fertilization or implantation, and (7) an abnormal uterine lining that may interfere with implantation of the

27

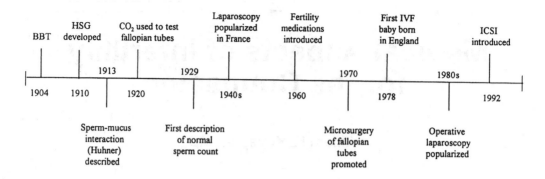

Figure 1 A time-line of the major advances in the diagnosis and treatment of infertility since 1900

embryo. The infertility work-up is designed to evaluate each of these major categories and to screen for the presence of underlying conditions or diseases. It is also important to note that an individual couple may have more than one reason for their infertility, and one should not assume that once an abnormality is found that there are no other contributing factors.

This chapter will:

- identify the etiology of infertility
- review diagnostic testing in evaluation of male and female infertility
- discuss current treatment options.

HISTORICAL OVERVIEW

The first written reference to infertility dates back to the Egyptians and the Kahoun papyrus (2200–1950 BC)[4]. The Egyptians described procedures to diagnose infertility (e.g., a failure to detect on the breath the odor of garlic after it had been placed in the vagina) and therapeutic measures (e.g., douching with garlic or wine). Hippocrates (460–370 BC) was the first Greek author to discuss infertility and believed that pregnancy was not likely to occur unless the penis actually entered the uterine cavity and the semen of the male mixed with a 'semen concentrate' produced by the female. The Roman author Soranus, who lived in the second century AD, and who is considered by some to be the father

of gynecology, believed that infertility was the result of the improper timing of intercourse and that the most fertile time of the menstrual cycle was just after the end of menstrual flow. He also believed that hot baths reduced fertility.

It was not until the 16th century that our understanding of fertility and infertility became more scientifically based when Vesalius (1514–1564) described the female reproductive tract and Spellanzani described the process of fertilization. In the 1800s, infertility was thought to be primarily a mechanical problem caused by disorders of the cervix or malposition of the uterus. As a result, the treatment of infertility was for the most part surgical with an emphasis on dilatation of the cervix, removal of pelvic adhesions, and surgical repositioning of the uterus.

Modern practice in infertility is based almost entirely on observations and insights gained during the 1900s (Figure 1). For example, the relationship between body temperature and the phases of the menstrual cycle was first described in 1904. The recording of the basal body temperature (BBT) has become the most commonly used and the most cost-effective method of detecting ovulation. Additional tests to document ovulation were introduced later this century, and today we commonly measure progesterone in the blood, look at the histological pattern of the lining of the uterus to determine if ovulation has occurred, or use ultrasound to assess follicular activity. Another example of the instrumental work of the early years of this century is the understanding of the interaction of sperm and cervical mucus. Though this interaction had been observed and described by J. Marion Sims[5] in 1888, its importance in achieving pregnancy was recognized by Huhner[6] in 1913.

Tests used to evaluate the fallopian tubes have changed very little in the past 60 years. In 1920, Isidor Rubin[7] described an office-based test in which oxygen was introduced through the cervix into the uterus and the resistance to flow measured. It was assumed that the fallopian tubes were open when there was little resistance and obstructed when there was a great deal of resistance. This test was later proven to be of little predictive value and has been replaced by the hysterosalpingogram (HSG), which was first described by Rindfleisch[8] in 1910. Hysterosalpingography involves the introduction of a radio contrast material into the cervix and uterus and gives a permanent radiological image of the shape and size of the uterine cavity and the fallopian tubes.

Evaluation of the fallopian tubes was limited to the HSG until the 1940s when Palmer[11], working in Paris, began to use laparoscopy to evaluate the pelvic organs. While this technique was soon popular in Europe and Great Britain, physicians in North America did not adopt laparoscopy in the evaluation of female infertility until the 1960s. During the 1970s and 1980s, not only was the laparoscope used to evaluate the pelvis and diagnose pelvic adhesions and endometriosis, but it became an important therapeutic tool as gynecologists learned to operate in the pelvis through it.

Evaluation of male infertility began with the microscopic observation of sperm by van Leeuwenhoek in the 17th century. However, the modern approach to the analysis of sperm can be traced to the description of what was thought to be a normal sperm count by Macomber and Sanders[9] in 1929. Much later in this century the World Health Organization published a manual that standardized the techniques of semen analysis, as well as the normal range of sperm and semen parameters such as sperm density (count), motility, and morphology[10]. During the past 20 years, several tests of sperm function have been developed, including the hamster egg penetration test, also referred to as the sperm penetration assay, hemizona assay, and zon binding assay.

Perhaps the most significant advance in the treatment of infertility occurred in 1978 when Robert Edwards and Patrick Steptoe announced the birth of the first baby conceived outside the human body. After almost a century of research on the process of fertilization, this announcement changed forever the evaluation and treatment of infertile couples. Now, 20 years later, over 6000 babies are born each year in North America after IVF. The process of IVF has quickly progressed from a medical curiosity to a cornerstone of infertility treatment.

During the 1990s, four major developments have occurred. The first is a technique known as intracytoplasmic sperm injection (ICSI), in which a single sperm is injected into a single egg (oocyte) to create a fertilized egg. This technique has been the most significant advance in the treatment of male-factor infertility because it has made it possible for men who produce only a few or dysfunctional sperm to father a child. The second major advancement has been the recent discovery of a means to freeze oocytes. Although not widely developed to date, this advance has the potential for dramatically changing the treatment of age-related and ovarian failure infertility in women. The third development has occurred in the field of medical economics, with the emergence of managed care and an emphasis on cost reduction. While a greater appreciation of the cost-effectiveness of infertility care may stream-line the evaluation of infertile couples, it also runs the risk that economic con-siderations will become the only factors considered in the choice among several therapeutic options. As a result, some couples may be forced by economic concerns to choose a therapy with which they may feel psychologically or ethically uncomfortable. Finally, the fourth major development in the 1990s has been the focus on the legal and ethical aspects of reproduction. As we have become techno-logically more sophisticated and capable of manipulating genes (as well as eggs, sperm, and embryos), society has become more interested in both the planning and oversight of artificial and third-party reproduction. (For a more detailed review, see reference 3.)

REVIEW OF LITERATURE

Only recently has there been an emphasis on well designed basic and research studies of infertility. During most of recorded history, reports and studies of fertility and infertility have consisted largely of anec-dotes, uncontrolled trials, and descriptive studies. This is rapidly changing, however, as metaanalyses and prospective random-ized trials have displaced opinions and case reports. With an increased need to justify diagnostic studies and therapeutic interventions, there has been increasing emphasis on 'evidence-based' medical care of infertility.

Clearly, the attempt to form a scientific basis for the clinical care of the infertile couple has begun to pay off, as those tests (e.g., postcoital tests) that have little productive value have been discarded, as have treatments that have been shown to be largely ineffective (e.g., thyroid hormone therapy).

Current areas of research include the following:

- Epidemiology of infertility: prevalence, role of life style, drifts in sperm production, influence of environmental toxins
- Predictive value of diagnostic tests: current interest in postcoital exam-ination, endometrial biopsy, lapar-oscopy and sperm function tests
- Clinical and cost-effectiveness of treatment options: tubal surgery, treatment of mild endometriosis, IVF
- Discovery of causes of 'unexplained infertility'; immunological, infections, and genetic factors
- Psychosocial factors as a cause or reaction to infertility: follow-up studies of assisted reproductive-technology babies, treatment of unexplained infertility with mind–body therapies
- Long term-complications of infertility treatments: relationship between infer-tility or ovulation-inducing agents (so-called 'fertility drugs') and cancer, complication rates of endoscopic surgery.

The results of these research efforts may change the content and style of infertility care in the future.

CLINICAL ISSUES
When Couples Should Seek Care

Based on the statistics presented earlier, couples should consider seeking medical care if they have not conceived after 12 months of unprotected sexual intercourse. However, some couples may benefit from earlier medical intervention[12]. For example, those who may be experiencing difficulty with sexual intercourse or have a known genetic disorder or a history of infertility in a previous relationship should consider medical evaluation before a year of unsuccessful attempts to conceive elapses. In addition, women should consider obtaining a medical consultation or evaluation either before the first attempts are made to conceive or after 6 months of unsuccessful attempts if they do not have regular menstrual periods, have had pelvic surgery or infections, have a history of cancer, or are attempting to conceive after age 35. Finally, men who have problems with ejaculation or are known to have a history of infections, surgery, or developmental abnormalities of the male reproductive tract should seek care prior to or soon after deciding to attempt conception. This recommendation to obtain medical care for infertility is based not only on the assumption that medical treatments may enhance a couple's chances of conceiving but also because infertility may be the presenting symptom of numerous underlying medical conditions. Individuals may be infertile because of diseases such as pituitary tumors, thyroid problems, endometriosis, or even cancer. The early detection of underlying diseases may simplify therapy and may improve not only the chance of conception but also the quality of an individual's life and, in rare instances, it can be life-saving. Thus, the treatment of infertility should not be seen as a purely elective process, for it clearly has potential health benefits.

Infertility Team

The care of the infertile man or woman should be provided by a team of professionals. While a family physician or internist can obtain an appropriate history and perform an adequate examination in a young woman with an uncomplicated history, the care of most infertile women is best provided by a general obstetrician–gynecologist or a specialist in female infer-

tility known as a reproductive endocrinologist. The specialist in female infertility is a general obstetrician–gynecologist who has taken an additional 2- or 3-year fellowship and passed written and oral examinations. The American Board of Obstetrics and Gynecology offers a certificate of special competence in the field of reproductive endocrinology to those who complete the fellowship and pass the examinations. The specialist should be involved early in the care of infertile women: older than 35 years who have had previous infertility; pelvic surgery, infection, or pain; cancer; congenital abnormalities of the reproductive tract; or infertility for greater than 2–3 years. A specialist should also be involved when previous diagnostic tests have demonstrated abnormalities that have not responded to simple, nonsurgical therapies.

The reproductive endocrinologist usually also has a nursing staff with special expertise in reproductive disorders and may have one or more nurses who have passed an examination qualifying them for a certificate of special knowledge in reproductive endocrinology/infertility nursing by the Nurses' Association of the American College of Obstetrics and Gynecology (NAACOG). While the physician establishes the treatment plan, supervises the care of the patient, and performs surgery and IVF, nurses provide much of the day-to-day care by answering questions, instructing and educating patients with respect to tests and treatments, and performing postcoital examinations and intrauterine inseminations. They also see and absorb much of the emotional reactions experienced by infertile couples. As a result, they must be knowledgeable about the impact of infertility, its tests, and treatments on emotions and relationships so that they can provide supportive care in an empathetic and nonjudgmental manner or make appropriate referral to an infertility counselor. Many infertility practices also have a part- or full-time mental health professional, such as a social worker or psychologist, who provides an array of services ranging from evaluation of couples' psychological and social background to counseling couples to better cope with the stress of the infertility work-up and treatment (see Chapter 26).

The infertile male usually is initially seen by the gynecologist who is providing care for his wife or female partner. The gynecologist usually orders the initial semen analysis and, if it is abnormal, refers the man to a urologist. While there are no formal fellowships for urologists, those who are interested or more knowledgeable about male infertility are called andrologists. There are some urologists who have a special interest in male infertility and even some who have had additional training beyond their residency in general urology. They may have sophisticated semen or hormone laboratories in their office, may conduct research into male infertility, and may be part of an IVF team, working side by side with the other team members listed above.

Most sophisticated infertility teams also have an embryologist on staff. The embryologist is a scientist with a masters or doctorate degree who is responsible for the fertilization of the eggs and the growth of the embryos, as well as the laboratory evaluation of the male and preparation of the sperm for intrauterine insemination, IVF, or gamete intrafallopian transfer. Some refer to this individual as an andrologist, even though he or she is not trained in urology.

The proper utilization of these professionals is essential to efficient and effective therapy. Because of the rapid expansion of new and highly technical options for therapy, designing the best 'game plan' for each couple is not easy. For nonspecialists in infertility, it is easy to overuse or misuse low-level technology in a misguided attempt to save money. It is also easy for specialists to suggest IVF or other sophisticated treatments before they are necessary. Just as there is no single best treatment plan for each infertile person, there is no ideal team either.

Initial Appointment

The initial visit is perhaps more important than any other visit that may follow because it establishes the foundation for all future visits. Ideally, it should involve both partners and focus on reviewing not only the medical but also the psychological and social aspects of the couple's infertility problem. The goal should be to develop a plan or outline for future care that will meet both the individual's and the couple's goals and needs. It is common practice to have infertile individuals or couples complete and return a detailed infertility questionnaire before the first visit. In addition, previous records and x-ray examinations or surgical videos are often obtained for review at the initial visit. During the initial interview, it is helpful to have a few minutes alone with each member of the couple, as well as interviewing them together. An individual may be more willing to share information about previous pregnancies, elective terminations, extramarital relationships, and/or sexually transmitted diseases if the other member of the couple is not present.

It is becoming more common for couples to seek the advice of several specialists before embarking on a program of evaluation or treatment. Infertile couples are commonly as interested in interviewing the infertility physician and team as the physician or team is in interviewing the couple.

The content of the initial interview should consist of a discussion of the following topics:

- Menstrual and gynecological history of infertility
- Medical history including a history of previous pregnancies, contraceptive techniques, surgeries, systemic diseases, medication use, pelvic infections, sexually transmitted diseases, abortions, sterilization, and infertility tests and treatments
- Previous relationships in which infertility may have been an issue
- Reasons why the individual or couple may be seeking medical care at the present time
- Goals and objectives, including the motives for seeking infertility care
- Lifestyle, including diet; exercise; use of alcohol, tobacco, or recreational drugs; exposure to environmental toxins; or occupational factors
- Sexual practices and the frequency and timing of intercourse, as well as the presence of pain with intercourse
- Beliefs about why they have not conceived and about the process of conception itself
- The unique psychosocial environment in which the couple is trying to conceive, including pressure exerted by a partner, extended family, or society, or other stresses
- The individual's psychosocial responses to his or her infertility and the possible need for referral for appropriate counseling
- The acceptability of tests and treatments such as donor insemination, IVF, selective reduction, and preimplantation genetic diagnoses
- Financial and other resources
- Family or personal history of genetic disorders.

In addition, in some practices the infertile couple may meet with an infertility counselor to discuss issues of concern, as well as strategies for coping with the stress associated with infertility and its evaluation and treatment. Once these issues have been addressed, the physician may outline a plan for evaluation and/or treatment and provide a decision-tree and time-line for the couple. Most couples will find the medical evaluation and treatments less stressful if they know in advance how the information gained from tests will be used and how long it will take to complete the evaluation or course of therapy. This approach establishes a partnership between the infertility team and the infertile couple or individual and may reduce the tension that is an inevitable part of the process. It is only after all these issues have been discussed that an appropriate plan can be outlined.

The initial visit to the gynecologist usually consists of a physical examination of the female. It should include height, weight, a general physical examination, blood pressure, hair distribution, breast development and an attempt to elicit breast secretions, and abdominal and pelvic examinations. If the male's history or semen analysis suggests a problem, he is usually referred to a urologist for a physical examination. If the individual or couple has decided to follow through with the infertility team, the visit should conclude with the discussion of a 'game plan', so that the individual or couple may return home to think about, discuss, and commit to additional care. It is advisable to write down the important points that have been discussed, so the couple can review them later. The plan should consist of an outline of tests and treatments, together with brief descriptions of their costs and odds of success. Some practices may also include a discussion about the insurance and financial aspects of infertility care. Finally, a bibliography or patient education brochures, available from the American Society for Reproductive Medicine and some pharmaceutical companies, may be of value to the infertile individual or couple.

Table 2 Evaluation of the infertile couple

Detection of ovulation
Basal body temperature
Serum progesterone
Endometrial biopsy
Serial ultrasound examinations
Semen analysis
Evaluation of fallopian tubes
Hysterosalpingogram
Infusion sonogram
Injection of dye at laparoscopy
Evaluation of pelvic cavity (adhesions, endometriosis)
Laparoscopy
Evaluation of transportation of sperm in female
Postcoital examination

Infertility Evaluation

As seen in Table 2, an infertility evaluation consists of some or all of the following tests: determination of ovulation, evaluation of the production and delivery of sperm, determination of patency of the fallopian tubes and size and shape of the uterine cavity, evaluation of the pelvic cavity with a search for endometriosis or adhesions, and evaluation of sperm transport within the female reproductive tract.

Detecting Ovulation

Detection of ovulation is extremely important because the treatment of infertility resulting from a failure to ovulate is among the most successful of all infertility treatments. The menstrual history is often by itself a reliable indicator of the presence or absence of ovulation. A history of regular, cyclic, predictable, and painful menstrual periods usually indicates that ovulation is occurring. However, the patient who is not ovulating is likely to have menstrual periods that occur less than every 35 days, at unpredictable intervals, and without uterine cramps. An inexpensive, convenient, and noninvasive approach to the documentation of ovulation is to chart the basal body temperature (BBT) each day through one or two menstrual cycles. A woman who is ovulating will have an early morning temperature usually less than 98°F (36.6°C) during the first half of the menstrual cycle and higher than 98°F during the second half of the menstrual cycle. However, the BBT does not give specific enough information to determine the day of ovulation, and it is not a good method for predicting which day ovulation will occur. However, because some women find it impractical and stressful to take their BBT, the measurement of progesterone within the blood can also be used to determine if ovulation has occurred. About the time of the ovulation, the ovary begins to produce progesterone, and once the level of progesterone exceeds 4 ng/mL, the temperature rises and one can be reasonably certain that ovulation has occurred[13]. The progesterone value is most reliable when testing occurs approximately 1 week after the assumed day of ovulation or approximately 1 week before the anticipated onset of the next menstrual period. Finally, some physicians will obtain a biopsy of the endometrium (lining of the uterus). The histological appearance of the endometrium will change after ovulation and in response to the secretion of progesterone. However, the biopsy is expensive and often uncomfortable for the woman. If it is determined that a woman is not ovulating, a search for specific causes of the ovulation disorder should then be performed. Over-the-counter ovulation predictor kits are often helpful in determining the day of ovulation in women with regular monthly periods. However, they are not a substitute for a BBT or blood progesterone test in women with irregular periods because they may occasionally produce false-positive or false-negative results and do not provide proof of ovulation.

Evaluation of the Numbers and Function of Sperm

It has been estimated that 40–50% of all couples with infertility have an identifiable cause that may be attributed to the male partner. Therefore, a semen analysis should be performed early in the course of the evaluation. A minimum of two analyses should be performed several weeks apart in order to properly assess male fertility. It is important that clinicians use a laboratory capable of performing an appropriate semen analysis. Laboratories usually perform a semen analysis and report the results according to the recommendations of the World Health Organization[10] (WHO). The parameters and normal values recommended by the WHO are seen in Table 3. Often, small hospital laboratories or independent laboratories may not utilize these standards, and consequently confidence in the results may be lacking. If a semen analysis report does not give the normal range of values and all of the parameters as outlined by the WHO, another semen sample should be obtained and evaluated in a more sophisticated laboratory. The semen analysis should be obtained through masturbation, after 2–5 days of abstinence, into a clean container that does not contain soap residue or other substances or residues that may be harmful to the sperm. For those men who have personal or ethical objections to the collection of a sample in this way, special condoms can be provided that may be used to collect the sample during intercourse. Standard, over-the-counter condoms used for contraception and prevention of disease transmission may be toxic to the sperm and should not be used.

If there is a consistent abnormality in the quality or numbers of sperm seen on two or more occasions, an evaluation of the male by a urologist is indicated. The urologist will take a general medical, surgical, reproductive, and sexual history,

Table 3 Normal semen analysis parameters from the World Health Organization

Volume	>2.0 mL
Count	>20 million/mL
Motility	>50%
Progressive motility	>25%
Morphology	>30% normal head forms

as well as a history of possible exposure to toxic substances, including medications and recreational drugs[14]. Various medications may interfere with normal sperm production by inhibiting the production of hormones by the pituitary or the testicles, by directly effecting the testicle itself, or by interfering with ejaculation. In addition, the use of tobacco, alcohol, and marijuana are associated with an abnormal sperm count, morphology, or function. Most infertile individuals are concerned that their diet, exercise program, or other aspects of their lifestyle may be the cause of their infertility. Although there is little evidence that common variations in lifestyle cause male infertility, the use of cigarettes or marijuana, excessive exposure to heat, and excessive masturbation near the time of ovulation may decrease fertility.

Physical examination of the male may detect systemic diseases, endocrine disorders, infections, or developmental abnormalities of the male reproductive system, including congenital absence of the vas deferens. Because congenital absence of the vas deferens may occur more often in men who carry a gene for cystic fibrosis, known as the cystic fibrosis transmembrane conductance regulator (CFTR), those in whom this abnormality is found should undergo genetic counseling and possibly CFTR mutation analysis before the start of any fertility treatments. They should also have an evaluation of their kidneys and ureters to look for congenital abnormalities of the urogenital system. In addition, abnormalities of the urethra may lead to the deposition of sperm outside the vagina during intercourse (see Chapter 11). Finally, infertile men may also have a collection of varicose veins within the scrotum known as a varicocele. Large varicoceles may interfere with both the number and quality of sperm. Surgical correction of a varicocele may occasionally have a dramatic impact on the number and quality of sperm.

Finally, as many as 18% of men with a decreased number of sperm that cannot otherwise be accounted for have a missing fragment of their Y chromosome (microdeletions)[15]. At this time, genetic testing for microdeletions is not routine because of the expense and the absence of a specific therapy.

Evaluation of the Fallopian Tubes

A potentially correctable cause of female infertility is obstruction or blockage of the fallopian tubes. While this may occasionally be congenital, it more often follows a pelvic infection or pelvic surgery. It has been estimated that approximately 15% of women who have a single episode of a pelvic infection caused by *Chlamydia* or *Neisseria gonorrhoeae* will have obstruction of the fallopian tubes[16]. As noted earlier, detection of an obstruction of the fallopian tubes is usually accomplished by hysterosalpingography (HSG). In this procedure, a colorless liquid, known as radiocontrast material, is injected into the opening of the cervix, and its flow through the uterus and the fallopian tubes is observed under an X-ray machine. A series of pictures is taken, and the location and type of obstruction may be detected. This procedure usually takes only 5–10 minutes to perform and is usually associated with mild-to-moderate menstrual-like cramps.

The cost of HSG has led to a search for less expensive office-based procedures to evaluate tubal patency. As a result, some physicians will perform a pelvic ultrasound examination while fluid is instilled into the uterine cavity through the cervix, a procedure known as an infusion sonography or sonohysterography. Ultrasound can detect the passage of fluid into and out of the fallopian tubes and can outline the shape of the uterine cavity. This procedure is not in widespread use, however, because it is slightly more complicated to interpret and to perform.

If abnormalities of the inside of the uterus are detected, hysteroscopy is often performed. This procedure consists of the introduction of a small telescope through the cervix into the uterine cavity. The walls of the uterus, as well as the shape of the uterine cavity, can be evaluated, and various operating instruments may be delivered through the hysteroscope to remove or destroy any abnormalities that are seen. A normal HSG is seen in Figure 2A; obstruction of the fallopian tubes with the presence of hydrosalpinges is seen in Figure 2B.

Postcoital Examination

The postcoital examination has long been a standard part of the infertility evaluation of a couple. It is designed to evaluate the transport of sperm within the female reproductive tract. However, there is a great deal of controversy regarding its validity. While an occasional study has demonstrated that the findings on postcoital examination are predictive of the ability to conceive, the majority of studies have found a very poor correlation between the result of this test and fertility[17]. During the test, which is usually performed on the day of ovulation or within 2 days prior to ovulation, a couple is instructed to have intercourse without the use of vaginal lubricants. The woman then comes into the office 2–12 hours after intercourse, and the nurse or physician obtains a sample of

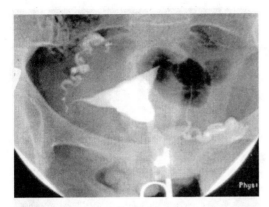

Figure 2a A normal hysterosalpingogram which shows the smooth-walled triangular uterine cavity

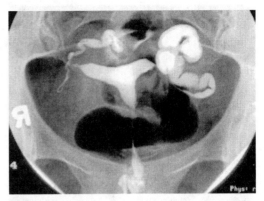

Figure 2b A hysterosalpingogram which shows swelling of the left fallopian tube because of obstruction of its distal end. The right tube is normal caliber and opens into the peritoneal cavity

mucus from the cervix. The quality of the mucus is then evaluated, and the sample is viewed through a microscope in the office. The sperm are counted and their motility determined. It is estimated that approximately $50 million a year is spent on the performance of the postcoital examination[17]. Given the lack of confidence in this test on the part of most clinicians, it is becoming a less important part of the infertility evaluation.

However, women who have had major cervical surgery may have an absence of cervical mucus with the consequent inability to transport sperm from the vagina into the fallopian tube. Infections of the cervix or the presence of antisperm antibodies in the cervical mucus may also interfere with the passage of sperm through the fallopian tubes. Unfortunately, at present we do not have a test that is considered to be better than the postcoital examination for the study of the interaction between sperm and cervical mucus or of transportation of the sperm in the reproductive tract.

Laparoscopy

Laparoscopy is an outpatient surgical procedure during which a telescope is placed through a small incision in the umbilicus or navel. The pelvic cavity is then visualized, and the various pelvic structures viewed. Figure 3 shows the appearance of a normal pelvis as seen through the laparoscope. Figure 4 shows adhesions within the pelvis. Laparoscopy is clearly indicated in women with infertility and either moderate-to-severe pain with their periods or pain with intercourse. In addition, women who have a history of pelvic surgery or pelvic infections may have pelvic scar tissue and often benefit from laparoscopy. Finally, women who have had an abnormal HSG with blockage of the fallopian tubes are also candidates for laparoscopy unless they choose to use IVF. However, laparoscopy is the most expensive of the diagnostic procedures, and many physicians are now delaying or omitting laparoscopy in women who have no significant pain and no history of pelvic infections or surgery if the HSG is normal. The role of laparoscopy in the evaluation of the infertile woman is evolving, and indications for its use are changing because of its expense and because often only clinically insignificant abnormalities are detected.

Once an evaluation has been completed, a course of therapy can be laid out for the

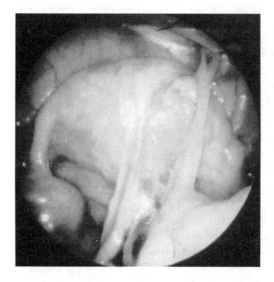

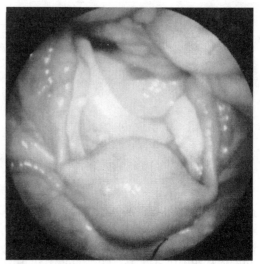

Figure 3 The appearance of normal pelvic organs as seen through a laparoscope

Figure 4 The laparoscopic appearance of pelvic adhesions

patient. The course of therapy will usually be dictated or determined by the results of the diagnostic tests. However, there are often several different options that may be provided.

THERAPEUTIC INTERVENTIONS

Using the tests described above, a possible reason for a couple's infertility will be found in approximately 85% of cases[3]. No explanation or reason will be found for the other 15%. The frequencies with which various reasons for infertility will be found are listed in Table 1. Once an explanation has been found, a treatment program can be presented to the infertile individual or couple.

Induction of Ovulation

Women who do not have monthly menstrual periods will almost always respond to ovulation-inducing drugs (so-called 'fertility drugs'), unless they have experienced ovarian failure (e.g., menopause). There are two commonly used classes of drugs to induce ovulation. The first are termed *antiestrogens* and consist of either clomiphene citrate or tamoxifen citrate. They are available in tablet form and are taken for 5 or more days during the early part of the menstrual cycle. Approximately 1 week after the last tablet is taken, ovulation will usually occur, and the couple should have intercourse several times during the week. The drugs may cause hot flashes but are usually free of other side effects, except for a multiple pregnancy rate of approximately 6–8%. If ovulation does not occur after use of clomiphene, the course of medication is usually repeated at a higher dose. Approximately 60–70% of women will ovulate on clomiphene, and 30–40% will conceive within 6 months of therapy.

The other class of ovulation induction medications are known as *gonadotropins*. These drugs are actually human hormones that are produced by the pituitary gland, extracted from urine, and purified for use. Brand-name examples of this class of drugs include Pergonal, Humegon, Repronex, Follistim, and Gonal-F. They are given by intramuscular or subcutaneous injection and tend to stimulate several follicles to grow and for several eggs to ovulate. Of those who conceive on these medications, 15–20% will have a multiple pregnancy. Because of the potential for multiple follicular development and a condition called *hyperstimulation syndrome*, close monitoring in the form of blood hormone tests and pelvic ultrasound examinations is commonly performed. In its most mild form, hyperstimulation syndrome is characterized by multiple ovarian cysts; its most severe form is marked by the production of a large amount of free fluid in the abdominal cavity and around the lungs. It may cause abdominal pain, marked weight gain, difficulty breathing, and, rarely, death. The syndrome is usually more severe if a woman conceives in the month in which she receives the gonadotropin. These medications are much more expensive and more potent than the antiestrogens.

Fallopian Tube Surgery

When the infertility investigation detects scar tissue or adhesions within the fallopian tubes, surgery may restore fertility to normal. The scar tissue may be limited to one small segment of the tube, and the rest of the tube may be remarkably normal. If the scar tissue is located at the junction of the tube and the uterus, the small segment of the tube containing the scar tissue can be removed and the healthy ends sewn back together. A relatively new procedure, transcervical balloon tuboplasty, uses small probes or catheters passed from within the uterus and out into the tubes to open the blocked area if the obstruction is due to delicate scar tissue or a plug of mucus wedged into the tube. Pregnancy rates following these procedures may approach 50% if the rest of the tube is normal and there are no other infertility factors.

In the case of a previous tubal ligation, surgery known as microsurgical tubal reanastomosis may restore fertility. The surgery requires magnification, very small sutures, and special training in gynecological microsurgery. If the previous tubal ligation has not removed or damaged the majority of the length of the fallopian tube and there are no other possible causes of infertility, an experienced microsurgeon can through this surgery achieve pregnancy rates of nearly 75%.

If scar tissue is blocking the distal end of the fallopian tube adjacent to the ovary, surgery may also be successful. This surgery is often performed through the laparoscope and may restore fertility in as few as 10% or as many as 60–70%, depending on the extent of scar tissue. Unfortunately, there is an increased risk of an ectopic or tubal pregnancy after restorative tubal surgery. The greatest advantage of tubal surgery is that the woman may have more than one pregnancy after a single successful tubal surgery.

Treatment of a Poorly Developed Lining of the Uterus

A successful intrauterine pregnancy requires a receptive and healthy uterine lining. Several therapies have been shown to improve the condition of the uterine lining. For some women who are extremely thin or engaged in extremely strenuous exercise, weight gain and restoration of normal eating habits along with a reduction in exercise may restore the lining of the uterus to normal by increasing the production of estrogen and progesterone by the ovaries. For others, fertility drugs such as clomiphene or a gonadotropin may be necessary to stimulate greater pro- duction of estrogen or progesterone by the ovaries, which will in turn improve the lining of the uterus. Finally, the admin- istration of progesterone by intramuscular injection or vaginal suppository or gel may restore fertility to normal in women with a thin uterine lining.

Treatment of Abnormal Sperm Transportation

If the number of sperm reaching the fallopian tubes after intercourse is inadequate because of the inability to deposit sperm into the vagina during intercourse or an abnormal interaction between the sperm and the cervical mucus, insemination of sperm directly into the uterus may lead to a successful pregnancy. The success of intrauterine insemination (IUI) requires processing of the sperm in the laboratory. Approximately 2 hours before the insemination is to be done, a semen sample is obtained through masturbation, and the sperm are separated from the semen by the use of a sperm 'washing' technique or the passage of the semen sample through a column of material that allows the sperm to swim out of the semen. Once prepared, the sperm are then placed into the uterine cavity using a thin catheter placed through the cervix during a pelvic speculum exam-ination at ovualtion. This process takes only 30–60 seconds and is usually painless. After lying on the examination table for 10–15 minutes, the woman leaves the office and goes about her usual daily activities. The other important factor in successful IUI is the appropriate timing. IUI may be performed approximately 14 days before the next anticipated menstrual period, within 18–36 hours of a positive ovulation detection test, or 36 hours after the administration of human chorionic gon-adotropin (hCG) given to trigger ovulation. Some physicians advocate two or more inseminations each month.

If poor transportation of sperm in the female reproductive tract is the result of an infection of the cervix, a course of antibiotic therapy may be successful. On the other hand, if the problem is the result of the production of antisperm antibodies, IVF may be more successful than IUI, as it avoids sperm interaction with secretions in the cervix, uterus, and fallopian tubes.

Treatment of Endometriosis

Endometriosis is defined as the presence of tissue that normally lines the inside of the uterus in locations outside the uterus. It is commonly found in and around the ovaries and fallopian tubes and may cause pelvic pain and infertility. While it is present in only 3–10% of all women of reproductive age, it is found in 30–35% of women with infertility. Exactly how endometriosis contributes to infertility is unknown, although it may cause infertility by stim-ulating the formation of ovarian cysts and scar tissue. Not all women with endometriosis will be infertile.

In cases of endometriosis, surgery, but not drug therapy, has been shown to improve pregnancy rates. Several medications are commonly used in the treatment of endometriosis, including birth-control pills, progesterone, danazol, and gonadotropin-releasing hormone (Gn-RH) agonists. These medications are most useful in treating the pain of endometriosis and, perhaps, prevent-ing its recurrence and less useful in treating infertility. By themselves, they have not been shown to improve fertility. They may, however, be useful in reducing the volume of disease before surgery or reducing the likelihood of adhesion formation or recurrence of endo-metriosis after surgery. While most women will tolerate and respond well to one or more of these medications, each has its own set of side effects that may be distressing to the woman and as a result limit its usefulness. Typical side effects include hot flashes, headaches, mood changes, vaginal dryness, acne, facial hair growth, and weight gain.

The most successful approach to the treatment of endometriosis appears to be surgery. The surgical removal or des-truction of mild endometriosis may not only improve fertility but is often useful in reducing pelvic pain. Surgical removal of extensive endometriosis and restoration of the normal anatomical relationships between the ovaries and the fallopian tubes may dramatically improve fertility so that as many as 50–60% of women will conceive after surgery. While most surgery for endometriosis can be performed on an outpatient basis through a laparoscope, occasionally a laparotomy and post-operative hospitalization are required.

Treatment of Uterine Abnormalities

Abnormalities of the uterine cavity may either prevent pregnancy or increase the chance of miscarriage. The most common abnormalities are fibroids, adhesions, polyps, and congenital abnormalities, such as a septum dividing the cavity into halves. Another abnormality of the uterine cavity occurs in women who were exposed to diethylstilbestrol (DES) during the first 3 months of their mother's pregnancy. The inside of the uterus in women with this abnormality has the appearance of the letter *T* instead of an inverted triangle. Women with a T-shaped uterus caused by DES-exposure may have more difficulty conceiving and carrying a pregnancy to term. In the past, adhesions or polyps were treated by performing a dilatation and curettage, and fibroids and congenital abnormalities were treated by performing a laparotomy and using a scissors to cut out the abnormal tissue. Today, however, almost all uterine surgery for infertility is performed through a hysteroscope.

Treatment of Male Infertility

A small number of infertile men may have a congenital or acquired deficiency in the secretion of the pituitary hormones, luteinizing hormone (LH) and follicle-stimulating hormone (FSH). As a result, there is inadequate stimulation of the testes and poor or no sperm production. Normal production of sperm and testosterone may be induced by administration of LH and FSH (by intramuscular injection using a preparation of human menopausal gonado-tropins), of a Gn-RH agonist to stimulate pituitary production of LH and FSH, or of hCG, which mimics the action of LH. One or more of these therapies are usually effective if the testes are normal.

There are numerous other hormonal therapies that have been studied and used in men who have a normal pituitary gland but produce sperm in reduced numbers. They include clomiphene, tamoxifen, low-dose testosterone, human menopausal gonadotropins, thyroid hormone, vitamins A, C, and E, and zinc. Unfortunately, while these treatments may benefit an occasional individual, none has been proven consistently successful in the treatment of low sperm production.

The surgical treatment of a varicocele has been shown to improve sperm count, motility, or morphology in 50–90% of men and is followed by pregnancy in 30–55% of previously infertile men[18]. However, 50% of men with varicoceles have normal fertility, and it is difficult to predict which infertile men will benefit from this surgery.

Finally, microsurgical procedures may restore fertility in men who have had a previous vasectomy or have accidental transection of the vasa during pelvic surgery or a previous hernia repair. Surgery may also be helpful when there is obstruction or other abnormalities of the ejaculatory duct. Unfortunately, fertility is not always restored after surgery because of either scar tissue formation in the vas deferens or antisperm antibodies in the testes. However, up to 75% of men may father children after surgical repair of a previous vasectomy.

Assisted Reproduction

While IVF was originally designed to overcome irreversible disorders of the fallopian tubes, it has become an appropriate treatment for virtually all forms of infertility. In addition, when coupled with the donation of eggs from younger women, it has been highly successful in helping women older than age 40 conceive.

IVF consists of several steps. The first step is the stimulation of the ovaries to produce multiple eggs or follicles. In response to clomiphene, human menopausal gonadotropins, pure FSH, or a Gn-RH agonist, most women will produce at least four to six and as many as 20–30 mature eggs. The goal is not to obtain the greatest number of eggs but to obtain 10–12 good-quality eggs capable of being fertilized. During stimulation with these medications, blood tests are obtained and pelvic ultrasound examinations are performed to monitor the response of the ovaries.

Once the eggs have reached an appropriate maturity, they are collected using a needle introduced into the pelvis through the vagina and guided by ultrasound. The eggs, once collected, are sent to an embryology laboratory, where they are mixed with large numbers of sperm in a small laboratory dish. Within 24 hours, evidence of fertilization can be observed through a microscope. The fertilized eggs are allowed to divide into 2-, then 4-, then 6–8-celled embryos over the next 48–72 hours. The embryos are graded according to their quality. Those embryos that divide rapidly and consist of individual cells that are round and equally sized are considered high quality and have a greater chance of implanting. At the time of embryo transfer, the couple is consulted and a decision is made regarding how many embryos will be transferred into the uterus. In women younger than 40, most IVF programs transfer two or three embryos. The transfer of a larger number of embryos may result in an unacceptable risk of multiple pregnancy without a significant improvement in pregnancy rate. As a result, some countries, but not the United States, have limited the number of embryos that can be legally transferred.

The transfer of embryos occurs during a pelvic examination using a thin, soft catheter. The embryos are loaded into the end of the catheter, and the catheter is passed painlessly through the cervix into the uterine cavity. After remaining quiet for a brief period, the woman returns home with instructions to remain relatively inactive for a day or two. She may then resume normal activity. During the weeks following the transfer of the embryos, most women receive progesterone by intramuscular injection or vaginal suppository or gel. Approximately 2 weeks later, a blood pregnancy test is done. Blood pregnancy tests are preferred to home pregnancy tests because of their reliability, sensitivity, and ability to quantify the pregnancy hormone hCG.

The success of IVF has recently improved, so that approximately one in every five IVF cycles will result in the birth of a baby[19]. However, some programs have recently reported success rates of 30–40% or even higher per attempt.

There are several variations of IVF that may be necessary or beneficial in selected couples:

Gamete intrafallopian transfer (GIFT). In this variation, the eggs collected from the ovaries are not fertilized in the laboratory but are mixed with sperm, and the mixture is placed into the fallopian tubes during laparoscopic surgery.

Zygote intrafallopian transfer (ZIFT). This technique involves the placement of embryos into the fallopian tubes at the time of laparoscopy, instead of into the uterus during pelvic examination. The success rates of GIFT and ZIFT are slightly higher than those of IVF, but it is not certain whether they are higher because the procedures are inherently more successful or because the procedures are performed in a younger or more fertile group of patients.

Intracytoplasmic sperm injection (ICSI). Instead of a simple mixture of eggs and sperm together in a laboratory dish, this procedure involves the injection of a single sperm into a single oocyte. ICSI dramatically improves the success rates of IVF when there are only a few motile sperm available or if the sperm lack the ability to penetrate the egg on their own. In the opinion of many, the introduction of ICSI has been the most single important advance in the treatment of male infertility. Fortunately, the occurrence of birth defects in the children conceived after ICSI is approximately 2.5–3.0%, which is no higher than that in children conceived after intercourse. However, there is some concern that some children conceived after ICSI may experience impaired fertility due to the presence of the same genetic abnormalities that caused their father's infertility.

Assisted hatching. Under some conditions, there is an impaired ability of embryos to implant in the uterine lining. Assisted hatching improves implantation by making a small opening in a clear membrane, called the zona pellucida, that surrounds the egg. This procedure takes place just minutes before the embryos are transferred to the uterus and allows them to make better contact with the lining of the uterus.

There are many ways to express the success rates for IVF, GIFT, and ZIFT. However, the most commonly quoted statistics report the percentage of clinical pregnancies or live births among those women who have had retrieval of eggs. The annual report of the Society of Assisted Reproductive Technology publishes the ratio of live births to egg retrievals for each of its member programs[19]. As stated in the introduction to the report, these statistics are published for the benefit of infertile individuals who may be considering IVF, GIFT, or ZIFT. However, the report states that these figures cannot be used to compare the quality of programs because of the differences between programs in the selection criteria, age of patients, and numbers of embryos transferred.

Third-Party Reproduction

Many persons who cannot produce their own sperm or eggs wish to have children. While adoption is one alternative, some couples may choose to use sperm or eggs from a known or anonymous donor. In the case of a woman without a fertile male partner, sperm from a donor can be inseminated into her cervix or uterus with a reasonable chance of success. There are many commercial sperm banks that provide sperm collected from donors who have been screened for genetic diseases, infections, and other undesirable traits. The sperm is frozen and quarantined for 6 months and then thawed for insemination at the time of ovulation each month. If the infertile woman has diseased or absent fallopian tubes, the donated sperm can also be used during an IVF cycle to inseminate her eggs in the laboratory.

In the case of a man whose wife does not produce eggs or have a uterus, conventional surrogacy is a useful option. In conventional surrogacy, the husband's sperm is used to inseminate a woman, called a surrogate, who has volunteered to become pregnant with, deliver a child, and then give the child to the infertile couple for adoption. This procedure is relatively uncomplicated medically and much simpler than the other option, oocyte donation, for the woman who does not produce eggs. In oocyte donation, a woman, referred to as an egg or oocyte donor, volunteers to receive fertility drugs and undergo the retrieval of her oocytes just as though she were undergoing IVF. Her eggs are then fertilized with sperm from the infertile woman's husband. The fertilized eggs are then transferred into the uterus of the infertile woman so that she may carry and delivery the baby.

Finally, in the case of a woman who does not have a uterus but has functioning ovaries, gestational carrier or surrogacy is an option. In gestational surrogacy, the infertile woman receives fertility drugs and undergoes egg retrieval as though she were undergoing IVF. Her eggs are fertilized by her husband's sperm, but the resulting embryos are transferred into the uterus of another woman, called a gestational carrier. After delivery of the baby, the infertile couple become the legal parents of the baby. This procedure is obviously more complicated than insemination of a surrogate, but it does make it possible for the infertile couple to have a child who is the product of their genes.

Thus, women without a uterus or functioning ovaries or men without sperm can still participate actively in overcoming their childlessness, using the new reproductive technologies and/or a third party.

FUTURE IMPLICATIONS

The past 10 years have been dominated by advances in medical technology. However, the next 10 years will not only see technological advances but also a much greater involvement by the nonmedical community in the economics and ethics of these new advanced reproductive technologies.

As we gain greater understanding of the role of the uterine lining in implantation and learn how to identify embryos with the greatest potential for implantation, we will be able to achieve higher success rates in IVF without the 20–25% risk of multiple pregnancies. In addition, not only will we be able to evaluate the genetic constitution of each embryo, but we will be able to correct some genetic abnormalities and prevent some types of birth defects.

The recent report of the successful cloning of a sheep in Scotland has stimulated interest in the options that may be available for infertile individuals in the future. While traditional cloning, involving a cell from an adult donor stimulated to create another individual who is genetically identical to the donor, will probably not be performed in humans in the next few years, other similar procedures may. For example, an embryo can be split into two embryos before implantation of the first embryo into the uterus. The second embryo can either be transferred into the uterus at that time or can be frozen and transferred into the uterus months or years later to create an identical twin.

The treatment of female-factor infertility due to advanced maternal age or ovarian incompetence may be dramatically changed by two recent developments: the report of successful oocyte freezing and the cryopreservation of ovaries or ovarian biopsies in conjunction with cancer treatment. In the future it may be possible for women to select oocytes from a commercial oocyte bank or even to cryopreserve their own oocytes for use later in their lives. In addition, women who must undergo chemotherapy for the treatment of cancer may have their ovaries biopsied or removed and frozen. After recovery from the chemotherapy and cancer, the ovaries may be thawed and the unstimulated eggs stimulated and matured in the laboratory.

In the future women with polycystic ovary syndrome who are unable to produce mature eggs for IVF may have unstimulated eggs retrieved from their ovaries and matured in the laboratory before insemination. We may even develop an artificial placenta, thus making it possible for a full-term pregnancy to take place in the laboratory.

Finally, we may separate the individual cells of a newly dividing embryo and place one of the cells into the uterus, while freezing the remaining cells. This would allow a woman to conceive again without undergoing another IVF cycle by having a thawed embryonic cell transferred to her uterus. Using this form of cloning, all of her children conceived in this way would have an identical genetic make-up and thus would be identical twins or triplets whose births were separated by several years.

None of these technological developments will take place in a social vacuum, however. Society is becoming increasingly involved through legislation, regulation, and the rationing of financial resources for artificial reproduction. Where in the past there has been little in the way of regulations (especially in the United States), in the future there will be a much greater government involvement in setting guidelines, regulations, and sanctions. Hopefully, regulation will develop as a positive force that will lead to a common agreement regarding the limits of artificial reproduction, as well as to an increased level of confidence and trust in the clinicians and scientists who provide such care.

The rationing of health care may pose the most serious threat to the treatment of infertility services in the future. To the fertile population, to adults past their reproductive years, and to medical practitioners in most medical specialties, utilizing limited financial resources for the treatment of infertility may not be a priority. Thus, minimal support and federal funds for reproductive research will probably continue. In addition, managed care organizations that offer infertility care as a benefit may dictate the type of care and therapeutic options based on their cost effectiveness, not on patient preference.

While the potential will exist for overcoming infertility for virtually every infertile individual, only time will tell how, when, and for whom these exciting technologies will be provided.

SUMMARY

- Infertility is defined as the inability to conceive during 12 months of sexual intercourse without contraception.
- Approximately 8% of couples will experience infertility.
- Causes of infertility include:
  Failure to ovulate
  Failure to produce or deliver
    adequate numbers of healthy
    sperm to the fallopian tubes
  Obstruction of the fallopian tubes
  Endometriosis or adhesions involving
    the ovaries or fallopian tubes
  Poor timing of technique of intercourse
  Possible infections of the reproductive
    tract
  Immunological barriers to fertilization or implantation
  An unreceptive lining of the uterus
  Genetic factors
- Efficient and effective delivery of care involves a multidisciplinary team consisting of physicians, nurses, a mental health professional, urologists, an andrologist, and embryologists.
- The medical work-up of the infertile couple consists of:
  Determination of ovulation
  Evaluation of the semen through a
    semen analysis and sperm
    function tests
  Evaluation of the uterus and fallopian tubes by hysterosalpingogram
  Evaluation of the pelvic organs by
    laparoscopy.
- Treatment options include:
  'Fertility drugs' to induce ovulation
    or enhance hormone production
  Surgery of the uterus or fallopian tubes
  Drug or hormone therapy to
    improve sperm production

> Surgery of the male reproductive tract to improve delivery of adequate numbers of sperm
> Insemination of sperm
> Assisted reproduction: IVF, ZIFT, GIFT, ICSI, and assisted hatching.

- Using third-party reproduction, women without a uterus, ovaries, or a partner who produces healthy sperm may 'have a baby'.

- In the future, the new reproductive technologies may include cloning, preimplantation genetic therapy, oocyte freezing, cryopreservation of ovaries from women prior to chemotherapy for cancer, and the freezing of eggs. The limitations and barriers to these technologies are likely to be more social and ethical than medical or technological.

REFERENCES

1. Olsen J. Subfecundity according to the age of the mother and father. *Dan Med Bull* 1990;37:281–2
2. Mosher WD. Infertility: Why business is booming. *Am Demogr* 1987;9:42–3
3. Taylor PJ, Collins JA. Overview of the prevalence of unexplained infertility and the investigations necessary to make the diagnosis. In: Taylor PJ, Collins JA, eds. *Unexplained Infertility*. Oxford: Oxford University Press, 1992: chapter 2
4. Shamma FN, DeCherney AH. Infertility: A historical perspective. In: Keye WR, Chang RJ, Rebar RW, Soules MR, eds. *Infertility: Evaluation and Treatment*. Philadelphia: Saunders, 1995: 3–7
5. Sims JM. Sterility and the value of the microscope in diagnosis and treatment. *Trans Am Gynecol Soc* 1888;77:886
6. Huhner M. *Sterility in the Female and Its Treatment*. New York: Robman Co, 1913
7. Rubin IC. Non-operative determination of fallopian tubes in infertility: Intrauterine inflation with oxygen and production of a subphrenic pneumoperitoneum, a preliminary report. *JAMA* 1920;75:661
8. Rindfleisch W. Darstellung des Cavum Utere. *Berl Klin Wochenschr* 1910;17:780
9. Macomber D, Sanders MR. The spermatozoa count. *N Engl J Med* 1929;200:981–4
10. World Health Organization. *WHO Laboratory Manual for the Examination of Human Semen and Sperm-Cervical Mucus Interaction*, 3rd edn. Cambridge: Press Syndicate of the University of Cambridge, 1992
11. Palmer R. Instrumentation et technique de la cœlioscopie gynécologique. *Gynecol Obstet* 1947;46:420–31
12. Keye WR Jr. Initial approach to the infertile couple. In: Keye WR Jr, Chang RJ, Rebar RW, Soules R, eds. *Infertility: Evaluation and Treatment*. Philadelphia: Saunders, 1995: 76–81
13. Cedars M. Prediction, detection and evaluation of ovulation. In: Keye WR Jr, Chang RJ, Rebar RW, Soules MR, eds. *Infertility: Evaluation and Treatment*. Philadelphia: Saunders, 1995: 107–14
14. Carter MD, Hollander MB, Lipschultz LI. Drug clues to male infertility. *Contemp Obstet Gynecol* 1994;27:30–44
15. Najmabadi H, Huang V, Yen P, *et al*. Substantial prevalence of microdeletions of the Y-chromosome in infertile men with idiopathic azoospermia and oligospermia detected using a sequence-tagged site-based mapping strategy. *J Clin Endocrinol Metab* 1996;81:1347–52
16. Westrom L. Influence of sexually transmitted diseases on sterility and ectopic pregnancy. *Acta Eur Fertil* 1985;16:21–4
17. Griffith CS, Grimes DA. The validity of the postcoital test. *Am J Obstet Gynecol* 1990; 162:615–20
18. Howards SS. Varicocele. *Infertil Reprod Med Clin North Am* 1992;3:428–41
19. Assisted Reproductive Technology and The American Society for Reproductive Medicine. Assisted reproductive technologies in the United States and Canada: 1994 results. *Fertil Steril* 1996;66:697–705

II. ASSESSMENT

3

Psychosocial Evaluation of the Infertile Patient

Susan Caruso Klock, PhD

Fear cannot be banished, but it be calm and without panic;
and it can be mitigated by reason and evaluation.

Vannevar Bush

HISTORICAL OVERVIEW

The role of the mental health professional in the evaluation and screening of infertility patients is relatively new, having evolved over the past 15–20 years. The use of a mental health professional either as a treatment team member or as a consultant is the norm in most academically based and large private practices. However, there are still some physicians who do not use a mental health professional to work with their patients. They generally believe that they are able to counsel their own patients about the psychosocial aspects of infertility treatment and feel that an additional psychological referral is (1) an added stress, (2) an unnecessary expense, and/or, (3) insulting to their patients. Nevertheless, mental health professionals continually work to demonstrate their utility in the reproductive medicine clinical setting. As their role continues to grow and develop, so too, hopefully, will outcome studies demonstrating the clinical utility of their role with infertility patients and the benefit to patients.

REVIEW OF LITERATURE

The goals of infertility treatment are to 'accomplish a thorough investigation, to treat any abnormalities that are uncovered, to educate the couple to the workings of the reproductive system, to give the couple some estimate of their fertility potential, to counsel for adoption when appropriate, and to provide emotional support'[1]. And while all team members contribute to patient care, it is the primary role of the mental health professional to address the psychosocial issues that emerge as the couple confronts infertility. The mental health professional evaluates, diagnoses, and treats psychological disorders, as well as providing patient education, an arena for facilitating decision-making, a forum for discussing ethical and cultural issues related to treatment, and emotional follow-up when the treatment results in a pregnancy and especially when it does not.

Typically, the initial psychosocial evaluation or consultation with the infertile couple is the first contact that the mental health professional has with the couple;

therefore, providing knowledgeable, compassionate care is imperative. It is well known that infertility and its treatment are psychologically stressful, with virtually hundreds of articles published on the psychological concomitants of infertility treatment[2]. The stressfulness of infertility can be related to numerous issues[3], including the blocking or postponement of an important life goal (having a child), marital discord related to infertility, the cyclical nature of treatment, the side effects of fertility medications, and the disappointment when treatment success rates do not match patient expectations. While it has been known for some time that infertility is stressful, it has been only recently that clinicians have acknowledged the need for psychosocial consultation as an integral part of infertility treatment[4]. To quote Christie[5], 'the physician needs to acquire a holistic perspective on infertility, so that he can assess somatic, psychological and social factors in each diagnostic work-up. Only then will he be in a position to evaluate and manage the complex human problems that can emerge during the diagnosis and treatment of a couple's infertility'.

Although the majority of patients do not develop overt psychiatric disorders in response to involuntary childlessness, investigators have documented the occurrence of anxiety and depressive symptoms[6–8], marital difficulties[8,9], and changes in sexual functioning[8,10] during or after infertility treatment. The results from several studies indicate that women report greater infertility-related psychological stress than men[11,12]. In addition, occasionally an infertile patient may present with a significant preexisting psychiatric disorder; for this patient, pregnancy may be contraindicated, based on concerns for both the patient and the potential child, or warrant special pretreatment preparation and care. For these reasons, many authors have recommended the routine provision of psychological services, both evaluation and treatment, to individuals and couples presenting for infertility treatment, especially those undergoing assisted reproductive technologies. Despite the expressed need for psychological services for infertile patients, there has been a paucity of information regarding the content of an initial psychosocial consultation and the identification of patient groups for whom a psychosocial consultation may be recommended or required. For example, some clinics may recommend a psychosocial consultation for all new patients, regardless of how much treatment they have previously received. Other clinics may recommend psychosocial consultations for subgroups of patients, depending on the type of treatment they are receiving, including in vitro fertilization (IVF), donor insemination (DI), oocyte donation (OD), and embryo donation (ED). Due to the nature of the treatment, there are several issues that need to be addressed with infertile patients that are not routinely covered in a typical first-visit psychological consultation.

The goals of this chapter are:

- to review the basic and specific areas that need to be addressed in the evaluation of an infertile couple
- address the use of psychological testing in the context of the evaluation.

THEORETICAL FRAMEWORK

The purpose of a psychological assessment is to gather information about an individual that describes their personal history and current level of functioning. The assessment can gather pieces of information in two ways: a clinical interview and psychological testing. In the clinical interview, specific questions are asked to obtain information about patients' history (family, education, occupation, social) and to ascertain their perception of the current event leading to the psychological consultation. The clinical interview is also essential for assessing mental status and general interpersonal style via direct experience with the interviewer. Psychological interviews are not standardized and are subject to the biases of the interviewer and the interviewee. Psychological tests, on the other hand, are used when one wants to gather information about patients in a standardized manner and compare their responses to a preestablished norm. The role of psychological testing in the evaluation of infertile patients will be discussed later in the chapter.

CLINICAL ISSUES AND THERAPEUTIC INTERVENTIONS

For the majority of men and women, having a child is an essential developmental milestone that cements their entry into adult social status. Most couples assume that they will be able to conceive effortlessly when they want to. When they try to conceive and are unsuccessful, many face, for the first time in their lives, the inability to meet a highly desired goal. This in turn begins to erode their previously held belief that they can do whatever they set their mind to, as long as they work hard enough. The couple then begins treatment and is exposed to a new world of technology, an invasion into their sexual and reproductive life, cyclical treatment demands, financial pressure, work absences, and relatively low per-cycle success rates. All of these factors over time can erode self-esteem, stress a previously solid marriage, and generally wreak havoc in a couple's life. For those less able to cope, these stresses can lead to the development of depression, anxiety disorders, obsessive/compulsive disorders, or sexual dysfunction. For those more able to cope, their life is still turned upside down, and they are forced to question

previously held beliefs about their life, their role in life, and their belief in a predictable, just world. The primary need for a psychological consultation is to aid in coping with the enormous psychological consequences of infertility and its treatment. A secondary reason that supports the use of a psychological consultation for infertility patients is patient satisfaction. It is the opinion and observation of many that patients are more satisfied when they believe that their psychological, as well as physical, health is being attended to by their physician. While some doctors continue to hold to the belief that they will insult their patients if they recommend a psychological consultation, it is the belief and experience of this clinician that the majority of patients welcome the opportunity and feel more satisfied with their overall care because of it.

Psychological Evaluation
Who Should Be Seen?

The question of who should have a psychological evaluation can be answered relatively easily. A psychological consultation with every infertile couple during the diagnostic work-up would be the ideal. While it may be impossible to see every infertile couple, the stakes become higher when patients begin to undergo an assisted reproductive technology procedure and/or make use of third-party reproduction options, such as DI, OD, or ED. In these situations, it is the growing opinion that a psychological evaluation of all parties should be mandated due to the extraordinary circumstances around the possible conception of a child[4,13]. In addition, Dennerstein and Morse[14] reported that any patient who is perceived by the physician to be 'psychiatrically at risk' should be referred. 'These include patients with psychosomatic symptoms or current psychiatric disorder; past psychiatric treatment; where there is concern about motivation; stability of the marriage and capacity of parenthood; and those with unrealistic expectations of treatment.' If psychosocial consultations remain on an 'as needed' basis, patients who are referred may feel stigmatized, which could result in increased attempts to mask or deny their difficulties. When operating on a routine basis, the role of the mental health professional is normalized, and the mental health professional is viewed as just another member of the treatment team whose goal it is to aid the patient.

Psychological consultation for infertility patients should be available to any individual or couple who is self-referred. For those patients undergoing IVF, DI, OD, or ED, a routine psychological consultation should take place at least 2 weeks prior to the start of treatment. This allows the couple time to consider the many psychological, social, and legal issues brought up during the psychological consultation. It may be indicative of a potential problem if patients want to rush through the evaluation process (both medical and psychological). They may be trying to push an unwilling partner through the treatment ('If I don't do it now, my husband won't do it'), deny their ambivalence ('I'd better do it now, or I'll lose my nerve'), or mask underlying pathology ('Let's get this over with'). When the medical and psychological evaluation happens over time, it tends to let the treatment team get to know the couple better, and issues or problems can emerge and be dealt with without the urgency and panic that might occur if a shortened timetable is used.

Who Should Do the Evaluation?

There are many different types of mental health practitioners, including psychiatrists, psychologists, social workers, psychiatric nurses, and a variety of therapists who have postgraduate training in a social science. Mental health professionals doing infer-

tility-related work should also meet the fundamental requirements described by the Mental Health Professional Group of the American Society for Reproductive Medicine (ASRM) (see Appendix 1). These guidelines provide the minimum training and experiential requirements for mental health practitioners in this area. An extremely important component of these guidelines is the recommendation that infertility-related mental health professionals have a thorough working knowledge of the medical aspects of the infertility work-up and treatment. Familiarity with procedures, medications, and various treatment protocols is a necessary foundation enabling the mental health clinician to work effectively with medical team professionals and communicate with patients. Patients seen by counselors without this background complain, with good reason, that they have to educate such counselors about the medical aspects of treatment, which is another hassle and expense for them. The interested reader should refer to Chapter 2 in this volume. Other excellent reviews are by Rein and Schiff[15] and Hardy and Fox[16] regarding the evaluation and treatment, respectively, of the infertile couple. For a more thorough understanding of reproductive endocrinology, the reader should review Speroff and colleagues'[1] *Clinical Reproductive Endocrinology and Infertility*. Last, clinicians can always update their fund of knowledge by attending one of the postgraduate courses sponsored by the ASRM at its annual meeting. These courses provide up-to-the-minute information on the rapidly developing infertility treatment techniques and their psychological consequences.

What is Being Assessed?

What is the mental health professional assessing during the psychological consultation with infertility patients? First, they are assessing all the usual content areas addressed in a psychological intake interview, such as presenting problem, psychological history, social history (including current relationship and sexual functioning), medical history, family history, and current mental status. In addition to these topics, the infertility assessment includes a review of the treatment about to be undertaken, the implications of the treatment, a discussion of the perceived stress of the treatment, social support for the treatment, legal and ethical issues, expectations of treatment success, and the treatment plan. These are typically covered in the first hour, with additional time scheduled as needed.

The goal of the psychological evaluation is:

- to prepare patients for the treatment that they are about to undergo
- to raise issues that they may not have considered thus far, so that these can be discussed prior to treatment
- to screen for individuals who may benefit from psychological treatment either before or during infertility treatment
- to evaluate patents for any preexisting psychopathology or social dysfunction that would preclude or impact infertility treatment.

Preparing for the Interview

Some logistics to consider prior to the interview include (1) boundaries of confidentiality, (2) clarification of the mental health professional's role, and (3) documentation of the consultation. The patient should be made aware of the nature of the information exchange between the psychologist and the treatment team. For example, if the mental health professional is part of the treatment team, he or she may be expected to provide relevant psychological information to the attending reproductive endocrinologist or other staff members. Consent from the patient is needed for this exchange of information and should be documented in the patient's chart after it has been obtained. The mental health professional must also be careful to maintain privacy boundaries for information that patients do not wish to be shared. A common example of information that a patient may not want her physician to know is previous sexual or reproductive trauma. As with any other type of consultation, the mental health professional's first obligation is to maintain patient confidentiality, but it is also to encourage patients to share any medically relevant information with their physician. In addition, the mental health professional should be aware of the laws governing the creation and storage of psychiatric records. For example, in some states, psychiatric and psychological reports and records are kept in a separate medical record to protect patient privacy. If this is the case, then only documentation of basic information (date, purpose, and time of interview; recommendation(s); plan) in a couple's medical chart is appropriate, and the major portion of the confidential information should be kept in a separate location. Some infertility counselors maintain this practice even if it is not legally mandated.

Preparation of a couple for the interview can be done by the physician or nurse on the team. In many practices, a couple is informed that the psychological consultation is a routine part of the diagnostic work-up; therefore, the couple learns early on that this is an expected part of the treatment process, just like an ultrasound examination or other procedure. In addition, the couple's primary nurse is responsible for helping schedule the psychological consultation appointment. Often it is helpful for a couple to briefly meet and say hello to the mental health professional prior to the interview, so that their anxiety about the interview can be minimized.

A couple can be told briefly about the purpose of the interview, which is to learn more psychosocial information about them that may impact their infertility treatment, to ease their psychological adjustment to the infertility diagnosis and treatment, and to act as a resource should they need one. In addition, the consultation provides a couple with the opportunity to discuss the ethical, religious, and moral issues related to treatment, to review treatment success rates, to ask questions about the informed-consent process, and to seek assistance in decisions about ending treatment and obtaining counseling regarding adoption or child-free living. It is often useful to encourage patients to come prepared with their own questions or concerns in order to make the best use of the interview.

Content of the Evaluation Interview

The foundation for the clinical interview for infertility patients is the same as a general psychological interview with elaboration and greater detail in obtaining information in areas related to reproductive history, marital history, sexual functioning, and cultural and religious issues. Given the nature of infertility (i.e., the majority of patients are married or in a committed relationship), the identified patient is most often the couple, not the woman alone. Therefore, the husband or partner's presence at the psychological evaluation is imperative. Not only does this give the clinician another source of information about the couple's history, but, more important, it can provide a snapshot of how the couple works (or does not work) together in conceptualizing and coping with infertility. The absence of the husband or partner on repeated occasions can indicate significant marital discord or ambivalence on his part.

A useful model for the structured clinical interview is the Comprehensive Psychosocial History for Infertility[17] (CPHI) (see Appendix 2). The CPHI provides clinicians with the structure for an interview that covers the needed content areas specific to infertile populations. As the authors note, the CPHI can be used by a variety of health professionals. It covers the spectrum of issues relevant to the emotional status of infertile patients, as well as issues relevant to a couple's functioning, and it can help identify 'red flag' issues that may be indicators that a couple is at risk for a poor adjustment to infertility treatment or that, in more serious cases, infertility treatment may need to be postponed or denied.

The content areas in the CPHI are self-explanatory. As a clinician goes through each section, information can be elicited from one or both partners about each area. It may be a good idea to begin by addressing the infertility history question to the woman because (1) she is usually the primary recipient of diagnostic and treatment interventions, (2) it is often easier for the woman to break the ice in the initial part of the interview, and (3) she can provide a role model for her husband or partner about how to talk about the emotionally sensitive issues related to infertility.

The first thing a clinician needs to determine is whether patients are accurate and reliable informants. Due to the high socioeconomic status of the majority of infertility patients, this is generally not a problem, but in some instances individuals may not be able to give reliable information or may be purposefully deceptive. A second fundamental cognitive prerequisite is that individuals fully understand the procedure(s) that are about to be performed and are cognitively able to provide informed consent. Patients must be able to understand procedures' risks, benefits, and chances for success. Occasionally, a patient with little education will come for treatment and may not comprehend the nature of the treatment and its risks and benefits.

An unfortunate but somewhat common clinical scenario is the couple seeking infertility treatment as a way to mend a faltering relationship or guarantee the continuation of a relationship. For example, an older woman in a relationship with a younger man may feel pressured to pursue infertility treatment to prove to her partner that she is still able to provide children or to ensure that he will not abandon her for a younger, fertile woman. Contingencies for the continuation of the relationship may rest on the outcome of the infertility treatment. In this situation, both partners will perceive an inordinate amount of pressure on the outcome of the treatment and want to begin treatment as soon as possible. However, it is advisable to slow the couple down and try to address this situation prior to beginning treatment.

In discussion of a couple's reproductive history, it is important to spend some time asking the infertile partner (if one has been identified) how he or she feels about being the 'one with the problem'. If the infertile partner has been identified, he or she may feel isolated, embarrassed, ashamed, and sad about the diagnosis but may be unable to talk to his/her partner about it. The infertile person often feels a huge sense of responsibility for being the one preventing a pregnancy and typically has fears that the fertile partner will leave or feel resentment. In the context of the consultation, it is useful to have both partners talk about their reaction to the infertility diagnosis and its impact on their self-esteem and marital equilibrium.

Marital or relationship history and the impact of the infertility are other topics to be addressed in the consultation interview. The circumstances surrounding courtship, marriage, and current marital situation can provide information about many aspects of the marriage, including how a couple handles relationship discord, emotional support of one another, division of labor, decision-making, and expression of emotional needs. During this discussion, the motivation of each partner to pursue infertility treatment and become a parent also emerges.

In addition to the social support supplied within the marriage, a clinician will also want to assess the availability and quality of the social support from family and friends. This is taken into consideration along with the tendency of a couple to be open or private regarding their infertility diagnosis and treatment. Often men and women differ in regard to how open they are with family and friends regarding their infertility. Problems can arise when one partner tells too many people too much about the infertility diagnosis and treatment or refuses to respect the other's need for privacy or support. This can cause a rift in the relationship, prompting unwanted intrusions or questions, albeit well-meaning, from family and friends. Therefore, initial discussion about a plan for the type and amount of disclosure is often helpful[18].

Infertility treatment is a less-than-perfect art. The per-cycle pregnancy and take-home-baby rates generally vary from clinic to clinic and procedure to procedure, depending on a couple's diagnosis. Therefore, it is important for mental health professionals to be aware of these rates for their clinic in order to talk candidly about a couple's expectations for treatment success. More often than not, a couple is not able to absorb all the information given to them during the medical consultation, including success-rate information[19]. Moreover, they may hear the statistics and inflate them, based on information specific to them. For example, a 30-year-old couple may have been told that they had a 35% chance of getting pregnant with use of a gonado-tropin and intrauterine insemination. They may tell themselves that since they are relatively young, have been in treatment a short time, and are 'good people', somehow their chances for success are higher. This increasing optimism sets up an inaccurate expectancy that can lead to a dysphoric or even depressive reaction in the event that the cycle is unsuccessful. In the course of the psychological consultation, it is important for mental health professionals to ask a couple about their perception of the chances for treatment success and help them maintain a cautiously optimistic attitude.

In the past 18 years since the advent of IVF, mental health professionals have had to talk to couples about their thoughts and feelings about extracorporeal creation of embryos, freezing and thawing of embryos, and disposition of unused embryos. Usually, within the context of this discussion, a couple also is made aware of the likelihood of a multiple pregnancy and the option of selective reduction. All of these issues are jarring to the couple who 'just wants to have a baby'. Couples, out of necessity, are forced to discuss and make decisions about things they never thought possible. In the psychological evaluation, mental health professionals can discuss each of these issues and elicit any religious or moral differences between the partners as well as acceptability of the options for patients. Some individuals may object to the cryopreservation of embryos; others may disagree with one another regarding the disposition of unused embryos. It is my opinion that mental health professionals can play a pivotal role in helping couples discuss their differences and come to a consensus regarding these important decisions. The decision can then be conveyed to the treatment team to allow greater clarity in clinical care and fewer last-minute decisions and/or misunderstandings.

Issues regarding multiple pregnancy and selective reduction are increasingly common. During the consultation, a couple may for the first time have the time to think about the implications of a multiple pregnancy and the possibility of parenting twins, triplets, or more. Couples often resist discussions of multiple pregnancy during the psychological consultation because they are solely focused on the goal of getting pregnant. They may dismiss these discussions by stating that they would be delighted with a 'family' instead of just one child and may minimize concerns about the welfare of the mother and infants in multiple pregnancies. It may take some redirection to help them understand the importance of preemptive discussion to aid in possible decision-making later on. It is a difficult clinical situation if there is a multiple pregnancy and the partners disagree with one another about their course of action. Again, as with the issue of cryopreservation of embryos, multiple pregnancy rates should be discussed with patients by their physician; while mental health professionals should focus on the partners' emotional and moral reaction to the possibility and aid in decision-making if a difference is identified.

Obtaining an accurate psychiatric history for both partners is essential. Due to the demographics of infertility patients, in general, partners are usually high-functioning, but this does not preclude the existence of a past or current psychiatric illness. The psychiatric history is important because it may impact the adjustment to pregnancy and the patient's ability to parent. For example, if a woman has major depression, discontinuation of antidepressants during infertility treatment and the possible reemergence of depression during pregnancy and the postpartum period need to be carefully considered. A psychiatric illness does not preclude the possibility of infertility treatment, but it needs to be assessed in order to make arrangements for the maintenance of psychiatric stability during treatment, pregnancy, and the transition to parenthood (see Chapter 4).

Although it is not included in the CPHI, it is a good idea to discuss a couple's legal history. It is extremely rare that a patient will have a legal history relevant to the infertility treatment, but legal history is relevant if it relates to instances of child neglect, endangerment, or abuse. Also relevant are legal entanglements indicating current alcoholism or drug addiction (e.g., 'Driving under the Influence' arrest), particularly in women. If such a history is found, then further information regarding the specific charges, reparation, or rehabilitation should be obtained.

During the course of the structured interview, the individuals' and couple's style of coping will become evident. Most infertility patients tend to use problem-focused coping, which may be a reason that they choose to seek infertility treatment. This style of coping is generally helpful, but couples need to understand that treatment outcome is not related to the amount of planning, medical compliance, and behavioral change that they undergo. This may be the first time that a couple experiences a situation in which the attainment of a highly desired goal is not related to the effort that they expend toward meeting that goal. This irony is one of the key components of the stressfulness of infertility treatment to otherwise highly effective and successful people.

After completion of the interview, clinicians can begin summarizing the information and coming up with impressions and recommendations. Most couples are high-functioning and psychologically aware. Therefore, mental health professionals may only need to remind the couple about adaptive coping skills, provide them with information or educational materials regarding the treatment, and offer further

follow-up as needed. Unfortunately, treatment may be contraindicated in a minority of cases. In general, infertility treatment is contraindicated and may be denied or postponed under certain circumstances. The contraindications for infertility treatment are listed in Table 1.

When one of these situations is found, the evaluating clinician has to carefully review his or her boundaries prior to making treatment recommendations. If further infertility treatment is contingent on the solution of a problem that requires psychotherapy and the evaluating clinician is an employee of the infertility program, it is probably a good idea for the evaluating clinician to refer the couple to a different treating clinician. In cases when a problem is identified but it is not serious enough to preclude treatment, then the conflict of interest between the evaluating and treating clinicians is not as great. If the

Table 1 Psychosocial contraindications to infertility treatment

---

Treatment or pregnancy may significantly worsen an active psychiatric illness

Active substance dependence with concomitant chaotic lifestyle

One partner is coercing the other to proceed with treatment

One or both partners are unable or unwilling to provide consent for the treatment

A legal history related to child endangerment is discovered

Infertility treatment is used to compensate for a sexual dysfunction

Decisions about privacy and disclosure in third-party reproduction cannot be resolved

Use of a family member gamete donor would cause significant familial discord

Custody arrangements for the potential child of a known gamete donor have not been agreed to by all parties

Serious marital discord

---

evaluating clinician feels that there is a conflict of interest between themselves, the couple, and the program, it is wise to refer to a colleague not affiliated with the infertility program and then obtain consent from the couple to receive information about their treatment progress when infertility treatment is desired in the future. This is often a time-consuming and difficult boundary to maintain, but for all concerned it is the best option for keeping couples' needs in the forefront and to reduce the likelihood of biased treatment.

Related to this issue is the communication of the results of the psychosocial evaluation to the team and the sharing of information obtained in the interview. Clinicians may want to write a note in the medical record indicating:

- date and time of the interview
- general content of the interview ('Reviewed couple's history and discussed the emotional concomitants of the treatment.')
- impression regarding the couple's preparedness for treatment ('The couple appear to be appropriate candidates for this treatment.' or 'Further clarification and treatment of marital difficulties need to be completed before initiation of treatment.')
- plan ('routine social support follow-up offered') or referral (e.g., for marital therapy)
- indication of full intake summary report and its location ('Full intake note dictated on ..., filed in separate psychological record.')

It is a good idea to inform couples that the recommendation will be shared with the team and that in the event of post-ponement or refusal of treatment the information will be shared with the attending physician. In keeping within the boundaries of confidentiality among mental health professionals, it is important for patients to know that specific information obtained in the history is not shared with the treatment team. This applies to all information but is especially important in cases in which there have been previous pregnancy termin-ations, sexual abuse, or legal problems.

The final purpose of the psychosocial evaluation is to provide couples with the feeling that they have an open door to a person with expertise in reproductive psychology who can be a resource to them in the future. Clinicians should leave time at the end of the interview for questions and long-term treatment planning. After the initial consultation, many couples find it useful to come in for a consultation when considering ending treatment and/or moving to adoption. Also, in cases of a pre-IVF egg donor or sperm donor evaluation, it is a good idea to call after the completion of the first treatment cycle to check in with the patients and see how they are feeling. This is usually a welcome opportunity to talk about their emotional reaction to treatment.

Psychological Testing
Role in the Evaluation of Infertility Patients

In general practice, the interview provides the majority of information gathered during the routine psychological evaluation of an infertile couple. This information is easy to obtain and is usually reliable. There may be cases in which the clinician wants a second source of information to provide confirmation or refutation of the interview material. In these cases, the use of psychological testing may be helpful.

Psychological cognitive tests were developed around the turn of the century as a way of assessing the skills and competencies of a large group of people on a uniform set of tasks. Personality tests were developed to get the unique response of an individual to standardized testing material in a controlled situation. The test results received from one individual can then be compared with the test's established norms for the representative sample to which the individual belongs. Testing is a useful source of additional information, but it is not a substitute for a clinical interview. Before discussion of the use of psychological tests with infertility patients, some basic background on the characteristics of psychological tests may be helpful.

Characteristics of Psychological Tests

Psychological tests can be either projective, such as the Rorschach inkblot test, in which a person's response to ambiguous stimuli is interpreted, or objective, such as the Minnesota Multiphasic Personality Inventory (MMPI), in which a person's answers to direct questions with a true or false response are scored via empirically derived scoring criteria. In both cases, responses are compared to preestablished norms. The difference between projective and objective tests is the degree to which the test administrator interprets the results: Projective tests are subject to greater interpretation than objective tests. Psychological tests can assess multidimensional characteristics, such as personality or intelligence, or a single psychological construct or attribute, such as anxiety or depression. The utility of either type of test is dependent on how well it answers the question that a clinician wants answered. For example, within the context of infertility, if it were known that a woman who had high levels of anxiety needed more anesthesia and nursing support during a laparoscopy, then pretreatment anxiety testing would be useful in determining which patients were more anxious in order to plan for greater anesthesia and nursing coverage. In this example, an anxiety test would be useful in helping plan the allocation of clinical resources. But before a test can be used to

predict behavior, two important characteristics about the test must be established: validity and reliability.

Validity and reliability are two key concepts in the theory of test construction[20]. In their simplest form, validity refers to how well a test measures what it purports to measure, and reliability refers to how consistently the measure assesses what it purports to measure. A test is essentially useless if it does not have moderate to high levels of validity and reliability. How do you know if a test is valid and/or reliable? There are several types of validity. One is called *content* validity, referring to the extent to which the items on a test assess the construct that it is trying to assess. For example, a test assessing depression should include items known to be symptoms of depression. A second type of validity is called *criterion-related* validity, referring to the process of checking to see whether a score on a test is correlated with an actual behavior hypothesized to be measured by the test. For example, scores on a depression test would be correlated with clinicians' ratings of depression. The extent to which the scores on the test and the clinicians' ratings corresponded would be the degree to which the test had criterion-related validity. A third type of validity is *construct* validity, referring to how well a test correlates with other measures of the same construct. For example, we would expect that a new measure of depression would be highly correlated with an older measure of depression. All these types of validity are usually investigated by the test constructors before a test becomes widely used. Prior to using a test, it is important for clinicians to understand the degree of validity the measure has in order to know its strengths and limitations in a given situation.

Reliability refers to the consistency of a test. There are two types of reliability, internal consistency and test–retest reliability. *Internal consistency* refers to the intercorrelation of items on a test and the extent to which they measure the same construct. For example, on a measure of depression, all the items should be related to the construct of depression and should correlate with one another. *Test–retest reliability* refers to the correlation of test scores over time. It reflects the extent to which the score on a test given at time 1 will be similar to the score obtained on the same test at time 2. A final word about reliability: Reliability is not necessarily correlated with validity. A test may be very reliable to the extent that it consistently yields the same result time after time, but it may not be valid to the extent that it does not measure the construct of interest.

Literature Review on Psychological Testing

In addition to the clinical interview, some clinicians working with infertile patients routinely use psychological tests, usually personality tests, to obtain further information. While numerous measures, including the MMPI, MMPI-2, Symptom Checklist 90 (SCL-90), Speilberger's State Trait Anxiety Inventory (STAI), and the Beck Depression Inventory (BDI), have been used to evaluate infertile patients in clinical research, their utility in the clinical context for predictive purposes has not been demonstrated.

Several researchers have used psychological tests with infertility patients. They have generally addressed one of the following points: (1) identification of psychopathology among idiopathic infertile women, (2) assessment of personality and other psychological constructs among IVF participants, and (3) assessment of depression, anxiety, locus of control, and/or coping among pregnant and nonpregnant infertility patients to determine if psychological variables correlate with pregnancy outcome. There have been no studies addressing the clinical utility of

psychological tests in predicting psychological outcome among general infertility patients.

IVF participants seem to be the most studied group of infertility patients[7,21,22]. During the mid to late 1980s, several studies reported the use of the MMPI[23] with IVF patients[24]. The MMPI-2 is the recent revision of the MMPI. It has 567 true/false items in 10 clinical scales and three validity scales that are designed to detect psychopathology[23]. Scale scores of 65 or higher on any of the clinical scales are indicative of psychopathology and may be indicative of a psychological disorder, but there is no one-to-one correlation between MMPI-2 scores and the presence of psychiatric illness. In a series of 200 IVF couples, Freeman and coworkers[7] found that 20% of men and women had at least one elevated clinical scale suggesting dysfunctional emotional distress or personality difficulties. Approximately 50% of the sample also had high levels of ego strength, indicating that they had a fair amount of emotional resilience to deal with the stress of the treatment. Alternatively, Haseltine and colleagues[21] reported no major personality disorders or psychological dysfunction on abbreviated MMPIs given to 75 couples in an IVF program. Keye and associates[25] found normal MMPI scores among all 22 women entering an IVF program, but 17% of the male IVF participants had abnormal MMPI profiles. In general, the MMPI has been used with IVF couples as a pretreatment screening tool to detect the small percentage of patients who may have preexisting psychopathology that might impact on their ability to participate in treatment. As Mazure and Greenfeld[22] noted, 'the single most important finding has been that, in general, IVF/ET participants score within normal limits on measurements of preexisting psychopathology. Furthermore, the data do not support the notion of an increased incidence of psychiatric diagnoses or psychosexual disorders in IVF participants'.

Other psychologically relevant constructs have also been studied among infertility patients, with again most studies focusing on IVF participants. Using a variety of measures, studies have looked at the incidence of depression[11,26,27], anxiety[6,11,21,26-29], marital adjustment[29,30], sexual functioning[7,8,31], and ways of coping[26,30]. These studies have helped characterize the psychological state of couples undergoing IVF treatment but are limited in generalization to other infertility patients because IVF patients represent a small, self-selected group who may differ from others who decide to stop treatment to pursue adoption or remain childless or those couples who get pregnant without assisted reproductive technologies.

The clinical recommendations regarding the use of psychological tests have been relatively sparse. The use of personality testing among infertility patients as a screening device seems to have indicated that infertility patients have no greater incidence of personality disorders than that found in the general population. Findings from other construct-specific tests, such as depression and anxiety inventories, have produced mixed results, indicating that infertility patients may be depressed or anxious at times during the treatment. Other tests have addressed coping styles, marital adjustment, and sexual functioning in relationship to infertility and, with the exception of a few studies[11,30,32,33], have not linked pretreatment test findings to posttreatment adjustment. In addition, there have been no studies comparing the predictive utility of clinical interview data with that of testing data in predicting outcome among infertility patients. Furthermore, numerous methodological flaws, such as limited patient selection, participation rates, and attrition, make generalization from these studies difficult. Finally, the relationship between a given test result at time 1 and its relationship to an outcome of interest at time 2 has not been demonstrated. If a measure such as a pretreatment depression instrument was helpful in identifying those women who would develop a clinical depression after their third cycle of infertility treatment, then that test would have a high clinical utility. There have been few studies addressing the relationship between pretreatment psychological status and posttreatment outcomes. Those that have been done have been interesting and have indicated that there are relationships between pretreatment coping style and posttreatment adjustment[30,32] and pretreatment depression and posttreatment depression[11], but further studies of this kind are needed to demonstrate the clinical utility of specific psychological measures.

In summary, recommendations for the use of psychological tests in conjunction with the structured interview for infertility patients would be premature due to the lack of methodologically sound research demonstrating their clinical utility. Further studies are needed with all infertility patients, not just convenient samples of IVF patients, to determine whether any standard measure can substantially add to the pretreatment screening information or can predict outcomes of clinical importance, such as the occurrence of depression, marital discord, length of treatment, or pregnancy. At present, the skilled clinician must determine whether additional testing information materially adds to the information collected during the interview.

SUMMARY

- Infertility treatment is psychologically stressful; therefore, many programs offer consultation with a trained mental health professional prior to treatment, 'as needed', or in the context of specific treatments.

- The Mental Health Professional Group of the American Society for Reproductive Medicine has developed guidelines for the qualifications for mental health professionals providing infertility-related services (see Appendix 1).
- The purpose of the interview is to educate and prepare couples for the treatment and to detect the presence of any psychosocial problem that would be a contraindication for infertility treatment or impact participation in treatment.
- The Comprehensive Psychosocial History for Infertility (CPHI) is an excellent structured interview to use with infertility patients (see Appendix 2).
- Criteria for exclusion from treatment include the presence of an active, major psychiatric disorder, severe relationship discord, cognitive impairment, or inability to resolve legal and ethical issues around third-party reproduction.
- While numerous psychological tests have been used with infertile samples, there is not yet enough research-based evidence to support the routine use of psychological tests to predict outcomes of interest among infertility patients.

REFERENCES

1. Speroff L, Glass RH, Kase NG. *Clinical Gynecologic Endocrinology and Infertility*, 4th edn. Baltimore: Williams & Wilkins, 1989
2. American Society for Reproductive Medicine, *Mental Health Professional Group Bibliography*. Birmingham, AL: American Society for Reproductive Medicine, 1996
3. Mahlstedt PP. The psychological component of infertility. *Fertil Steril* 1985;43:335–42
4. Klock SC, Maier D. Guidelines for the provision of psychological services at the University of Connecticut Health Center. *Fertil Steril* 1991;56:680–5
5. Christie GL. The psychological and social management of the infertile couple. In: Pepperell RJ, Hudson B, Wood C, eds. *The Infertile Couple*. New York: Churchill Livingstone, 1980: 229–47
6. Mazure CM, Del'Aune W, De Cherney AH. Two methodological issues in the psychological study of in vitro fertilization/embryo transfer participants. *J Psychosom Obstet Gynaecol*, 1988;9:17–21
7. Freeman E, Boxer AS, Rickels K, *et al.* Psychological evaluation and support in a program of in vitro fertilization and embryo transfer. *Fertil Steril* 1985;43:48–53
8. Baram D, Tourelot E, Muechler E, Huang K. Psychosocial adjustment following unsuccessful in vitro fertilization. *J Psychosom Obstet Gynaecol* 1988;9:181–90
9. Micioni G, Jeker L, Zeeb M, *et al.* Doubtful and negative psychological indications for AID: A study of 835 couples. *J Psychosom Obstet Gynaecol* 1987;6:89–99
10. Downey J, Yingling S, McKinney M, *et al.* Mood disorders, psychiatric symptoms, and distress in women presenting for infertility evaluation. *Fertil Steril* 1989;52:425–32
11. Newton CR, Hearn MT, Yuzpe AA. Psychological assessment and follow-up after in vitro fertilization: Assessing the impact of failure. *Fertil Steril* 1990;54:879–86
12. Nachtigall RD, Becker G, Wozny M. The effect of gender-specific diagnosis on men's and women's response to infertility. *Fertil Steril* 1992;57:113–21
13. Klock SC. Psychological aspects of donor insemination. *Infertil Reprod Med Clin North Am* 1993;4:455–70
14. Dennerstein L, Morse C. A review of psychological and social aspects of in vitro fertilization. *J Psychosom Obstet Gynaecol* 1988;9:159–70
15. Rein MS, Schiff I. Evaluation of the infertile couple. In: Ryan KJ, Berkowitz, RS, Barbieri RL, eds. *Kistner's Gynecology: Principles and Practice*, 6th edn. St. Louis, MO: Mosby-Yearbook, 1995;278–304

16. Hardy RI, Fox J. Infertility treatment. In: Ryan KJ, Berkowitz, RS, Barbieri RL, eds. *Kistner's Gynecology: Principles and Practice*, 6th edn. St. Louis, MO: Mosby-Yearbook, 1995;305–30

17. Burns LH, Greenfeld DA, for the Mental Health Professional Group. *CPHI: Comprehensive Psychosocial History for Infertility*. Birmingham, AL: American Society for Reproductive Medicine, 1990

18. Klock SC. Privacy and disclosure in infertility treatment. In *Session: Psychotherapy in Practice* 1996;2:55–71

19. Reading AE, Kerin J. Psychologic aspects of providing infertility services. *J Reprod Med* 1989;34:861–71

20. Mazure C. What can we learn from psychological testing? In: *Clinical assessment and counseling in third-party reproduction*. Presented at the 26th annual meeting of the American Society for Reproductive Medicine, Montreal, Quebec, Canada, October 3, 1993

21. Haseltine FP, Mazure CM, Del'Aune W, et al. Psychological interview in screening couples undergoing in vitro fertilization. *Ann N Y Acad Sci* 1985;442:523–32

22. *Mazure* CM, Greenfeld DA. Psychological studies of in vitro fertilization/embryo transfer participants. *J In Vitro Fertil Emb Transfer* 1989;6:242–56

23. Graham, JR. *MMPI-2: Assessing Personality and Psychopathology*, 2nd edn. New York: Oxford University Press, 1993

24. Garner CH, Kelly M, Arnold ES. Psychological profile of IVF patients. *Fertil Steril* 1984;41(suppl):57S

25. Keye WR, Bensch RL, Jones KP, et al. The psychosocial evaluation of couples undergoing in vitro fertilization. *J In Vitro Fertil Emb Transfer* 1984;1:119–26

26. Shatford LA, Hearn MT, Yuzpe AA, et al. Psychological correlates of differential infertility diagnosis in an in vitro fertilization program. *Am J Obstet Gynecol* 1988;158:1099–107

27. Hearn MT, Yuzpe AA, Brown SE, Casper RF. Psychological characteristic of in vitro fertilization participants. *Am J Obstet Gynecol* 1987;156:269–74

28. Thiering P, Beaurepaire J, Jones M, et al. Mood state as a predictor of treatment outcome after in vitro fertilization/embryo transfer technology. *J Psychosom Res* 1993; 37:481–91

29. Shaw P, Johnston M, Shaw R. Counselling needs, emotional and relationship problems in couples awaiting IVF. *J Psychosom Obstet Gynaecol* 1988;9:171–80

30. Litt MD, Tennen H, Affleck G, Klock S. Coping and cognitive factors in adaptation to in vitro fertilization failure. *J Behav Med* 1992;15:171–87

31. Leiblum S, Kemmann E, Lane MK. The psychological concomitants of in vitro fertilization. *J Psychosom Obstet Gynaecol* 1987;6:65–78

32. Morrow KA, Toreson RW, Penney LL. Predictors of psychological distress among infertility clinic patients. *J Consult Clin Psychol* 1995;63:163–7

33. Boivin J, Takefman JE. Stress level across stages of in vitro fertilization in subsequently pregnant and nonpregnant women. *Fertil Steril* 1995;64:802–10

4

Psychopathology and Psychopharmacology in the Infertile Patient

Katherine E. Williams, MD

Fortunately psychoanalysis is not the only way to resolve inner conflicts.
Life itself still remains a very effective therapist.

Karen Horney

HISTORICAL OVERVIEW

Prior to advances in medical evaluation techniques, many researchers believed that a woman's psychological problems caused many forms of infertility, including ovulatory dysfunction, recurrent miscarriage, and unexplained infertility. In her classic and influential article, 'Infertility as a Psychosomatic Defense', Benedek[1] postulated that 'underlying ambivalence' and 'rejection of motherhood' caused infertility. Infertility patients were frequently described as emotionally immature and psychologically conflicted, and researchers expected to find high rates of psychiatric morbidity in this population. However, studies over the years have not confirmed these earlier theories, and it is now known that the psychopathology found in this population is usually a result of the stresses and losses associated with infertility or exacerbation of pre-existing conditions rather than a primary cause of infertility.

The goals of this chapter are:

- to review the literature regarding the prevalence, clinical course, and treatment of psychiatric disorders in infertility patients
- to discuss the known effects of typically used infertility medications on mood
- to clarify potential drug interactions between infertility treatment medications and psychotropic medications.

REVIEW OF LITERATURE

There has been considerable research on psychopathology and infertile patients (most commonly women); however, most of it was based on the hypothesis that infertility was caused by psychopathology, which, if treated, would thereby improve fertility. Most of this 'research' involved anecdotal case studies. Ultimately, the findings or conclusions of this research were not supported by more scientifically rigorous research. More recently, research has focused on the development of psychopathology in response to infertility diagnosis and treatment and, even more recently, the impact of preexisting psychopathology and its treatment on infertility diagnosis and treatment. The review of the literature that follows will address current research on the incidence and treatment of psychopathology in infertile patients and the impact of medications for the treatment of infertility on mood and psychological functioning.

Psychopathology in Infertility Patients

Affective Disorders

Grief reactions are common in both men and women undergoing infertility treatment, since infertility represents a loss on so many levels: from the loss of a sense of self and belief in the creative powers of one's own body to the loss of the chance to have and nurture one's biological child. Several studies have shown that many women identify infertility treatment as the most distressing event in their lives—more upsetting than the loss of a loved one or divorce[2,3]. Many men, as well, report significant emotional distress associated with the diagnosis and treatment of infertility[4,5]. However, studies suggest that there are gender differences in the prevalence, intensity, and duration of grief reactions and most agree that women suffer more than men after the diagnosis of infertility[6,7].

It is important, then, that clinicians be able to differentially diagnose the expected grief reaction seen in most infertility patients[8] from the less common and serious complication of pathological grief. As described in Chapter 1, *normal grief* includes the classic symptom complex of initial shock and numbness followed by intense sadness and distress, frequent anger and hostility, guilt and self-reproach. Grief reactions are commonly classified as *Adjustment Disorders* in the *Diagnostic and Statistical Manual of Mental Disorders*[9] (DSM-IV). It is normal for infertility patients to experience some measure of grief, and it is believed that the mourning process is important for the final resolution of the crisis of infertility[10,11]. In contrast, *pathological grief* is considered a psychiatric illness that requires immediate evaluation and treatment. Pathological grief is consistent with the DSM-IV definition of major depression, and it is characterized by marked vegetative symptoms such as appetite, sleep, and psychomotor disturbances; anhedonia; suicidal ideation; and memory and concentration problems. Pathologic grief may also include psychotic features, such as paranoid or somatic delusions and excessive punitive thoughts.

The prevalence of major depression in infertility patients appears to be higher than previously thought. Many earlier studies failed to define important population variables such as length of infertility treatment, diagnosis, and medication usage, all of which are now known to be important contributors to depression[12]. For instance, Hearn and colleagues[13] and Downey and colleagues[14] reported that Beck Depression Inventory (BDI) scores in female infertility patients did not differ from scores in a group of healthy female controls; however, the infertility patients were pre–in vitro fertilization (IVF) treatment, and studies have shown that there may be a honeymoon period of optimism prior to the first IVF cycle[6]. More recent studies suggest that major depression is in fact more common in women undergoing infertility treatment than in fertile controls. Domar and associates[15] evaluated 338 infertility patients with the BDI and the Center for Epidemiological Studies Depression Scale (CES-D), comparing them to 39 healthy controls, and found that depression was twice as common in the infertility patients: 37% scored in the depressed range on the BDI compared to 18% of controls. BDI scores were correlated with length of treatment. Women with a history of infertility of 2–3 years had higher BDI scores than women in treatment for less than 1 year or greater than 6 years. Several other studies demonstrated increased emotional distress over time in both male and female infertility patients due to repeated treatment failures[5,16]. Domar and coworkers[17] also found that symptoms of anxiety and depression in infertile women were as prevalent as in patients with other chronic medical conditions, such as hypertension and cancer.

No studies have investigated the prevalence or the emergence of bipolar disorder in infertility patients. Prevalence rates of bipolar disorder in the general population are low (0.7–1.6%), compared to prevalence rates of major depression (25%)[18]. However, the peak years for onset of bipolar disorder coincide with a woman's reproductive years; consequently, clinicians working with infertility patients can expect to treat women with this disorder.

Anxiety Disorders

Several studies have reported that anxiety levels are often elevated in both male and female infertility patients[17,19]; thus, it is expected that there is a high incidence of Adjustment Disorder with anxiety in this population. The prevalence of other anxiety disorders, such as obsessive compulsive disorder, in this population is unknown. Anxiety disorders, especially phobias, are quite common in the general population. Six-month prevalence rates for specific phobias range from 4.5% to 11.8%[20]. Blood-injury and needle phobia can lead to significant impairment in infertility treatment. Couples in whom one or both partners suffer from these specific phobias can be expected to have significant difficulty with injections, as well as greater emotional distress associated with preparation for and recuperation from surgery and other medical procedures. During treatment planning, clinicians should inquire about both a personal and a family history of blood-injury or needle

phobias, since these anxiety disorders appear to have a very strong genetic link[21].

Eating Disorders

Anorexia nervosa and bulimia are common causes of ovulatory dysfunction, yet eating disorders are frequently overlooked in women presenting for infertility evaluation. In a study of 66 women consecutively presenting to an infertility clinic, Stewart and colleagues[22] found that 7.6% met DSM-III criteria for anorexia or bulimia and 16.7% for an eating disorder, not otherwise specified, as measured by the Eating Attitudes Test and a structured clinical interview. When women with menstrual irregularities were studied separately, 58% were found to have an eating disorder. Active eating disorders are associated not only with diminished fertility but with increased perinatal morbidity, including intrauterine growth retardation and increased congenital anomalies[23]. Women with menstrual irregularities should be carefully screened for the presence of an underlying eating disorder, which should be treated before proceeding with infertility treatment[22–24].

Personality Disorders

Large population studies using standardized psychometric tests such as the Minnesota Multiphasic Personality Inventory (MMPI or MMPI-2) and the Eysenck Personality Inventory showed no increased prevalence or pattern of preexisting personality disorders in women undergoing infertility treatment[25]. Nevertheless, because of the prevalence of these disorders in the general population, clinicians can expect to be faced with personality-disordered patients, who can represent major challenges to the treatment team. The borderline, narcissistic, and histrionic personality disorders are

Table 1 Psychiatric effects of infertility medications

Drug	Use	Psychological effects
Bromocriptine	hyperprolactinemia	antidepressant effects hypomania psychosis
Leuprolide acetate	hypothalamic 'downregulation'	depression cognitive problems fine motor problems
Progesterone	endometrial support	depression decreased libido irritability
Estradiol	endometrial support	antidepressant effects induction of rapid cycling

especially difficult to manage, and the treatment of these 'cluster B' patients will be discussed later in the chapter.

Infertility Medications and Mood

Many of the medications prescribed for the treatment of infertility have effects on the neurotransmitter systems involved with affective regulation. Surprisingly, very few studies have investigated the psychiatric side effects of infertility medications. A brief review of the effects of gonadal hormones on mood and a review of the reports of the effects of infertility medications on mood will follow. It is important for clinicians to understand the potential effects of infertility medications on mood in order to help patients in their decision-making regarding the risks and benefits of infertility treatment (Table 1).

Neurotropic Effects of Gonadal Hormones

Estrogen and progesterone are steroid hormones that directly and indirectly affect central nervous system neurons involved in the regulation of mood and cognition. Animal studies have shown that these hormones can influence the production of neurotransmitters and modulate the affinity of receptors for substrates[26]. Studies suggest that estradiol affects dopamine receptors and has neuroleptic properties in both animals and humans[27]. Several authors report that women with psychotic disorders such as schizophrenia improve during pregnancy[28,29], and it is presumed that this is due to enhanced dopamine blockade with increased estrogen levels[30].

Recent studies of estrogen use in perimenopausal women suggest that estrogen may improve mood in women whose anxiety or depression is not severe enough to meet the criteria for major depression[31]. Estrogen has been shown to increase serotonin bioavailability in several ways, including displacing its precursor tryptophan from albumin-binding sites, thereby allowing more tryptophan to be converted to serotonin[32], and decreasing monoamine oxidase, an enzyme that degrades serotonin[33,34]. Estrogen also promotes norepinephrine release[35], which may further improve mood; however, this enhanced noradrenergic function has also been associated with the emergence or exacerbation of anxiety disorders in some women. New-onset panic attacks have been reported in women initiating estrogen replacement therapy[36], and some women experience increased anxiety during the second and third trimesters of pregnancy when estrogen levels are highest[37].

In rats, progesterone treatment decreases serotonin accumulation in the brain[38]. In humans, progesterone in oral birth control pills has been shown to decrease tryptophan oxygenase and this decreased tryptophan metabolism has been correlated with depression[39]. Progesterone metabolites act in a similar manner to barbiturates to modulate γ-aminobutyric acid (GABA) receptor complexes and have sedative effects[40,41]. Consequently, many women report improvement in anxiety disorders, such as panic disorder, during pregnancy[31].

Clomiphene Citrate

Clomiphene citrate (Clomid, Serophene) is a synthetic estrogen used to induce ovulation in anovulatory women, improve luteal phase deficiency, and increase follicle number in women with unexplained infertility[42]. Clomiphene is usually taken on days 3 to 5 of the menstrual cycle; however, it has a metabolite that can be found in the circulation for up to 30 days after the last dose[43]. Clomiphene acts directly on the hypothalamus[44] to increase gonadotropin-releasing hormone (Gn-RH) pulse frequency and amplitude[45]. Subsequent increases in luteinizing hormone (LH) and follicle-stimulating hormone (FSH) lead to the development of multiple ovarian follicles and significant increases in midcycle estradiol in clomiphene-treated cycles, as compared to control cycles, which may persist into the luteal phase and is often accompanied by increased levels of progesterone[46].

Clomiphene is associated with menopausal symptoms, and 10% of women taking the medication complain of hot flashes[47]. No large prospective studies using validated, standardized measurements have yet been published that evaluate the effect of clomiphene on mood. However, many women report that this medication is associated with mood changes, including irritability, emotionality, and increased symptoms of premenstrual syndrome[48]. In a small pilot study, Williams and Casper[49] reported that clomiphene is associated with decreased fatigue at midcycle, at the time when the estradiol levels are highest. They hypothesized that clomiphene may be associated with more mood changes in women with a history of affective lability at times of hormonal change, such as women with a history of premenstrual dysphoric disorder (PDD), since several studies suggested that increased estrogen levels in the luteal phase leads to increased psychiatric symptoms in women with PDD[50,51].

Human Menopausal Gonadotropins

Human menopausal gonadotropins, including menotropins (Humegon, Pergonal, Pregova) and urofollotropin (e.g., Metrodin), are composed of purified FSH and LH in varying combinations. They act directly on the ovary to stimulate folliculogenesis; but unlike clomiphene, they have no direct hypothalamic effects. While the potential physical side effects of these medications, such as hyperstimulation syndrome, are well documented, the psychiatric side effects have been overlooked. Since these medications lead to extremely elevated estrogen levels during the follicular and midluteal phase, it can be expected that they affect mood in some women in a manner similar to clomiphene. Williams and Casper[49] are currently investigating the effects of these medications on mood and anecdotally report that many women feel a burst of energy and improved mood when their estrogen levels are rising.

Bromocriptine Mesylate

Bromocriptine mesylate (Parlodel) is an ergot alkaloid structurally related to the neurotransmitter dopamine[52]. It inhibits prolactin release from the lactotroph cells of the anterior pituitary and is used in infertility treatment to treat hyper-prolactinemia (elevated levels of prolactin), which is associated with ovulatory dys-function[42]. Because of its effects on mono-amine systems associated with affective regulation, bromocriptine has been used as an antidepressant for over 20 years. It has been shown to be as effective as imipramine and amitriptyline in the treatment of depression in several double-blind, placebo-controlled studies[52]. Bromocriptine is also an effective adjunctive treatment, turning tricyclic antidepressant nonresp-onders into responders[53].

The bromocriptine dosages used in these antidepressant studies ranged from 40 mg/day to 220 mg/day, which is considerably higher than the 1.25– 5 mg/day dosing commonly used in hyper-prolactinemia. Nevertheless, patients with hyperprolactinemia suffer from irritability, decreased libido and depressive symptoms that improve with low-dose bromocriptine treatment but not with placebo[54].

Infertility patients should be counseled about the potential psychiatric side effects of bromocriptine treatment, and women on antidepressants or with a history of bipolar disorder should be cautioned about the possible emergence of hypomania or mania[55], when taking this medication for fertility treatment. Other adverse psychiatric side effects include hallucin-ations, delusions, confusion, and behavioral changes[52].

Gonadotropin-Releasing Hormone Agonists

Gn-RH agonists, such as Lupron and triptorelin (Decapeptyl), are used to downregulate the pituitary to prevent premature ovulation during IVF cycles[42]. Usually, these medications are begun in the midluteal phase of the preceding cycle and continued during the stimulation phase of the treatment cycle. Gn-RH agonists lead to acute hypoestrogenism, a pharmacological menopause[42], and women frequently complain of mood changes and physical symptoms, such as hot flashes and headaches[56,57].

Toren and colleagues[58] compared depression scores in IVF patients pretreated with the Gn-RH agonist triptorelin to scores in a control group undergoing IVF without downregulation. Triptorelin caused a 40% reduction in estradiol levels during the pretreatment phase, and this hypo-estrogenism was associated with a significant increase in depression and anxiety, compared to controls. All subjects entering the study were euthymic, and despite significant increases in mood symptoms in those on triptorelin, no patients developed symptoms severe enough to meet criteria for major depression or anxiety disorder. This is the first study of its kind, and it is not known what effect Gn-RH-induced hypoestro-genism has on women with preexisting mood disorders. From our knowledge of the interaction of gonadal hormones with the neurotransmitters associated with depression, it is theorized that these medications may aggravate preexisting psychopathology, and patients with mood disorders should be carefully monitored for the emergence of depression and anxiety while on Gn-RH agonists.

Many women taking Gn-RH agonists also complain of cognitive changes, such as poor memory and concentration, that may or may not be accompanied by symptoms of a mood disorder. Varney and associates[59] compared neuropsychiatric tests in women prior to pre-IVF treatment with the Gn-RH agonist leuprolide, during leuprolide treatment, and at ovulation, approximately 10 days after leuprolide administration. Each woman served as her own control. A significant proportion of women demonstrated impairment in performance on one or more memory tests while taking leuprolide. Similarly, Sherwin and Tulandi[60] demonstrated significant decreases in verbal memory scores in women on leuprolide that were reversed in a group receiving 'add back' estrogen but not in the control group.

Progesterone

Progesterone is frequently used during infertility treatment to improve luteal phase endometrial lining in both clomiphene and IVF cycles[42]. Progesterone in the oral birth control pill has been associated with the onset of depression in women[61], and there have been reports of the emergence of major depression with suicidal ideation and panic disorder in women using synthetic progesterones such as levonorgestrel subdermal implants (Norplant)[62]. However, some women report improvement in anxiety symptoms while on progesterone because of the sedative properties of its metabolites[40,41].

Oral Birth Control Pills

Oral birth control pills are frequently used in infertility patients prior to an IVF cycle to downregulate the hypothalamus. Prevalence rates of depression in women taking oral birth control pills range from 5% to 50%, depression being most common in progesterone-dominant pills[63]. However, because of the estrogen in oral birth control pills, there have been some case reports of the induction of rapid cycling mood in women taking these medications[63].

THEORETICAL FRAMEWORK

The theoretical approach most applicable to psychopathology, psychopharmacology, and infertile patients is a medical model of psychiatric illness and its medical treatment. In this approach, a distinction is made between psychological disorders with emotional etiology and psychiatric illness of primarily physical etiology, such as inherited disorders or neurological changes. As brain research has increased, it has become increasingly apparent that a significant proportion of psychiatric illnesses are probably the result of physical factors, such as altered brain chemistry. Psychopathology may be related to social, environmental, or personal history, although physical factors can always be a mediating influence. As a result, psychiatry has seen a shift away from the psychological treatment of psychopathology (as initiated by the father of psychiatry, Sigmund Freud) to a greater emphasis on the psychopharmacological treatment of psychiatric illness, with psychotherapy as adjunctive care.

CLINICAL ISSUES AND THERAPEUTIC INTERVENTIONS

It is difficult to separate the clinical issues of psychiatric illness and psychopathology from therapeutic interventions, especially those involving psychopharmacological treatment. For this reason, clinical issues and therapeutic interventions will be combined for practicality and greater efficiency. The clinical issues and interventions to be addressed include psychopathology, including disorders of mood and personality, and drug interactions in which the interaction of psychotherapeutic medications and infertility treatment medications are reviewed.

Psychopathology

Psychopathology is generally defined as the science dealing with diseases and abnormalities of the mind, while psychopharmacology is the treatment of psychiatric illness with psychotropic medications, such as antidepressants. Although the exact mechanism of treatment is not completely understood, it is thought that psychotropic medications affect levels of brain chemicals (e.g., serotonin) or the effective operation of brain cells (e.g., neurotransmitters), which in turn impact mood and behavior.

Affective Disorders

Depressive reactions to the diagnosis or treatment of infertility are common, and treatment decisions should be based on symptom severity and past psychiatric history. Adjustment disorders, not accompanied by pronounced vegetative symptoms, are best treated with supportive psychotherapy. The treatment of choice for depression in infertility patients is psychotherapy rather than pharmacotherapy. Behaviorally oriented group psychotherapy has been found to decrease anxiety and depression in female infertility patients in several studies[64,65] (see Chapter 8).

If a patient has a history of rapid relapse of depression after antidepressant discontinuation or a history of severe depression with suicidality, psychosis, or dangerous vegetative symptoms, maintenance on antidepressants may be recommended or unavoidable even during medical treatment for infertility. While some women may feel better during pregnancy, studies do not support the popular belief that pregnancy 'protects' against depressive episodes. The prevalence of major depression during pregnancy is similar to that in nonpregnant women: 10%[66]. Furthermore, risk factors for depression (e.g., prior depressive episode, reproductive loss, genetic predisposition) must be considered.

Tricyclic antidepressants have been in use for over 20 years, and to date studies do not suggest significant increases in congenital malformations in prenatally exposed infants[67]. Most studies have been retrospective and included small numbers of patients. However, a recent prospective study of over 600 patients reported that tricyclics are not associated with increased rates of major fetal malformations[68]. The long-term neurobehavioral effects of these medications on offspring have only recently been studied. The two published investigations report no differences in cognitive and behavioral measures between tricyclic-exposed infants and controls at up to 3 years[69] and 6 years[70] of age. These drugs should be used with extreme caution, and pregnant women should always be maintained on the lowest possible dose of medication. However, Wisner and colleagues[71] reported that tricyclic antidepressants required dosage increases during the second and third trimesters of pregnancy; so if a patient is nonresponsive, it is important to check tricyclic antidepressant blood levels.

Serotonin-reuptake inhibitors (SSRIs) appear to be relatively safe as well in pregnancy, since preliminary reports do not suggest an increased risk of major congenital malformations in women exposed to fluoxetine (Prozac)[72,73]. However, Chambers and coworkers[73] reported that the prevalence of minor malformations may be increased with in-utero fluoxetine exposure, which may represent occult major malformations. The postnatal effects of in-utero fluoxetine exposure remain controversial. While Goldstein[74] reported no increased incidence of postnatal complications in 112 infants exposed to fluoxetine during the third trimester, Chambers and colleagues[73] did report an increased risk of complications such as premature delivery and respiratory and feeding problems in their series of 228 infants exposed to fluoxetine. No studies have yet been published of the long-term neurodevelopmental effects of in-utero fluoxetine or SSRI exposure.

Women taking fluoxetine and planning to discontinue medication once they have a positive pregnancy test should be switched to another SSRI such as sertraline (Zoloft) or paroxetine (Paxil), which have shorter half-lives. Fluoxetine's active metabolite, norfluoxetine, remains in the body for nearly 2 weeks after the last dose, which prolongs the period of fetal exposure to the medication[75]. Women who plan to abruptly discontinue their SSRI should be cautioned about the possible emergence of a flu-like syndrome with antidepressant withdrawal, which does not appear to be dangerous but may exacerbate pregnancy symptoms such as nausea, malaise, and headaches[76].

Infertility patients taking an SSRI should also be warned about recent reports of sertraline-associated galactorrhea (excessive milk production). Several case reports have recently emerged in the literature, suggesting that sertraline may induce the onset of galactorrhea[77,78]. The mechanism of action is not clear, but it is postulated that SSRIs may elevate serum prolactin through serotonergic activation of prolactin-releasing factors. Since galactorrhea is associated with subfertility, it is important that women on SSRIs examine themselves for the onset of breast discharge, have their prolactin levels carefully checked, and consider switching to a tricyclic antidepressant.

Finally, it is important that clinicians warn all infertility patients considering antidepressant continuation or initiation about the ongoing controversy regarding the association between antidepressants and spontaneous abortion. When Pastuszak and colleagues[72] compared pregnancy outcomes in women following first-trimester fluoxetine exposure, women with tricyclic-antidepressant exposure, and women with no teratogen exposure, they found that women who had been on antidepressants had a higher incidence of miscarriage (approximately 13% in medication-exposed vs. 6.8% in controls). However, Chambers and colleagues[73] did not find an increased risk of spontaneous abortion in women exposed to fluoxetine as compared to antidepressant-free controls (10.5% vs. 9.1%, respectively). Furthermore, while the incidence of spontaneous abortion was twice as high in antidepressant-exposed patients as compared to controls in Pastuszak and associates'[72] study, it is important to point out that the miscarriage rates in the medication group were still lower than many of the recently quoted rates for spontaneous abortion in the general population, which range from 15% to 25%[42]. Finally, in the largest prospective study to date of antidepressants in pregnancy, McElhatton and colleagues[68] did not find an increased risk of miscarriage in women using tricyclic antidepressants.

Another conundrum in counseling women regarding risks versus benefits of antidepressant exposure is the question of whether underlying depression is associated with an increased risk for infertility. Lapane and coworkers[79] reported that a history of depression was associated with an increased risk for later infertility; however, this was a retrospective report and therefore subject to problems of recall and validity of retrospective diagnoses of depression. Thiering and colleagues'[80] prospective study of IVF patients reported that women with elevated depression scores at the start of treatment had significantly lower pregnancy rates than women who were not depressed. As Rubinow and Roca[81] hypothesized, depression may affect behaviors associated with fertility, such as loss of libido leading to decreased sexual activity, or the underlying hypothalamic dysregulation associated with depression may compromise reproductive mechanisms and events. Whether depression is associated with infertility remains controversial, and further studies are needed to evaluate this question. At this time, we can only counsel patients that the long-term effects of untreated depression on fertility are not known, but clearly affect behavior and quality of life.

Women taking mood stabilizers, such as lithium for bipolar disorder, should be counseled about the high rates of relapse with abrupt medication withdrawal[67]. In addition, abrupt changes in hormones postpartum and premenstrually have been shown to be associated with increased risk for bipolar relapse[29,82,83]. While no studies have yet been done evaluating the effects of infertility medications on mood in women with bipolar disorder, it may be expected that hormonal changes during IVF may increase relapse risk. Mood stabilizers such as lithium have been associated with an increased risk of congenital malformations, so the risks of maintaining a woman on medication should be carefully weighed against the risk of withdrawing medication[71]. Women without a history of severe illness can be tapered off their medication, while women with a history of dangerous relapses may be maintained on the lowest possible dose of lithium. The risk of cardiac defects with lithium is less than previously thought, approximately 0.1%; however, this estimate is still 10–20 times greater than the risk in the general population[67].

Since valproic acid is now a first-line treatment for mania in bipolar disorder[84,85], clinicians may increasingly see women on these medications presenting for infertility treatment. First-trimester exposure to valproic acid is associated with a 1–5% risk of spina bifida, while exposure to carbamazepine is associated with a 1–1.5% risk. Therefore, it may be safest to switch women taking these anticonvulsant mood stabilizers to lithium[67].

It has been repeatedly documented that the postpartum period is associated with an increased risk of relapse in bipolar disorder patients[29,82,83], so patients should be counseled about the benefits of resuming medication immediately postpartum and relinquishing breast feeding[86,87]. This is also true of women with a history of major depressive episode, particulary if she has a history of multiple episodes.

Anxiety Disorders

The effect of infertility treatment on anxiety disorders has not been studied. Since anxiety disorders, such as obsessive-compulsive disorder (OCD), increase during times of stress, it can be expected that patients with these disorders will experience exacerbations of their symptoms during the process of infertility diagnosis and treatment. Patients with contamination obsessions and cleaning rituals may experience increased anxiety due to the responsibility of sterile technique associated with injections. These patients may find that they experience excessive hand washing before and after injections, and they will need extra guidance and reassurance regarding sterile technique. Behavioral strategies for managing their symptoms should be implemented, such as strict time limits on hand washing prior to and after injections and thought-stopping for obsessive, intrusive thoughts.

Infertility treatment with the Gn-RH agonists requires injections; therefore, it may be an overwhelming proposition to a patient with needle phobia. Since needle phobia is the most common specific phobia in the general population[20], clinicians should inquire about the presence of this disorder prior to assuming that a patient or her partner can assume responsibility for injections. If a patient does experience needle phobia, treatment should consist of desensitization exercises.

The effect of anxiety disorders on pregnancy remains controversial. As previously discussed, progesterone metabolites interact with the GABA receptors in a manner similar to barbiturates[40], so theoretically the increased progesterone in pregnancy may be associated with decreased anxiety. However, not all women report an improvement in anxiety during pregnancy, and studies have shown that panic and OCD symptoms may in fact emerge or worsen during pregnancy[31]. As with bipolar disorder, the postpartum period appears to be the time of greatest risk for relapse or escalation of symptoms in panic disorder and OCD patients[31,88].

Infertility patients taking benzodiazepines for their anxiety should attempt to taper off these medications because therapeutic doses have been associated with an increased risk of cleft abnormalities[89]. Tricyclic antidepressants or SSRIs may be substituted for anxiolytics in women who are unable to manage without medications. Cognitive behavior therapy should always be the first-line treatment in infertility patients, pregnant women, and nursing mothers[90].

Personality Disorders

Borderline Personality Disorder

The most common and troubling personality disorders challenging the infertility treatment team and therapist are the 'cluster B' patients: borderline, narcissistic, and histrionic personality disorders. The use of primitive defenses by individuals with borderline personality disorder can be a major obstacle to infertility treatment. Projection of poor self-esteem and fears of abandonment may disrupt patients relationship with infertility caregivers. Patients may perceive rejection in a clinician's hurried appointment or delayed call-back, which leads to intense, disruptive rage reactions and splitting. Frequently, the physician will remain the 'good object', since these patients often have intense, idealized transference reactions to the caregivers who they believe have the ultimate power over

their fertility. Clinic support staff, such as nurses, receptionists, and administrative personnel, more often bear the brunt of the angry outbursts. It is extremely important that infertility treatment personnel become educated about these primitive defenses so that they can approach these patients in a dispassionate, clinical manner in order to minimize splitting. Angry rebuttals to such patients' rage will only fuel the projective fires and lead to canceled or disrupted cycles and staff disturbances.

Persons with borderline personality disorder have problems with boundaries and entitlement that may also pose major problems for medical staff. These patients desperately need clear, articulated, and immutable boundaries. For instance, if they keep calling after hours for questions that could be addressed earlier in the day, they need to be reminded in a calm, caring way that the on-call staff is only for emergencies, and criteria for emergencies should be reviewed. These boundaries often need restating several times.

Because they are already emotionally labile and frequently suffer comorbid depression, borderline patients may be especially sensitive to the effects of infertility medications on mood[91]. The dysphoria, increased anxiety, and irritability associated with some infertility medications may be frightening to these patients. Similarly, the 'rollercoaster' of emotions associated with infertility treatment may further destabilize this group of affectively labile women.

Finally, in borderline personality disorder, patients have a high prevalence of history of sexual abuse[92], and the infertility evaluation and treatment process include many invasive, frequently painful procedures that may trigger increased anxiety, flashbacks, and intrusive memories. These patients should be carefully educated about all of the steps involved in treatment. If care is being provided at a teaching hospital, it is best that examinations and procedures be performed by one caregiver and his or her team, rather than by a 'revolving door' of students and residents, which may heighten anxiety and threaten the fragile sense of bodily integrity that these patients have. Some women who have been victims of sexual abuse prefer female gynecologists, and their requests should be met with understanding and accommodation, if possible.

Borderline patients may enter a mental health practice in two ways: self-referral because of emotional distress or referral by the infertility team because of disruptive behavior in the clinic. In both situations, mental health clinicians must adhere to a fundamental treatment principle with these patients: compassionate limit-setting, since they will often attempt to engage their therapists in their battles with the clinic, furthering the splitting process. Initially, psychotherapy with borderline patients undergoing infertility treatment should be extremely supportive and educational. Once stabilized, these patients may benefit from the use of other treatment modalities, such as dialectical behavioral therapy, a form of cognitive-behavioral therapy[93]. Psychopharmacological interventions may be necessary for the management of comorbid major depression and anger.

Narcissistic Personality Disorder

Because infertility is by its nature a 'narcissistic injury', patients with narcissistic personality disorder can be expected to be at risk for decompensation during infertility evaluation and treatment. Common reactions include narcissistic rage and devaluation of caregivers. Narcissistic patients may have trouble following directions because they are so humiliated at being in such a dependent position. For instance, they may choose their own treatment plan (e.g., taking more or less of a medication than recommended) to assert their autonomy and authority, and they may fail to ask questions when they are confused. When faced with such patients, infertility clinicians must continually remind themselves that these patients, at their core, suffer from tremendously low self-esteem[94]. Therapeutic management of a narcissistic patient includes friendly acknowledgment of their intelligence and fund of knowledge about infertility, but clear and firm recommendations regarding treatment plans. Clinicians can expect that angry confrontation or disavowal of a narcissist's ideas will lead to rage reactions and should be avoided, if possible. Psychopharmacological treatment is typically not helpful in these patients.

Histrionic Personality Disorder

Patients with histrionic personality disorder will challenge infertility clinicians with their somatization of affect. They are less likely than borderline or narcissistic patients to split their caregiving team into adversarial positions, but they may create chaos and confusion and, in so doing, disrupt their care. For instance, the histrionic amplification of symptoms may lead to excessive testing, unnecessary changes in medication dosage, excessive phone calls, and extra appointments. Clinicians will be called on to differentially diagnose histrionic complaints from true, potentially life-threatening, treatment-emergent side effects, such as ovarian hyperstimulation syndrome. Infertility clinicians can help these patients by redirecting their somatic preoccupations and facilitating the expression of their psychological distress through referral to a mental health professional. Therapy necessarily focuses on exploration of underlying psychodynamic and interpersonal conflicts and more effective methods of communicating. Psychopharmacological interventions are not useful, although these patients prefer a medical explanation for their distress.

Obsessive-Compulsive Personality Disorder

The disruptive nature of infertility treatment represents extended torture to many patients with OCD. Patients with this disorder long for a sense of control in their lives and normally rely on a devotion to work, schedules, and productivity to manage anxiety. Infertility diagnosis and treatment signify a loss of control, since despite multiple attempts to control patients' chances for conception through ritualistic procedures, the end result is ultimately out of the control of both patients and clinicians. Consequently, OCD patients can be expected to experience significantly increased stress and anxiety during infertility procedures, which may lead to increased irritability, anger, and a need to control the medical team or treatment protocol. Providing a predictable medical environment will alleviate some of the stress for these individuals. Clinicians working with OCD patients should attempt to provide consistent, timely information and engage them in clinical decision-making, when appropriate. Psychopharmacological treatment is highly recommended in these patients, particularly SSRIs.

Avoidant and Dependent Personality Disorder

Patients with avoidant and dependent personality disorder can challenge the infertility medical team as well, although their interpersonal style is usually more subtle and insidious than the disorders just discussed. These patients may engender maternal and paternal feelings in their caregivers, which may lead to exceptional dependence. They may leave all medical decisions up to their clinicians, and caregivers should be careful to involve these patients in medical plans.

In summary, personality disorders and traits may have important effects on infertility patients' ability to cope and comply with treatment. It is extremely important for infertility clinicians to be aware of the varying personality types and their defensive behaviors as outlined in Appendix 3.

Drug Interactions

Drugs used in infertility treatment may interact with psychotropic medications, influencing their bioavailability and thus potentially affecting both infertility and psychiatric treatment. Synthetic estrogens are metabolized by the cytochrome P-450 system in the liver; consequently, they affect psychotropic drugs that are also metabolized by this system. As reviewed by Jensvold[63], in general, oral birth control pills stimulate metabolism of drugs metabolized conjugatively and by glucuronidation, such as the benzodiazepines lorazepam and oxazepam, which may be associated with decreased serum levels of these drugs. Oral birth control pills impair clearance of oxidatively metabolized drugs, such as the alprazolam, triazolam, and imipramine, thus potentially leading to increased serum levels[63].

The mood stabilizer carbamazepine induces cytochrome P-450, leading to increased oral birth control metabolism; thus, this medication combination may lead to failure of ovulation suppression[63]. Women taking carbamazepine should be counseled to inform their reproductive endocrinologists about their medication so that higher doses of an oral birth control pill may be used for pre-IVF down-regulation.

Bromocriptine is a dopamine agonist; therefore, combining it with other dopaminergic agents such as bupropion (Wellbutrin) or venlafaxine (Effexor) may lead to symptoms of dopaminergic toxicity (e.g., hypertension, stereotypy, and confusion). Women taking bromocriptine who are started on a tricyclic antidepressant should be warned about the increased risk of orthostatic hypotension with the combination of these two medications.

FUTURE IMPLICATIONS

Recent decades have seen a growing interest among clinicians and researchers in psychiatric disorders in women, their etiology, biology, and the impact of reproductive hormones on psychological symptomology in childbearing and menopause. As this research has begun to indicate, women appear to be under the unique influence of reproductive hormones, so that when these hormones are artificially increased (as they typically are during infertility treatments), alterations in mood or cognition may be seen. In addition, the dramatic increase and wide variety of psychotropic medications providing more effective and efficient psychopharmacological treatment have improved the health and quality of life of individuals, allowing them (in some instances) to pursue reproductive choices they may have been denied in the past. As research on the reproductive biology of women, the brain, and the biology of psychiatric disorders increases, the understanding of the unique effect or interaction of hormones and psychiatric symptomology (e.g., mood, cognition), particularly regarding reproduction, will become an area of increasing interest and concern to mental health practitioners working in the field of reproductive medicine.

SUMMARY

- Personality disorders do not appear to be more common in infertility patients, but when they do occur, they may be very disruptive to infertility treatment. Clinicians should be educated regarding the diagnosis and management of primitive defenses, such as splitting and projection, in borderline, narcissistic, and histrionic patients.

- Grief reactions are common in infertility treatment. Major depression is more common in infertility patients than previously recognized; it is as prevalent as in other chronic medical conditions.

- Antidepressants should be used only when the risk of not treating with medication is greater than the risk of treating—in conditions such as suicidality, psychotic depression, and severe vegetative depressions.

- Infertility medications affect the neurotransmitters involved with regulation of mood and cognition. Bromocriptine is a dopamine agonist that has been shown to be an effective antidepressant. Ovulation-induction medications may be associated with affective instability due to their induction of rapid hormonal shifts. Gonadotropin-releasing hormone agonists are associated with depressive symptoms and cognitive problems due to their induction of hypoestrogenism. In women with a history of anxiety disorder, progesterone may be anxiolytic due to barbiturate-like metabolites. In women with a history of depression, progesterone may be depressogenic. Oral birth control pills, especially progesterone-dominant pills, are frequently associated with the onset of depression.

- Women taking antidepressants or considering starting these medications should be warned that antidepressant exposure during the first trimester may be associated with an increased incidence of spontaneous abortion. However, the two existing studies in the literature are contradictory. The increased risk, if it does exist, appears to be very small.

REFERENCES

1. Benedek T. Infertility as a psychosomatic defense. *Fertil Steril* 1951;3:527–41
2. Freeman EW, Boxer AS, Rickels K, *et al.* Psychological evaluation and support in a program of in vitro fertilization and embryo transfer. *Fertil Steril* 1985;43:48–53
3. Mahlstedt PP, Macduff S, Bernstein J. Emotional factors and the in vitro fertilization and embryo transfer process. *J In Vitro Fertil Emb Transfer* 1987;4:232–6
4. Newton CR, Hearn MT, Yuzpe AA. Psychological assessment and follow-up after in vitro fertilization: Assessing the impact of failure. *Fertil Steril* 1990;54:879–86
5. Baram D, Tourtelot E, Muechler E, Huang K. Psychological adjustment following unsuccessful in vitro fertilization. *J Psychosom Obstet Gynaecol* 1988;9:181–90
6. Leiblum SR, Kemmann E, Lane MK. The psychological concomitants of in vitro fertilization. *J Psychosom Obstet Gynaecol* 1987;6:165–78
7. Laffont I, Edelmann RJ. Psychological aspects of in vitro fertilization: A gender comparison. *J Psychosom Obstet Gynaecol* 1994;15:85–92
8. Greenfeld DA, Diamond MP, Decherney AH. Grief reactions following IVF treatment. *J Psychosom Obstet Gynaecol* 1988;8:169–74
9. American Psychiatric Association. *Diagnostic and Statistical Manual of Mental Disorders*, 4th edn. Washington DC: American Psychiatric Association, 1994
10. Menning BE. The emotional needs of infertile couples. *Fertil Steril* 1980;34:313–19
11. Rosenfeld DL, Mitchell E. Treating the emotional aspects of infertility: Counseling services in an infertility clinic. *Am J Obstet Gynecol* 1979;135:177–80
12. Golombok S. Psychological functioning in infertility patients. *Hum Reprod* 1992;7:208–12
13. Hearn MT, Yuzpe AA, Brown SE, Caspar RF. Psychological characteristics of in vitro fertilization participants. *Am J Obstet Gynecol* 1987;156:879–86
14. Downey J, Yingling S, McKinney M, *et al.* Mood disorders, psychiatric symptoms, and distress in women presenting for infertility evaluation. *Fertil Steril* 1989;52:425–32
15. Domar AD, Broome A, Zuttermeister PC, *et al.* The prevalence and predictability of depression in infertile women. *Fertil Steril* 1992;58:1158–63
16. Boivin J, Takefman J, Tulandi T, Brender W. Reactions to infertility based on extent of treatment failure. *Fertil Steril* 1995;63:801–7
17. Domar AD, Zuttermeister PC, Friedman R. The psychological impact of infertility: A comparison with patients with other medical conditions. *J Psychosom Obstet Gynaecol* 1993;14:45–52
18. Robins LN, Regier DA, eds. *Psychiatric Disorders in America: The Epidemiological Catchment Area Study*. New York: The Free Press, 1991
19. Lalos A, Lalos O, Jacobson L, *et al.* Psychological reactions to the medical investigation and surgical treatment of infertility. *Gynecol Obstet* 1985;20:209–17
20. Stoudemire A, ed. *Clinical Psychiatry for Medical Students*, 2nd edn. Philadelphia: Lippincott, 1994
21. Fyer AJ, Mannuzza S, Gallops MS, *et al.* Familial transmission of simple phobias and fears: A preliminary report. *Arch Gen Psychiatry* 1990;47:252–6
22. Stewart DE, Robinson GE, Goldbloom DS, Wright C. Infertility and eating disorders. *Am J Obstet Gynecol* 1990;163:1196–9
23. Stewart DE. Reproductive functions in eating disorders. *Ann Med* 1992;24:287–91
24. Abraham S, Mira M, Llewellyn-Jones D. Should ovulation be induced in women recovering from an eating disorder or who are compulsive exercisers? *Fertil Steril* 1990;53:566–8
25. Mazure C, Greenfeld DA. Psychological studies of in vitro fertilization/embryo transfer participants. *J In Vitro Fertil Emb Transfer* 1989;6:242–56
26. McEwan BS. Neural gonadal steroid actions. *Science* 1981;211:1303–10
27. Van Hartesveldt C, Joyce JN. Effects of estrogen on the basal ganglia. *Neurosci Biobehav Rev* 1986;10:1–14
28. Chang SS, Renshaw DC. Psychosis and

pregnancy. *Compr Ther* 1986;12:36–41

29. McNeil TF, Kaij L, Malmquist-Larsson A. Women with non-organic psychosis: Pregnancy's effect on mental health during pregnancy. *Acta Psychiatr Scand* 1984; 75:140–8

30. Seeman MV, Lang M. The role of estrogens in schizophrenia gender differences. *Hosp Community Psychiatry* 1990;16:185–94

31. Williams KE, Casper RC. Reproduction and psychopathology. In: Casper RC, ed. *Women's Health: Hormones, Emotions and Behavior*. Portchester, NY: Cambridge University Press, 1997:14–35

32. Aylward M. Plasma tryptophan levels and mental depression in postmenopausal subjects: Effects of natural piperazine oestrone sulphate. *J IRCS Med Sci* 1973; 1:30–4

33. Luine VN, Khylchevskaya RI, McEwen BS. Effect of gonadal steroids on activities of monoamine oxidase and choline acetylase in rat brain. *Brain Res* 1975;86:293–306

34. Klaiber EL, Broverman DM, Vogel W, Kobayashi Y. Estrogen therapy for severe persistent depressions in women. *Arch Gen Psychiatry* 1979;36:50–4

35. Etgen A, Karkanias GB. Estrogen regulation of noradrenergic signaling in the hypothalamus. *Psychoneuroendocrinology* 1994;19:603–10

36. Price WA, Heil D. Estrogen induced panic attack. *Psychosomatics* 1988;29:433–5

37. Verburg C, Griez C, Meijer J. Increase of panic disorder during second half of pregnancy. *Eur Psychiatry* 1994;9:260–1

38. Krey LC, Luine VN. Effect of progesterone on monoamine turnover in the brain of the estrogen-primed rat. *Brain Res Bull* 1987;19:195–202

39. Shaaraway M, Fayad M, Nagui AR, *et al.* Serotonin metabolism and depression in oral contraceptive users. *Contraception* 1985; 26:193–204

40. Majewski M, Harrison N, Schwartz R, *et al.* Steroid hormone metabolites are barbiturate-like modulators of the GABA receptor. *Science* 1986;232:1024–7

41. Morrow A, Suzdak P, Paul S. Steroid hormone metabolites potentiate GABA receptor mediated chloride ion flux with nanomolar potency. *Eur J Pharmacol* 1987;142:483–5

42. Speroff L, Glass RH, Kase NG. *Clinical Gynecology, Endocrinology and Infertility*, 5th edn. Baltimore: Williams & Wilkins, 1994

43. Glasier AF. Clomiphene citrate. *Baillières Clin Obstet Gynaecol* 1990;4:491–501

44. Kerin JF, Liu JH, Phillipou G, Yen SSC. Evidence of a hypothalamic site of action of clomiphene citrate in women. *J Clin Endocrinol Metab* 1985;61:265–8

45. Martikainen H, Ronnberg L, Ruokonen A, Kauppila A. Gonadotropin pulsatility in a stimulated cycle: Clomiphene citrate increases pulse amplitudes of both luteinizing hormone and follicle stimulating hormone. *Fertil Steril* 1991;56:641–5

46. Randall JM, Templeton A. The effects of clomiphene citrate upon ovulation and endocrinology when administered to patients with unexplained infertility. *Hum Reprod* 1991;6:659–64

47. Glasier AF. Clomiphene citrate. *Baillieres Clin Obstet Gynaecol* 1990;4:491–501

48. Brenner JL. Clomiphene-induced mood swings. *J Obstet Gynecol Neonatal Nurs* 1991; 20:321–7

49. Williams KE, Casper RC. Personal communication

50. Hammarbachk S, Damber JF, Backstrom T. Relationship between symptom severity and hormone changes in women with premenstrual syndrome. *J Clin Endocrinol Metab* 1989;68:125–30

51. Dhar V, Murphy GE. Double-blind randomized cross-over trial of luteal phase estrogens (Premarin) in the premenstrual syndrome (PMS). *Psychoneuroendocrinology* 1990;15:489–93

52. Sitland-Marken PA, Wells BG, Froemming JH, *et al.* Psychiatric applications of bromocriptine therapy. *J Clin Psychiatry* 1990;51: 59–82

53. Inoue T, Tsuchiya K, Miura J, *et al.* Bromocriptine treatment of tricyclic and heterocyclic antidepressant–resistant depression. *Biol Psychiatry* 1996;40:151–3

54. Koppelman MCS, Parry BL, Hamilton JA, *et al.* Effect of bromocriptine on affect and libido in hyperprolactinemia. *Am J Psychiatry* 1987;144:1037–41

55. Diehl DJ, Gershon S. The role of dopamine in mood disorders. *Compr Psychiatry* 1992;33:115–20

56. Henzl MR. Gonadotropin-releasing hor-

mone (GnRH) agonists in the management of endometriosis: A review. *Clin Obstet Gynecol* 1988;31:840–56

57. Erickson LD, Ory SJ. GnRH analogues in the treatment of endometriosis. *Obstet Gynecol Clin North Am* 1989;16:123–45

58. Toren P, Dor J, Mester R, *et al.* Depression in women treated with a gonadotropin-releasing hormone agonist. *Biol Psychiatry* 1996;39:378–82

59. Varney NR, Syrop C, Kubu CS, *et al.* Neuropsychologic dysfunction in women following leuprolide acetate induction of hypoestrogenism. *J Assist Reprod Genet* 1993;10:53–7

60. Sherwin BB, Tulandi T. 'Add-back' estrogen reverses cognitive deficits induced by a gonadotropin-releasing hormone agonist in women with leiomyomata uteri. *J Clin Endocrinol Metab* 1996;81:2545–9

61. Culberg J. Premenstrual symptom patterns and mental reactions to medication—a latent profile analysis. *Acta Psychiatr Scand Suppl* 1972;236:9–86

62. Wagner KD, Berenson AB. Norplant-associated major depression and panic disorder. *J Clin Psychiatry* 1994;55:478–89

63. Jensvold MF. Nonpregnant reproductive age women. Part II: Exogenous sex steroid hormones and psychopharmacology. In: Jensvold MF, Halbreich U, Hamilton JA, eds. *Psychopharmacology and Women: Sex, Gender and Hormones.* Washington DC: American Psychiatric Press Inc., 1996;171–90

64. Domar AD, Siebel MM, Benson H. The mind/body program for infertility: A new behavioral treatment approach for women with infertility. *Fertil Steril* 1990;53:246–9

65. Domar AD, Zuttermeister PC, Seibel M, Benson H. Psychological improvement in infertile women after behavioral treatment: A replication. *Fertil Steril* 1992;58:144–7

66. O'Hara MS, Zekoski EM, Phillips LH, Wright EJ. Controlled prospective study of postpartum mood disorders: A comparison of childbearing and non-childbearing women. *J Abnorm Psychol* 1990;99:3–15

67. Altshuler LL, Cohen L, Szuba MP, *et al.* Pharmacologic management of psychiatric illness during pregnancy: Dilemmas and guidelines. *Am J Psychiatry* 1996;153:595–606

68. McElhatton PR, Garbis HM, Elefant E, *et al.* The outcome of pregnancy in 689 women exposed to therapeutic doses of antidepressants: A collaborative study of the European Network of Teratology Information Services (ENTIS). *Reprod Toxicol* 1996;10:285–94

69. Misri S, Sivertz K. Tricyclic drugs in pregnancy and lactation: A preliminary report. *Int J Psychiatry Med* 1991;21:157–71

70. Nulman I, Rovet J, Stewart DE, *et al.* Neurodevelopment of children exposed in utero to antidepressant drugs. *N Engl J Med* 1997;336:258–62

71. Wisner KL, Perel JM, Wheeler SM. Tricyclic dose requirements across pregnancy. *Am J Psychiatry* 1993;150:1541–2

72. Pastuszak A, Schick-Boschetto B, Zuber C, *et al.* Pregnancy outcome following first-trimester exposure to fluoxetine. *JAMA* 1993;269:2246–8

73. Chambers CD, Johnson KA, Dick LM, *et al.* Birth outcomes in pregnant women taking fluoxetine. *N Engl J Med* 1996;335:1010–15

74. Goldstein DJ. Effects of third trimester fluoxetine exposure on the newborn. *J Clin Psychopharmacol* 1995;15:417–20

75. Schatzberg AF, Cole JO. *Manual of Clinical Psychopharmacology.* Washington DC: American Psychiatric Press Inc., 1991

76. DeBattista C. *Medical Management of Depression.* Durant, OK: Emis Inc, 1997

77. Bronzo M, Stahl S. Galactorrhea induced by sertraline. *Am J Psychiatry* 1993; 150:1269–70

78. Lesaca T. Sertraline and galactorrhea (letter). *J Clin Psychopharmacol* 1996;16:333–4

79. Lapane KL, Zierler S, Thomas M, *et al.* Is a history of depressive symptoms associated with an increased risk of infertility in women? *Psychosom Med* 1995;57:509–13

80. Thiering P, Beaurepaire J, Jones M, *et al.* Mood state as a predictor of treatment outcome after in vitro fertilization/embryo transfer technology (IVF/ET). *J Psychosom Res* 1993;37:481–91

81. Rubinow DR, Roca CA. Editorial comment: Infertility and depression. *Psychosom Med* 1995;57:514–16

82. Braftos O, Haug J. Peurperal disorders in manic depressive females. *Acta Psychiatr Scand* 1966;42:285–94

83. Reich T, Winokur G. Postpartum psychoses

in patients with manic depressive disease. *J Nerv Ment Dis* 1970;152:60–8

84. Keck PE, McElroy SL, Tugrul KC, Bennet JA. Valproate oral loading in the treatment of acute mania. *J Clin Psychiatry* 1993; 54:305–8

85. Kaplan HI, Saddock BJ, Grebb JA. *Synopsis of Psychiatry*. Baltimore: Williams & Wilkins, 1994

86. Stewart DE, Klompenhauwer JL, Kendell RE, Brockington I. Prophylactic lithium in peurperal psychosis: The experience of three centers. *Br J Psychiatry* 1991;158:393–7

87. Cohen LS, Sichel DA, Robertson LH, Heckscher E, Rosenbaum JF. Postpartum prophylaxis for women with bipolar disorder. *J Clin Psychiatry* 1995;55:289–92

88. Williams KE, Koran L. Obsessive compulsive disorder in pregnancy, premenstruum and postpartum. *J Clin Psychiatry* 1997;58:330–4

89. Casper RC. Gender differences in psychopharmacology. In: Casper RC, ed. *Women's Health: Hormones, Emotions and Behavior*. Portchester, NY: Cambridge University Press, 1997:192–218

90. Miller LJ. Psychiatric medication during pregnancy: Understanding and minimizing the risks. *Psychiatr Ann* 1994;24:69–75

91. Perry JC. Depression in borderline personality disorder: Lifetime prevalence at interview and longitudinal course of symptoms. *Am J Psychiatry* 1985;142:15–21

92. Herman JL, Perry C, van der Kolk BA. Childhood trauma in borderline personality disorder. *Am J Psychiatry* 1989;146:490–5

93. Linehan MM. *Cognitive-Behavioral Treatment of Borderline Personality Disorder*. New York: Guilford Press, 1993

94. Kohut H, Wolff ES. The disorders of the self and their treatment: An outline. *Int J Psychoanal* 1978;59:413–25

95. Goldfarb JM, Rosenthal MB, Utian WH. Impact of psychological factors in the care of the infertile couple. *Semin Reprod Endocrinol* 1985;3:93–9

III.   TREATMENT MODALITIES

5

Individual Counseling and Psychotherapy

Linda D. Applegarth, EdD

*... the success of all forms of psychotherapy depends more on the personal influence
of the therapist than do medical and surgical procedures.*

J.D. Frank[1]

The rapid scientific and medical advances in the assisted reproductive technologies and the growth of fertility clinics throughout this country and others have led to a greater understanding and appreciation of the psychosocial concerns and emotional needs of individuals who suffer from infertility. As the available technology has developed along with the vicissitudes of fertility treatment, patients have turned to mental health professionals for help in dealing with the many stresses inherent in the treatment and for assistance in decision-making relative to treatment protocols and parenting options.

This chapter focuses on three general areas:

- a historical perspective of infertility counseling and a brief consideration of some key psychological issues that also are commonly a part of the infertility struggle. The literature review is intended to provide some basic educational and theoretical constructs on which individual counseling and psychotherapy can most effectively occur;
- several theoretical treatment approaches that may be particularly appropriate to infertile individuals. These approaches

will be presented in some detail with discussion of their clinical applicability to infertility;

- a discussion about the infertility counselor per se, with emphasis on the need for solid knowledge of medical treatments and parenting options and focus on specific qualities of the therapist. Regardless of one's theoretical background and treatment style, it is imperative to recognize countertransference issues that may come up for psychotherapists working with patients whose powerful and painful desire for a child can be especially palpable.

HISTORICAL OVERVIEW

The pioneering work of Barbara Eck Menning[2,3] and her establishment over 20 years ago of RESOLVE, a national organization offering emotional support and education to infertile persons, have led to increased attention by health and mental health professionals to the important psychological issues inherent in this condition. As RESOLVE chapters sprang up around the country, mental health professionals, often those who themselves had had personal experience with infertility, were called on by the infertile community to lead or facilitate self-help groups for individuals and couples. Gradually, mental health clinicians and researchers in medical and academic settings also began to consider the psychological components of the infertility experience and to recognize patients' need for emotional support.

More recently, the Mental Health Professional Group (MHPG) of the American Society for Reproductive Medicine (formerly the American Fertility Society) was formed in 1986 to provide a forum for professionals working in reproductive medicine to exchange theories, research findings, and clinical experiences. Continuing education programs were also developed by the MHPG as a means of providing more formalized instruction to mental health specialists within or entering the field. Ultimately, a primary goal has been to enhance theoretical understandings, as well as to fine tune the clinical skills of mental health practitioners as they work with this special population. In recent years, the role of the mental health professional has been clarified and expanded within the area of reproductive medicine[4-6]. The primary functions delineated include assessment, treatment, education and consultation, and research. The field of infertility counseling presents new and continuing challenges to mental health practitioners and offers limitless rewards in working with health professionals as well as with patients (see Chapter 26).

REVIEW OF LITERATURE

There are literally thousands of papers, articles, and books written about individual counseling and psychotherapy; however, infertility counseling is a new area and the data needed to guide psychological

intervention and treatment recommendations are not readily available. Leiblum[7] pointed out that the role of the mental health clinician in counseling individuals and couples seeking treatment with the assisted reproductive technologies is complicated. She noted that 'it often feels like negotiating rocky terrain without a map or without any certainty of arriving at a desirable destination'[7]. Although the experience of infertility is not uncommon, Leon[8] suggested that there appears to be something about it that interferes with undertaking both long- and short-term psychoanalytic psychotherapy. He added that even when medical interventions have ended and emotional wounds endure, psychoanalytic psychotherapy is rarely chosen as a treatment option. Rather, it seems that most infertility patients enter counseling or psychotherapy to obtain symptom relief, to develop better coping mechanisms, to obtain assistance with decision-making, or to deal with issues of loss. They may choose a more cognitive-behavioral approach or seek out grief counseling rather than ask for intensive psychotherapy aimed at personality change.

As recently as 1987, there has been psychiatric and gynecological literature pointing to a dynamic psychogenic basis for infertility[9-11]. This condition was thought to be the result of intrapsychic conflicts around femininity or a conflicted or ambivalent relationship with the 'maternal object'. Others[12] suggested that infertility was a sign of an intrapsychic conflict between motherhood and career for some women. Men and women were both seen as experiencing psychosexual maladjustments that resulted in the inability to conceive[13]. More recently, data have appeared that question these ideas about psychogenic causes of infertility[14,15]. Downey[16] pointed out that the significant decrease of so-called psychogenic infertility from over 50% of cases to less than 5% over the past 30 years underscores how what was originally attributed to psychological disturbances can now be explained by physical causes. The latest research in fact indicates that there are a number of predictable and apparently normal emotional responses to infertility and its treatment for which counseling can be especially helpful. Leiblum and Greenfeld[17] noted in fact that, from a counseling perspective, attention has shifted most recently to supporting infertile individuals and minimizing the destructive emotional components of this medical condition.

The Meaning of Reproduction

To better understand the context in which counseling or psychotherapy occurs, it is important to explore the range of psychological and emotional sequelae that individuals experience after their expect-ations, values, and beliefs are challenged by difficulties in achieving reproduction. It has been pointed out that, for most people, to have a child is to continue the human life cycle; it is seen as a renewal of life, as a form of immortality[5]. The inability to bear a child precipitates a generally unantici-pated life crisis for which many individuals and couples lack sufficient coping skills.

For most women and men, the ability to conceive and give birth to a child is paramount to their lifelong notions of femininity and masculinity, to gender identity, and ultimately to the meaning of life. Bearing children and parenting reflect Erickson's[18] concept of 'generativity' and are often one of the foundations around which a couple builds a relationship. Benedek[19] and Bibring[20] also described how pregnancy brings with it a new develop-mental phase and that deprivation of the opportunity to parent because of infertility may lead to a break in development, resulting in stagnation. When efforts to

achieve parenthood fail, life is put 'on hold', and many infertile people are left with deep personal feelings of guilt, self-blame, and inadequacy. There is often a fruitless but constant review of past life events that are seen as having led to the infertility. This retrospective may be coupled with private dialogues with the self that frequently commence with the phase, 'If only ...'.

For women, Klempner[21] suggested that, in psychoanalytic thinking, maternal identification provides a background for parenting and infertility disrupts the opportunity to recapitulate or make reparation for early maternal failures. She added that when identifications with maternal objects are disrupted for women, there is an alteration of self and object representations. Notman and Lester[22] noted that a woman's knowledge that she is able to bear children is essential for the development of a notion of femininity, gender identity, and self-esteem. Conversely, Bassin[23] pointed out that although the use of reproductive tech-nology can be a situational trauma for a woman, it need not have destructive symbolic meaning for her. The dependency on reproductive medical technology can be a temporary insult to a woman's narcissism in that it interferes with her expectation of the natural unfolding of a life process within her body; nonetheless, we are also told that women may respond differently to the infertility experience depending on their internal psychological organization or sense of themselves as female[23].

In addition, many women both consciously and unconsciously feel that motherhood can be reparative. Benedek[24] pointed out that parenthood allows adults to reexperience and gain mastery over early developmental states as they go through them with their children. For some women, the act of creation and the process of motherhood lead to a reidentification with positive aspects of their mothers that were denied during earlier attempts to separate from them.

Data suggest that as fertility problems arise, women worry more, are more self-blaming, and take a more active responsibility to solve problems[25]. In addition, during the various phases of infertility, men and women seem to use different coping strategies.

Lee[26] stressed that men also have special psychological issues and feelings about male infertility that must be better understood and addressed. Certainly much has been written about the female psychosocial experience of infertility[27-29] but little about the male viewpoint. Lee posited that men do not enter psychotherapy to work on crisis or bereavement but rather to get help in dealing with the stresses of treatment. It is also this author's opinion that men seek out counseling because of difficulties in understanding and effectively managing their partner's angst and emotionality about the infertility. It is therefore not the crisis of infertility itself, but the resulting crisis in the relationship that then lead men to an initiation of psychotherapy.

Nonetheless, when struggling with male-factor infertility, men also may suffer from low self-esteem, loss of self-confidence, and feelings of incompetence, isolation, loneliness, guilt, fear, anger, shame, frustration, and so on[26,30]. Not only is the diagnosis of male infertility a shock, but also male ideology is challenged. Thus, the entire idea of being a man (manhood) is challenged, and a man's belief system is threatened, thereby placing him in a state of emotional crisis.

In spite of advances in the feminist movement, there continues to be clear cultural and social factors that influence women's and men's views of themselves as parents. Regardless of other chief goals and expectations, the social message is clear:

Motherhood is the primary job in a woman's life. For men, the expectations regarding fatherhood and family have been more ambiguous. Newton and Houle[25] and others[31,32] stated that men appear to be more accepting of possible childlessness and more willing than women to consider an end to treatment, even when infertility is the result of a male factor. It seems that male responses to infertility approximate those of women only if infertility is attributed solely to a male factor[33].

Infertility: Attachment and Loss

We are told that the concepts of attachment and loss are integral to the infertility struggle[34]. The attachments can be to a fantasy child or to the gestating fetus, and they are enhanced as a person dreams about the ways that a baby will change one's lifestyle, envisions the physical characteristics that a child may have, or anticipates the impact that a new baby will have on the lives of and relationships with extended family members. These kinds of fantasies and others can occur well before a baby is conceived[35]. Women clients, for example, will often describe their girlhood in terms of fantasies about future motherhood. The interruption of the emotional attachment to a dream child either through infertility or pregnancy loss can be devastating.

This loss of fertility or the loss of an unborn child generally goes unrecognized in our society[34]. Thus, infertility is a silent loss, usually lacking rituals to legitimize the grief of a couple who mourn their dream child. In addition, many find that the attachment to the unconceived or unborn child is often not shared by anyone else. Shapiro[34] suggested that as soon as there is a realization that infertility is a real problem, a process of *anticipatory* mourning begins for the offspring that may never be. Anticipatory mourning thus represents an emotional distancing from those initial attachments to the fantasy child. This type of mourning can lead to depression. Mahlstedt[36] also pointed to research that has categorized the losses occurring in adulthood as factors causing depression. These include real or potential losses of a relationship, health, status or prestige, self-esteem, or self-confidence, as well as the loss of a fantasy, the hope of fulfilling an important fantasy, and the loss of someone or something of a great symbolic value. The author delineated how the experience of infertility involves *each* of these losses.

It is not surprising therefore that most infertility patients are depressed and anxious. They have lost a sense of control over their lives and life plans. Infertility is a life crisis. It is frequently this crisis state (usually prolonged) that precipitates a movement into psychotherapy to obtain emotional relief and regain some sense of psychological equilibrium.

Counseling and Psychotherapy

Although the terms *counseling* and *psychotherapy* may be differentiated by some writers and mental health practitioners, they are used interchangeably in this chapter. Some may view psychotherapy as a more in-depth form of treatment aimed at significant psychiatric disorders using a broad variety of techniques. On the other hand, counseling may be considered as supportive work or as a venue for providing advice or guidance to clients. No such distinction will be made here, and the reader may determine which term is preferable or most appropriate based on his or her professional training, theoretical orientation, and/or treatment approach.

THEORETICAL FRAMEWORKS

Many infertile persons seek out counseling because their circumstances create feelings, thoughts, and actions that are frequently restrictive, painful, or repetitive. Primarily through talk, psychotherapy provides support, understanding, and new experiences that can result in learning and behavioral changes. There is no debate here about whether psychotherapy works; rather, it is more important for the reader to consider which psychotherapy (or combination thereof) is best for which infertile patient.

All individual counseling or psychotherapies share a general definition: a two-person interaction, primarily verbal, in which one person is designated as the help-giver and the other the help-receiver. The goal is to elucidate the patient's characteristic problems of living, with the hope of achieving behavioral change[37].

Different psychotherapy orientations target different aspects of psychological functioning for change. The duration of treatments can be from hours to years, depending on the therapist's own theoretical orientation, as well as the patient's request for treatment, financial resources, description of the problem(s), and mental health status.

This section will summarize a large body of information regarding a number of treatment approaches:

- psychodynamic psychotherapy
- cognitive-behavioral therapy
- strategic/solution-focused brief therapy
- crisis intervention
- grief counseling.

Because of space limitations, this means forgoing more comprehensive reviews of these psychotherapies. In addition, this chapter is not intended as a substitute for the knowledge and skill that come from professional experience and training in a specific mental health field and as an infertility counselor.

Psychodynamic Psychotherapy

In psychodynamic psychotherapy, behavioral change occurs primarily through two processes of the treatment: (1) under-standing the cognitive and affective patterns (defense mechanisms) derived from childhood and (2) understanding the conflicted relation(s) one had with significant childhood figures as it is reexperienced in the therapist–patient relationship (transference)[37]. Of great importance to the success of psycho-analytically oriented psychotherapy is the need for patients to feel engaged in the work and to trust the relationship with the therapist.

The losses associated with the inability to conceive or give birth to a child often can reawaken unresolved issues and conflicts from the past. Patients may describe themselves as feeling under-appreciated for their efforts to conceive or misunderstood with respect to their emotional pain, or they may relate to people (spouses, friends, medical person-nel) partly on the basis of expectations formed by early childhood experience. Clarifying character styles and restructur-ing defense mechanisms may become part of the therapist's focus in psychodynamic treatment relative to how patients react to their infertility.

Psychodynamic therapy can be brief or long-term, but much of the treatment intervention is based on psychoanalytic principles. Cooper[38] stressed, however, that the concepts of 'brief' and 'long-term' therapy are routinely ill-defined solely in terms of elapsed calendar time or total number of visits. He noted that 'in practice, long-term treatment is often intermittent; while technically brief therapies may occur episodically over years with challenging problems such as severe abuse or trauma'[38]. More specifically, brief psychodynamic psychotherapy relies more heavily than longer-term therapy on patients' ability to generalize and apply what is gained in the therapeutic work to expand the therapy's effects.

From a psychodynamic viewpoint, the importance of the therapist's role is also underscored. Psychotherapists treating infertility patients can effect healing of both the narcissistic wound and the object-relational loss if they serve as consistently empathic figures who depend less on interpretation of unconscious conflicts than on resonating with conscious and pre-conscious affective states. Clearly, this is a less ambitious treatment form than psycho-analytic psychotherapy.

Interestingly, Freud's early work involved analyses that lasted 3–6 months. Over time, however, treatment became a much longer process. Franz Alexander was one of the first clinicians to describe brief psychodynamic psychotherapy. More recently, the works of David Malan, Peter Sifneos, James Mann, and Habib Davanloo form the basis of this treatment theory. It has also been emphasized that long-term and brief treatments share many common processes. These include specific therapist activities such as the use of interpretation and a clear treatment focus, as well as nonspecific factors such as support and reassurance[39]. The brief psychotherapies can be especially difficult to describe and define because currently over 50 forms exist[38,39]. Yet most brief psychotherapies share some essential characteristics and a common value system along with several common principles[38–41] which will be discussed in a later section and elucidated in relation to infertility.

Historically, the growth in the demand for counseling and psychotherapy, the community mental health movement, and the cost-consciousness of managed mental health care has lead to a greatly increased demand for brief psychotherapy. We are told in fact that 'brief psychotherapy is now a necessary part of every clinician's skills'[37].

In general, long-term psychotherapy seems less applicable to the needs of patients suffering from infertility and

pregnancy loss. In psychoanalytic psychotherapy, the patient's task of developing a
working alliance with the therapist,
learning free association, recognizing the
'disappointment' of the opening phase of
treatment, developing an understanding of
transference, defenses, and resistance, and
learning how to work with dreams may feel
overwhelming, as well as unnecessary. As
Leon[8] speculated,

> Ultimately, people seeking emotional
> help in the midst of reproductive loss
> are not looking—unconsciously as
> well as consciously—to change in
> fundamental ways who they are.
> They have endured so much recent
> upheaval in their self-definition and
> self-esteem—and essentially have
> changed so much in that process—
> that they long to regain some earlier
> sense of well-being and stable
> identity. They are less receptive to
> analyzing conflictual parts of
> themselves than seeking and
> needing to feel whole again ... a
> flexible approach seems to work best
> with this population.

With this in mind, the short-term dynamic
psychotherapies may offer infertility
patients an opportunity for reflective
exploration and a search for meaning in
experience. Self-awareness, understanding,
and personal control are promoted rather
than a resolution of symptoms, although
symptomatology often recedes with the
resolution of internal and interpersonal
conflicts and the growth of insight[42].

Cognitive-Behavioral Therapy

In contrast to psychodynamic psychotherapy, cognitive-behavioral theories
emphasize assessment and relief of current
problems and use a number of empirically
based techniques to achieve mutually
determined goals[43]. The brief therapies

associated with Aaron Beck and Albert Ellis
primarily stress the importance of changing
cognitive processes and structures to
achieve a desired outcome. Cognitive-
behavioral therapy strives for self-efficacy
and relief of problems through challenging
faulty cognitions and their behavioral
correlates[38]. It can be a particularly
appropriate treatment for infertility
patients who present as anxious, depressed,
and/or fearful of medical interventions.

Essentially, cognitive-behavioral therapy
bases its theory on an interactionist
perspective regarding the determinants of
human behavior and psychological well-
being[44]. The core belief of this perspective
is that the interaction between the
individual and the environment continuously determines behavior, cognitions,
and affect. Private thoughts and intrapersonal factors act on the environment,
just as environmental factors influence
these same intrapersonal factors. Further,
intrapersonal factors affect an individual's
perception of environmental forces. What
emerges therefore is a three-factor model—
environment/person/behavior—that in turn
affects the person/situation interaction.
Bandura[45] labeled this *reciprocal determinism*.
Understanding and accepting the principle
of reciprocal determinism within the
cognitive-behavioral perspective vastly
increases the range of available therapeutic
options and enhances the therapist's
sensitivity to a wide variety of data.

Cognitive-behavioral therapy emphasizes the learning process and encourages
clients to acquire new skills during the
course of therapy[46]. Coping skills in
particular are stressed; patient problems
can often be understood as stemming from
inadequate coping skills.

Lehman and Salovey[44] emphasized the
primary goals of this treatment approach
and pointed to the importance of client–
therapist collaboration to attain these
goals. They include the following:

- providing cost-effective treatment for a wide range of client problems
- altering clients' interpretations of themselves and their environment by changing their behavior, their environment, or their cognitions directly
- increasing clients' available store of coping skills
- increasing the likelihood that therapeutic gain will be maintained once therapy is terminated.

Given the integrative framework of cognitive-behavioral therapy, a therapist working with infertility patients can effectively attend to thoughts, feelings, and behaviors and can intervene at any point in the person/environment/behavior triangle. Counselors working in this capacity can therefore establish an effective rapport with their infertile clients.

In sum, cognitive-behavioral therapy is currently accepted across a wide range of health and mental health settings. The emphasis on cognition in a number of therapy approaches has lead to a new interest in understanding and assessing the processes of change that occur throughout all forms of psychotherapy. Interestingly, we are told that 'a new rapprochement between behavioral and psychodynamic perspectives appears to be underway, taking its strength from the interactive approach afforded by cognitive-behavior therapy'[44].

Strategic and Solution-Focused Psychotherapy

Strategic therapy has built a great deal of its foundation on the works of Milton Erikson, Gregory Bateson, and Jay Haley. Erikson deemphasized psychopathology and used a directive (and metaphorical) style based on hypnotic paradigms. These paradigms were further elaborated in Haley's pragmatic, problem-solving approach. Cooper[38] added that Haley has solid ties to Minuchin, whose 'structural' approach to family treatment emphasizes resolution of specific immediate problems by 'altering the transactional process that reveals and maintains them'.

The term *strategic* refers to the therapist's task of developing a strategy, or a plan, to interpret the unsuccessful attempted solution, and a primary task is to motivate clients to implement it. The purpose of this counseling approach is to resolve the original complaint to a patient's satisfaction[47]. Change is therefore effected principally through treating a specific symptom. The treatment is implicitly systemic and interpersonal.

Rosenbaum[48] reported that strategic therapy is not a particular orientation or therapy; rather, it can refer to any therapy in which the counselor willingly assumes responsibility for influencing people and takes an active role in planning a strategy for promoting change. He adds, however, that strategic psychotherapy *does* have major distinguishing characteristics that are particularly relevant. Some of these characteristics are the following:

- Strategic therapists work with a systemic epistemology.
- Strategic therapy focuses on problems and their solutions.
- Strategic therapists tend to see client problems as maintained by their *attempted* solutions.
- Only a small change is necessary.
- Strategic therapists utilize whatever clients bring, in order to help them make a satisfactory life.
- Strategic therapy is brief therapy.

Solution-focused therapy is an important variation of strategic therapy[38] that has been described by deShazer, O'Hanlan and Weiner-Davis, Berg and Miller, Quick, and Walter and Peller. This therapy approach emphasizes building on exceptions to the presenting problem and making transitions rapidly to the identification and development of solutions intrinsic to the client or problem.

As opposed to considering the question 'What maintains the problems?' often asked in the strategic therapy mode, the solution-focused counselor asks, 'How do we construct solutions?' Walter and Peller[49] pointed out that the presuppositions within this question are:

- that there are solutions
- that there is more than one solution
- that they are constructible
- that 'we' (therapist and client) can do the construction
- that we 'construct' and/or 'invent' solutions rather than discover them
- that this process or these processes can be articulated and modeled.

There are essentially three steps to constructing solutions in this treatment approach[49]:

1. Define what the client wants rather than what he or she does not want.
2. Look for what is working and do more of it.
3. If what the client is doing is not working, have him or her do something different.

Solution-focused brief therapy is seen as a total model. It is not a collection of techniques or an elaboration of a technique; rather, it reflects fundamental ideas about change, interaction, and reaching goals[47–49].

A strategic solution-focused approach to working with infertility patients may involve the use of 'coping questions'. Quick[47] stated that coping questions ask how the client goes on in the face of a difficult, painful situation. An example of a coping question might be: 'Given what this past year of failed infertility treatment has been like for you, how have you managed to get through it?' Clients then may answer by describing simple behaviors or say, 'I just do it'. Thus, even if the coping behavior did not seem to be the result of an active choice, the therapist may gently point out that the client *did* have a choice and that he or she chose a 'coping' alternative[47]. Identifying coping behaviors and encouraging and amplifying them are an important tool in solution-focused therapy intended to help patients continue the coping and increase the tolerance for distress. This treatment process can be extremely helpful to infertility patients, particularly when the therapist is also able to 'interrupt' unsuccessful coping solutions by redirecting clients' efforts into more productive and satisfying behaviors.

Crisis Intervention

The term *crisis intervention* originated in relation to people with stable personalities and a history of adequate coping resources who are facing important but transitory difficulties[50]. Although infertility patients fall into this general category, it is also clear that, in most cases, the difficult infertility experience is seldom transitory. However, infertile individuals often experience 'crises within the crisis', particularly when they are confronted by an unexpected event such as failed fertilization, premature ovarian failure, a pregnancy loss, or the sudden recommendation to end treatment.

Although the precise goals of crisis intervention depend on the specific nature of the crisis, crisis-oriented treatments do share a number of general goals[51]:

- relieving the client's symptoms
- restoring the client to his or her previous level of functioning
- identifying the factors that precipitated the crisis
- identifying and applying remedial measures
- helping the client connect the current stresses with past life experiences

- helping the client develop adaptive coping skills that can be used in future situations.

According to Rapoport[51], the first four goals are the minimum goals of all types of crisis intervention, while the last two are considered 'optional' or feasible only in certain situations. Understanding and developing coping behaviors appear to be a key component of crisis intervention. Lazarus and Folkman[52] suggested that coping should be depicted as a process and stressed that much coping behavior is situation specific.

Infertility patients are known to use a combination of coping mechanisms, but in certain circumstances, they often fail to do so because of a number of factors: The infertility problem may seem too overwhelming or too unfamiliar; the person may use maladaptive coping methods; coping may be limited by physical or mental illness; or support from friends or family that would otherwise enable a person to cope is unavailable.

When coping fails, one may observe what Caplan[53] described as four phases of crisis:

I Arousal and efforts at problem-solving behavior increase.

II With increased arousal or 'tension', functional impairment ensues with associated disorganization and distress. Arousal reaches a point at which coping is hindered: The person is too anxious or too angry or unable to sleep properly and so on.

III Emergency resources both internal and external are mobilized and novel methods of coping tried.

IV Continuing failure to resolve the problem leads to progressive deterioration, exhaustion, and 'decompensation'.

Psychotherapeutic intervention can be made at any point during these four phases.

Bancroft and Graham[50] noted that there is much scope for skill and experience in practicing crisis intervention. It requires empathy and sensitivity; therapists also often rely on the skillful use of common sense rather than highly specialized techniques. Although it has been difficult to reach a conclusion about the effectiveness of crisis intervention because of the range of approaches for which the term is applied, this should not deter the counselor from using an approach that is based on both caring, common sense, and practical suggestions[50]. Infertility patients appear to respond well to crisis intervention and often benefit from having the opportunity to mobilize their coping skills and support systems. (Further discussion of coping mechanisms can be found in Chapter 8.)

Grief Counseling

Because bonds of attachment often develop before a child is conceived or delivered, it is important to acknowledge that the breaking of these bonds either through loss or disruption can create intense emotional pain. In the face of these reproductive losses, many infertility patients need to grieve or mourn. In this section, grief and mourning are defined as the intellectual and emotional processes that gradually lessen the psychological bond to the lost loved one, enabling the bereaved to accept the loss and move forward[54].

Grief counseling for individuals unable to conceive takes a different form from that of individuals who have experienced a pregnancy loss or perinatal death. For both groups, it is imperative that the reality of the loss be acknowledged: The loss of a child, real or fantasized, is a brutal shock and feels like an assault on self-worth. The counselor's role is to encourage patients to accept the loss.

Second, bereaved infertility patients must also be helped to experience the pain of grief. This crucial aspect of grief consists of expressing in words the intense feelings that accompany the loss[54]. Leon[8] added that, in working with the bereaved, it is also necessary to challenge directly the therapist's own discomfort with and pathologizing of grief.

Third, the counselor can be helpful in assisting individuals who have experienced a perinatal death to commemorate the loss. Often, these people need assistance in finding an acceptable way to honor and remember the baby's death. This can be particularly important when there is a significant burden of guilt in relation to the death[54].

Fourth, the therapist may also play an important role in helping bereaved persons 'let go' of the loss. The bereaved ultimately must withdraw their emotional investment in the loss in order to go forward with life.

Lastly, the therapist may also be called on to assist bereaved individuals to 'move on'. Crenshaw[54] pointed out that this can be very difficult because it involves relinquishing the hopes, dreams, plans, and aspirations that revolved around the lost dream child. At times, the resistance to moving on may result from anger that life has dealt the bereaved a cruel blow. Similarly, some grievers tend to identify themselves as 'tragic figures', gaining gratification from the solicitations of family and friends. As a result of these secondary gains, they have difficulty again becoming active participants in life.

In sum, grief counseling can be a very meaningful intervention for patients who experience reproductive loss. Often, the feelings of pain can be extremely heavy to bear and must be shared, in part, by the therapist and managed supportively. In this way, the counseling intervention provides a secure base and a normalizing experience for the bereaved.

CLINICAL ISSUES AND THERAPEUTIC INTERVENTIONS

We are told that although theoretical differences in treatment approaches definitely exist, it is unclear as to the extent to which these differences are 'purely' applied in practice. Experienced clinicians are likely to use interventions that are similar in utility and intent, if not form, but that also reflect their own unique personalities and experience, as well as situational demands[38].

Energetic efforts to distinguish approaches from one another also risk unfairly dichotomizing and limiting them. For example, the highly interpersonal and implicit nature of strategic therapy is often ignored in favor of its technical components. Similarly, most psychodynamic approaches now consider interpersonal factors in psychotherapy to be as important as intrapsychic ones.

Because it appears that infertility patients primarily seek out short-term or brief counseling or psychotherapy, it is important to outline some essential characteristics and common principles. It is also useful to point out a common value system that most brief psychotherapies share[38–40,55]. These include:

Technical features:

- maintenance of a clear, specific treatment focus
- a conscious and conscientious use of time
- limited goals with clearly defined outcomes
- emphasis on intervening in the present
- rapid assessment and integration of assessment within treatment
- frequent review of progress and discarding of ineffective interventions
- high level of therapist–patient activity
- pragmatic and flexible use of techniques

Shared values:

- emphasis on pragmatism, parsimony, and least intrusive treatment versus 'cure'
- recognition that human change is inevitable
- emphasis on client strengths and resources and the legitimacy of presenting complaints
- recognition that most change occurs outside of therapy
- commitment that a patient's outside life is more important than therapy
- a stance that therapy is not always helpful
- a belief that therapy is not 'timeless'.

Leon[56] noted that of 20 cases of women presenting with emotional problems following pregnancy loss, six women left treatment during the consultation or soon after therapy began. Of the six, five were also dealing with infertility before or after their loss. Most remarkably, however, those five who left treatment early were the only infertile women in his total sample. Other clinicians appear to have had similar experiences with infertility patients. For this reason, it would seem especially important to emphasize the significance of the first session, because it may be the *only* session.

Cooper[38] pointed out that it is helpful if the clinician considers each session as a whole in itself. To do this effectively, he described at least six 'first-session tasks' that can serve multiple purposes:

1. Form a positive working relationship:

Spend a few moments constructively getting acquainted.
- Do some therapy education.
- Ask how you can be helpful.
- Use active listening, empathy, and language that demonstrates respect for each client's point of view.

- Find a one-sentence summary to repeat to clients that reflects your understanding of their problem.
- Find at least one thing to like or respect about each patient or his or her coping and call attention to it.
- Create an expectation of improvement.

2. Find a treatment focus:
- Ask what brought the patient to treatment *now* rather than earlier or later.
- Ask what improved since the appointment was made that patients would like to continue improving.
- Determine at the *beginning* what would be tangibly different for clients at the *end* of successful treatment.
- Define problems in specific terms conducive to change.
- Determine the meaning or significance of a problem to a patient.
- If multiple problems are identified, focus first on the most important to the client.

3. Negotiate criteria for a successful outcome:
- Put solutions in positive, specific, achievable terms, using client language to facilitate change.
- Make goals/solutions achievable, and place goals within the patient's control.

4. Distinguish clients from non-clients. Not every person who presents in therapy is a candidate for change:
- Clients are characterized by the acknowledgment of a problem and a willingness to work on it.
- Nonclients will acknowledge a problem exists but do not see themselves as part of the solution.

5. Identify patient motivational levels, and tailor interventions accordingly.

Table 1 Personality types and infertility

Personality structure	Reaction to infertility
Obsessive: orderly, systematic, perfectionist, inflexible	infertility is seen as punishment for letting things get out of control
Narcissistic: self-involved, angry, independent, perfectionist	infertility is seen as an attack on autonomy and perfection of self
Borderline: demanding, impulsive, unstable	infertility is seen as a threat of abandonment
Dependent: long-suffering, depressed, submissive	infertility is seen as expected punishment for worthlessness
Avoidant: remote, unsociable, uninvolved	infertility and its procedures are seen as a dangerous invasion of privacy
Paranoid: wary, suspicious, blaming, hypersensitive	infertility is seen as annihilating assault coming from everywhere outside of self

See Appendix 3. (Reproduced from Goldfarb JM, Rosenthal MB, Utian WH. Impact of psychologic factors in the care of the infertile couple. *Semin Reprod Endocrinol* 1985;3:97; with permission)

6. Do something that makes a difference immediately:

- Listen actively and empathetically.
- Help patients understand that most of their reactions to infertility are normal and predictable.
- Discuss the process of achieving desired solutions.
- Conceptualize or *reframe* problems in ways that suggest solutions.

The focus of treatment in individual counseling with infertility patients can be collaboratively developed with them and is closely related to the ideas of assessment and diagnosis. It is therefore important to have sound diagnostic skills, while working within an infertility patient's perception of the problem. A helpful diagnostic framework describing personality structures and reactions to infertility is presented in Table 1. Along with understanding the psychological components of infertility, it is also imperative to assess the presence of personality disorders, substance abuse or dependency, sexual abuse, domestic violence, sociopathy, and so on.

It is clear that individual counseling with infertility patients requires special expertise and an understanding of and appreciation for the many psychosocial and medical components relative to this condition. Appendix 1 delineates qualification guidelines for mental health professionals working in reproductive medicine and stresses the need for a solid knowledge of family-building options, such as adoption, third- and fourth-party reproduction, child-free living, and so on.

Countertransference and the Role of the Counselor

Although transference and countertransference are intrinsic parts of every patient–therapist relationship, it is crucial for infertility counselors to be mindful of powerful and compelling countertransference issues when working with patients experiencing infertility and pregnancy loss.

It is not uncommon, for example, for counselors working in this field to have had some form of personal experience with infertility and its associated losses. This position can have very positive, as well as negative, effects. Countertransference, broadly defined as the therapist's total response to a patient, both conscious and unconscious, can be useful in understanding the experience of the patient[57]. The infertility crisis can be laden with profound feelings for both counselors and clients about gender identity, self-image, and wishes for nurturance. The feelings that arise within therapists vary greatly depending on how they have resolved their own issues about infertility. Unless there is some form of resolution about this aspect of a therapist's life, it seems that it would be difficult to explore childbearing problems and decisions with patients, while maintaining a 'neutral' stance. Subtle and not-so-subtle conflicts can therefore come into play in clinicians' relationships with clients. As a therapist personally struggles with painful, unresolved issues around becoming a parent, his or her guilt, ambivalence, and anger can interfere with patients' efforts at working through their conflicts and concerns about infertility and loss.

Self-disclosure by therapists is another important countertransference issue in infertility counseling. The question often arises regarding how much to self-disclose, if at all, and to which patients. The issue must be carefully considered because revealing personal pain can potentially be manipulative and self-indulgent rather than serving to further a patient's growth. Leibowitz[58] believed that the key to self-revelation to a patient is based on a sense of how open a therapist and patient have been with one another and how much trust and connection have been established in the therapy. In any case, self-disclosure by therapists must be used in a thoughtful, purposeful way so as to benefit or assist a client. A therapist's personal experience with infertility may in some cases increase his or her ability to empathize with clients'

pain and anger. Self-disclosure can also be a way to model effective behaviors and to close the perceived distance between therapist and client, thereby facilitating greater trust and openness[59]. In other cases, however, a therapist's own infertility issues may be projected onto clients and potentially interfere with their coping abilities and/or efforts to resolve this difficult and painful experience.

In sum, the treatment modalities discussed in this chapter can be extremely useful when counseling infertile patients. Most psychotherapists employ a combination of interventions to meet clients' needs in the most effective and efficient way. These theoretical approaches, however, are only as effective as the therapist who makes use of them. Kottler[59] pointed out a number of common characteristics or qualities of successful psychotherapeutic outcomes, including a counselor's personality, skillful thinking processes and communication, and the establishment of an intimate and trusting relationship.

FUTURE IMPLICATIONS

There is a clear future for mental health professionals treating infertile individuals. At the same time, one of the goals of this chapter has been to emphasize the importance of having a sound knowledge of the psychosocial experience of infertility and an appreciation of the numerous medical interventions available, the high financial costs involved, and the range of parenting alternatives from which patients might ultimately choose. It is only with this solid background that a psychotherapist can best apply his or her theoretical and clinical expertise to assist individuals struggling with losses and concerns associated with infertility.

In light of the complexities of all forms of reproductive loss, it appears that professional training programs and postgraduate courses may, in the future, choose to incorporate or develop specific curricula that address the psychosocial components of infertility. The rapid growth of the assisted reproductive technologies and the psychological and ethical implications inherent in them require that formal clinical programs be established to provide training in this increasingly important arena. Subspecialties can be developed that focus on reproductive health, as well as on perinatal issues including not only pregnancy loss but also pregnancy and parenting after infertility.

SUMMARY

- Historically, infertility and reproductive loss were often considered by mental health professionals as having a dynamic psychogenic basis. More recently, there has been a significant shift to supporting infertile individuals and minimizing the destructive emotional components of this medical condition.
- The five theoretical treatment approaches presented may be useful in working with individuals struggling with infertility. These include psychodynamic psychotherapy, cognitive-behavioral therapy, strategic and solution-focused psychotherapy, crisis intervention, and grief counseling.
- Many infertile individuals request and/or require only brief psychotherapeutic intervention.
- All infertility counselors can apply several specific tasks when meeting a new client for the first time. These tasks can serve several important purposes and include:
  forming a positive working relationship
  finding a treatment focus
  negotiating criteria for a successful outcome
  distinguishing clients from non-clients
  identifying patient motivational levels and tailoring interventions accordingly
  doing something that makes a difference immediately.
- The treatment approach is only as effective as the therapist who employs it.
- Issues of countertransference and the role of the therapist who works with this special population need to be understood, especially since many therapists working in the field have had personal experience with infertility.
- Individual counseling and psychotherapy with infertility patients is an area that deserves our special attention. The psychosocial needs of those who struggle to build families are compelling and require clinical expertise and a clear understanding of the underlying emotional issues involved.

REFERENCES

1. Frank JD. What is psychotherapy? In: Bloch S, ed. *An Introduction to the Psychotherapies*, 3rd edn. New York: Oxford University Press, 1996;1–9
2. Menning BE. RESOLVE: A support group for infertile couples. *Am J Nurs* 1976; 76:258–9
3. Menning BE. Counseling infertile couples. *Contemp Obstet Gynecol* 1979;13:101–8
4. Applegarth LD. The psychological aspects of infertility. In: Keye WR, Chang RJ, Rebar RW, Soules MR, eds. *Infertility: Evaluation and Treatment*. Philadelphia: Saunders, 1995;25–41
5. Applegarth LD. Emotional implications. In: Adashi EY, Rock JA, Rosenwaks Z, eds. *Reproductive Endocrinology, Surgery, and Technology*. Philadelphia: Lippincott-Raven,

1996;2:1954–68

6. Covington SN. The role of the mental health professional in reproductive medicine. *Fertil Steril* 1995;64:895–97

7. Leiblum SR. Introduction. In: Leiblum SR, ed. *Infertility: Psychological Issues and Counseling Strategies.* New York: Wiley, 1997;3–19

8. Leon IG. Reproductive loss: Barriers to psychoanalytic treatment. *J Am Acad Psychoanal* 1996;24:341–52

9. Jeker L, Micioni G, Ruspa M, Zeeb M, Carnpana A. Wish for a child and infertility in 116 couples. 1. Interview and psychodynamic hypothesis. *Int J Fertil* 1987;33: 411–20

10. Benedek T. Infertility as a psychosomatic defense. *Fertil Steril* 1952;3:527–35

11. Deutsch H. *The Psychology of Women.* New York: Grune & Stratton, 1944

12. Sandler B. Infertility of emotional origin. *J Obstet Gynaecol Brit Emp* 1961;68:809–15

13. Seibel MM, Taymor ML. Emotional aspects of infertility. *Fertil Steril* 1982;37:137–45

14. Mai FM, Munday RN, Rump EE. Psychiatric interview comparisons between infertile and fertile couples. *Psychosom Med* 1972;12:46–59

15. Paulson JD, Haarmann BS, Salerno RL, Asmar P. An investigation of the relationship between emotional maladjustment and infertility. *Fertil Steril* 1988;49:258–62

16. Downey J. The new reproductive technologies: Psychological issues for female patients. Presented at the 35th winter meeting of the American Academy of Psychoanalysis, New York, December, 1991

17. Leiblum SR, Greenfeld DA. The course of infertility: Immediate and long-term reactions. In: Leiblum SR, ed. *Infertility: Psychological Issues and Counseling Strategies.* New York: Wiley, 1997;83–2

18. Erickson E. *Childhood and Society.* New York: Norton, 1950

19. Benedek T. Parenthood as a developmental phase. *J Am Psychoanal Assoc* 1959; 7: 389–417

20. Bibring G. Some consideration of the psychological processes in pregnancy. *Psychoanal Study Child* 1959;14:113–21

21. Klempner L. Infertility: Identification and disruptions with the maternal object. *Clin*

Soc Work J 1992;20:193–8

22. Notman MT, Lester EP. Pregnancy: Theoretical consideration. *Psychoanal Inq* 1988;8:139–45

23. Bassin D. Woman's shifting sense of self—the impact of reproductive technology. In: Offerman-Zuckerberg J, ed. *Gender in Transition: A New Frontier.* New York: Plenum, 1989:191–202

24. Benedek T. Parenthood as a developmental phase: A contribution to libido theory. *Psychoanal Study Child* 1960; 15:60–76

25. Newton CR, Houle M. Gender differences in psychological response to infertility treatment. *Infertil Reprod Med Clin North Am* 1993;4:545–58

26. Lee S. *Counseling in Male Infertility.* London: Blackwell Science, 1996

27. Crawshaw M. Offering woman-centered counseling in reproductive medicine. In: Jennings S, ed. *Infertility Counseling.* Oxford: Blackwell Science, 1995;38–65

28. Freeman EW, Rickels K, Tausig J, *et al.* Emotional and psychosocial factors in follow-up of women after IVF-ET treatment. *Acta Obstet Gynecol Scand* 1987;66:517–25

29. Lalos A, Lalos O, Jacobson L, Von Schoultz B. Depression, guilt and isolation among infertile women and their partners. *J Psychosom Obstet Gynaecol* 1996;5:197–206

30. Mason MC. *Male Infertility—Men Talking.* London: Routledge, 1993

31. Greil AL, Porter KL, Leitko TA. Sex and intimacy among infertile couples. *J Psychol Hum Sex* 1989;2:117–23

32. Ulbrich PM, Tremaglio Coyle A, Llabre MM. Involuntary childlessness and marital adjustment: His and hers. *J Sex Marital Ther* 1990;16:147–58

33. Nachtigall RD, Becker G, Wozny M. The effects of gender-specific diagnosis on men's and women's response to infertility. *Fertil Steril* 1992;57:113–21

34. Shapiro CH. *Infertility and Pregnancy Loss: A Guide for Helping Professionals.* San Francisco: Jossey-Bass, 1988

35. Raphael B. *The Anatomy of Bereavement.* New York: Basic Books, 1983

36. Mahlstedt PP. The psychological component of infertility. *Fertil Steril* 1985; 43:335–46

37. Ursano RJ, Sonnenberg SM, Lazar SG. *Psychodynamic Psychotherapy*. Washington, DC: American Psychiatric Association Press, 1991

38. Cooper JF. *A Primer of Brief Psychotherapy*. New York: Norton, 1995

39. Koss MP, Butcher JN. Research on brief therapy. In: Garfield SL, Bergin AE, eds. *Handbook of Psychotherapy and Behavior Change*, 3rd edn. New York: Wiley, 1986; 627–70

40. Bloom BL. *Planned Short-Term Psychotherapy: A Clinical Handbook*. Boston: Allyn & Bacon, 1992

41. Wells RA. Clinical strategies in brief psychotherapy. In: Wells RA, Gianetti VJ, eds. *Casebook of the Brief Psychotherapies*. New York: Plenum, 1993;3–17

42. Hobbs M. Short-term dynamic psychotherapy. In: Bloch S. ed. *An Introduction to the Psychotherapies*, 3rd edn. New York: Oxford University Press, 1996; 52–83

43. Peake TH, Borduin CM, Archer RP. *Brief Psychotherapies: Changing Frames of Mind*. Beverly Hills, CA: Sage, 1988

44. Lehman AK, Salovey P. An introduction to cognitive behavior therapy In: Wells RA, Gianetti VJ, eds. *Handbook of the Brief Psychotherapies*. New York: Plenum, 1990; 239–59

45. Bandura A. The self in reciprocal determinism. *Am Psychol* 1978;33:344–58

46. Mahoney MJ. Personal science: A cognitive learning theory. In: Ellis A, Grieger R, eds. *Handbook of Rational Psychotherapy*. New York: Springer, 1977;3–33

47. Quick EK. *Doing What Works in Brief Therapy: A Strategic Solution-Focused Approach*. San Diego, CA: Academic, 1996

48. Rosenbaum R. Strategic psychotherapy. In: Wells RA, Gianetti VJ, eds. *Handbook of the Brief Psychotherapies*. New York: Plenum, 1990;351–403

49. Walter JL, Peller JE. *Becoming Solution-Focused in Brief Therapy*. New York: Brunner/Mazel, 1992

50. Bancroft J, Graham C. Crisis intervention. In: Bloch S, ed. *An Introduction to the Psychotherapies*, 3rd edn. New York: Oxford University Press, 1996;134–47

51. Rapoport L. Crisis intervention as a mode of brief treatment. In: Roberts RW, Nee RH, eds. *Theories of Social Casework*. Chicago: University of Chicago Press, 1970; 77–98

52. Lazarus RS, Folkman S. *Stress, Appraisal, and Coping*. New York: Springer, 1984

53. Caplan G. *An Approach to Community Mental Health*. London: Tavistock, 1961

54. Crenshaw DA. *Bereavement: Counseling the Grieving Throughout the Life Cycle*. New York: Continuum, 1990

55. Pekarik G. Rationale, training, and implementation of time-sensitive treatments. Presented to the executive directors, MCC Companies, Inc., Minneapolis, MN, January, 1990

56. Leon IG. *When a Baby Dies: Psychotherapy for Pregnancy and Newborn Loss*. New Haven: Yale University Press, 1990

57. Tansey MJ, Burke WF. *Understanding Countertransference—From Projective Identification to Empathy*. Hillsdale, NJ: Analytic, 1989

58. Leibowitz L. Reflections of a childless analyst. In: Gershon B, ed. *The Therapist as a Person: Life Crises, Life Choices, Life Experiences and Their Effects on Treatment*. Hillsdale, NJ: Analytic, 1996;71–87

59. Kottler JA. *The Compleat Therapist*. San Francisco: Jossey-Bass, 1991

6

Counseling the Infertile Couple

Christopher R. Newton, PhD

There can be no disparity in marriage
like unsuitability of mind and purpose.

Charles Dickens

The advent of assisted reproductive techniques such as in vitro fertilization (IVF) placed much of the burden for treatment on women, and, not surprisingly, much of what has been written about treatment stress and infertility has been derived from the experience of women. In contrast, attention has only recently been directed toward the male response, and men's reactions to infertility remain less understood. Studies assessing infertile couples have typically compared male and female levels of psychosocial distress[1] but rarely have examined the ways in which couples' relationships are affected. Similarly, in terms of counseling, a review of the literature revealed only one published evaluation of intervention with infertile couples. As a result, this chapter draws on a growing body of experimental literature about the individual effects of infertility. It also incorporates current marital theory and approaches to marital therapy from what has been described as 'a social learning theory–cognitive perspective'[2]. An important premise of this approach is that skills are required to maintain a satisfactory relationship over an extended period of time. Love and attraction are assumed not to be enough to sustain a relationship in the face of various obstacles in life's path. This seems partic-

ularly apropos with respect to infertility. House-sized boulders seem to pepper the trail of unwary couples, who often need to learn a variety of new skills in order to cope with the sometimes unique demands placed on their relationship.

This chapter will:

- review current research on the impact of treatment on couples and assessment tools
- provide a framework for assisting couples with problems created or exacerbated by infertility.

HISTORICAL OVERVIEW

Thirty years ago, the field of marital therapy was described as 'a technique in search of a theory'[3], where therapy with couples consisted of a hodgepodge of clinical interventions based on partial and sometimes tenuous theories[2]. Therapy with infertile couples today appears to be at a similar preliminary stage and faces many of the same challenges.

Early theories of infertility were heavily influenced by psychodynamic and psychoanalytic formulations, and in the 1960s 50% of infertility cases were believed to be caused by psychological factors[4]. In this context, early couples therapy often consisted of attempts to uncover unconscious conflicts and work through unresolved emotional issues that might be affecting fertility. For example, Sarrel and DeCherney[5] randomly assigned 20 couples with unexplained infertility to either a single psychotherapeutic interview, in which a psychodynamic formulation of conflict was offered, or to a no-contact control group. At 18 months follow-up, 60% of interviewed couples had achieved pregnancy in comparison to 11% of controls. While the identification of previously unrecognized conflict was suggested as the mechanism of change, it was unclear to what extent other important issues concerning the marriage or the sexual relationship might also have been addressed in therapy, thereby facilitating pregnancy.

THEORETICAL FRAMEWORKS

A theoretical framework that seeks both to explain and to make testable hypotheses about the impact of infertility on couples' relationships is currently lacking. Instead, theoretical descriptions of the impact of infertility on couples are often, in reality, theories of the individual, that are assumed to apply generally but that ignore gender differences and add little to our understanding of important interactional patterns.

For example, in the 1970s, the causal relationship between stress and infertility was challenged by Menning[6] and others, who argued that psychological distress observed in this population, rather than causing infertility, was largely a consequence of infertility and accompanying treatment. In the past 20 years, concepts of grief and loss, together with stage theories, have heavily influenced thinking about the infertility experience. Individuals (and therefore couples) are assumed to move through certain emotional stages, for example, shock, denial, anger, guilt, grief, and resolution[7].

In conjunction with treatment, couples have been described as moving through phases of engagement (dawning of awareness, facing a new reality), immersion (intensified treatment efforts, growing emotional distress), and disengagement (ending treatment, finding a new focus)[8]. Infertility has also been characterized as involving a 'transition to non-parenthood'[9]. On the basis of this model, therapeutic suggestions often involve helping couples 'work through' the grief process[10]. Unfortunately, despite its theoretical and clinical appeal, the stage theory of grief has received little empirical support. Response to loss may be more variable than has been acknowledged, and assumptions that distress is necessary and that loss must always be 'processed' to achieve effective recovery and resolution may be incorrect[11]. The danger therefore is that clinicians may either create or reinforce inaccurate expectations for a couple about appropriate ways to react and respond to each other.

At this stage, much of the published experimental literature on infertility has been quite atheoretical, although work on control[12], coping and appraisal[13], and social support[14] is beginning to highlight both the complexity in couples' reactions and the need to recognize gender differences in planning treatment interventions. (For further discussion of theoretical approaches see Chapter 1.)

REVIEW OF LITERATURE

Effects of Infertility

There is a considerable body of evidence illustrating that men and women are affected differently by the experience of infertility. Women are more likely to worry that something is wrong even before seeking treatment, more likely to initiate discussion with their partners, and more likely to assume personal responsibility when efforts to conceive prove unsuccessful[15]. A recent review found that during infertility investigations or treatment women reported higher levels of distress than men on measures of anxiety (7 of 13 studies), depression (4 of 7 studies), self-esteem (3 of 4 studies), and psychological adjustment (6 of 14 studies)[16]. In terms of the above measures, none of the studies found infertile men to be more distressed than infertile women.

How the couple as a unit is affected remains more unclear. As a group, infertile couples reported levels of marital adjustment in the normal range[17-19]. However, some couples complained of a deterioration in marital functioning[20], while others reported that the crisis of infertility improved marital communication and consequently emotional intimacy[21]. Still others suggested that sexual functioning may be disturbed but that marital satisfaction remained intact[22].

Impact of Treatment

In the assessment of the impact of infertility on a couple's relationship, it appears that the stage of medical treatment may be a contributing factor. While the initial phase of infertility diagnosis and treatment is often characterized as an acute stress, research findings on the impact of this stage are mixed. For example, Daniluk and associates[23] presented data on 43 couples attending an infertility clinic. The couples reported marital and sexual functioning in the normal range and no change from the first visit to 6 weeks postdiagnosis. However, a similar study described a decrease in marital adjustment over the diagnostic period[24]. The results of studies examining the effects of longer infertility treatment on a couple's relationship are similarly ambiguous. In a longitudinal study, Benazon and colleagues[25] followed 165 infertile couples over the course of 18 months of treatment.

Although women who failed to conceive reported increased sexual dissatisfaction over this time period, marital satisfaction remained normal and unchanged for both sexes. The fact that 8% of couples separated and were lost to the study is striking but, in the absence of a comparative control group, difficult to interpret. However, prolonged infertility treatment may well be a source of chronic relationship strain. Berg and Wilson[19] compared 104 couples with varying lengths of treatment experience and found that, overall, marital and sexual satisfaction indices were in the normal range. However, in those couples in advanced stages of treatment (greater than 3 years), these indices were at the lowest overall level, and marital adjustment scores were near the maladjusted range.

Rather than the length of time spent in treatment, the repeated experience of treatment failure may be more important. Boivin and coworkers[26] presented data on 91 women with varying amounts of treatment failure. Women who had experienced a moderate amount of treatment failure reported greater marital distress than women who had never experienced treatment failure, and more distress than those who had experienced the most treatment failure. These findings were seen as support for a stage theory, that is, that the experience of infertility is a process and individual and marital distress (at least for women) is a necessary part of an evolution toward acceptance and improved marital functioning.

Unfortunately, after multiple treatment failures, when marital distress is likely to be at a peak, couples may be least able to achieve consensus on the need for conjoint counseling. McCartney and Wada[27], in a large survey of 486 male and female infertility patients found, not surprisingly, that women expressed greater openness to counseling than men. Interestingly, the greatest gender disparity occurred among men and women who had ended infertility treatment without pregnancy, compared to couples still active in treatment, couples who were pregnant, and couples who had experienced a pregnancy loss[27]. In devising a treatment plan acceptable to the couple, these findings highlight the importance of identifying and addressing partners' potentially disparate levels of motivation for counseling.

Assessment

In assessing the effects of infertility on a relationship, clinicians need to be mindful of several factors that may influence a couple's presentation. Couples referred for medical treatment employing assisted reproductive technologies such as IVF may have suffered a series of demoralizing treatment failures in the recent past, resulting in both increased emotional turmoil and relationship tension. However, referral to these new programs can produce an upsurge of optimism and a temporary sense of well-being[28]. As a result, couples may portray both the stress of infertility and its impact on the relationship as a past problem, now largely resolved. Similarly, couples may engage in positive-impression management, minimizing or denying difficulties in order not to jeopardize their acceptance into the program. Even when couples seek counseling, relationship problems may be relatively circumscribed, and couples may maintain a reserve of good-will toward each other. This may lead some couples to try to protect each other by engaging in self-blame and avoiding overt criticism of the other's behavior. Finally, most couples (infertile or not) have difficulty thinking of a problem in systemic terms and, as a result, offer rather vague definitions—often in terms of 'communication difficulties'. Rather than asking a couple to more clearly define a communication problem, it is often more effective to have the couple demonstrate. This can be accomplished by asking the couple to discuss and try to solve a 'moderate' problem in the therapist's presence.

Unfortunately, standardized measures that are infertility-specific are not yet available to provide an objective measure of relationship problems. Alternatively, more general measures of marital relationship functioning often lack sensitivity to infertility concerns. However, tests with good reliability, validity, and norms for comparison can be useful both in determining the severity of relationship complaints and in offering clinical leads for further inquiry. Among tests used primarily by psychologists and marriage/family therapists, the following measures can contribute to the assessment.

Locke-Wallace Marital Adjustment Scale

Locke and Wallace's[29] Marital Adjustment Scale (MAS) is a 15-item self-report instrument that inquires about the extent of disagreement on eight subareas (e.g., mutual activity, mutual decision-making). The lack of a conceptual plan in selecting items raises doubts about the comprehensiveness (content validity) of the MAS. Item wording is dated, and the 'husband' and 'wife' format is not suitable for other dyads.

Dyadic Adjustment Scale

A 32-item self-report scale, the Dyadic Adjustment Scale (DAS)[30] taps marital satisfaction in four areas: (1) consensus on matters important to the relationship, (2) degree of tension, (3) agreement over affection/sex, and (4) satisfaction with verbal communication and companionship activities. The DAS is probably the best brief screening device available and is a good indicator of overall relationship stress.

Marital Satisfaction Inventory

The Marital Satisfaction Inventory (MSI)[31] is a 280-item self report inventory developed to assess global marital satisfaction and individuals' attitudes and beliefs regarding specific areas of the relationship. It is suitable for couples with or without children. The 11 scales were constructed on a rational basis and tap areas of the relationship such as: affective communication, problem-solving communication, time together, sexual dissatisfaction, and disagreement over finances. A validity scale assesses the tendency to describe the marriage in socially desirable terms. Particularly in cases where problems seem to extend beyond the bounds of infertility-related concerns, the MSI provides useful information in terms of areas of the relationship needing change. While its comprehensiveness is a strength, couples may be reluctant to complete such a lengthy instrument, unless they have serious concerns about their relationship.

CLINICAL ISSUES AND THERAPEUTIC INTERVENTION

Initial Consultation

Many infertility treatment programs, particularly those offering assisted reproductive technologies such as IVF, either provide the opportunity for or require couples to be psychologically assessed prior to treatment. Assessment provides the opportunity to screen for individual problems (anxiety, depression, substance abuse) or relationship concerns that might compromise a couple's ability to cope, comply with, or agree about treatment.

At this stage, counseling often has a significant psychoeducational component in terms of ensuring that couples understand the treatment process and helping them identify and solve potential problems associated with treatment procedures. Issues might include understanding treatment success rates, arranging time away from work, whom and how much to tell about treatment, the possible impact of medications on the woman's mood and hence the relationship, dealing with treatment failure, and couple agreement on the nature and extent of infertility treatment.

While most couples may not report marital dissatisfaction or conflict at this stage, it represents an important opportunity to prevent or minimize potential future problems. This may be particularly important if couples have markedly contrasting coping styles. Among infertile couples, women are more likely to reach out for social support and to use certain escape/avoidance strategies (wishing, hoping, fantasizing, social avoidance) than men. Men, by contrast, are more likely to engage in distancing through cognitive distraction, to engage in emotional self-regulation, and to view infertility in a pragmatic, problem-solving fashion[13]. Couples who fail to recognize and adjust to such differences may misinterpret each other's reactions and give negative attributions to their partner's response. For example, a husband may cope through cognitive avoidance, emotional distancing, and self control, while his wife may cope by seeking discussion and expressing her feelings. As a result, when treatment fails, he may perceive her as overreacting and conclude that she is too preoccupied with infertility and undervalues their relationship. She in turn may regard him as emotionally unaffected and therefore insensitive, uncaring, or uninvolved. Rather than simply resigning themselves to this difference and accepting an emotional distance between them, couples can better support each other by learning to accommodate to their partner's coping strategies.

Reversing Reinforcement Erosion

Because women are more likely than men to utilize social support as a means of coping, complaints about communication difficulties are often made by female partners. As counseling implicitly assumes a relationship model, when such a complaint is made, it is tempting to immediately provide a venue for more open discussion. Although this model is likely to be attractive to women, when a husband is clearly a reluctant participant and/or uncomfortable with 'talking' therapy, this approach might be a strategic error. An immediate and unskilled discussion of infertility may simply serve to perpetuate the negative interactional cycle already played out at home. Instead, it may be worthwhile to adopt a wider perspective.

For example, a couple may be experiencing 'reinforcement erosion'. Unlike the early stages of a relationship, when simply being with a partner was likely to be exciting and rewarding in itself, most couples find that over time pleasing a partner and ensuring that positive shared activities occur require a degree of effort and planning. The protracted nature of infertility, accompanied by repeated treatment failures, can accelerate this erosion. Over time, physical and emotional energy is increasingly taken up in coping with treatment and its disappointments. As a result, the time and effort needed to nurture the relationship assume secondary importance. Vacation time is used to participate in treatment programs, and holidays such as Christmas, or Halloween where children have a central role, may become aversive. The couple may begin to avoid previously enjoyed recreational or social activities with friends and family as a result of reminders or questions about their infertility. In turn, family and friends, unsure how to respond, may circumvent attempts to discuss infertility or avoid the couple. While understandable, avoidance on the part of infertile couples has been correlated with greater overall levels of distress for both men and women[13]. As a result, the couple may need help (e.g., through role playing and rehearsal) in developing new ways to give a public face to their infertility, together with encouragement to resume previously enjoyed activities.

In a related vein, there appears to be a relationship between an ability to identify positive aspects of infertility and adjustment. In one study, wives who characterized infertility as an opportunity for growth or strengthening of the relationship had husbands who reported less global and infertility-specific stress[39]. Although the authors cautioned against telling patients to 'look on the bright side' as countertherapeutic, helping couples rediscover positive aspects of their relationship appears to be important. With some couples, this might involve a direct form of cognitive restructuring in terms of identifying and altering cognitive distortions (e.g., all-or-none thinking, ignoring positives, magnification). For others, a positive cognitive shift might better be achieved indirectly by first having the couple experiment with new or neglected positive relationship behaviors. However, restoration of positive relationship behaviors needs to be targeted explicitly because the expression of positive and negative behaviors appears to be largely independent. In other words, changing negative behaviors that create tension or unhappiness does not necessarily lead to an increase in positive interactions[3]. In contrast, increasing positive relationship behaviors has been found to decrease negative interactions.

Increasing the frequency of positive exchanges[40] or devising what has been termed *perception-shifting* tasks designed to get couples to attend to other positive aspects of their situation[38] has several therapeutic advantages. By encouraging couples to refocus some of their efforts on pleasing each other, the focus of therapy shifts from problems and complaints toward finding solutions. If couples can achieve some rapid and early gains in therapy, this can foster positive expectancies about further treatment, a willingness to persist if setbacks occur, and a spirit of collaboration necessary before asking couples to engage in more difficult therapeutic tasks, such as altering patterns of communication.

Communication Skills Training

'I feel like I'm talking to a brick wall.'
'In the beginning I understood and accepted her unhappiness. But it never seemed to stop. Gradually I withdrew because I didn't know what to say and I couldn't stand to watch her crying all the time'[32].

When an infertile couple seeks counseling, one party (more typically the woman) may complain that when it comes to infertility, her partner avoids discussions, fails to listen, or fails to self-disclose. As a result, the complainant feels angry, isolated, unloved, or a burden on the relationship. This pattern, in which one spouse ('the pursuer') attempts to engage in problem discussion, often resorting to pressure and demands, while the other spouse ('the distancer') attempts to withdraw from the discussion, has been identified as a particularly destructive style of marital interaction[33,34]. Interestingly, the potential seriousness of this problem depends on which partner engages in withdrawal. While husbands' withdrawal has been shown to be predictive of wives' hostility, wives' withdrawal did not predict husbands' hostility[35].

Similarly, among infertile couples, it appears that discussion needs to meet a certain threshold of frequency for women's marital satisfaction but it need not be balanced. For example, women more frequently report initiating communication about infertility with husbands than men report initiating such discussions with their wives. Women also report receiving more emotional support from husbands than husbands report receiving from them. Nevertheless, both sexes describe satisfaction with this arrangement[36]. At the same time, women's and men's perceptions of the amount of support and disregard given and received from a spouse have been found to be only moderately related, suggesting that many couples are not communicating effectively with each other[37].

Improving a couple's ability to offer each other effective support can involve striking a balance between meeting women's needs for discussion and men's needs to maintain distance and emotional control. Discussion can be improved by teaching couples to employ better active-listening skills. Basic nonverbal skills (posture, facial expressions, eye contact, tone of voice), if neglected, leave a partner feeling unheard and often negate any other efforts made by the listener to provide support. Because men are more likely to utilize problem-solving strategies, they often offer support in terms of suggesting solutions to the problem or ways in which women can regain emotional control. Although well-intended, such efforts can be perceived as ignoring important feelings or as an attempt to abbreviate the discussion. Over time, men may feel increasingly helpless to provide effective support, but subsequent avoidance of discussion then produces increasing emotional disengagement. Learning to summarize ideas heard and to reflect feelings not only provides couples with better listening skills but also affords the opportunity for them to give effective support without having to generate solutions to a problem over which they have little control.

At the same time that communication is encouraged, men's needs for distance and control can be incorporated by emphasizing the importance of mutual agreement on the time and place for discussion. Couples can also agree to set specific time limits on such discussions and may follow these by sharing a mutually enjoyable activity.

Once both partners feel better heard and understood, it may be easier for each to accept that the other is affected quite differently by infertility. In therapy, couples have a tendency to tell stories about each other and then to argue about their accuracy. Instead, partners need to acknowledge each other's experience without trying to change it[38]. By learning the skill of emotional validation (showing empathy for a partner's feelings without necessarily being in agreement), couples can hold quite different perceptions of the infertility experience but still be mutually supportive.

Problems of Anger

The occurrence of infertility may be perceived by one or both partners as arbitrary and unfair, while the lack of control over a solution can trigger a rising tide of frustration. Couples may disagree on the need for treatment or the appropriate course of action. A man may feel helpless in his inability to reduce his partner's intense emotional distress and worry about her emotional stability. However, the expression of vulnerability is difficult for many men, and instead feelings may be manifested as anger. In fact, men's use of confrontative coping strategies involving impulsive and hostile blaming appears to be a predictor of poorer adjustment to infertility and to suggest the unskilled expression of anger[13].

Any expression of frustration and anger is likely to be interpreted by a partner as unfair blaming, if not expressed clearly. In these situations, couples may need help in identifying and conveying feelings more accurately, expressing complaints more constructively, and developing better conflict-resolution skills. Couples can learn to translate vague complaints into specific behavioral descriptions by encouraging the use of 'videotalk'[38]. In other words, complainants are taught to describe a partner's behavior minus attributed meanings or interpretations. For example, the therapist might ask, 'What kinds of things would I see him doing when he is acting "insensitive"?' In expressing complaints, couples can learn to incorporate positive statements about a partner, to avoid derogatory labels, to talk about specific behavior, to incorporate 'I' language rather than 'you' in statements of feelings, and to accept partial responsibility for problems.

In addition to the targeting of negative interactional patterns for change, the use of cognitive-behavioral techniques can assist couples in examining certain beliefs that seem to underlie feelings of anger. Briefly, this approach assumes that an individual's perceptions of her- or himself, the circumstances, or the future can trigger and maintain certain emotional responses[11]. Clients learn to identify and challenge self-defeating, irrational thoughts and to replace these with more accurate and adaptive thinking. For example, couples might be encouraged to consider the costs and benefits of maintaining a belief that infertility is 'unfair' and are then invited to consider the pros and cons of behaving as if they rejected this view.

Problems of Guilt and Self-Blame

In reacting to a diagnosis of infertility, women seem to be affected more personally than men. Women describe feelings of role failure[21] and diminished self-esteem[42] regardless of the locus of impairment, whereas men's reactions seem to be similar to women only when infertility is due to a male factor. Even when one partner is the sole diagnosed cause of the problem, women report a greater sense of responsibility than men[12]. As a result, when infertility treatment fails, intense feelings of guilt and self-blame can place some rather unique strains on a couple's relationship.

Due to guilt feelings and/or altruistic beliefs that a partner would be better off seeking a new mate, an infertile partner may openly encourage separation, sabotage the relationship by deliberately provoking conflict, or, in the extreme, engage in open marital infidelity. In this situation, cognitive-behavioral techniques can help the guilt-ridden partner distinguish between 'illegitimate guilt' (based on unrealistic expectations and standards) and 'legitimate guilt', (where a direct cause–effect relationship between the person's behavior and infertility exists)[13]. If guilt is legitimate, then it must be accommodated, and the 'guilty party' in conjunction with her or his partner can explore other, more constructive ways of atoning. Interventions might also include challenging idealistic predictions that separation will ensure a partner's happiness or helping the guilty partner listen to and accept her or his partner's actual relationship priorities.

In situations of actual infidelity, motivations may be more complex. It is assumed that such behavior can occur in reaction to guilt, in an effort to repair wounded sexual self-esteem, as a means to punish an infertile partner, or due to general marital dissatisfaction. However, the incidence of such behavior is hard to determine, and without a comparison group of fertile same-aged couples, it is difficult to know to what extent such behavior is a specific reaction to infertility.

Although women's tendency to accept responsibility (even when infertility is unexplained) can be problematic; in some situations it may reflect an adaptive coping response. In attributing the cause of infertility to herself, a woman may be achieving what has been described as 'interpretive control', that is, giving a threatening, largely uncontrollable, situation meaning or purpose[12]. While the fact that some women feel 'relieved' when perceiving themselves as responsible for a fertility problem might suggest an attempt to protect a partner. It also might reflect a degree of success in reestablishing some sense of control. Thus, men and women may not need to hold identical explanations for a fertility problem, and a therapist might need to weigh the importance and benefits of trying to change such attributions.

Decision-making

The decision to end unsuccessful medical treatment for infertility can trigger a complex series of issues for a couple. One partner may be ready to end treatment before the other. Couples may be in disagreement about the acceptability of alternative methods to build a family, such as adoption. Similarly, the prospect of remaining childless may be more acceptable and/or attractive to one partner. Helping couples identify and acknowledge their feelings about available options and assisting them to clarify their current priorities are usually facilitative. However, if one partner is coping by means of cognitive avoidance and/or denial, a cognitive-behavioral approach to challenge maladaptive beliefs, gentle confrontation, or communication skills training may be needed.

Facilitating Long-Term Adjustment

When the decision is made to discontinue treatment and other options to build a family are rejected, couples confront a future without children. Stage theories characterize this phase as one of grief, as individuals acknowledge the permanence of their infertility and fully confront the loss of pregnancy, childbirth, and parenting experiences. Currently, there seems to be general agreement among clinicians that the final stages of acceptance and resolution are achieved when grief feelings are acknowledged and expressed, while avoidance of such feelings may prevent resolution. However, the stages of a grief reaction have not been clearly validated, and there is some evidence that effective recovery can occur without prior apparent emotional processing[11]. In addition, the process by which couples reach a degree of closure on treatment efforts seems to be more lengthy and difficult for women than men[44]. As a result, one partner may be having greater difficulty adjusting to this new reality than the other, and the clinician must decide whether to recommend individual or conjoint counseling. To what extent the presence in therapy of the less distressed partner is facilitative is unclear, and at present there is no body of information to guide this decision. As a compromise, the clinician might recommend individual therapy for the partner in distress, with his or her partner included for discussion of particular relationship issues. When both partners are experiencing significant emotional distress and/or if problems in adjustment are creating concerns that threaten the relationship, therapy as a couple would be more clearly indicated.

Deconstruction

If stage theory is correct, helping couples deconstruct the infertility experience by encouraging them to discuss their loss and to express the full range of feelings associated with grief should facilitate the mourning process. Counseling tasks might include helping couples understand feelings of loss and lack of control, recognize and accept gender differences in ways of coping, and communicate with each other effectively and constructively[15]. Similarly, from a cognitive-behavioral perspective, there is evidence that repeated exposure to a traumatic event through recall can be beneficial. Through emotionally processing (i.e., repeated access and partial reexperience of difficult emotions), certain experiences have been shown to lose their emotional impact[46]. While such interventions have proved effective in cases of morbid grief[47], their utility in managing normal grief has not been demonstrated.

Reconstruction

As couples deconstruct the old reality, there is a need to construct a new reality and a new future together. The therapist must strike a balance between validating a couple's experience, while not ignoring the possibilities for change. Too much emphasis on acknowledging emotional pain may either encourage preoccupation with negative feelings or give a message that the situation cannot improve. At the same time, premature emphasis on making changes could give the impression that the therapist is insensitive to the couple's distress[38]. Solution-focused approaches to therapy[48,49] offer interesting, but as yet untested, ways in which the therapist can validate the couple's distress, while at the same time encouraging progression. Perceptions of infertility as global and unchangeable can be challenged by highlighting and amplifying exceptions that often go unnoticed by the couple. Problems can be restated as specific to certain times or places rather than generally present, and problem statements can be recast as preferred or future goals.

Because infertility can be such a blow to self-esteem, one or both partners may exhibit what has been termed a 'spoiled identity'[49]. Rather than having a problem, the individuals define themselves *as* the problem; that is, 'we are infertile'. In this situation, the clinician can assist the couple in externalizing and localizing a 'fertility problem' that then creates possibilities for the couple to generate solutions. The appropriate use of metaphor with the couple can facilitate this perceptual shift; for example, infertility has been characterized as 'a hurricane' that threatens 'the marital home', with a consequent need to 'strengthen it' (via communication skills) so that the home can weather the storm[50]. Alternatively, couples (women in particular) have a history of struggling long and hard to overcome infertility, and this history can be used to encourage a different 'hero' identity in which the person is valued for his or her strengths and for standing up to the fertility problem[49].

In constructing a new reality, couples often need to reexamine the basis for their relationship. At the time of marriage, a couple may have held certain assumptions about their individual roles and the role of children in their marriage. This is a time when the infertile partner may have unexpressed fears of abandonment, or fears that feelings of blame and resentment may create a permanent distance in the relationship. The therapist can elicit these concerns and help the couple share and discuss their future priorities. Sometimes, it is beneficial to have the couple step back and evaluate the personal qualities that triggered the initial mutual attraction and the actual reasons underlying their choice of a marital partner.

Ritual

Finally, in order to mark and facilitate a transition from infertility patient to what is sometimes termed 'childfree status'[51], the use of a special ceremony or ritual is often advocated[52]. In the design of a ritual with the couple, 'linked objects' (symbols physically associated with infertility) can be used to generate rituals of passage[38]— medications for disposal, baby items to be given away. Alternatively, couples sometimes wish to create symbols that facilitate mourning (a letter to the unrealized child) or to memorialize their loss (making regular donations to a certain charity, planting a tree).

However, if the ritual is to accomplish a sense of ending, couples need to feel that enough discussion, emotional expression, and exploration of feelings has first taken place. As yet, the optimal timing of such rituals is not well defined. In addition, because infertile couples use diverse and at times contrasting coping strategies, it remains unclear which couples are likely to benefit from ritual and to what extent men and women find this process similarly helpful.

FUTURE ISSUES

Based on a combination of research findings and clinical observation, this chapter has argued that certain factors (e.g., length of treatment, ineffective social and emotional support, noncomplementary coping skills) can give rise to relationship problems. However, at this stage, a number of questions remain. First, it is unclear whether relationship distress among infertile couples differs in any important ways from more general relationship distress. Second, while we have identified external risk factors, such as treatment experience, it is still unknown whether there are critical relationship factors that reliably differentiate distressed couples from nondistressed couples. Similarly, it is unknown whether there are aspects of a relationship that serve to buffer infertile couples from marital distress and increase the likelihood of successful long-term adjustment. Efforts to answer these questions would certainly be aided by the development of psychological and/or marital measures that are infertility-specific.

Despite the stress of infertility and treatment involvement, marital satisfaction scores for infertile couples generally fall within the normal range. However, these findings are derived largely from studies of couples before and during infertility treatment, and a clear picture is still lacking of posttreatment marital adjustment and the incidence of marital breakdown.

Finally, while stage theories have proved extremely useful in conceptualizing both infertility and the medical treatment experience, they are unable to incorporate the complexities of a couple's relationship or to account for gender differences in adjustment to infertility. At this time, there is a need to examine the potential contribution of other theoretical models for understanding and counseling infertile couples.

SUMMARY

- Clinical understanding of an individual's adjustment to infertility has been heavily influenced by stage theories, and similar theoretical assumptions are being utilized in approaches to counseling infertile couples.

- Until empirically tested theories emerge, clinicians need to be cognizant of gender differences and remain flexible in their clinical approach to counseling infertile couples.

- Assessment tools for the study of infertile couples are currently lacking, and clinicians will need to rely on more general instruments to evaluate relationship functioning.

- Both length of time in treatment and the frequency of experience with treatment failure appear to be important risk factors in predicting relationship satisfaction.

- Counseling objectives can vary considerably according to a couple's degree of experience with infertility and infertility treatment.

- Infertile couples in conflict are often characterized by their inability to understand and accept gender differences in reaction to infertility, together with an inability to provide each other with effective social and emotional support.

- In assisting couples facing final treatment failure, clinicians need to strike a balance between validating feelings of loss and inviting couples to be future-oriented and to focus on solutions.

REFERENCES

1. Wright J, Allard M, Lecours A, et al. Psychosocial distress and infertility: A review of controlled research. Int J Fertil 1989;34:126–42
2. Gurman AS, Jacobson NS. Marital therapy: From technique to theory, back again, and beyond. In: Jacobson NS, Gurman AS, eds. Clinical Handbook of Marital Therapy. New York: Guilford Press, 1986;1–9
3. Manus GI. Marriage counseling: A technique in search of a theory. J Marriage Fam 1966;28:449–53
4. Moghissi KS, Wallack EE. Unexplained infertility. Fertil Steril 1983;39:5–20
5. Sarrel PM, DeCherney AH. Psychotherapeutic intervention for treatment of couples with secondary infertility. Fertil Steril 1985;43:897–900
6. Menning BE. The infertile couple: A plea for advocacy. Child Welfare 1975;4:454–61
7. Menning BE. The emotional needs of infertile couples. Fertil Steril 1980;34:313–19

8. Blenner JL. Passage through infertility: A stage theory. *Image J Nurs Sch* 1990;22:153–5
9. Mathews R, Mathews AM. Infertility and involuntary childlessness: The transition to non-parenthood. *J Mar Fam Ther* 1986; 48:641–9
10. Mahlstedt PP. The psychological component of infertility. *Fertil Steril* 1985;43:335–46
11. Wortman CB, Silver RC. The myths of coping with loss. *J Consult Clin Psychol* 1989;57:349–57
12. Tennen H, Affleck G, Mandala R. Causal explanations for infertility: Their relation to control appraisals and psychological adjustment. In: Stanton AL, Dunkel-Schetter C, eds. *Infertility: Perspectives from Stress and Coping Research*. New York: Plenum, 1991;109–31
13. Stanton A. Cognitive appraisals, coping processes, and adjustment to infertility. In: Stanton AL, Dunkel-Schetter C, eds: *Infertility: Perspectives from Stress and Coping Research*. New York: Plenum, 1991;87–108
14. Abbey A, Andrews FM, Halman JL. The importance of social relationships for infertile couples' well-being. In: Stanton AL, Dunkel-Schetter C, eds. *Infertility: Perspectives from Stress and Coping Research*. New York: Plenum, 1991;61–86
15. Newton CR, Houle M. Gender differences in psychological response to infertility treatment. *Infertil Reprod Med Clin North Am* 1993;4:545–8
16. Wright J, Duchesne C, Sabourin S, *et al*. Psychosocial distress and infertility: Men and women respond differently. *Fertil Steril* 1991;55:100–8
17. Freeman EW, Rickels K, Tausig J, *et al*. Emotional and psychosocial factors in follow-up of women after IVF-ET treatment. *Acta Obstet Gynecol Scand* 1987;66:517–21
18. Newton CR, Hearn MT, Yuzpe AA. Psychological assessment and follow up after in vitro fertilization assessing the impact of failure. *Fertil Steril* 1990;54:879–86
19. Berg BJ, Wilson JF. Psychological functioning across stages of treatment for infertility. *J Behav Med* 1991;14:11–26
20. Leiblum SR, Kennan E, Lane MK. The psychological concomitants of in vitro fertilization. *J Psychosom Obstet Gynaecol* 1987;6:165–78
21. Greil AL, Leitko TA, Porter KL. Infertility: His and hers. *Gender Soc* 1958;2:172–99
22. Lalos A, Lalos O, Jacobson L, *et al*. The psychosocial impact of infertility two years after completed surgical treatment. *Acta Obstet Gynecol Scand* 1985;64:599–604
23. Daniluk JC, Leader A, Taylor P. Psychological and relationship changes of couples undergoing an infertility investigation: Some implications for consultants. *Br J Guid Couns* 1987;15:29–36
24. Takefman JE, Brender W, Boivin J, *et al*. Sexual and emotional adjustment of couples undergoing infertility investigation and the effectiveness of preparatory information. *J Psychosom Obstet Gynaecol* 1990; 11:275–90
25. Benezon N, Wright J, Sabourin S. Stress, sexual satisfaction, and marital adjustment in infertile couples. *J Sex Marital Ther* 1992;18:273–84
26. Boivin J, Takefman J, Tulandi T. Reactions to infertility based on extent of treatment failure. *Fertil Steril* 1995;63:801–7
27. McCartney CF, Wada CY. Gender differences in counseling needs during infertility treatment. In: Stotland NL, ed. *Psychiatric Aspects of New Reproductive Technologies*. Washington, DC: American Psychiatric Press, 1990;141–54
28. Reading AE, Kerin J. Psychologic aspects of providing infertility services. *J Reprod Med* 1989;34:861–71
29. Locke HJ, Wallace KM. Short marital adjustment and prediction tests: Their reliability and validity. *Marriage Fam Living* 1959;21:251–5
30. Spanier GB. Measuring dyadic adjustment: New scales for assessing the quality of marriage and similar dyads. *J Marriage Fam* 1976;38:15–28
31. Snyder DK. Multi-dimensional assessment of marital satisfaction. *J Marriage Fam* 1979;41:812–23
32. Salzer LP. *Infertility: How Couples Can Cope*. Boston: GK Hall, 1986
33. Heavy C, Layne C, Christensen A. Gender and conflict structure in marital interaction: A replication and extension. *J Consult Clin Psychol* 1993;61:16–27
34. Notarius CI, Pellegrini DS. Differences

between husbands and wives: Implications for understanding marital discord. In: Hahlweg K, Goldstein MJ, eds. *Understanding Major Mental Disorder: The Contribution of Family Interaction Research.* New York: Family Process, 1987: 231–49

35. Gottman JM, Krokoff LJ. Marital interaction and satisfaction: A longitudinal view. *J Couns Clin Psychol* 1989;57:47–52

36. Berg BJ, Wilson JF, Weingartner PJ. Psychological sequelae of infertility treatment: The role of gender and sex role identification. *Soc Sci Med* 1991;33:1071–80

37. Abbey A, Andrews, FM, Hartman J. Provision and receipt of social support and disregard: What is their impact on the marital life quality of infertile and fertile couples? *J Pers Soc Psychol* 1995;68:455–69

38. O'Hanlon-Hudson P, Hudson-O'Hanlon W. *Rewriting Love Stories: Brief Marital Therapy.* New York: Norton, 1991

39. Stanton AL, Tennen H, Affleck G, et al. Cognitive appraisal and adjustment to infertility. *Women Health* 1991;17:1–15

40. Jacobson NS, Margolin G. *Marital Therapy: Strategies Based on Social Learning and Behavior Exchange Principles.* New York: Brunner/Mazel, 1979

41. Beck AT, Rush JA, Shaw BF, Emery G. *Cognitive Therapy of Depression.* New York: Guilford, 1979

42. Nachtigall RD, Becker G, Wozny M. The effects of gender-specific diagnosis on men's and women's response to infertility. *Fertil Steril* 1992;57:113–21

43. Rando T. *Grieving: How to Go on Living When Someone You Love Dies.* Lexington, MA: Lexington, 1988

44. Baram D, Tourtelot Z, Eberhard M, et al. Psychosocial adjustment following unsuccessful in vitro fertilization. *J Psychosom Obstet Gynaecol* 1988;9:181–90

45. Myers M, Weinshel M, Scharf C, et al. An infertility primer for family therapists: II. Working with couples who struggle with infertility. *Fam Process* 1995;34:231–40

46. Rachman S. Emotional processing. *Behav Res Ther* 1980;18:51–60

47. Sireling L, Cohen D, Marks I. Guided mourning for morbid grief: A controlled replication. *Behav Ther* 1988;19:121–32

48. De Shazer S. *Keys to Solution in Brief Therapy.* New York: Norton, 1985

49. O'Hanlon WH, Weiner-Davis M. *In Search of Solutions: A New Direction in Psychotherapy.* New York: Norton, 1988

50. Atwood JD, Dobkin S. Storm clouds are coming: Ways to help couples reconstruct the crisis of infertility. *Contemp Fam Ther* 1992;14:385–403

51. Carter JW, Carter M. *Sweet Grapes: How to Stop Being Infertile and Start Living Again.* Indianapolis, IN: Perspectives Press, 1989

52. Becker G. *Healing the Infertile Family: Strengthening Your Relationship in the Search for Parenthood.* New York: Bantam, 1990

7

Group Counseling

Constance Hoenk Shapiro, PhD

We are held in place by the pressure of the crowd around us.
We must all lean upon others. Let us see that we lean gracefully
and freely and acknowledge their support.

Margaret Collier Graham

HISTORICAL OVERVIEW

Historically, the use of groups with infertile persons had its beginnings in the early 1970s when a small group of women in Boston began having monthly discussions to explore the feelings generated by their infertility. From this small core, the group increased its membership and the frequency of meetings and eventually developed beyond informal discussions to being a support group. Since that initial group that formed the seeds of RESOLVE, many groups have formed to meet the needs of infertile persons. Some of these groups are affiliated with RESOLVE and its many chapters, other groups are affiliated with clinics and medical facilities, and still other groups are facilitated by mental health professionals or infertile consumers. Different as these groups may be, one cannot help but be impressed with the ways in which infertile persons seek out one another at a time in their lives when they need respite from the all-too-familiar feelings of isolation and alienation.

This chapter will:

- outline the history of group counseling for infertility
- describe the remedial model, mediating model, and developmental models of group counseling
- address management issues of group counseling for infertility
- discuss the important most common themes of group counseling for infertility.

REVIEW OF LITERATURE

Current literature on groups for infertile individuals reminds us that they provide opportunities for peer support, new learning, personal insight, and stress reduction[1-4]. Research on the effectiveness of groups reveals its capacity for positive impact in areas of belongingness, education, and the strength to go on[5,6]. The reduction of self-reported distress and depression has also been noted as a result of participation in an infertility support group[7]. Specialized support groups, such as those dealing with premature ovarian failure[8], diethylstilbestrol exposure[9], and other topics, provide both information and psychological support for women and their partners. Most RESOLVE chapters have at least one support group, and larger chapters also have groups for special concerns common to infertile couples such as: pregnancy loss, pregnancy after infertility, child-free living, and adoption exploration. Although RESOLVE has not conducted any formal research on the effectiveness of these groups, their continued proliferation in cities across the country speaks to the need felt by infertile people for a connection with others sharing their diagnosis and the accompanying emotional responses. The spectrum among groups for infertile people ranges from RESOLVE groups that focus on helping to strengthen members' coping capacities and advocacy skills through peer support to behavioral programs that are highly structured in terms of content, with a focus on learning relaxation techniques and cognitive restructuring of negative thoughts.

THEORETICAL FRAMEWORKS

The theoretical models applicable to the use of groups vary considerably. However, even though there are distinct theoretical orientations, it is common for therapists and group facilitators to utilize an eclectic approach, depending on their expertise and the needs of group participants. Middleman and Wood[10] suggested that a mainstream model of work with groups should include the counselor

- helping members develop a system of mutual aid
- understanding, valuing, and respecting group processes as powerful dynamics for change
- helping members become empowered for autonomous functioning within and outside the group
- helping members reexperience their groupness at the point of termination.

The following models draw upon a wealth of influential theories, in addition to systems theory, which most group workers believe to be basic to all group work practice. Psychoanalytic theory, learning theory, field theory, and social exchange

theory all have been used by group workers to frame their interventions with group members, depending on the needs and purposes of the groups. Let us now examine those models and identify examples of infertility groups that might be especially appropriate for each.

Remedial Model

This perspective, closely allied with the medical model, utilizes the group as a context and a means for altering dysfunctional patterns of behavior. Developed by Vinter and colleagues at the University of Michigan, this approach tends to place the group leader in a position of authority and expertise, with relatively little emphasis on the contribution of environmental factors to individuals' distress. This approach might be most appropriate for consideration with infertile individuals whose depression, low self-esteem, or alienation is perceived to be intrapersonal and whose need for change in the external environment is minimal. The remedial model, with its focus on the individual, is less appropriate for couples than other models.

Mediating Model

Developed by William Schwartz, the mediating model draws extensively from systems theory, humanistic psychology, and an existential perspective to encourage group members to confront the environmental barriers to solving their problems. In this model, both individuals and the social environment provide opportunities for the group facilitator to encourage interactions. This approach is especially well-suited to infertile consumers who are experiencing frustration with health professionals, medical settings, work colleagues, family members, or others who are perceived as barriers to smooth resolution of infertile clients' problems. In this model, the facilitator encourages the group to develop goals for action and to seek to resolve conflict with the external social forces.

Developmental Model

Having its roots at Boston University, the developmental model is based primarily on the dynamics of intimacy and draws on a knowledge base of ego psychology, group dynamics, and conflict theory. In this model, the therapist encourages members to struggle with how to implement their goals at the same time that they continually assess thoughts, feelings, and behaviors. Infertile persons who are grappling with feelings of loss, stagnation, and confusion are likely to find a developmental model to be of relevance to their needs.

CLINICAL ISSUES AND THERAPEUTIC INTERVENTIONS

Whether the person who convenes a group of infertile people is called a group worker, a group leader, a group facilitator, or a group therapist is determined by the purpose of the group. Being clear about the purpose of the group is critical to the role of the professional in the group, as that person must help the group develop goals, foster a sense of group cohesion, encourage the expression of emotions that often are painful, yet ultimately help the group to be of assistance to its members. Both support groups and therapeutic groups face a number of clinical challenges as they strive to help their members become resilient during their struggle with infertility.

Support Versus Therapy Groups

The major distinctions between support groups and therapeutic groups have to do with purpose and sponsorship. Generally, a

therapeutic group strives to change behaviors that its members consider dysfunctional. The therapist's role is to encourage group members to use strategies ranging from insight to behavioral change to improve their ways of coping with the stress of infertility. Therapeutic groups are likely to be run through an agency, a health care setting, or a mental health professional's private practice. In some cases, they are targeted for specific agency clientele (couples hoping to adopt, individuals and couples undergoing assisted reproductive technologies, or people being treated in a particular infertility clinic); in other cases, the therapist may specify the focus of the group (for individuals in a particular stage of infertility, grappling with specific losses, or experiencing a dysfunctional emotional response to infertility). It is common for fees to be charged for participation in a professionally run group. The professional facilitator brings a knowledge and skill base to the group experience that guides his or her actions with the group. The professional is likely to be attentive to group dynamics, to the phases of group development, and to individuals and their special issues in the group. Likewise, the professional has some familiarity with professional ethics and usually introduces issues such as confidentiality for discussion in the group. A professional may or may not have had personal experience with infertility and is likely to keep the group discussion focused on members of the group rather than to disclose personal experiences. Although therapeutic groups may be open-ended, it is more common for them to have a specified membership over a time-limited period.

In contrast, a support group is very likely to have been formed by infertile individuals who have a strong commitment to fostering communication and support but who may not have had much experience working with groups. Support groups may be led by a person who initially convenes the group, with subsequent leadership evolving to other group members as they feel able to assume this role. In some support groups, the leader takes responsibility for making the physical arrangements for the group meeting, while encouraging other members to take responsibility for maintaining group discussion. The content of support group discussions is likely to be both informational and cathartic, with less attention to group dynamics than would be found in a therapeutic group. Personal disclosure by both the facilitator and the group members is a common experience in the group. Open-ended support groups are open to new membership on a continual basis and terminate only when the interest of the members wanes. Support groups often meet in the homes of members, although some select a convenient-to-access community location.

A special word needs to be said here about the distinction of support groups sponsored through RESOLVE. RESOLVE support groups are usually facilitated by a professional whose background may be in social work, psychology, nursing, or counseling. Because these are support groups and not therapy groups, the professional facilitators screen self-referrals to ascertain that prospective members are generally normally functioning and are not massively depressed or disturbed, do not have a distorted sense of reality, or do not have deep-seated issues of loss that have been reactivated by their infertility. RESOLVE groups are time-limited and issue-oriented, although many participants continue relationships with one another long after the formal group has disbanded.

Management Issues

The group facilitator needs to attend first to the purpose of the group, which in turn will influence other organizational issues. The first question to address is whether the group will be *open* (admitting new members on a continual basis) or *closed* (with membership established on the first group meeting). The open-group model is especially well-suited to informal or educational groups in which agendas evolve in response to members' needs and that are comfortable with a changing membership. In contrast, a closed-group model is often preferred by groups that seek a level of intimacy and trust in which they can share painful feelings and handle confrontation and corrective feedback or have a structured format. The frequency of meetings is usually an issue that the group addresses at its first meeting; weekly meetings may be appropriate for time-limited groups, but more long-term groups tend to prefer a monthly format.

Decisions about group size should take into consideration that not all members will be able to attend all sessions. Attendance will be more stable at time-limited groups or at groups in which fees are being paid by participants. Open-ended groups, on the other hand, may find that attendance varies depending on the topic to be addressed in the group at a particular session, on the level of emotional exhaustion that members feel regarding their infertility, and on how connected members feel to the group at a given point in time. The ideal group size tends to be about eight participants[1,3], which allows for trust to develop and for members to be able to participate at a level that is comfortable for them.

Most group meetings last 1½ to 2 hours. Depending on the type of group, refreshments may be served, and many groups prefer to have time for informal conversation either just before or just after the group meeting. The duration of a group is not an issue for open-ended groups, since they continue to meet as long as there are enough members to contribute to the vitality of the group. However, for time-limited groups, the duration is likely to be set in advance by the facilitator, depending on the purpose of the group. An initial plan to meet from 8 to 12 sessions is reasonable for most groups; group members wishing to continue after that period may renegotiate with the facilitator or may decide to reassemble as an open-ended group, with or without the group leader.

The location of the group has the potential to influence feelings of physical and emotional comfort of group members. Ideally, the location should be easily accessible to all group members and remain the same for the duration of the group. The safety of the neighborhood will be a special concern to women attending meetings in the evening; the facilitator may need to make special efforts to encourage carpools, to provide escorts to and from parking lots, and to address other safety concerns. Whether in an agency or in a group member's home, the meeting room should be as aesthetically pleasing as possible and should have comfortable furniture that can be moved into a circle. The facilitator should avoid a room that is too small; in addition to being physically cramped, members may also feel that the tight quarters force a sense of intimacy before it has evolved naturally within the group[11].

Confidentiality

The capacity for the group to develop intimacy and trust will be influenced by the way in which the group treats information that is shared among themselves. The group facilitator's explanation of confidentiality might be along these lines[3]:

> Many of us are at different points in our struggles with infertility. We also have made different kinds of decisions about how public or private to be in sharing information about our infertility with others. It is my hope that we can foster a spirit of openness in the group, since we all share the common bond of infertility and have a great deal to offer one another. However, no matter how open we will be in this group, it is important to keep the information discussed here confidential. That means that, although we may choose to share the information about our participation in this group with friends, we must never violate the confidentiality of others by revealing that they are members of this group, or by revealing anything that they discuss with the group. Do any of you have any questions or comments on the group's respect for the confidentiality of its members?

Group members may need clarification on how confidentiality impacts their conversations with members between group meetings. The most reasonable response is that the work of the group should be carried on inside the group, so it is not appropriate to discuss the content or dynamics of a meeting with anyone else, even a group member, outside of the group. However, group members who wish to socialize, which may include sharing information about their infertility outside of the group, should feel free to do so as they would with any friend, assuming that the group agrees to its members' socializing apart from group meetings.

Pregnant Group Members

The presence of pregnant women in a group is an issue that must be anticipated by the group facilitator and discussed in the group[2]. It is entirely possible that a much-wanted pregnancy will occur during the life of the group, and members need to have decided in advance whether a pregnant member will remain in the group or whether her pregnancy would feel too threatening or distracting to other group members. There is no right or wrong answer to this potential dilemma; groups have reached different resolutions, depending on the needs of their members. What is important, however, is the capacity of the group to grapple with this issue in advance of its occurrence and to reach a general consensus about what would be in the best interest of their particular group[3].

Group Themes

The group leader is likely to encounter several themes that are common to people in an infertility group.

Loss

All members of the group are likely to refer to their issues of loss during the life of the group[12]. The loss of their dream child is often the most frightening one, but members may also perceive other losses: the role of being a birth parent, trust in their reproductive capacities, sense of control over life plans, and the feeling of normalcy in a predominantly fertile world. Losses may also be family members or friends who fail to provide support, financial or career (e.g., failure to get a promotion due to reduced productivity). Group members should be helped to identify their losses, so they can articulate the emotions associated with each loss.

Anger

Anger is a common emotion associated with infertility. At the same time that the group facilitator validates members' feelings of entitlement to anger, there is also the need to identify how members are channeling their anger. This emotion may

be very rational, as occurs when friends, relatives, or coworkers are unable to offer the support that the infertile person needs; at other times, the feelings of anger may be less rational or may be displaced onto others (partners, parents, medical professionals) or turned against the self, which typically results in depression. The group experience can provide a safe place to explore feelings of anger, to express anger without fear of being negatively judged, and to share coping strategies with other group members.

Grief

As the feeling of hopelessness builds, some group members will acknowledge profound sadness and will need to talk about the impact on their lives of the losses that they are experiencing. Society does not provide comforting rituals for the losses that infertile people experience, so members often will look to the group for the comfort they need at a time when tears flow readily, when life has lost its meaning, and when emptiness is overwhelming. The facilitator needs to acknowledge that these feelings are a predictable part of coming to terms with one's infertility, and to encourage other group members to support and comfort members who are working through their grief. The facilitator familiar with techniques of grief counseling will find many opportunities to apply this knowledge when issues of grief arise in a group.

Powerlessness

Not only do infertile group members feel powerless against the situation of their infertility, but they also feel powerless in specific situations: family and work situations involving infants and pregnant women, medical environments that are emotionally unsupportive or stressful in other ways, and interactions with their partners, where problems in communication are common. The group facilitator can guide group members away from their self-identification as victims and turn their attention to ways in which they can confront difficult situations assertively[3].

Feeling Out of Control

Whether this feeling relates specifically to members' inability to improve their fertility (which is now very much in the hands of medical professionals) or whether it relates to other life plans that are disrupted by infertility, members' responses are usually to struggle to maintain control—only to find that the all-consuming effort to conceive is in itself disruptive[3]. Vacations are postponed, employment or educational opportunities are deferred, and business trips are synchronized with doctors' appointments and ovulation schedules. A useful defense against feeling out of control is information. People who become knowledgeable in their special areas of concern are able to feel like active participants in the process, thereby regaining some measure of intellectual mastery over previously intimidating medical procedures and baffling emotional reactions connected with infertility. The group can be an excellent source of information, as the facilitator encourages members to compare experiences, share resources, introduce educational materials, and offer suggestions of coping strategies.

Gender Issues

All of the scholars who have researched the question of gender as it relates to infertility have reached virtually the same conclusion: that men and women in American society interpret and react to infertility in different ways and that understanding the influence of gender on infertility is crucial to understanding how couples experience it[13,14]. In a

study of 22 infertile couples, it was found that the wives experienced infertility as a cataclysmic role failure that spoiled their ability to live normal lives. They tended to retreat from interaction with the fertile world and to become very focused on the problem of infertility. Husbands tended to see infertility as a disconcerting event, but not a tragedy. They were likely to feel that it was something they could accept and put into perspective, and were chagrined that their wives could not do this as well. While wives tended to be interested in overcoming infertility no matter what it took, their husbands were more interested in returning to normalcy, whether this implied pursuing treatment or ceasing treatment. These gender-specific patterns were found regardless of which partner had the reproductive impairment. Furthermore, because it was wives who were more treatment-oriented and who experienced more profound role failure, couples tended to see infertility as a problem for wives[13]. In a study of 185 infertile couples, it was found that wives, as opposed to their husbands, perceived their fertility problem as more stressful, felt more responsible for and in control of their infertility, and engaged in more problem-focused coping. Infertile husbands experienced more home life stress than did their wives[14]. It is common for women to be the initiator of efforts to get help for their emotional pain[8]; and husbands' participation in counseling is often framed in terms of a wish to support their wife rather than to access help for themselves. The challenge for the group facilitator who has couples within the group is to understand the differing needs and perceptions that men and women may have, even though they may be presumed to be sharing the same infertility situation.

Termination

The ending of a time-limited group is likely to reawaken issues of isolation for many

123

group members. Even though members know on a factual and an intellectual level that the group will end, the facilitator should make every effort to help members acknowledge the meaning of the group's ending. The facilitator should prepare the group for termination issues by mentioning periodically during the life of the group the amount of time remaining before the last session. As the last sessions approach, the facilitator might take the lead by asking members what it feels like to anticipate the ending of the group. Most will feel the loss of a safe place to share their struggles; many will identify new relationships formed as a result of participating in the group; still others will articulate their feelings that they are not yet ready to continue their infertility struggle without the support of the group. And, finally, since infertility itself is a series of losses, the loss of the group can feel to some members like an especially poignant and emotion-laden sadness. When the one relationship they covet, that of themselves and a baby, seems elusive, the sadness of losing the group relationship is even more compelling. The expression of grief by group members may be fleeting or intense, depending on the group and the comfort of the facilitator with the expression of painful feelings.

While acknowledging the feelings of sadness that permeate the group as its last sessions approach, the facilitator will want to focus on how new learning from the group may have prepared members to deal with the ongoing challenges of their infertility. Members can be encouraged to reflect on the hard work they have done and their feelings of accomplishment. While members may wish that the group could continue, they may also feel some relief about termination in that a considerable amount of time, energy, and, perhaps, money was committed to the group experience. As they explore their ambivalence about ending, members often become willing to look at other endings with energy and courage, knowing that they have done all that they can and there comes a time when one must move forward[3].

Many groups have a special ritual or ceremony at their last group meeting. This idea may come from the group itself, or it may be suggested by the facilitator. After the challenging emotional work of anticipating the ending of the group, the ritual itself may offer an opportunity for lightheartedness and sociability, while at the same time enabling the group to end with warm memories of their last time together. The group may choose to meet in a member's home or other sociable setting, a group picture may be taken, and there may be some closing remarks by the facilitator and group members. The planning of the ending ritual should be shared to ensure that it represents the needs of the group. Termination in an infertility group is a crucial process for the consolidation of gains by group members. Struggling with the ongoing challenges of infertility, members may find the ending of the group both symbolically and realistically painful. Since one of the greatest challenges in infertility is to move forward and look ahead, the sensitive termination of a group can contribute dramatically to its members' readiness to see in endings the promise of new beginnings[3].

FUTURE IMPLICATIONS

Infertile individuals and couples experience both medical quandaries and emotional quagmires. It is virtually impossible to separate the physiological condition of infertility from the emotional process that accompanies it. Yet many infertile people find medical services more accessible than the emotional support they need concurrently. In addition, if there are costs associated with infertility counseling or support groups, many individuals will need to choose between medical and emotional treatment because of depleted finances and limited insurance coverage. Professionals who recognize the importance of integrating the medical and emotional responses to infertility can find several creative responses to the current consumer dilemma.

First, infertility clinics and other clinics providing assisted reproductive technologies should recognize the advantages of employing a social worker, a psychologist, or a psychiatric nurse to work with individuals and couples seeking treatment. This individual should be a part of the initial intake process, at which time patients can be alerted to the predictable stressors of pursuing infertility treatment. In addition to providing individual counseling, the professional in the clinic setting is in an ideal position to facilitate support or therapy groups for clinic patients. These groups should be considered an integral part of the medical services of the clinic and should be free of charge for clinic patients. Not only will patients feel that their infertility is being addressed in many dimensions, but the professional providing psychological support is in an ideal position to advocate for patients, to encourage more positive communication by medical professionals, and to access medical information promptly and accurately.

Second, for those clinics located many miles from their patients' homes, there is a need to ascertain available emotional supports when patients return to their home communities. One such clinic, which drew its patients from seven surrounding rural counties, identified a counselor in each of the seven counties who would provide infertility counseling to clinic clients[15]. Orientation was provided by the clinic for the county counselors, who were then free to provide individual or group

services to clinic patients on request. The advantage of this clinic outreach service is that it was geographically accessible to patients, local community supports could be coordinated by the county counselor, the counselor could advocate on behalf of patients, even at a distance, and the costs associated with the long-distance emotional support were assumed by the infertility clinic.

A third creative response by counselors is to serve as *pro bono* consultants to individuals wishing to start support groups in the community. Many infertile consumers are eager to connect with others in similar circumstances but will need some initial guidance about recruiting group members and, ultimately, about facilitating a support group for interested individuals. The professional counselor is in an ideal position to provide both information and periodic consultation during the meetings of the open-ended group. The group members might ultimately decide to affiliate as a RESOLVE chapter, thereby giving them access to even greater resources than their locality could provide.

A fourth creative response is one that is consumer-initiated. With the increasing availability of computer technology, not only are infertility services and resources available on the World Wide Web, but chat rooms for infertile people are an additional resource on the Internet. In addition to being accessible at the convenience of the consumer, free of charge and anonymous, such chat rooms may be the only acceptable channel for some infertile persons to connect with others. The potential disadvantages of chat rooms as sources of group support include inaccuracy of information that may be conveyed, the lack of a professional who can assist people's efforts to sort out their emotions constructively, and the dependence on a technological 'connection' at a time when medical technology may already cause the infertile person to feel nameless and faceless. On the other hand, for people who live in isolated or rural areas or those who need to gradually expose themselves to the mutual support that can come from a chat room, this experience may be a real lifeline at a time of emotional isolation.

SUMMARY

- Research on the effectiveness of groups with infertile people reveals the capacity for increasing feelings of belongingness, relieving depression, providing education, and maintaining the strength to go on.
- Models that may guide professionals in their work with groups may include the *remedial model*, which alters dysfunctional patterns of behavior *mediating model*, which encourages group members to confront barriers to solving their problems *developmental model*, which encourages personal growth through intimacy with group members.
- Important therapeutic issues that the group facilitator must consider have to do with support versus therapeutic groups; management issues such as group structure, size, frequency, duration, and location; confidentiality; the presence of pregnant members in the group; gender issues; and the sensitive termination of time-limited groups.
- Group themes that are likely to emerge in the course of a group include loss, anger, grief, powerlessness, feeling out of control, and reactions to the termination of the group.
- Future challenges include how to make emotional support available to infertile people who may feel financially depleted, geographically isolated, or unaware of how to access a consumer-led support group.

REFERENCES

1. Menning B. RESOLVE: Counseling and support for infertile couples. In: Mazor M, Simons H, eds. *Infertility: Medical, Emotional, and Social Considerations.* New York: Human Sciences Press, 1984;53–60
2. Goodman K, Rothman B. Group work in infertility treatment. *Soc Work Groups* 1984; 7:79–97
3. Shapiro C. *Infertility and Pregnancy Loss.* San Francisco: Jossey-Bass Publishers, 1988
4. Domar A, Seibel M, Benson H. The mind/body program for infertility: A new behavioral treatment approach for women with infertility. *Fertil Steril* 1990;53:246–9
5. Lentner E, Glazer G. Infertile couples' perceptions of infertility support-group participation. *Health Care Women Int* 1991; 12:317–30
6. O'Moore A. Counseling and support systems for infertile couples. *Irish J Med Sci* 1986;155 (Supplement 12):12s–16s
7. Stewart D, Boydell K, McCarthy K, Swerdlyk S, Redmond C, Cohrs W. A prospective study of the effectiveness of brief professionally-led support groups for infertility patients. *Int J Psychiatry Med* 1992;22:173–82
8. Berson A. Quality of life issues for patients with reproductive loss. *Clin Consult Obstet Gynecol* 1994;6:100–8
9. Apfel R, Fisher S. Emotional aspects of DES exposure. In: Mazor M, Simons H, eds. *Infertility: Medical, Emotional and Social Considerations.* New York: Human Sciences Press, 1984;173–9
10. Middleman R, Wood G. Reviewing the past and present of group work and the challenge of the future. *Soc Work Groups* 1990;13:3–20
11. Sommer R. *Personal Space.* Englewood Cliffs, NJ: Prentice-Hall, 1969

12. Mahlstedt P. The psychological component of infertility. *Fertil Steril* 1985;43:335–46
13. Greil A, Leitko T, Porter K. Infertility: His and hers. *Gender Soc* 1988;2:172–99
14. Abbey A, Andrews F, Halman L. Gender's role in responses to infertility. *Psychol Women Q* 1991;15:295–316
15. Shapiro C. Integrating medical and psychosocial services for rural infertility clients. Presented at the annual meeting of the American Public Health Association, October, 1990

8

Behavioral Medicine Approaches to Infertility Counseling

Annette L. Stanton, PhD, and Linda Hammer Burns, PhD

*The trouble about always trying to preserve the health of the body
is that it is so difficult to do without destroying the health of the mind.*

G.K. Chesterton

HISTORICAL OVERVIEW

Evolving over the past several decades, behavioral medicine is 'the interdisciplinary field concerned with the development and integration of behavioral and biomedical science knowledge and techniques relevant to health and illness and the application of this knowledge to prevention, diagnosis, treatment, and rehabilitation'[1]. Similarly, within the field of psychology, health psychology has developed as a specialty that involves the aggregate of the specific educational, scientific, and professional contributions of the discipline of psychology to the promotion and maintenance of health, the prevention and treatment of illness, the identification of etiologic and diagnostic correlates of health, illness, and related dysfunction, and the analysis and improvement of the health care system and health policy formation[2].

In recent decades, behavioral medicine and health psychology have enjoyed rapid expansion, owing in part to burgeoning scientific evidence linking psychosocial factors with important aspects of health and illness, as well as empirically demonstrated successes of psychosocial

interventions applied to disease treatment and health promotion. In this chapter, we:

- provide a brief historical overview of the psychosomatic approaches to the psychology of infertility
- outline illustrative theoretical frameworks of behavioral medicine and health psychology as they apply to the psychology of infertility
- describe several stress management and coping interventions
- discuss clinical applications of stress and coping theory for aiding couples as they confront infertility's many psychosocial demands.

Early psychosomatic approaches to infertility, which assumed a connection between psychological conflicts and somatic functioning, focused on infertility caused by intrapsychic conflicts in men and women, more commonly women. So-called *psychogenic infertility* was thought to result from deep-seated neurotic anxiety, given that the female genital tract was assumed to be the most 'hysterical' portion of a woman's anatomy, under both nervous and hormonal control[3]. At a time when infertility of unknown etiology was significant, theories of neurotic personality structure, conflicted feelings about parenthood, sexuality, and adult roles, fears of childbirth, and intrapsychic conflict regarding one's own mother were considered feasible explanations for infertility. Psychic conflict was considered a cause of physiological changes and stress a contributory factor in psychological disturbances related to infertility. For example, 'Emotional stress, either directly or by releasing adrenaline, was thought to centrally inhibit or prevent the secretions of oxytocin or counteract its action'[4]. Sandler[5] considered personality factors and a recurring pattern of 'situation-stress-symptom' as a cause of infertility. He presented as evidence his investigation of 268 infertile marriages, concluding that 67 of the marriages experienced stress-provoked incidents of infertility resulting from emotional immaturity, impotence, ignorance of sex technique, and vaginismus/frigidity. Pregnancy after adoption and pregnancy after the initial diagnostic work-up were considered further evidence supporting psychogenic infertility, with Sandler concluding that adoption facilitated conception by relieving emotional distress.

Beginning in the 1970s, however, psychoanalytic and psychosomatic approaches fell into disfavor, with increasingly successful medical diagnosis of infertility and emerging findings such as the lack of significant relation between adoption and subsequent conception. Psychological distress was no longer thought to be the *cause* of infertility, but rather the *result* of the stress of infertility and its medical treatment. Research began to focus on assessing typical psychological responses to infertility, reactions to particular medical treatments (e.g., assisted reproductive technologies), individual and gender differences in response to infertility,

and the development of coping skills interventions for individuals experiencing infertility. Coping and stress management interventions for infertility were emphasized, fueled in part by the consumer advocacy movement. Recent research has addressed the interaction between stress and medical outcomes (e.g., increased pregnancy rates or improved sperm production), the impact of fertility medications on psychological well-being, and the development or adaptation of treatment techniques to improve psychosocial adjustment and quality of life for infertile men and women.

Behavioral medicine and health psychology have been useful in exploring the mind–body connection in infertility. Both approaches facilitate the understanding of emotional consequences of infertility, development of coping and stress management interventions, research design, and theory development.

REVIEW OF LITERATURE

Early investigations of the psychology of infertility focused on intrapsychic conflicts in infertile women that would account for their infertility. Some of this literature centered solely on psychological factors or emotional responses associated with infertility, whereas other studies focused on physical manifestations of emotional distress, such as impotence, anovulation, or altered hypothalamic functioning. Wright and colleagues[6] offered a review of 30 published articles on controlled research regarding psychosocial distress and infertility. They examined three hypotheses regarding potential links between infertility and psychosocial distress: (1) Psychosocial problems trigger infertility; (2) infertility triggers psychosocial distress; and (3) an interactive causal relationship between infertility and psychosocial distress exists. They concluded that, as a whole, patients diagnosed and treated in infertility clinics showed significantly higher levels of psychosocial distress than did control groups and that female patients were more distressed than males. However, they also concluded that much of the research had flawed designs that failed to control crucial variables, thus preventing conclusive empirical tests of the three hypotheses.

Although the specific links between psychosocial and biomedical aspects of infertility have yet to be delineated, it is clear that the experience of infertility taxes the psychosocial resources of some couples. Several studies have focused on assessing stressful aspects of assisted reproductive technologies, such as in vitro fertilization (IVF). Baram and associates[7] used questionnaires to evaluate 86 couples following failed IVF cycles. The couples were asked to rate the experience of IVF compared to nine other stressful life events on a scale of 1 to 10 (1 for the least stressful and 10 for most stressful). Women reported higher stress levels than men at every stage of infertility evaluation and IVF treatment; they ranked IVF fourth on a list of stressful life events, whereas men ranked IVF as seventh. Both men and women found that the most stressful points of the IVF process were waiting to see whether IVF had worked and discovering that IVF had not been successful; the least stressful were deciding to undergo IVF and the period after IVF had been completed. Collins and colleagues[8] evaluated 200 couples entering IVF treatment and found that women anticipated more stress in IVF treatment than men but women also had more social support than men. Both partners overestimated chances of success in IVF. They also found that the factors influencing anticipated stress were the same for both partners: Intense focus on having a child was the predominant factor in anticipated stress of IVF for both men and women. In a study of 117 women following IVF and IVF failure, Laffont and Edelmann[9] found that men and women agreed that a negative outcome and waiting for the results were the most stressful aspects of IVF, and that women reported experiencing more stress than men across the stages of treatment.

Certainly, infertility potentially presents many stressors for couples. However, most do not evidence clinically significant elevations on measures of psychological distress or psychopathology. Dunkel-Schetter and Lobel[10] reviewed research on psychological reactions to infertility, evaluating both descriptive and empirical articles on observable responses to infertility. Their review was updated by Stanton and Danoff-Burg[11]. Both reviews concluded that empirical evidence from scientifically rigorous research on the psychological effects of infertility did not support the contention that there are specific reactions to infertility that are common and predictable. The authors found that methodologically rigorous research suggested that the majority of people do not experience clinically significant emotional reactions, loss of self-esteem, or adverse marital and sexual consequences associated with infertility. These findings indicated that the majority of infertile men and women maintain adequate psychosocial functioning. Even though most individuals remain psychologically resilient in the face of infertility, there is wide variability in response. Some infertile individuals experience extreme distress and life disruption, and others may experience peaks in distress at particular points in the process (e.g., a failed IVF attempt). Psychosocial interventions can aid individuals and couples in managing both the acute and chronic stresses of infertility.

THEORETICAL FRAMEWORKS

A strength of the field of health psychology is its focus on development and testing of theories to understand psychosocial issues in health and disease. Careful theory development allows integration of findings and systematic accumulation of knowledge. Research on psychosocial aspects of and intervention in infertility can benefit from theoretical frameworks in health psychology and other areas. Two such frameworks, stress and coping theory and the biopsychosocial model, will serve as illustrations of the utility of applying such theories to infertility.

Stress and Coping Theory

Stress and coping theories[12] have been applied in order to understand adjustment to many health-related problems, including infertility[10,13]. According to these theories, stress is experienced when one encounters demands perceived as taxing or exceeding one's resources. The cognitive appraisal and coping process are central to these accounts, as individuals assess the potentially harmful and beneficial aspects of the stressful experience (i.e., primary appraisal), as well as their potential ability to influence its outcome (i.e., secondary appraisal). Appraisal-focused coping involves attempts to define the meaning of the stressful situation and includes logical analysis, cognitive redefinition, and cognitive avoidance. Problem-focused coping is the modification or elimination of the source of stress and involves seeking information or advice, taking problem-solving action, and developing alternative rewards. Emotion-focused coping is defined as responses to stress in which the primary function is managing emotions aroused by stressors, thereby maintaining affective equilibrium. Emotion-focused strategies include affective regulation, resigned acceptance, and emotional discharge[14].

Infertile couples typically perceive infertility as carrying the potential for both harm (e.g., loss of a central role) and benefit (e.g., strengthening of the marital relationship)[15]. They also perceive some aspects of infertility as relatively uncontrollable (e.g., attaining conception) and others as more controllable (e.g., engaging in diagnostic tests and treatments)[16]. Appraisal may influence psychosocial adjustment directly. For example, Litt and colleagues[17] found that women experienced more depressive symptoms after IVF failure when they perceived a general loss of control over their lives as a result of infertility.

Stress and coping theories also suggest that personal and situational attribution, in conjunction with this appraisal process, guide the individual's initiation of coping strategies, which are cognitive, emotional, and behavioral efforts to alter the problem itself (i.e., problem-focused coping) or the associated negative affect (i.e., emotion-focused coping). Appraisal and coping processes in turn influence psychological and social outcomes. For example, coping through avoidance and self-blame are related to greater distress in infertile individuals, while garnering emotional support is associated with more positive adjustment[15]. One recent study[18] that assessed severity of psychological distress and coping strategies used by infertile men and women, found significant distress in 10% of women and 15% of men. Interestingly, of the three ways of coping with stress (self-blame and avoidance, informational and emotional-support seeking, and cognitive restructuring), the use of self-blame and avoidance was found to be the most highly correlated with increased psychological distress.

In general, coping responses are neither uniformly adaptive nor maladaptive, although some coping strategies (e.g., denial, behavioral disengagement) are most often associated with maladjustment. Coping is most effective when the strategy is responsive to contextual demands and individual attributes. For example, problem-solving strategies may be most effective for alterable aspects of the stressful situation, such as the decision to engage in a diagnostic test. Emotion-focused coping strategies may be more useful for uncontrollable aspects of a stressor, such as when one receives a negative pregnancy result.

The application of stress and coping theories to infertility has provided greater understanding of the determinants of distress experienced by infertile women and men, as well as suggesting research directions. In addition, findings from stress and coping theories can guide professionals in their attempts to target specific appraisal and coping strategies for therapeutic intervention, tailoring them to specific patient needs, contexts, and resources.

Biopsychosocial Model

The biopsychosocial model of illness and health[19,20] represents an alternative to the traditional biomedical model in that it recognizes biological, psychological, and social influences on the onset, course, and treatment of disease. It goes beyond a focus on the individual to acknowledge cultural, familial, and other interpersonal influences on health, and assumes a complex and reciprocal interplay among body, mind, and environment. This model has been successfully applied to a variety of chronic illnesses, including infertility.

The biopsychosocial model is relevant for infertility in several ways. First, the possibility that environmental stress or other psychosocial factors may influence fertility status for some individuals is consistent with a biopsychosocial model. Domar and associates[21] described mechanisms by which stress may impair fertility. Functioning of the hypothalamic-pituitary-adrenal axis is influenced by stressful conditions in humans and other animals[22,23], and investigation is warranted of environmental conditions, such as a lack of social support[24], that may compromise fertility. Furthermore, personal, social, and environmental factors that influence susceptibility to sexually transmitted diseases, thereby affecting fertility status, are other areas for study[25].

Second, a biopsychosocial approach may aid in understanding outcomes of particular medical procedures. For example, Boivin and colleagues[26] reported associations among the demands of a diagnostic procedure (i.e., postcoital test), sexual response, and medical outcomes for women. Harrison and coworkers[27] demonstrated a link between stress and semen quality during IVF attempts. Researchers are currently investigating the psychological side effects of ovulation-inducing medications, as well as serotonin imbalance as a factor in anovulation (see Chapter 4).

Third, the biopsychosocial model implies that optimal patient care involves an interdisciplinary approach. Such an approach fosters attention to both the biological and psychosocial realms, as well as promoting active, collaborative involvement of the interdisciplinary team with patients. Aims of this approach are to bolster patients' sense of control and self-efficacy, promote health-enhancing behaviors, and recognize cultural and other contextual influences on patients' orientation toward treatment.

The biopsychosocial model requires greater attention as applied to infertility. However, it certainly should not be equated with older theories that attributed infertility to characterological factors and unconscious conflicts residing in women. Rather, application of this approach is warranted to acknowledge reciprocal interactions of environmental, psychosocial, and biological factors that may affect fertility status and treatment response in some individuals.

CLINICAL ISSUES AND THERAPEUTIC INTERVENTIONS

Measures of Stress and Coping During Infertility

The assessment measures most often used in behavioral medicine and health psychology include questionnaires, self-monitoring, behavioral observation, and psychophysiological measurement. Although validated questionnaires are also used, much infertility research has used researcher-developed questionnaires that do not have established reliability and validity. Further development of reliable and valid measures tailored to infertile samples or adaptation of current measures for the infertile are warranted. Self-monitoring measures, used in assessment and treatment of medical conditions such as headache and obesity, have been used infrequently by infertility researchers. Boivin[28] and Takefman[29] developed the Daily Record Keeping Sheet (see Appendix 15) to assess emotional, physical, and coping responses across an infertility treatment cycle. Depression, anger, anxiety, and uncertainty are monitored, and coping is assessed using an adaptation of the Ways of Coping Questionnaire[12], tapping confrontative, distancing, self-controlling, social-support-seeking, responsibility-accepting, escape/avoidance, planful-problem-solving, and positive-reappraisal coping techniques. Physical well-being is assessed through rating of symptoms such as nausea, ovulation pain, weight gain, abdominal discomfort, abdominal bleeding, breast tenderness, and headaches. Boivin[30] has validated this measure using 500 women, so that it can be used as a research or clinical instrument to assess emotional well-being and coping effectiveness before, during, and after a treatment cycle.

Clinical Applications of Stress and Coping Theory

Stress and coping theories and associated findings carry implications for psychosocial intervention with infertile couples. The central place of cognitive appraisal in these theories suggests the utility of exploring personal meanings that infertility holds for individuals. For some individuals, the experience of infertility may violate deeply held beliefs about the world and their place in it. Infertility can challenge stable assumptions that the world is benevolent, predictable, and just and that the self is worthy. Some may fear that life holds no meaning or that they have no worth if they cannot bear a child. Because infertility involves a potential loss of control over an important outcome, appraisals of control also deserve therapeutic attention. High perceived control in areas that actually are amenable to influence, such as becoming an active participant in medical treatments or seeking parenting alternatives, is associated with better adjustment[16,31]. If the uncontrollable aspects of infertility are generalized to yield a perception that life itself is uncontrollable, high distress is likely.

Cognitive interventions, which are components of Domar and associates'[32] and McQueeney and colleagues'[33] programs described below, may be useful in addressing individuals' appraisals that contribute to distress. Such approaches involve eliciting personal meanings and cognitions regarding the stressor, promoting understanding of the connection between cognitions and resultant emotions, and engaging a variety of techniques to challenge unhelpful cognitions, thereby decreasing distress[34,35]. For example, a therapist might help a woman who associates infertility with a generalized loss of control over life differentiate the controllable and uncontrollable aspects of infertility, and encourage her to perform personal experiments demonstrating that some facets of life remain under her control and to explore alternative sources of control and meaning.

As a second example, women who perceive some potential for benefit in their infertility report better adjustment[16]. Understandably, infertile couples may perceive the didactic suggestion that benefits arise from infertility as a minimization of their plight. However, a more favorable response may result from gentle and appropriately timed questioning regarding potentially positive consequences coupled with acknowledgment of the losses that may accompany the experience (e.g., 'Has anything positive come out of this experience for you?' 'Has going through this experience together strengthened your relationship in any way?' 'Has anything happened during this very stressful time that made you feel fortunate?'). Such questioning may also prompt couples to consider alternative meanings of the infertility experience.

Intervention strategies for altering appraisal involve helping an infertile person or couple understand and find a pattern of meaning for their infertility experience. Over the course of medical treatment for infertility, a couple enters a process of appraisal and reappraisal in their attempts to gain understanding and meaning. Examples of appraisal-focused interventions include the separation of overwhelming aspects of infertility into manageable facets, the use of positive appraisals of the experience and one's management of it, and the comparison of one's fertility problem and experiences with those of real or imagined others who are worse off. Working with couples to define and address systematically the central adaptive tasks for managing the stresses of

Table 1 Adaptive tasks for managing crisis and stress of infertility

---

Establish meaning and personal significance of infertility for each partner and for couple

Confront reality of infertility and respond to requirements of medical treatment and psychosocial distress

Sustain relationships with family members, friends, or others who may be helpful

Maintain reasonable emotional balance

Preserve a satisfactory self-image and sense of competence

(Adapted from Moos RH, Schaefer JA. Life transitions and crises: A conceptual overview. In: Moos RH, ed. *Coping with Life Crisis: An Integrated Approach*. New York: Plenum, 1986;3–28; with permission)

infertility is another means of helping couples boost their sense of control and mastery over the infertility experience (Table 1). For some couples, giving meaning to infertility involves religious or spiritual examination, whereas for others meaning is found in relationship rewards or compensations in other aspects of their lives.

In addition to exploring the appraisal process, stress and coping theories suggest that bolstering couples' adaptive coping skills represents a productive therapeutic goal. According to these theories, coping techniques are inherently neither maladaptive nor adaptive. As an example, for some women, avoiding baby showers may represent a positive means of self-protection, whereas for others it may indicate a broader pattern of avoidant coping that short-circuits valuable sources of support and gratification. As McQueeney and colleagues'[33] intervention study demonstrated, coping skills training directed toward both problem-solving and palliation of negative emotions surrounding infertility may be useful, although perhaps in the service of different goals and at different points in the infertility process. Avoidant coping may be useful as a temporary strategy but over time becomes less helpful, eventually contributing to more distress than that experienced by those who initially confronted the problem.

Finally, what women find to be a useful coping strategy may not necessarily be what men find most successful. For example, Collins and colleagues[8] found that women were more likely to discuss their feelings about infertility with others such as close friends, parents, and siblings, whereas men were more likely to discuss their infertility only with their spouse. Attending support groups may be another gender-linked coping strategy: Although both partners may find support groups helpful, the majority of attendees are women[8,31]. In a metaanalytic study of gender differences in coping with infertility, Jordan and Revenson[36] found gender differences in four of eight coping strategies: seeking social support, escape/avoidance, planful problem-solving, and positive reappraisal, with wives using these strategies to a greater degree than husbands. Women also reported greater levels of infertility-specific distress.

Two studies serve as illustrations that women and men may use different coping strategies. Davis and Dearman[37] interviewed 30 infertile women who were asked to describe actions that they had taken to help them cope with feelings and experiences of infertility. They identified six coping strategies used by infertile women: (1) increasing the space or distancing oneself from reminders of infertility, (2) instituting measures for regaining control, (3) acting to increase self-esteem by being the best (e.g., control weight and appearance), (4) looking for hidden meaning in infertility, (5) giving in to feelings, and (6) sharing the burden with others. By comparison, Snarey and colleagues[38] investigated 52 men who had experienced infertility and identified styles of coping across three longitudinal phases: initial substitutes, subsequent parenting resolutions, and final marital outcomes. The authors found that the infertility coping strategy used by men in earlier phases of infertility was predictive of men's later parenting resolutions, marital outcome, and midlife achievement of psychosocial generativity. Men were found to use three coping strategies during infertility: (1) substitution of self by treating himself as if he were his only child (e.g., preoccupation with personal body building, health foods, macho sexuality), (2) substitution of a nonhuman object by treating it as if it were his pride and joy (e.g., parent-like devotion to house, pet, garden, or car), and (3) substitution of a child or other appropriate human by becoming involved in vicarious child-rearing activities with the children of others (e.g., leading youth group, teaching religious school). None of the men who used self-centered substitutes achieved clear generativity by midlife. In contrast, 24% of those who substituted an object and 75% who substituted a child were clearly generative (and parents) by midlife.

Potential gender differences in coping with infertility need further evaluation with regard to their impact on individual and marital functioning, as well as their implications for psychosocial interventions for women and men. What may be perceived as useful to one partner may actually be irritating or stressful to the other partner, thereby influencing effectiveness of coping and overall marital satisfaction. Given gender differences in coping, what are the couple-focused coping strategies that meet the needs of both partners and yet are comforting and helpful to the individuals? The use and effectiveness of coping techniques also may be influenced by several other factors, including the specific point in the infertility process and the existence of a gender-specific infertility diagnosis. Again, different coping processes may be useful at different points during the course of infertility.

Clinical Applications of the Biopsychosocial Model

The biopsychosocial model has long been applied to chronic illness and specific somatic conditions. Increasingly, this model is being applied to infertility; it offers a perspective that considers interactions of multiple systems, including biological, psychological, marital, family, community, and cultural systems. The biopsychosocial model, as applied to infertility, provides a multispeciality approach that considers the medical treatment and the infertility condition within the social and psychological context of the patient and offers an array of treatment interventions.

A biopsychological model of infertility leads one to question whether psychosocial interventions might affect fertility status and outcomes of medical treatment. Certainly, this remains an open question. Although some findings[32,33] suggest that such interventions might facilitate becoming a parent, a determination of this association is not definitive until truly random assignment to appropriate control groups is conducted. Even if such associations are found, further investigation will be required to specify mechanisms for the effects. For example, a psychosocial intervention's contribution to active pursuit of excellent medical treatment or parenting options (e.g., adoption), rather than to biological mediators of fertility, may explain any obtained effects on parental status. Certainly, psychological interventions can be valuable owing to benefits accrued in quality of life alone, but any suggestion that they also confer biological advantage must be interpreted cautiously.

Stress Management Interventions

In reviewing stress management interventions as applied to chronic illness, Parker[39] suggested that four categories of approaches are most often applied: (1) patient education, (2) cognitive-behavioral treatment, (3) psychophysiological interventions, and (4) eclectic psychotherapy. Each of these approaches is represented in the empirical literature on psychosocial interventions for infertile individuals. However, as is true of much of the broader literature on stress management, examination of the infertility-specific literature reveals that the approaches are often combined in multimodal treatment formats, rather than being evaluated for their unique contribution to stress reduction. Also immediately apparent is that only a few controlled studies have been conducted to test the effectiveness of these approaches for women and men confronting infertility. The following is a review of the handful of controlled and uncontrolled studies designed to aid individuals managing the stresses of infertility.

Patient Education

An assumption of patient-education approaches is that if health care professionals can assist individuals in knowing what to expect regarding diagnostic or treatment procedures, patients will benefit as a result of an enhanced sense of control and more informed decision-making. Certainly, some infertile individuals diligently seek information regarding their diagnoses and available treatment options. However, as Parker[39] pointed out, information alone often is insufficient for decreasing stress. Its effects may vary substantially as a function of characteristics of the information offered (e.g., information regarding the medical procedure itself, the expected sensory experience of the patient, or recommended coping strategies), the nature of the stressor (e.g., its controllability), and patient characteristics (e.g., preference for information). This seems particularly important in that patients pursuing IVF have been consistently found to *overestimate* personal likelihood of success, despite patient education about treatment success rates.

Although a no-treatment control group was not included, suggestive evidence that information provision is useful comes from Connolly and colleagues[40]. Couples undergoing a first IVF attempt were assigned randomly to a single session of oral and written information provision regarding IVF treatment procedures or to information plus three sessions of nondirective counseling across a treatment cycle. State anxiety dropped significantly over the course of treatment; however, counseling did not enhance anxiety reduction over information provision alone. Takefman and colleagues[41] randomly assigned 39 couples beginning medical investigation of infertility to one of three interventions: (1) informational videotape regarding procedural aspects of diagnostic tests only, (2) videotape on diagnostic procedures, as well as the emotional strains of the investigation, and (3) videotape on diagnostic procedures and emotional strains, as well as a pamphlet on sexual relationship issues. Those receiving the procedural information alone evidenced significantly decreased infertility-specific negative feelings and increased infertility knowledge, whereas groups that received the enhanced information did not demonstrate significant benefit across the course of the medical investigation. Perhaps the additional information created a sense of overload in couples just beginning the diagnostic work-up, or specific training in coping strategies to manage the psychological strains illustrated in the videotape would have produced more beneficial effects.

Further evidence of positive effects of patient education, at least when combined with other interventions, was provided by Newton and associates[42]. Highly anxious women preparing for oocyte retrieval were assigned randomly to relaxation training alone or to relaxation training plus education (including a booklet) regarding the retrieval procedure, the accompanying sensory experience, and coping mechanisms. Those who received relaxation training along with information reported less anxiety and pain surrounding the retrieval procedure than did women who received relaxation training alone. This study design does not allow us to know what specific aspect of the information provision was helpful and whether the benefits might be attributed simply to the enhanced professional attention provided to those in the more comprehensive intervention rather than to the specific treatments themselves. However, these results suggest that information to enhance infertile patients' understanding of particular medical procedures, offered within the context of training in techniques to cope with the procedure, may yield benefits.

It is interesting to note the growing variety of available patient education resources for infertility. Patient education materials have become a small industry that includes videotapes, audiotapes, and self-help books addressing both the medical and psychological aspects of infertility; pamphlets from pharmaceutical companies; materials from support organizations, such as RESOLVE; and booklets from professional organizations, such as American Society for Reproductive Medicine. Patients are also educating themselves through radio, television, telephone help-lines, and the Internet. Because some information obtained through some of these sources (e.g., the Internet) may be inaccurate or misunderstood by patients, it is always useful to review carefully patients' information sources and understanding of the information.

Cognitive-Behavioral Interventions and Psychophysiological Approaches

Cognitive-behavioral and psychophysiological approaches are discussed together because they have often been combined in the infertility intervention literature. Cognitive-behavioral approaches often involve several techniques, including training in coping skills and problem-solving, modification of dysfunctional cognitions, and role-playing and behavioral rehearsal (Table 2). Psychophysiological interventions are designed to modify a client's physiological response to stress, including acute and prolonged neurochemical, hormonal, and neuroanatomical changes. The specific psychophysiological approach that has been investigated with regard to infertility is relaxation training. Several approaches are effective in inducing relaxation, such as progressive

Table 2 Strategies for coping with infertility

Appraisal-focused coping

Be mentally prepared

Accept and redefine

Keep busy, avoid, and deny

Problem-focused coping

Seek information and support

Take action to be a problem solver

Look to alternative rewards

Emotion-focused coping

Calm acceptance of emotions

Emotional discharge

Resigned acceptance

(Reproduced from Callan VJ, Hennessey JF. Strategies for coping with infertility. *Br J Med Psychol* 1989; 62:343–54; with permission)

muscle relaxation (i.e., systematic tensing and releasing of muscle groups[43]). Cognitive and behavioral approaches have been demonstrated to be effective in reducing stress and improving coping with a variety of chronic health-related stressors[35,36,39,44], as have psychophysiological approaches involving relaxation training[45].

With regard to infertility, O'Moore, and colleagues[31] offered autogenic training, composed of exercises in body awareness, passive concentration, and physical relaxation to 11 infertile couples over 8 weeks, with an additional 2 months for self-directed practice. Assessed at the end of the 2-month practice, a significant reduction in state anxiety was documented for women and men, although trait anxiety evidenced no significant change. Plasma prolactin (but not urinary free cortisol) also declined significantly for women participants.

Domar and coworkers[21,32] developed a 10-week group behavioral treatment program for infertile women based on the elicitation of the relaxation response, which is assumed to be an integrated hypothalamic response associated with a generalized decrease in sympathetic nervous system activity. In addition to training in relaxation, several additional techniques were administered over approximately 27 hours of treatment, including stress management training, cognitive restructuring, gentle stretching exercise, discussion of nutrition, and promotion of self-empathy. Group support was also encouraged, and women's partners were involved in a small portion of the treatment. The intervention in these reports, involving 54[21] and 41[32] self-referred women in active medical treatment for infertility of approximately 3 years' duration, resulted in significant decreases in state and trait anxiety and depressed mood, as well as an increase in vigor over the 10-week period. Additional benefits of decreased fatigue, confusion, and anger expression were documented in individual reports. In the women for whom conception was physically possible, pregnancy rates within 6 months of program completion were 34% in the 1990 report[21] and 32% in the 1992 report[32].

As the authors acknowledged, these studies did not involve random assignment to psychological intervention versus a control group, and thus it cannot be inferred that the intervention or particular aspects of the intervention produced the reported benefits. In addition, definitive interpretation of the pregnancy rate is not possible. As a result, several factors must be considered. First, 29.4% of the women in the group were infertile due to male-factor infertility, indicating that pregnancy may be the result of the husband's successful treatment rather than psychological interventions. Second, perhaps women who elected to volunteer for the 10-week behavioral medicine program were also those who very actively pursued excellent medical treatment, thus bolstering their chances of pregnancy. Perhaps the intervention promoted a more persistent approach to medical treatment. That some aspect of the intervention conferred biological benefit facilitating conception is feasible, but it certainly cannot be concluded that the intervention produced a higher pregnancy rate than would be found in similarly motivated women receiving similar medical treatment or that any specific facet of the psychological intervention was responsible for enhancing the likelihood of pregnancy.

McQueeney and associates[33] examined training in emotion-focused versus problem-focused coping skills in 29 women who had been experiencing fertility problems for an average of 4 years. Conducted in group format over six sessions, the problem-focused intervention centered on bolstering perceived control over infertility through providing infertility-focused information, increasing assertive and effective communication skills with medical personnel and significant others, and teaching problem-solving strategies. The emotion-focused intervention involved encouraging emotional expression surrounding fertility concerns, promoting pleasurable activities and relaxation, and reducing negative affect associated with dysfunctional cognitions surrounding infertility. Women were assigned randomly to treatment conditions; the control group was composed of women who volunteered for treatment but could not attend owing to group scheduling constraints. Both problem- and emotion-focused groups evidenced significantly reduced distress at treatment termination relative to controls. At a 1-month follow-up, only the emotion-focused group evidenced significantly better psychological adjustment than controls (i.e., lower depressive symptoms and greater infertility-specific well-being) and in fact showed continued gains from treatment termination through 1 month. At 18 months after treatment, a significant between-groups difference emerged on parental status. Eight of 10 problem-focused participants had become mothers (four biological, four adoptive) versus two of eight emotion-focused members and three of eight controls.

These results suggest that coping skills training is beneficial in decreasing distress and increasing well-being in women with fertility problems. However, truly random assignment to the control group was not conducted, rendering replication essential. Emotion-focused training appeared to yield more enduring psychological gains; however, this finding may be dependent on the nature of the sample. On average, women had been attempting conception for almost 4 years. Perhaps, problem-focused intervention is more effective for those who are just beginning the diagnostic and treatment process, whereas emotion-focused treatment is relatively beneficial for those confronting the chronic stress of infertility. The most parsimonious explanation of the apparent effectiveness of problem-focused intervention in promoting parenthood at 18 months is that such training bolsters effective communication and persistent attempts directed toward becoming a parent. However, replication of findings from this relatively small sample and examination of mechanisms for the obtained effects are essential. Further extension of this study to testing the effects of combined coping skills approaches and of coping skills interventions for couples is warranted.

Cognitive-behavioral interventions and psychophysiological approaches, conducted in group sessions or with individuals, can offer infertile patients a variety of strategies for improving coping skills, managing stress, and enhancing quality of life. Specific stressful situations or chronically stressful aspects of infertility may be the focus of intervention. Self-management strategies directed toward stress management and healthful self-care may also be taught (see Table 3). It appears that both problem- and emotion-focused coping are beneficial to infertile couples, but which coping strategies are most effective for specific individuals may be contingent on a number of factors, such as the phase of the infertility experience or the person's gender. Finally, patient selection for both cognitive-behavioral and psychophysiological strategies is important in that these interventions may be more effective for patients who are highly motivated, who can concentrate and focus readily, and who are not so anxious that they cannot tolerate the training[46].

Eclectic Psychotherapies

A few studies are available that involve other psychotherapeutic orientations or a group support approach to managing the stresses of infertility (see Chapter 7). Lukse[47] conducted six sessions of structured group counseling with 14 couples and one woman, in which counseling focused on management of grief surrounding infertility. Women participants evidenced significant decreases in depressive symptoms and anger, as well as an increase in positive self-concept, whereas the data for men revealed no significant change. No significant changes emerged in marital and sexual satisfaction. No comparison group was included in this study.

Stewart and colleagues[48] compared 64 (39 female, 25 male) patients at a university hospital infertility program who elected support group participation to 35 consecutive patients who were not offered participation. Led by a psychiatrist and infertility nurse, the 8-week program focused on topics raised by the patients but also involved stress reduction techniques and promotion of collaborative decision-making. Program participants evidenced significant reductions in distress and depressive symptomatology, as well as decreases in avoidant coping and increases in active cognitive-behavioral coping. Patients not offered the program reported levels of psychological symptoms similar to group participants at the first assessment, but these levels did not change significantly over the 8-week period. As acknowledged by the authors, in addition to the possibility that the support program produced the reported benefits, motivational differences in the participant group versus the comparison group may in part account for the findings.

Table 3 Sample patient coping strategies suggested by clinical or empirical literature

Use relaxation audiotapes, videotapes, compact disks

Improve decision-making and problem-solving skills

Take treatment holidays

Learn and use self-hypnosis or guided imagery

Learn the benefits of physical well-being (e.g., exercise and massage)

Pay attention to nutrition and eating a balanced diet

Eliminate recreational drugs and tobacco; eliminate or cut down on caffeine and alcohol

Get plenty of sleep

Learn and practice positive reappraisal

Use relaxing music during specific medical procedures

Reduce daily hassles and minor stressors (e.g., improve time management)

Get assertiveness training if needed

Increase pleasurable activities

Seek information on infertility and/or coping through books, videos, organizations, or the Internet

Enhance spirituality (e.g., prayer, meditation, religious services, classes, or pastoral counseling)

Learn to manage hostility and anger

Expand support system by confiding in a trusted friend or joining a support group

Find enjoyment in the company of loved ones and friendships

Learn to decrease worry and anxiety through relaxation, meditation, or progressive relaxation

Laugh more and look for humor

Try to maintain a realistic yet positive and hopeful attitude

Get a pet or spend time with animals

Refute irrational ideas

Learn thought-stopping and how to refute illogical fears

Turn to nature for comfort (e.g., plant a garden, visit parks)

Volunteer and find time for kindness to others

Structure infertility treatment (i.e., manage what you can)

Find ways to soothe yourself

Take frequent brief weekends to relax and enjoy life and one's partner

Establish realistic goals and expectations of treatments or success rates

Improve management of financial matters

Identify stress responses and successful coping techniques

Conclusions from the Empirical Intervention Literature

Given that so few researchers have tested the effectiveness of stress management interventions for infertile individuals and that most of the available studies are uncontrolled, it is difficult to reach firm conclusions regarding the effectiveness of these interventions. To this point, cognitive and behavioral interventions, perhaps coupled with relaxation training, hold promise with regard to reducing the stresses of infertility. Conducted with groups of participants, relatively structured sessions that focus on the development of emotive, cognitive, and behavioral coping skills appear useful in decreasing distress and increasing well-being of infertile individuals. However, it is possible that the simple sharing of experiences surrounding fertility within a supportive group context is sufficient for benefit to occur. Clearly, controlled studies are needed to elucidate the most effective stress management interventions for those confronting infertility.

In general, women are more likely than men to participate in support groups for a variety of problems. Lentner and Glazer[49] in a survey of 16 men and 22 women currently attending community-based infertility support groups reported that fewer men than women initially wanted to join the groups. There was some indication that, compared to women, men perceived information provision and education as more important group components. Nevertheless, women and men perceived similar benefits of group participation, and all respondents concluded that the groups were helpful. Delineation of the most effective strategies for women and men requires study. Relatedly, because many therapists today use a combination of techniques representing cognitive-behavioral interventions, psychophysiological approaches, and patient education, it is difficult to sort out which technique is most beneficial to infertility patients in a given setting under specific circumstances.

FUTURE IMPLICATIONS

The role of behavioral medicine and health psychology in medical care has grown in recent years, with relevant techniques applied to an increasingly wide array of medical conditions. This movement has been fueled in part by the consumer health movement and, increasingly, by traditional medicine. The National Institute of Mental Health and the Health and Behavior Coordinating Committee of the National Institutes of Health have suggested that the application of behavioral medicine should be extended to disease processes, bio-behavioral risk factors, treatment interventions, and disease prevention/ health promotion[46], as well as to the integration of behavioral and relaxation approaches in the treatment of various medical disorders[50]. The application of relevant theories and intervention strategies to infertility is helpful to consumers and caregivers alike. Whether considering stress, coping strategies, stress management training, or the examination of health behaviors in general, behavioral medicine and health psychology provide models for both medical and psychological care of infertile patients.

A priority for infertility counselors and medical caregivers is the need to identify the most effective therapeutic techniques for infertile couples and the conditions under which specific interventions are most helpful. It is understandable that most psychological studies have focused on infertile women because women are more likely than men to initiate fertility treatment, undergo a greater proportion of medical treatment for infertility, and are more distressed by fertility problems or involuntary childlessness. However, this focus on women has left a deficit: Do different psychological approaches carry differential effectiveness for women versus men? Because infertility is a shared stressor, it is important to determine effective approaches for couples, as well as for individuals, seeking infertility treatment. Finally, it would be helpful for clinicians to know which interventions are most effective for couples versus individuals, during initial phases of diagnosis and treatment versus chronic or permanent infertility; and during specific stressful medical procedures.

Understanding of the psychology of infertility has increased considerably since the days when infertility was considered a psychosomatic response to psychological instability. Patients' psychological and tangible resources, environmental influences, and medical factors (e.g., prognosis) are thought to play important roles in psychological outcomes for infertile couples. Increased understanding of adaptive and maladaptive cognitive appraisals and coping strategies also is accruing. However, the complex interactions of psychological, social, and biological factors influencing health and well-being remain a challenging puzzle for infertile women and men, as well as for their care providers.

SUMMARY

- The relationship of stress and infertility remains complex such that : (1) psychosocial problems may trigger infertility in some cases; (2) infertility may trigger psychosocial distress; or (3) a reciprocal causal relationship between infertility and psychosocial distress may exist[51].

- Stress management interventions include patient education, cognitive-behavioral therapies, psychophysiological interventions (e.g., relaxation training), and eclectic psychotherapy. All of these have been applied to aid individuals in managing the stresses of infertility, although few controlled intervention studies exist.

- Cognitive and behavioral coping skills interventions appear to hold promise with regard to reducing the stresses of infertility and increasing well-being of infertile individuals. However, it is impossible to conclude based on current research that these interventions actually improve conception or produce other physiological changes that improve fertility.

- Men and women appear to react differently to infertility, and as such may find different coping techniques useful, although this has not been tested.

- Both problem-focused and emotion-focused coping skills training appear to reduce significantly the distress of infertile women.

- Stress management techniques may help patients take a more active role in their health care and in pursuing parenting options, perhaps facilitating attainment of parenthood. Whether or not parenthood is achieved, such psychosocial interventions appear to enhance quality of life for those who confront infertility.

REFERENCES

1. Schwartz GE, Weiss SM. Behavioral medicine revisited: An amended definition. *J Behav Med* 1978;1:249–51
2. Matarazzo JC. Behavioral health's challenge to academic, scientific, and professional psychology. *Am Psychol* 1982; 37:1–14
3. Kroger WS, Freed SC. Psychosomatic aspects of sterility. *Am J Obstet Gynecol* 1950; 59:867–74
4. Karahasanoglu A, Barglow P, Growe G. Psychological aspects of infertility. *J Reprod Med* 1972;9:241–7
5. Sandler B. Emotional stress and infertility. *J Psychosom Res* 1968;12:51–9
6. Wright J, Allard M, Lecours A, *et al.* Psychosocial distress and infertility: A review of controlled research. *Int J Fertil* 1989;34:126–42
7. Baram D, Tourtelot E, Muechler E, *et al.* Psychological adjustment following unsuccessful in vitro fertilization. *J Psychosom Obstet Gynaecol* 1988;9:181–90
8. Collins A, Freeman EW, Boxer AS, *et al.* Perceptions of infertility and treatment stress in females as compared to males entering in vitro fertilization treatment. *Fertil Steril* 1992;57:350–6
9. Laffont I, Edelmann RJ. Psychological aspects of in vitro fertilization: A gender comparison. *J Psychosom Obstet Gynaecol* 1994;15:85–92
10. Dunkel-Schetter C, Lobel M. Psychological reactions to infertility. In: Stanton AL, Dunkel-Schetter C, eds. *Infertility: Perspectives from Stress and Coping Research.* New York: Plenum, 1991;29–57
11. Stanton AL, Danoff-Burg S. Selected issues in women's reproductive health: Psychological perspectives. In: Stanton AL, Gallant SJ, eds. *The Psychology of Women's Health: Progress and Challenges in Research and Application.* Washington DC: American Psychological Association, 1996;261–305
12. Lazarus RS, Folkman S. *Stress, Appraisal, and Coping.* New York: Springer, 1984
13. Stanton AL, Dinoff BL. Infertility. In: Friedman HS, ed. *Encyclopedia of Mental Health.* San Diego, CA: Academic Press, 1998:561–9
14. Moos RH, Billings AG. Conceptualizing and measuring coping resources and processes. In: Goldberger L, Breznitz S, eds. *Handbook of Stress: Theoretical and Clinical Aspects.* New York: Free Press, 1982; 218–19
15. Stanton AL. Cognitive appraisals, coping processes, and adjustment to infertility. In: Stanton AL, Dunkel-Schetter C, eds. *Infertility: Perspectives from Stress and Coping Research.* New York: Plenum, 1991;87–108
16. Campbell SM, Dunkel-Schetter C, Peplau LA. Perceived control and adjustment to infertility among women undergoing in vitro fertilization. In: Stanton AL, Dunkel-Schetter C, eds. *Infertility: Perspectives from Stress and Coping Research.* New York: Plenum, 1991;133-56
17. Litt MD, Tennen H, Affleck G, *et al.* Coping and cognitive factors in adaptation to in vitro fertilization failure. *J Behav Med* 1992;15:171-87
18. Morrow K, Thoreson R, Penney L. Predictors of psychological distress among infertility clinic patients. *J Consult Clin Psychol* 1995;63:163-7
19. Engel GL. The need for a new medical model: A challenge for biomedicine. *Science* 1977;196:126–9
20. Nicassio PM, Smith TW, eds. *Managing Chronic Illness: A Biopsychosocial Perspective.* Washington, DC: American Psychological Association, 1995
21. Domar AD, Seibel MM, Benson H. The mind/body program for infertility: A new behavioral treatment approach for women with infertility. *Fertil Steril* 1990;53:246–9
22. Berga SL. Stress and reproductive compromise. Presented at the Biopsychology of Infertility Workshop, sponsored by the National Institute of Child Health and Human Development and the National Institutes of Health. Betheseda, MD, September, 1995
23. Rivier C. Stress-induced infertility: Role of the hypothalamic-pituitary-adrenal axis and influence of interleukins. Presented at the Biopsychology of Infertility Workshop, sponsored by the National Institute of Child Health and Human Development

and the National Institutes of Health, Betheseda, MD, September, 1995

24. Wasser SK, Sewall G, Soules M. Psychosocial stress as a cause of infertility. *Fertil Steril* 1993;59:685–9

25. Kramer DG, Brown ST. Sexually transmitted disease and infertility. *J Gynaecol Obstet* 1984;22:19–27

26. Boivin J, Takefman JE, Brender W, *et al.* The effects of female sexual response in coitus on early reproductive processes. *J Behav Med* 1992;15:509–18

27. Harrison KL, Callan VJ, Hennessey JF. Stress and semen quality in an in vitro fertilization program. *Fertil Steril* 1987; 48:633–6

28. Boivin J. *Daily Record Keeping Sheet.* 1995

29. Takefman J, Boivin J. *Daily Record Keeping Sheet.* 1990

30. Boivin J. Personal communication

31. O'Moore AM, O'Moore RR, Harrison RF, *et al.* Psychosomatic aspects in idiopathic infertility: Effects of treatment with autogenic training. *J Psychosom Res* 1983; 27:145–51

32. Domar AD, Zuttermeister PC, Seibel M, *et al.* Psychological improvement in infertile women after behavioral treatment: A replication. *Fertil Steril* 1992;58:144–7

33. McQueeney DA, Stanton AL, Sigmon S. Efficacy of emotion-focused and problem-focused group therapies for women with fertility problems. *J Behav Med* 1997;20: 313–31

34. Meichenbaum D. *Stress Inoculation Training.* Elmsford, NY: Pergamon, 1985

35. Meichenbaum D, Fitzpatrick D. A constructivist narrative perspective on stress and coping: Stress inoculation applications. In: Goldberger L, Breznitz S, eds. *Handbook of Stress: Theoretical and Clinical Aspects,* 2nd edn. New York: Free Press, 1993;706–23

36. Jordan C, Revenson TA. Gender differences in coping with infertility: A meta-analysis. Poster presentation at Psychosocial and Behavioral Factors in Women's Health: Research, Prevention, Treatment, and Service Delivery in Clinical and Community Settings. Washington DC, September 18–21, 1996

37. Davis DC, Dearman CN. Coping strategies of infertile women. *J Obstet Gynecol Neonatal Nurs* 1991;20:221–8

38. Snarey J, Son L, Kuehne VS, *et al.* The role of parenting in men's psychosocial development: A longitudinal study of early adulthood infertility and midlife generativity. *Dev Psychology* 1987;23:593–603

39. Parker JC. Stress management. In: Nicassio PM, Smith TW, eds. *Managing Chronic Illness: A Biopsychosocial Perspective.* Washington, DC: American Psychological Association, 1995;285–312

40. Connolly KJ, Edelmann RJ, Bartlett H, *et al.* An evaluation of counselling for couples undergoing treatment for in-vitro fertilization. *Hum Reprod* 1993;8:1332–8

41. Takefman JE, Brender W, Boivin J, *et al.* Sexual and emotional adjustment of couples undergoing infertility investigation and the effectiveness of preparatory information. *J Psychosom Obstet Gynaecol* 1990;11:275–90

42. Newton CR, Sherrard W, Houle M. Preparing women for oocyte retrieval (OR): A comparison of psychological interventions. *Fertil Steril* 1994;S27 [abstract]

43. Bernstein DA, Borkovec TD. *Progressive Relaxation Training.* Champaign, IL: Research Press, 1973

44. Woolfolk RL, Lehrer PM, eds. *Principles and Practices of Stress Management.* New York: Guilford, 1984

45. Hyman RB, Feldman HR, Harris RB, *et al.* The effects of relaxation training on clinical symptoms: A meta-analysis. *Nurs Res* 1983;8:216–20

46. Benson H. The common physiological events that occur when behavioral and relaxation approaches are practiced by patients. Presented at NIH Technology Assessment Conference: Integration of Behavioral and Relaxation Approaches into the Treatment of Chronic Pain and Insomnia, Bethesda, MD, October 16–18, 1995

47. Lukse MP. The effect of group counseling on the frequency of grief reported by infertile couples. *J Obstet Gynecol Neonatal Nurs* 1985;14:67s–70s

48. Stewart DE, Boydell KM, McCarthy K, *et al.* A prospective study of the effectiveness of brief professionally-led support groups for infertility patients. *Int J Psychiatry Med* 1992;22:173–82

49. Lentner E, Glazer G. Infertile couples' perceptions of infertility support group participation. *Health Care Women Int* 1991; 12:317–30

50. Blumenthal SJ, Matthews K, Weiss SM, eds. *New Research Frontiers in Behavioral Medicine: Proceedings of the National Conference.* Washington, DC: NIH Health and Behavior Committee and NIMH, 1994

51. Elstein M. Effect of infertility on psychosexual functioning. *Br Med J* 1975;3:296–9

9

Sexual Counseling and Infertility

Linda Hammer Burns, PhD

The child will never lie in me, and you will never be its father. Mirrors must replace the real image, make it true so that the gentle lovemaking we do has powerful passions and a parents' trust.

Elizabeth Jennings

Sex is an important means of expressing feelings of sharing and commitment, as well as strengthening the bonds between a man and a woman. Sexuality and sexual activity represent a unique combination of physical, emotional, and social expression bringing individuals together to be close, procreate, and play, as well as to express lust, desire, and need. Sexuality is influenced by social mores, religious beliefs, laws, emotions, relationships, and a myriad of physical factors, not the least of which is the brain. In addition, sexual activity is influenced by health and well-being, availability of a partner, self-concept, sexual stimuli, social setting, and prior sexual experiences. Sexuality also represents one of the most unique, intimate, and rewarding of human experiences.

However, for many infertile couples, the pleasurable experience of sexual intimacy is altered so that sex becomes methodical, predictable, and unexciting. No longer a way of communicating intimacy and sharing, the meaning of sex focuses on procreation only. Frequently, self-perceptions are impacted: Research indicates that men may feel less virile and women less feminine or incomplete when they are infertile[1]. Common feelings of infertility, such as loss, anger, guilt, despair, depression, shame, and anxiety, often overshadow the usual feelings of warmth, affection, and emotional connection that are the natural prerequisites of enjoyable sexual encounters. Furthermore, infertility can be a melancholy reminder of the child that should be, past procreative failures, and the myriad 'insults' imposed by medical treatment. Gone is lovemaking that is primarily spontaneous, adventuresome, tender, and thrilling.

Sexual health is a multidimensional phenomenon that generally encompasses three essential elements: (1) capacity to enjoy and control sexual and reproductive behavior in accordance with social and personal values; (2) freedom from fear, shame, guilt, false beliefs, and other psychological factors that inhibit sexual response and impair sexual relationships; and (3) freedom from organic disorders, diseases, and deficiencies that interfere with sexual and reproductive functions[2]. In short, sexual health is considered the physical and emotional state of well-being that enables sexual enjoyment and acting on sexual feelings.

By contrast, sexual dysfunction involves an interruption in an individual's or couple's enjoyment or performance of sexual activity. Sexual dysfunction is defined as any impairment or disturbance in one or more of the phases of the sexual response cycle: desire, arousal, orgasm, and satisfaction. A *primary* (lifelong) dysfunction has always been present, while a *secondary* (acquired) dysfunction is one that occurs after a period of normal, healthy sexual functioning. Dysfunctions are further specified as *generalized* when they occur in all situations and with all partners or *situational* when the sexual problem is limited to certain situations or partners. The three categories of sexual dysfunctions are: disorders of sexual desire, disorders of arousal, and disorders of orgasm.

At times, infertility highlights long-standing sexual or marital problems, which existed before infertility. In some instances, sexual difficulties may be the *cause* of the inability to conceive by either preventing or interrupting coitus, thereby preventing conception. However, most often sexual difficulties for infertile individuals are the result of scheduled sex and the pressure to perform on demand, often with the psychological presence of the medical team in the bedroom.

This chapter will:

- provide an outline of sexual dysfunctions within the context of infertility
- identify etiology and treatment for men and women.

It does not include issues related to homosexuality or marital problems, which are addressed in Chapters 6 and 14 respectively.

HISTORICAL OVERVIEW

Sexual functioning and infertility have not until recently been the subject of scientific study. Early analyses of sexual functioning and infertility were most often based on unique clinical cases and/or theoretical speculations that focused on emotional barriers (especially in women) as an explanation for impaired fertility. At a time when 50% of infertility could not be explained by a medical diagnosis, it was the contention of early psychoanalytic theories that infertility was caused by psychological or emotional disturbances. Termed *psychogenic infertility*, it was thought to be caused by a woman's unconscious fear of pregnancy; history of frigidity, childhood timidity, or unsocial behavior; poor psychosexual development; rejection by or hatred of her mother; and fear that the infertile woman would kill her child if she had one[3-7]. In a man, psychogenic infertility was thought to be due to a controlling, unaffectionate, rigid, and moralistic mother; ambivalence about parenthood; insecure masculinity; and anger toward his spouse[8-11]. These theories contended that a man or woman's psychological problems either directly caused infertility or interrupted sexual activity sufficiently to impair reproduction. In fact, one early researcher[12] concluded that tubal spasming in tense and nervous women (a 'relatively permanent' condition) resulted in sexual dysfunction and infertility because infertile women were extremely preoccupied 'with female sex organs in a disturbed way'. Although these theories have fallen into disfavor over the last 20 years, different versions continue to resurface in various forms, influencing theory, practice, and research.

With the burgeoning of medical treatments for infertility and the consumer movement of the 1970s, the psychogenic model fell into disrepute, as it was more widely accepted that emotional distress was most often the *result* of infertility than the *cause* of it. In the 1970s, Walker[9] was one of the first to suggest that 'sexual functioning is subject to disruption from physical, cultural, and psychological forces ... and as well as *causing* infertility, sexual dysfunction may *result* from the work-up and treatment procedures such as sex on demand'. Riddick[13] expanded on this premise, suggesting that sexual impairment in infertile couples was due to planned sex, extensive and painful tests, intense feelings of anxiety, and the highly personal matter of sexuality being turned over to the external control of a physician. The interactive effect of infertility treatment and sexual functioning appears to provide the best understanding of the complexities of infertility: Severe sexual dysfunction can cause infertility, just as psychological disturbance often impairs sexual functioning, as well as responses to infertility treatment (Table 1).

Table 1 Impact of infertility on sexual practices and function

Effect on sexual practices

Increased frequency at midcycle

Decreased frequency in luteal phase

Decreased variety of sexual expression

Change in who initiates sex

Effect on sexual function

Occasional periovulatory impotence or retarded ejaculation

Occasional periovulatory orgasmic dysfunction due to 'spectatoring'

(Reproduced from Keye 1984, with permission)

REVIEW OF LITERATURE

Early research on sexual functioning in infertile couples focused on evidence of neurotic conflicts or personality traits that prevented normal sexual functioning. More recently, research has focused on the incidence and type of sexual dysfunctions in infertile couples, the impact of infertility on sexual functioning in women or in comparison to men, and the impact of specific infertility diagnosis or treatments (most often assisted reproductive technologies) on sexual functioning. Elstein[14] described the causes of sexual dysfunction in infertile couples as

- psychosexual problems masquerading as cases of infertility
- incidental findings of psychosexual disturbances in cases of infertility
- infertility causing psychosexual problems.

This is a good framework for evaluating the sexual dysfunctions with which infertile couples and individuals present. In addition, the prevalence of sexually transmitted diseases as a cause of infertility and the overall incidence of sexual dysfunction in infertile couples will be examined.

Sexually Transmitted Diseases as a Cause of Infertility

Although often overlooked, the most common preventable cause of infertility for both men and women is infection due to sexually transmitted diseases (STDs). In some parts of the world, infection-related infertility is so widespread that it constitutes not only a personal health problem but a public health crisis[15]. Although research has progressed on the prevention and treatment of STDs, patient barriers still include misconceptions about the impact of STDs on fertility, silent (asymptomatic) infections, shame and embarrassment, reluctance to seek medical care and support, fear of the impact on partner(s), and lack of ready access to medical care[16]. Infertility due to STDs has not only significant reproductive health consequences but also significant psychosocial ramifications, often highlighting an individual's lifestyle and personal history.

STDs adversely affect fertility through three primary mechanisms: (1) pregnancy loss, (2) neonatal deaths, and (3) obstruction of either male or female

151

reproductive ducts[17,18]. STDs cause infertility by infecting the genital tract of men and women, although this is a less frequent mechanism of infertility in men. Portals of entry for STDs include genitalia, urinary tract, mouth, rectum, and skin[18]. The most common STDs resulting in infertility are syphilis, gonorrhea, chlamydiosis, human papilloma virus (HPV), mycoplasmosis, genital herpes, trichomoniasis, and human immunodeficiency virus (HIV)[18,19].

STDs resulting in infertility require examination of personal decisions, especially those regarding sexual behavior, partner choice, cultural circumstances, domestic environment, drug and alcohol use/abuse, social life, and availability/usage of quality medical care[19]. While it is widely recognized that the distress of infertility results in feelings of anger, depression, isolation, guilt, self-reproach, and diminished self-esteem, these feelings can be significantly intensified when infertility is caused by sexual behavior and was therefore preventable. Not only is the individual vulnerable to significant feelings of loss, guilt, and self-reproach, but the marital relationship may be disturbed or threatened by the diagnosis, especially if it intimates extramarital sexual contacts.

Incidence of Sexual Dysfunction in Infertile Couples

The incidence of sexual dysfunctions in the general population is: 5–10%, inhibited female orgasm; 4–9% male erectile disorder; 4–10%, inhibited male orgasm; and 36–38%, premature ejaculation[20]. Sexual desire disorders in both men and women are the most common problem, representing 55% of sexual dysfunction, with the majority of the presenting patients being *male*.

A number of studies have found no evidence of higher incidences of sexual disturbance in infertile couples than in the general population. Daniluk[21] reported normal scores on a measure of marital and sexual satisfaction, although a percentage of couples with no identified infertility diagnosis were more dissatisfied with their sexual relationships than couples with identified infertility diagnosis. Van Balen and Trimbos-Kemper[22] found sexual functioning was within normal range and had no effect on overall well-being. While some researchers found that marital relationships deteriorated and encountered difficulties later in the treatment process, others found that the crisis of infertility enhanced intimacy and improved couple communication[23,24]. Berg and Wilson[25] found both genders were generally satisfied with their sexual relationship, although advanced-stage patients experienced lower levels of sexual satisfaction than either early- or intermediate-stage patients.

One early study[26], comparing fertile and infertile couples, found that infertile women reported significantly less satisfactory sexual relationships than fertile men and women. In a similar finding[9], infertile women reported significantly lower correlations with their husbands on stated intercourse and frequency: 22% of women reported difficulty or dissatisfaction with their sexual relationship. Andrews and associates[27] found that fertility-problem stress increased marital conflict and decreased sexual self-esteem, satisfaction with their individual sexual performance, and frequency of sexual intercourse.

In a study of over 500 infertile couples, Keye[28] determined that sexual problems arose for the following reasons: dyspareunia, progesterone-inhibited sexual desire, sex on demand, unrealistic sexual demands, rigid or routinized approach to sex, poor body image, depression, guilt, and ambivalence. The three areas of sexual difficulty were (1) the actual physical condition causing infertility or resulting from treatment, (2) sexual intercourse becoming only a means of reproduction rather than intimacy or pleasure, and (3) the global psychological impact of the infertility experience.

In an intriguingly different approach to sexual dysfunction among infertile couples, van Zyl[29] in a study of South African infertile couples found that general ignorance about sex (81% of men and 56% of women had received no sex education from their parents) resulted in unfavorable attitudes toward sex that adversely affected their fertility. For example, to facilitate intercourse, 18% of couples with severe psychosexual problems used lubricating substances that had a deleterious effect on sperm survival.

Sexual Dysfunction Causing Infertility

For a small percentage of infertile couples, sexual problems in one or both partners will be the primary cause of infertility. Sexual difficulties are the cause of infertility when sexual dysfunction prevents or interrupts coitus, preventing conception. The exact number of men and women impacted by this type of infertility is not known, primarily because these patients may not seek infertility treatment or disclose the problem to caregivers, or because caregivers fail to investigate it and little research has been devoted to it. Aribarg and Aribarg[30] found that 4% of infertile patients had psychosexual causes of their infertility, which included impotence, retarded ejaculation, vaginismus, and nonconsummation of marriage. Dubin and Amelar[31] in an examination of male infertility secondary to sexual problems found the following sexual dysfunctions contributing to infertility: impotency (both general and organic), and sexual activities that were too frequent (resulting in reduced sperm count) or too infrequent (no ejaculation, premature ejaculation, and failure of intromission). Additional reported causes of infertility due to sexual dysfunction include unconsummated marriage (failure to ever have sexual intercourse), vaginismus (vaginal muscle spasms that prevent penile penetration), infrequent sexual intercourse, midcycle male impotency, inability to achieve coitus for postcoital examination, or refusal (inability) to submit a semen sample[32,33]. In addition, some sexual practices related to a sexual dysfunction may cause infertility, such as use of vaginal lubricants that are spermicidal or religious customs such as *mikva* (Orthodox Jewish custom prohibiting sexual intercourse when the wife is 'unclean', a period of time that includes menses and 7 days after the last sign of vaginal bleeding)[34].

Psychological problems or psychiatric disorders as an antecedent or contributing factor to sexual dysfunctions causing infertility may also be a consideration. In a study that evaluated the incidence of sexual dysfunction (anejaculation) as a primary cause of infertility, Hamer and Bain[35] evaluated 11 men with ejaculatory incompetence presenting at a urology clinic, nine of whom presented for infertility treatment. Two of the nine men refused referral for sex therapy. Three men chose to pursue artificial insemination by husband (AIH), and two of the three men who accepted referral to a sex therapist achieved pregnancy through sexual intercourse. The authors concluded that sexual functioning should be investigated in cases of infertility and that sex therapy is an effective treatment, as opposed to AIH.

Although rare, deviant sexual activities may cause infertility; these include exclusively oral sex, bondage, cross-dressing, fetishism, sadomasochism, or partner swapping[31]. Conflicted gender identity, homosexuality, and bisexuality are other potential causes of infertility, especially if a partner is unaware or unwilling to acknowledge his or her sexual orientation, sexual identity problems or is attempting to be deceptive. However these issues arise, they usually contribute to personal crisis, serious marital disruption, and interference with infertility treatment.

Incidental Sexual Dysfunction with Infertility

Several studies have assessed the incidence and type of sexual dysfunction in men undergoing treatment for infertility or requesting infertility treatment. Van Zyl[29] found that 27% of infertile men attributed their sexual difficulties (low libido, premature ejaculation, and impotence) to infertility. Pepe and Byrne[36] found that during infertility treatment, sexual relationships encountered serious difficulties (particularly in the areas of initiation and partner's embarrassment). Although women reported that their sexual relationships improved after the discontinuation of medical treatment, it did not return to its pretreatment level even two years following treatment termination when there was no pregnancy. Slade[37] found that infertile women had generally more restrictive attitudes and greater guilt levels regarding sexual activity, as well as perceptions of sex as primarily for reproductive purposes.

In a study comparing infertile women to other groups of women, Benazon[38] found that after 12 months, nonpregnant women showed higher levels of stress and lower levels of sexual satisfaction than did women who had become pregnant. Keye and Deneris[39] used a survey to compare infertile women with a control group of asymptomatic women attending a gynecology clinic. Although they found that no differences existed between the groups, 18% of the infertile women attributed their sexual problems to infertility, and 37% reported sexual dissatisfaction that they

attributed to infertility and the loss of spontaneity.

In a study evaluating the impact of stress on semen quality, Hammond and colleagues[40] studied men undergoing in vitro fertilization (IVF) and AIH to assess semen quality in infertility treatments associated with heightened performance anxiety. The researchers found no significant differences in either group of men. In fact some of the men who had begun health-seeking behaviors (reduced hot baths, and use of recreational drugs) had noted improved semen quality, leading the researchers to conclude that performance anxiety does not appear to be detrimental to semen quality.

Infertility Causing Psychosexual Problems

Common sexual dysfunctions in women resulting from the stresses of medical treatments (most often directed at women regardless of the etiology of the infertility) include problems with loss of libido, anorgasmia, and disturbance of sexual identity[41]. Several researchers have found that infertility treatment contributed to feelings of loss of control, intimacy, privacy, and esteem and decreased sexual desire, response, and activity in women[23]. In an Italian study[42] of infertile women, researchers determined that there was no change in the level of sexual fulfillment but there was a decrease in frequency of sexual intercourse and in sexual desire. Keye[43] found the rates of sexual dysfunction in women to be comparable to fertile women, although 58% of infertile women reported decreased sexual enjoyment due to scheduled intercourse.

In a study of infertile women, Boivin and colleagues[44] found that one-third experienced feelings of discomfort and nervousness during postcoital testing and 20% with normal sexual functioning reported an unfavorable sexual response to sexual intercourse prior to postcoital testing. Furthermore, the majority of the women reported lower levels of postcoital sexual satisfaction as compared to sexual relations at other times. The authors concluded that the inherent pressure of the postcoital situation may be stressful for women, contributing to decreased sexual enjoyment and poor sexual response, resulting in poorer physiological results. Interestingly, they found no significant relation between erectile difficulties and female sexual satisfaction, arousal, and orgasm. Van Zyl[29] reported that 43% of women felt that their inability to conceive had serious negative effects on their lives, particularly their sexual relations. Women reported severe marital strain, as well as sexual inhibitions, anorgasmia, and reduced interest in sex. Andrews and associates[27] found that fertility-problem stress had a stronger negative impact on women's sense of sexual identity and self-efficacy than it did on men.

A few studies have investigated the impact of a specific infertility diagnosis or a treatment protocol on male sexual functioning. In an investigation of infertile couples in which the husband had been diagnosed with azoospermia, Berger[45] found that 63% of the men experienced a period of impotence following the diagnosis. In addition, 87% of their wives reported significant psychological distress following the diagnosis, such as rage toward their husband, psychological symptoms, and/or dreams that incorporated three themes: concern for husband, wish to be rid of him, and guilt over this wish. However, this research has not been replicated. Interestingly, wives of men who did not experience erectile dysfunction were symptom-free. In a study of infertile couples, Drake and Grunert[46] found acute midcycle sexual dysfunction in a majority of the men, attributing this to:

(1) 'This is the night' syndrome, (2) change in purpose of sexual intercourse, (3) stress of clinical testing by a third party, and (4) self-doubt of adequate future performance. In a study assessing stigma in infertile couples with male-identified infertility, Nachtigall and coworkers[47] reported that men with male-factor infertility experienced greater stigma than men who did not have it. Berg and Wilson[25] evaluated couples across different stages of the infertility investigation (years 1, 2, and 3) and found that over time infertile couples experienced increased marital and sexual problems, with men reporting less ability to control ejaculation and less satisfaction with their sexual performance in general. In a study comparing infertile men and a control group, Kemer and associates[48] found that infertile men reported lower self-esteem, higher anxiety, more somatic symptoms, and greater sexual inadequacy, as well as more depression, which, in turn, impacted erectile functioning.

A few researchers have evaluated sexual dysfunction in couples requesting or completing IVF, an interesting approach since the success or failure of the IVF protocol is not contingent on sexual intercourse, thereby eliminating the pressure and marital strain that many infertile couples experience as a result of other infertility treatments. Baram and colleagues[49] studied the responses to failed IVF in couples and found that a minority (20% of women and 17% of men) felt that the IVF experience had an adverse effect on their sexual relationship by decreasing communication and emotional closeness, contributing to sexual difficulties and blaming. Women complained of dyspareunia or difficulty with arousal and/or achieving orgasm, whereas men experienced impotence or premature ejaculation. Although a majority of patients (58% of women and 67% of men) reported no change in sexual function following IVF, a significant number of both men and women noted decreased spontaneity and satisfaction. Fagan and colleagues[50] found similar levels of sexual difficulties in their study assessing sexual functioning and psychological status in married couples requesting IVF. Sexual dysfunction was found in 15.5% of the couples (an additional 14.4% were given DSM-III psychiatric diagnoses) and was more common in couples with unexplained infertility. This study also found that approximately 20% of IVF participants began the procedure with measurable degrees of psychological or sexual distress. In a study[51] comparing perceptions of men and women following IVF, researchers found fewer gender differences regarding couples' sexual relationship and that both men and women felt that IVF decreased the female partner's sexual desire. In short, the high-technology treatment of IVF does not appear to dramatically affect sexual functioning in couples as a whole or in men in particular, but women (who receive the greatest portion of treatment during IVF) may experience a slight increased risk of diminished sexual satisfaction or desire.

THEORETICAL FRAMEWORKS

The Human Sexual Response

Sexuality is a term used to refer to a person's gender identity, feelings, sexual orientation, and attitudes, and is distinct from sexual behavior. It encompasses the most intimate feelings of individuality, the need for emotional closeness to another human being, and a fundamental aspect of one's humanity. Sexual health includes a knowledge of sexual functioning; a positive body image; self-awareness about attitudes regarding sex; understanding and appreciation of one's sexual feelings; a well developed and usable value system; the ability to create effective and rewarding relationships; and emotional comfort, interdependence, and stability within sexual encounters. It is these qualities of personal awareness, values, and relationships that contribute as much to sexual health and well-being as hormones, genitalia, and brain centers.

The human sexual response is not much different from other human interactions: It follows a pattern of response involving biological responses to psychological and sensory input. It represents the interplay of physiological, psychological, and social influences that determine behavior. The three phases of human sexual response cycle are *desire, arousal,* and *orgasm*[52,53]. The *desire phase* is influenced by a wide variety of environmental stimuli, including psychosocial and cultural factors and physiology, allowing initiation or receptivity to sexual activity. During the *arousal phase* of sexual response, various factors come together, allowing one to either initiate or respond to sexual activity. Vaginal lubrication in women and penile erection in men are the most noticeable signs of increased excitement of the arousal phase. In women, this phase also involves internal vaginal expansion (ballooning) and erection of the nipples and clitoris. Vasocongestion results, in women, in swelling of the outer portion of the vagina and the labia and, in men, an increase in scrotal size and its pulling up against the body. *Orgasm* in both men and women involves a series of muscular contractions that diminish in intensity and rapidity. In women, these contractions involve the vagina, uterus, and anal sphincter, while in men orgasm involves the prostate and seminal vesicles and the contractions are followed by ejaculation. Following orgasm, the body returns to its resting or preexcitement state as vasocongestion is relieved. In men, this is marked by loss of erection, while in women it involves decrease in clitoral size and diminished vaginal width and length.

While men have a refractory period after orgasm during which ejaculation and orgasm cannot occur, this is not the case for women. Failure to experience orgasm in both men and women can result in pelvic and genital discomfort when vasocongestion is not relieved. Contrary to popular belief, orgasmic response in women is the same whether it is the result of clitoral or vaginal stimulation.

Assessment of Sexual Dysfunction

The most commonly used assessment strategy is the sexual history interview developed by Masters and Johnson[52]. It is a semistructured, extended face-to-face interview, often lasting several hours. Masters and Johnson's approach focuses on exploration of the current sexual problem with attention to environmental influences on sexual functioning. Kaplan's[53] adaptation of this method provides a means of evaluation and consideration of sexual dysfunctions that uses a 'conflict-oriented' approach for investigating psychodynamic phenomena (Table 2). An adaptation of this evaluation technique for infertile men and women is the Comprehensive Psychosocial History for Infertility by Burns[54] and Greenfeld (see Appendix 2), a semistructured interview tool that includes sections on sexual dysfunction and marital adjustment. The Infertility Questionnaire[55], a short instrument with 8 of its 21 items devoted to sexual functioning, was developed for research purposes. It has not

Table 2 Taking a sexual history

Chief complaint
Sexual status examination
Assessment of medical status
Assessment of psychiatric status
Family and psychosexual history
Evaluation of the relationship

(Reproduced from Kaplan 1983, with permission)

been shown to have reliability or validity, nor has it been adapted for clinical practice. Most researchers and clinicians using assessment measures of sexual adjustment rely on available standardized measures, even though none to date has been adapted to the infertility population (see Chapter 6).

CLINICAL ISSUES

Sexual Dysfunctions in Both Men and Women

Loss of sexual desire or libido, also referred to as *hypoactive sexual desire disorder*, is shared by both men and women, representing dysfunction in the first phase of the sexual response (desire, arousal, orgasm)[56]. Low libido may be an isolated sexual problem that is episodic or situational, a long-standing malady, or a symptom of a problem that is not primarily sexual in nature, such as depression, physical illness (e.g., heart disease, hypertension), or social problems (e.g., job stress, social isolation). The proportion of sexual desire disorders has risen steadily and dramatically over the past decades and now accounts for the largest group of complaints voiced by patients seeking sex therapy[20,57]. Traditionally, loss of sexual desire was more common in women, but today low libido is more prevalent in men.

The desire phase of sexual functioning represents interest in sexual contact and the need for sexual intimacy in both men and women. Diagnostic criteria of disordered sexual desire include presence or absence of sexual fantasies, masturbation, noncoital sexual activity, coitus with the partner, any nonpartner-related sexual activity, and initiation of sexual activity versus partner receptivity[56,57]. Sexual desire disorders rarely occur in isolation; the context and mediating factors include age, number of years married, socioeconomic status, religiosity, marital happiness, physical well-being, previous sexual appetite, and current social stressors.

Hypoactive sexual desire disorder is low libido, loss of sexual interest or mood, and diminished desire or sexual appetite, which may be *generalized* to all real or potential sexual partners or specific to one's current partner, usually indicating relationship problems or dissatisfaction with this partner. *Primary* hypoactive sexual desire disorder is the total absence of sexual desire, feelings, thoughts, fantasies, or interest, and typically becomes apparent in adolescence or early adulthood. It is generally a lifelong problem that is very difficult to treat, as its etiology is usually a combination of physical and psychological factors. *Secondary* hypoactive sexual desire disorder, occurring after a period of normal sexual desire, is marked by absence of sexual desire, feelings, thoughts, fantasies, or interest.

Low libido or diminished sexual desire may be the result of relationship problems, alcohol or other drugs, illness, sexual boredom, inadequate sexual information, restrictive upbringing, or body-image problems. Sometimes, loss of sexual interest is due to psychological problems such as depression, stress, history of traumatic sexual experiences, or insecurity about one's psychosexual role—all influencing sexual responsiveness and enjoyment. For infertile men and women, disorders of sexual desire are usually episodic or situational responses to the emotional distress or physical strains of infertility or a specific medical treatment. As the focus of sexual activity continues to emphasize procreation, infertile men and women may feel depressed, lose interest in sex-on-demand, or find it difficult to feel sexual when they feel frustrated and unhappy much of the time. Chronic health problems or the invasiveness of medical treatment for infertility often dampen erotic thoughts and feelings, resulting in

sexual intercourse becoming a less appealing source of affection and more a necessary reproductive chore. Finally, another common culprit in loss of sexual interest in men and women is medications such as oral contraceptives, medroxy-progesterone contraceptive injection (Depo-Provera), gonadotropin-releasing hormone agonists, ovulation-induction medications, antihypertensives, and anti-depressants that interfere with sexual response and/or interest by changing hormone levels, affecting sexual appetite or arousal, or altering the experience of orgasm.

Relationship problems such as poor communication, anger, rejection, avoidance of commitment, and confused priorities often masquerade (or at least present) as sexual complaints regardless of the presence or absence of infertility. Intra-psychic issues such as concealed homo-sexuality, participation in extramarital sex, excessive masturbation, or compulsive sexual activity are not problems of sexual desire as they are presented, but actually represent problems within the individual or the relationship. Persistent marital difficulties in infertile couples may be indicative of earlier conflicts either within the marriage or within the individuals[45]. In some couples, partners blame themselves or each other for infertility (irrespective of actual etiology), resulting in anger that interferes with sexual desire and functioning[58]. Lack of emotional closeness may masquerade as sexual problems when the actual problem is inappropriate or destructive behaviors such as violence, abuse, or boundary violations. In such cases, treatment for sexual dysfunction is less important than resolution of more significant marital issues (see Chapter 6).

One approach for determining whether a presenting sexual complaint is primarily sexual or relationship-related was designed by Sanderson and Maddock[59] and includes

Table 3 Sexual problem diagnostic grid

Influencing factors	Focus of problem		
	Orgasm	Arousal	Desire
Contextual	1	1	1,2
Relational I (simple conflict communication)	1,2	2	2,3
Relational II (underlying structural issues)	2,3	3	3,4
Relational III (commitment)	3	3,4	4
Intrapsychic	3,4	4	4

Key: 1, low severity: educational/behavioral treatment, including self-help methods; 2, moderate severity: behavioral treatment with additional counseling likely; 3, high severity: behavioral treatment by a sex therapist in conjunction with personal or relational counseling; 4, extreme severity: behavioral treatment only an adjunct to intensive personal and/or relational psychotherapy
(Reproduced from Sanderson and Maddock 1989, with permission)

a diagnostic and treatment planning guide, as well as a helpful taxonomy of relationship difficulties (Table 3). The sexual complaint is assessed in terms of the phase of sexual functioning (desire, arousal, orgasm) and three 'influencing variables': *context* (immediate context of the erotic contact), *relationship* (general interaction of the partners), and *intrapsychic* (psychological makeup of the individual). As a general rule, the longer the duration of sexual complaints, the more resistant they are to treatment. Relationship difficulties are defined in terms of three subgroups: (1) problems involving minor difficulties that may affect sexual interaction but do not threaten the overall structure of the relationship (e.g., simple conflicts or stylistic communication differences), (2) more severe conflicts impacting every aspect of the overall relationship, as well as relationship dynamics (e.g., inability to trust each other, power struggles, or differing levels of need for intimacy), and (3) problems involving partner commitment and psychological presence in the relationship affecting the fundamental stability of the relationship.

Even couples who never encounter major or disrupting sexual problems often experience periodic diminished sexual desire and satisfaction at some point during medical treatment for infertility. Episodic loss of libido in one or both partners is not particularly disruptive and can usually be addressed with minimal education and reassurance. However, consistent and extensive diminished sexual desire in infertile men and women is more problematic and usually multifactorial: a common side effect of feelings of sexual unattractiveness or defectiveness, guilt or shame, depression or anger. Loss of libido may be the result of the conditions contributing to infertility or the result of a specific medical treatment for infertility. Or it may be due to the stresses and demands infertility place on the marriage, social relationships, work life, or financial resources. All these factors contribute to loss of sexual desire or interest in infertile men and women, resulting in diminished sexual functioning. Individuals may respond with silent resignation; anger or blame directed at self, spouse, infertility, or medical caregivers; help-seeking; or self-treatment. Silent resignation is the abandonment of sexual satisfaction or desire by one or both partners, who learn *not* to expect physical or emotional rewards from their lovemaking and consider sexual intercourse a reproductive duty to be endured. This is often more common and easier to disguise in women. Self-treatment for lack of sexual desire includes not only a variety of over-the-counter medical remedies or gadgets but also various self-defeating sexual behaviors such as excessive masturbation, additional intimate relationships, obsessive search for sexual thrills, sexual release without emotional entanglement, or parenthood without one's infertility partner. Rarely do infertile men or women actually seek help for sexual problems, unless the difficulty is clearly interfering with their reproductive agenda or treatment plan. This lack of help-seeking behavior may represent a desire to avoid further boundary violations (maintaining as much of the privacy around their intimate relationship as possible), or a belief that sexual problems are unimportant to their caregivers or that their caregivers cannot provide assistance.

Response to treatment of a sexual desire disorder is contingent on its etiology, whether it is generalized or situational, and how long the desire disorder has continued without treatment. Disorders of sexual desire have traditionally been notoriously difficult to treat, primarily because men and women have learned to involuntarily and automatically focus on negative or distracting thoughts that suppress sexual feelings. Research on the treatment of sexual desire disorders has shown that standard sex therapy usually fails to raise sexual desire[60]. However, treatments that focus specifically on low sexual desire have been found to be more effective, especially those using a combination of cognitive-behavioral treatment programs involving the following principles: (1) Affectional awareness helps patients become aware of negative attitudes, beliefs, and cognitions regarding sex; (2) insight-oriented therapy helps patients gain understanding of their negative thoughts or feelings; (3) cognitive therapy assists alteration of irrational thoughts that inhibit sexual desire; and (4) behavioral interventions focus on behavioral assignments that help evoke feelings during experiential/sensory awareness and change nonsexual behaviors that may be maintaining the sexual difficulty[57]. Successful treatment involving behavioral tasks and a nondemanding, reassuring environment removes common obstacles to sexual pleasure such as poor communication, anxiety, unrealistic expectations, or mechanical sex. Other treatment suggestions include hormonal therapy (testosterone) or medications (e.g., Viagra) for both men and women, anxiety reduction, increasing sensory awareness, enhancing sexual/sensual experiences, modifying the inhibition of erotic impulses, and facilitation of erotic responses.

Sexual Dysfunction in Women

Regardless of the cause of infertility, research has consistently shown that in response to infertility women experience greater emotional distress than men and often assume personal responsibility, while enduring a disproportionate share of medical treatment. More often women initiate medical treatment for infertility and are more invested in having a child, more aware of the limits of their reproductive life, and more willing to consider extreme or alternative measures to achieve parenthood. For women, reproduction and sexuality may be more intrinsically intertwined than they are for men, so that disturbances in one area necessarily reverberate into the other. In short, infertility clearly impacts the sexual functioning and sexual health of women in myriad ways.

Current research indicates that the most common female sexual dysfunction is arousal phase disorders, followed by orgasm phase disorders of vaginismus and dyspareunia[20]. Sexual dysfunction in women may be due to hormonal changes, anatomical or physical factors (e.g., endometriosis, ovarian cysts, or uterine fibroids), or organic conditions (e.g., illness and diseases impacting general well-being and sexual health). Medications, disease, or physical problems can, and often do, affect sexual pleasure and sexual functioning. *Hormonal changes*, including loss of hormones with menopause, premature ovarian failure, or surgical removal of the ovaries, may lead to diminished sexual appetite, loss of vaginal lubrication, painful intercourse, decreased sexual sensation and arousal, and less intense orgasms. *Anatomical* reasons for sexual dysfunction include surgical outcomes and congenital malformations of the reproductive tract, such as congenital absence of the vagina or biforate uterus. *Organic conditions* include endometriosis, ovarian cysts, pelvic disorders, STDs (e.g., herpes or HPV infection), myomas, diabetes, alcoholism, neurological conditions, or other illnesses that can cause painful intercourse and sexual dysfunction.

Arousal Phase Disorders

The arousal phase of sexual excitement occurs in response to sexual stimuli and results in vaginal lubrication and expansion. Arousal disorders are defined as impaired female excitement or the persistent and recurrent lack of response to sexual stimuli and activity, resulting in lack of vaginal lubrication and engorgement. Estimates of the prevalence of arousal disorders in the general population vary between 11% and 48%[60]. Causes of arousal problems include pelvic vascular disease, neurological conditions, hormonal changes, and psychosocial factors, such as stress, prior history of sexual trauma, painful intercourse, or relationship problems.

Arousal disorders in women are often difficult to treat. Cognitive restructuring can be helpful in changing involuntary,

automatic negative thoughts that suppress sexual feelings[53]. Other treatment suggestions include sensate-focus exercises (see Table 6), anxiety reduction, education about normal physiological sexual responses, increased sensory awareness, enhancing sexual/ sensual experiences, facilitation of erotic responses, increased use of fantasy and/or erotica, and masturbation[61].

Orgasm Phase Disorders

Impaired or inhibited orgasm, or anorgasmia, is the total absence or persistent, recurrent delay of orgasm following normal and sufficient arousal. The inability to achieve orgasm is an orgasm phase disorder in women that is present in about a one-third of young women. Historically referred to as frigidity, disorders of orgasm were once considered the most common sexual problem in women. *Primary* anorgasmia is never having experienced orgasm either alone or with a partner following any kind of stimulation. *Secondary* anorgasmia is the absence or delay of orgasm after previously having been orgasmic. Most often, a woman can achieve orgasm with masturbation, manual stimulation, or oral sex but is unable to do so with intercourse. In the past, there was some controversy about whether failure to orgasm with intercourse alone was actually a 'dysfunction' in women, however this issue is less of a concern today.

Orgasmic dysfunction in infertile women is common, at least episodically, and is attributable to several factors including medical conditions (e.g., diabetes, estrogen deficiency, anatomical problems, and gynecological conditions), medications (including psychotropic drugs, alcohol, 'recreational' drugs, and certain pain medications), and psychosocial factors (e.g., depression, marital conflict). Although anorgasmia is frequently attributed to psychological disturbances, there are few psychological factors that consistently relate to the ability to achieve orgasm. Since orgasm is not necessary for natural procreation in women, preoccupation with pregnancy and a willingness to relinquish orgasm often impact sexual responsiveness during infertility. This is more likely to become a marital problem than a psychosexual problem for the woman. Women may surrender orgasm as penance for past sexual misdeeds, in trade for the 'baby at any price', or for the sake of minimizing the impact of infertility on their own or their partner's life. Sometimes women and their partners, in an attempt to proceed with intercourse and circumvent natural sexual response, use various commercial lubricants (all of which are spermicidal) to facilitate intercourse.

Treatment techniques for anorgasmia in women focus on increasing sexual response by providing increasing awareness of arousing environmental cues and her body's responses to sensation, often with the assistance of masturbation. Treatment must necessarily address the issue of 'relinquishing orgasm' for procreative purposes, and the woman's willingness to recognize and alter this practice. Treatment that focuses on satisfying her male partner is usually not successful, although attention to relationship and interaction issues and her partner's sexual response and sensitivity to her are usually beneficial. Additional treatment techniques include relaxation training, cognitive restructuring, pelvic exercises, relaxation and biofeedback, and increased tolerance for normal feelings of arousal and excitement. Treatment of female orgasm disorders has been quite successful, although the definition of success has been an issue: If orgasm with their partner is the criterion, the success rate is 85–95%, but only 30–50% if orgasm during intercourse is the criterion.

Vaginismus

Vaginismus is defined as recurrent and persistent involuntary vaginal spasms or muscle contractions that make entry into the vagina impossible or painful. Although the woman is sexually aroused and capable of experiencing an orgasm, the vaginal muscles close tightly, preventing penile or digital entry into the vagina. Vaginismus may be localized to sexual intercourse or may be generalized to include any attempt to enter the vagina, including digital foreplay, cunnilingus, self-examine with fingers, tampon insertion, or pelvic examinations by a physician. Vaginismus may be *primary* (inability to tolerate penetration and present in all encounters) or *secondary* (occurring in specific relationships or situations). Women with vaginismus typically experience sexual arousal and sexual pleasure in response to foreplay and are often able to have pleasurable and plentiful sexual activity, even though they are unable to have sexual intercourse.

Vaginismus may be caused by physical problems, emotional trauma, or psychosocial stressors but is less likely to be due to physical etiology. However, while this condition generally is thought to be psychological in nature, physical factors cannot be ruled out. Possible causal factors include congenital deformity of the vagina, infections, hormonal abnormalities, sexual trauma, insufficient lubrication as a result of inadequate foreplay or poor sexual technique, allergic reactions, or other physical etiology[62]. Understandably, vaginismus often causes significant relationship problems, sometimes triggering erectile dysfunction in partners, particularly if he becomes impatient, angry, or guilty, or feels responsible for his partner's problem.

Treatment of vaginismus usually involves a comprehensive program of psychotherapy and behavioral interventions aimed at modifying or altering the

Table 4 Success rates for treatment of sexual dysfunction

Premature ejaculation and vaginismus	90–95%
Absolute female orgasmic dysfunction (no orgasm ever)	85–95% if orgasm with partner is criterion, but only 30–50% if orgasm during intercourse is criterion
Partial female orgasmic dysfunction (patient seldom orgasmic or orgasmic only with solo masturbation)	70–80%, but only 30–50% if criterion is during intercourse
Secondary erectile dysfunction (patient has had erections in past)	60–80%
Primary erectile dysfunction (no erections ever in sexual situations)	40–60%
Retarded or blocked ejaculations	50–82%
Low or inhibited sexual desire	no reliable outcome studies of sex therapy; sporadic success at best after much longer therapies

(Reproduced from Heiman, LoPiccolo and LoPiccolo 1981, with permission)

immediate cause of the conditioned response (tightening of the vaginal muscles)[63]. Treatment often includes pelvic exercises, dilators, biofeedback, psychotherapeutic interventions, or physical therapy. Finally, treatment for vaginismus can take a fair bit of time, requiring the woman's commitment and compliance, as well as the cooperation of her partner. The time demand can be an additional stressor for infertile couples who often do not want to take the time away from their pursuit of pregnancy to treat a problem they may already have lived with for a time. However, vaginismus has the highest rates of treatment success (Table 4).

Dyspareunia

Painful intercourse, or dyspareunia, may be the result of lack of arousal but is most often due to physical factors such as pelvic infection, anatomical conditions, congenital deformities, or vaginal atrophy due to inadequate estrogen exposure. Female sexual pain disorder can or may become the *cause* of infertility, if not the result, when pain is so intense as to limit or halt sexual intercourse[62]. Other factors causing painful intercourse include side effects of medications, insufficient hormones, scarring from pelvic infections or surgeries, myomas, cancer, and STDs such as HPV infection and genital herpes. In infertile women, dyspareunia may be the result of ovarian cysts, side effects of ovulation-induction medications, ovarian hyperstimulation, infection, surgical adhesions, and endometriosis. Lubrication problems, or failure of the vaginal walls to provide adequate secretions to moisten the vagina and facilitate penile penetration, can be another common cause of painful intercourse and may be due to inadequate hormone levels, injury to the vaginal walls, lack of adequate sexual arousal, or poor sexual technique. Inadequate lubrication may also be due to attempts to proceed with sexual intercourse when a woman is not sufficiently aroused, an all too common occurrence in infertile couples who wish to get the reproductive chore over.

The optimum treatment for dyspareunia is contingent on etiology and involves a multimodal assessment and treatment protocol that addresses the following: behavior, affect, sensation, imagery, cognition, interpersonal relations, and drugs[62]. Pain during intercourse can be treated medically (e.g., pain medications, leuprolide for endometriosis, hormone-replacement therapy) or surgically (e.g., removal of pelvic adhesions or myomas). Psychotherapy involves relaxation techniques, desensitization, pain management, biofeedback, specialized physical therapy, and reeducation focusing on recognition of pelvic, genital, and muscular sensations. Alteration or adaptation of sexual positions, with the woman taking more control of the sexual encounter, has also been found helpful, especially for women with endometriosis or other pelvic conditions.

Sexual Dysfunction in Men

Myths about male sexual functioning—such as men are ready, willing, and able to engage in sexual activity at any time or any place—have contributed to cavalier and unrealistic expectations regarding sexual functioning in men, and infertile men in particular. Such assumptions and perfunctory attitudes toward male sexuality are often the biggest impediment in the identification and treatment of sexual dysfunction in infertile men. Traditionally, sexual functioning in infertile men has focused on sexual disorders preventing impregnation or impacting infertility treatment plans, and less on sexual satisfaction or men's feelings about sexual performance or reproductive ability. However, infertility (especially male-factor infertility) frequently triggers feelings of failure, sexual inadequacy, diminished masculinity, loss of potency or power, and altered sense of self—all contributory factors in male sexual dysfunction[47]. During infertility, sexual intercourse for many men becomes obligatory, repetitive, and routine,

providing few emotional rewards and little excitement. Many men develop performance anxiety, sexual avoidance, or aversion to sex, especially if sex is for 'procreation purposes only' and his partner is sexually unresponsive or impassive. Frequently, infertile men complain of feeling like 'stud service' (that all his partner wants from him is his sperm) or of the 'queen bee syndrome' (his sole importance is to fertilize his partner)[64]. Such feelings can be further intensified if the man equates sperm production with ejaculation, even though the two are distinct physiological functions.

The most common sexual dysfunctions in men are erectile dysfunction, traditionally referred to as impotence (inability to achieve or maintain an erection adequate for sexual intercourse), premature ejaculation (inability to exert voluntary control of ejaculatory reflex), and retarded or inhibited ejaculation (inhibition, delay, or absence of ejaculation). For men, erectile disorder is the most common presenting problem in sex therapy clinics, whereas premature ejaculation is more widespread in the community[65]. Inhibited male orgasm is less common both in community and clinical settings. Causes of sexual dysfunction in men include hormonal changes (e.g., diminished testosterone with age,) physical factors (e.g., injury or congenital anomaly), or organic conditions (e.g., illness and diseases such as diabetes or hypertension).

Erectile Dysfunction

Primary erectile dysfunction is never having had the ability to achieve and/or maintain an erection sufficient for vaginal penetration or successful coitus. This is a very rare condition most often due to physical or organic factors but, in rare situations, to psychological factors as well. Although rare, when it does occur, primary erectile dysfunction due to psychological factors is a direct cause of infertility. Treatment success rates for primary erectile dysfunction are the lowest among all sexual disorders in men and women. *Secondary* or *acquired* erectile dysfunction is partial or weak erections, total absence of an erection, or the inability to sustain an erection long enough for vaginal penetration or sexual intercourse. Most men experience some form of episodic, transient erectile dysfunction at some point in their lifetime. A significant number of men suffer from chronic erectile dysfunction especially as they age, although it affects men of all ages. In the past, it was believed that 90% of erectile dysfunction disorders were due to psychological factors, but it is now believed that this is an overestimate and that 50% of erectile dysfunction problems are due to physical (or organic) etiology[66]. Causes of impotence include organic factors (e.g., endocrine or neurological problems, antidepressant or antihypertensive medications, and alcohol and recreational drugs), hormonal changes (e.g., hormonal therapy including medications used to treat infertility), physical factors (e.g., injury, urological, or vascular problems), and psychological or relationship difficulties.

Erectile dysfunction is the most important cause of male-factor infertility due to sexual dysfunction, although men rarely disclose this problem to caregivers[27]. This may be because many men generally have difficulty discussing their sexual problems or because it is difficult to discuss these problems with infertility physicians (who are often gynecologists). Erectile dysfunction due to psychological factors is generally believed to be the result of the man's blocking sexual arousal and focusing instead on nonsexual or antisexual cues[67]. A variety of psychosexual issues may account for erection problems in men, involving not only his feelings about himself but his feelings about his health, relationships, sexuality, and life situation. Relationship issues, especially those involving conflict and anger, have been found to be a major factor in erectile dysfunction[68]. Intrapersonal dynamics, such as ambivalence about parenthood, threatened masculinity or self-esteem, or fear of intimacy or commitment, can surface during the crisis of infertility and become influential issues in the man's sexual functioning.

Erectile dysfunction, like vaginismus in women, often contributes to considerable marital tension, especially in terms of infertility, in which the husband's healthy sexual functioning is a prerequisite to many infertility treatment protocols. Inability to sexually perform (intercourse or produce a sperm specimen) may not be simply embarrassing but financially expensive, emotionally distressing, and relationship-damaging. Conflicts or disagreements about medical treatments, family-building options, personal agendas, or relationship dynamics can, and often do, contribute to erectile dysfunction problems in infertile couples.

Treatments for secondary erectile dysfunction have had mixed success rates, although new medical treatments (e.g., Viagra) have shown considerable promise. Treatment usually begins with a physical examination that evaluates hormone levels, nerves, and blood vessels and assesses nocturnal tumescence (rigidity of the penis during sleep). There are two general types of nocturnal tumescence devices: the snap gauge cuff and the nocturnal penile tumescence monitor. When erectile dysfunction is determined to be organic and not reversible (e.g., in the case of injury or disease), treatment usually involves medical (oral or injectable medications) or surgical interventions such as penile injections, penile prostheses, and/or penile implants. Medications, penile injections, penile prostheses, and penile implants all facilitate erections and sexual intercourse, thereby improving quality of life. However, these treatments usually do not and cannot improve or restore fertility.

Psychological treatments for erectile dysfunction include decreasing performance anxiety, eliminating spectatoring, increasing awareness of erotic sensations, and disputing irrational beliefs and myths. Psychodynamic-depth approaches that do not include behavioral or cognitive interventions have been found to be ineffective in the treatment of erectile dysfunction[67], while guided imagery and sensate-focus exercises (see Table 6) have been found to be helpful in deemphasizing sexual performance and refocusing on sensation and pleasure. Cognitive restructuring, sexual education, and relaxation techniques are successful for redirecting negative and automatic thoughts while increasing comfort with feelings of sexual arousal. For infertile couples, marital counseling addressing relationship issues, husband's sexuality, and couple sexual functioning can be beneficial. Whether erectile dysfunction is due to physical or emotional factors, counseling can help the man and his partner maintain realistic expectations about treatment outcomes and provides a supportive environment for discussing the problem.

Premature Ejaculation

Premature ejaculation, or inadequate ejaculatory control, is the inability to exert voluntary control over the ejaculatory reflex, so that once a man reaches a certain level of sexual arousal or excitement, he ejaculates reflexively and rapidly soon after or even before vaginal penetration. It has also been defined as the inability to delay ejaculatory reflex for sufficient time during intercourse to satisfy a responsive partner during 50% of their coital experiences[68].

Premature ejaculation is usually not situational; it occurs with *all* partners because the man has not learned to voluntarily control his ejaculatory reflexes. Diagnostic criteria for premature ejaculation are contingent on the length of coitus, sexual attitudes of both partners, and sexual expectations often defined by sociocultural issues. Although rare, there can be physical causes for premature ejaculation, especially when loss of control is not associated with significant stress or a change in the man's sexual relationship[53]. Organic causes of premature ejaculation involve congenital conditions, neurological problems, side effects of medications, and other health problems, including hormonal changes (especially those used for infertility treatment). Psychological factors (apart from learned response) may be related to infertility with its emphasis on sex for procreation, the man's attempts to make the sexual encounter as brief as possible, or habituated rapid ejaculation to provide specimens for infertility treatment.

Premature ejaculation has the highest rates of treatment success (see Table 4). Psychological interventions in which couples are taught either the stop-start or squeeze technique have had fairly high success rates, although they are less successful when both partners are overconcerned with reproduction and underconcerned with sexual pleasuring or lovemaking. Medical treatment of ejaculatory problems is often difficult, although there are numerous medications that can sometimes delay ejaculation. Other treatment interventions include promoting couple communication and couple cooperation, teaching the man to concentrate on his genital sensations, and facilitating his mastery of a series of tasks that progressively provide more intense genital stimulation while he learns to control his ejaculatory response.

Inhibited or Delayed Ejaculation

Inhibited or delayed ejaculation or orgasm (traditionally called retarded ejaculation) is the persistent and recurrent inhibition of orgasm, manifested by delay or absence of ejaculation following adequate sexual excitement. It is commonly defined as a difficulty or inability to ejaculate during sexual intercourse or masturbation. Although failure to orgasm is fairly common in women, delayed or absence of orgasm in men is fairly rare. Inhibited male orgasm or delayed ejaculation ranges from mild situational delays in ejaculation to excessively long periods of intravaginal thrusting without orgasm. Historically, physical causes have been rare, although delayed ejaculation may be symptomatic of underlying medical conditions or due to physical conditions such as spinal chord injury. Recently, delayed ejaculation has been identified as a common side effect of some antidepressant medications, such as fluoxetine (Prozac). Psychological etiology may be due to performance anxiety, depression, anger, guilt regarding sex in general or with certain partners, relationship problems, traumatic sexual history, religious orthodoxy, prolonged fear of pregnancy leading to conditioned response, history of withdrawal method of birth control, gender identity issues, and/or partner unresponsiveness.

Treatment of inhibited male orgasm or delayed ejaculation has been notoriously difficult and time-consuming, with success often followed by relapse. Medical treatment for delayed ejaculation usually entails addressing underlying medical problems or the removal of medications. Psychological treatment of delayed ejaculation using sensate-focus techniques have been successful by increasing the man's awareness of his sexual sensations and arousal responses. Psychological interventions in which couples are taught either the stop-start or squeeze technique have had fairly high success rates, although they are less successful when both partners are overconcerned with reproduction and under-concerned with sexual pleasuring or lovemaking. Other psychological interventions aim at overcoming ejaculatory inhibitions, reducing fear and anxiety, improving couple interactions, and resolving underlying psychological conflicts, aggression, and problems. When delayed ejaculation affects fertility, electroejaculation or testicular biopsy can be used to obtain sperm for insemination of the female partner or use in IVF. However, this solution is only recommended when psychosocial causes have been ruled out or successfully treated, something many infertile couples resist in their relentless pursuit of pregnancy and their aversion to 'wasting time' in that pursuit.

Sexual Pain Disorders in Men

Disorders in men involving any form of pain during sexual activity (also termed male dyspareunia) are usually categorized on the basis of the point in the sexual act during which pain occurs: pain with erection, pain on intromission, or pain accompanying ejaculation. Sexual pain disorders in men are typically uncommon and are usually due to physical factors such as infection, tight foreskin, or spasm of the perineal muscles[66–68]. When no physical etiology can be identified, treatment usually consists of empirical medical remedies, reassurance of anatomical normalcy, and investigation of psychological factors[68]. Psychological interventions focus on adaptation to physical factors in pain disorder, the secondary gains of pain, illness behaviors, relaxation and behavioral-cognitive interventions, and relationship issues.

THERAPEUTIC INTERVENTIONS

Treatment of Sexual Dysfunction

Most couples are reluctant to discuss the private sexual aspects of their relationship, but even more so when sexual functioning may be problematic and/or involve behavior that is embarrassing or atypical for either one or both partners[69]. Infertile couples appear to be even more reluctant to discuss sexual dysfunction if they fear that it will interrupt medical treatment. Even so, no clinician working with infertile couples should *assume* that a couple is having regular sexual intercourse sufficient for reproduction or ignore the possibility of unusual sexual practices that interfere with conception. The first issue in any sexual history, especially regarding infertility, must address whether or not the couple is having sexual intercourse that involves penile ejaculation into the vagina on a regular basis.

Treatment success rates vary according to the specific sexual dysfunction: Premature ejaculation and vaginismus have the highest rates of treatment success, while primary erectile dysfunction has the lowest (see Table 4). Female orgasm disorders can be treated with considerable success, but the definition of success is often an issue: 85–95% success rate if orgasm with partner is the criterion but only 30–50% success rate if orgasm during intercourse is the criterion. Erectile dysfunctions have mixed success rates, with secondary erectile dysfunctions having higher rates of success than primary erectile dysfunction (no erections in any sexual situation). Mixed success is also the case for delayed ejaculations. In general, the most difficult sexual dysfunction to treat is low or inhibited sexual desire because of the intransigent nature of the disorder and the multifactorial nature of its etiology[63]. Finally, successful outcomes in sex therapy have been found to be influenced by the diagnosis of sexual dysfunction, the

Table 5 P-LI-SS-IT model

P	permission to talk about sexual issues, reassurance and empathy, and the acknowledgment that we are sexual beings
LI	limited information, including sex education; clarification of sexual myths and stereotypes; and bibliography with suggested related books
SS	specific suggestions, such as Kegel exercises, squeeze technique, or sensate focus
IT	intensive therapy, individual or conjoint, including focus on relationship dynamics and psychological concerns and other complex issues

(Reproduced from Annon and Robinson 1981, with permission)

pretreatment quality of a couple's general relationship, the quality of their pretreatment sexual relations, their motivation, medical diagnosis of infertility, type of sex therapy, and extent of progress made by the third treatment session[53].

Clinicians treating sexual problems can intervene on several different therapeutic levels. Annon and Robinson's[70] P-LI-SS-IT model of sexual counseling identifies four levels of intervention: (1) permission, (2) limited information, (3) specific suggestions, and (4) intensive therapy (Table 5). This behavioral therapy model is based on less intense to increasingly intensive interventions. The initial interventions involve encouraging discussions of the sexual problem and either providing basic information about sexual functioning and definition and explanation of the specific sexual problem, or educating about the particular situation, such as how infertility impacts sexual functioning. More intense therapeutic interventions and formal treatment may involve referral to a trained sex therapist or collaborative work between an infertility counselor and sex therapist.

Almost all approaches for the treatment of sexual dysfunction incorporate strategies of sexual reeducation designed to eliminate sexual myth and misinformation, attitude-changing techniques, marital and communication enhancement methods, and specific prescriptions for behavior change[71]. The basic behavioral techniques include:

- *anxiety-reduction techniques*: progressive relaxation, systematic desensitization, methohexital sodium (Brevital; a fast-acting muscle relaxant), and assertiveness training procedures
- *directed masturbation*: treatment for both anorgasmia and impotence
- *orgasmic reconditioning*: directed fantasy in conjunction with masturbation to modify the kinds of sexual stimuli associated with arousal
- *imagery techniques*: assessment and rehearsal of desired sexual responses
- *explicit homework assignments*: massage, self-stimulation, or couple communication exercises
- *sensate-focus technique*: exercises designed to help couples enrich their ways of touching each other initially and increasing their awareness of pleasurable feelings. Touch is initially nongenital, eventually leading to genital touching (Table 6).

At times, sex therapy includes the use of various devices, such as the vacuum constriction device and penile prosthesis for impotence and vaginal dilators or vibrators for vaginismus. Devices may be used alone or in combination with medical or surgical therapies, couples counseling, or interpersonal therapy. In all treatment of sexual dysfunction, religious proscriptions against masturbation, foreplay, and timing of sexual intercourse should be considered, as well as persistent marital difficulties, including preexisting marital disturbance, unrealistic sexual expectations, prior sexual trauma or victimization, and performance

Table 6 Sensate-focus exercises

Pleasuring without direct attempts to produce arousal/erection
Penile erection/arousal through genital pleasuring
Extravaginal orgasm
Penetration without orgasm
Full coitus with orgasm

pressures[7]. In truth, individuals often find the suggestions of homework, reading, or devices alarming or offensive. Finally, the success of treatment is contingent on diagnosis, motivation of the patient and his or her partner, the type of therapy, and the qualifications of the therapist, as well as the fundamentals of sexual intimacy—equality, mutuality, and reciprocity.

Prevention of Sexual Dysfunction in Infertile Couples

One of the goals of infertility counseling is the prevention of disturbance whenever possible, a goal that is particularly important to an infertile couple's sexual relationship (see Table 7). Prevention of sexual dysfunction may involve targeting either issues related to the medical treatment or the couple's relationship. Demands of medical treatment that strain sexual functioning include producing a sperm specimen for medical treatments, the requirement of midcycle sexual intercourse, and sexual intercourse followed by postcoital testing. It is important to carefully assess with a couple (and medical caregivers) the pros and cons of a treatment procedure in terms of its potential for contributing to or exacerbating sexual difficulties. For example, if a couple already has problems with sexual intercourse, the medical information provided by postcoital testing may be

Table 7 Tips for infertile couples on keeping sex enjoyable

For female sexual disorders: change sexual positions (woman on top or side by side), use over-the-counter pain medication before sexual intercourse, try preintercourse relaxation exercises, and/or hot baths

For problems with sperm collection: bring an audiotape player with ear plugs or ask to use the clinic video machine and bring own videotape with ear phones

Discuss sexual problems with physician or other caregivers

Educate oneself about normal sexual functioning and typical sexual problems of infertility

Don't 'sacrifice' rewarding sexual encounters or intimacy for infertility treatment

For marital problems (in addition to sexual difficulties): seek help from qualified infertility counselor

Take turns planning special sex 'dates' at nonfertile times

Practice 'nonintercourse' sexual pleasuring

Plan treatment 'holidays' with focus on renewing physical intimacy and warmth

Plan a hotel date or special time away from home for 'distraction-free' sex

Renew commitment to each other

Devote time to activities and interests you as a couple really enjoy

Try sexual 'play', as you did early in your relationship

Be creative and inventive

Take your time

When interest wanes, try erotic books, board games, or videotapes

---

minimal, compared to the deleterious effect on their sexual relationship. By the same token, every effort should be made to accommodate a couple's sexual problems and religious proscriptions. For men with problems producing a sperm sample,

assistance may involve allowing his wife to assist, providing special sperm collection condoms to be used during intercourse, or making environmental accommodations (e.g., providing erotica, more secluded 'collection' room). For example, some clinics use a regular examination room for specimen collection, and men complain of difficulty concentrating because they overhear normal clinic conversations ('Paging Dr. Jones' or 'Mrs. Doe is here for her pregnancy testing'). Short of renovating the clinic, it may be useful for these men to bring a tape player with ear plugs to block out clinic sounds. For couples with female pain problems (perhaps related to endometriosis or ovulation induction), changing sexual positions, the use of over-the-counter pain medication *before* sexual intercourse, or preintercourse relaxation exercises, massage, and hot baths may be beneficial.

Sometimes, the most effective means of preventing sexual dysfunction is simply addressing with the couple their sexual relationship and specifically asking each partner about common sexual problems, such as painful intercourse, sex on demand, and problems with specimen production. Couples usually respond with relief at being given permission to discuss these problems, especially men who are often embarrassed by problems such as shyness about specimen production, midcycle sexual problems, or sex causing or increasing pain in their partners. For these couples, preventing problems may involve basic education, offering helpful tips, or encouraging them to discuss the problems with their physician or infertility counselor. This can also normalize sexual problems for the infertile couple, minimizing guilt and stigma, while helping them understand the nature of common sexual problems in infertility. In this manner, the importance of their sexual relationship is validated, and they are encouraged not to 'sacrifice' sexual rewards for the sake of a pregnancy or infertility treatment.

Prevention of sexual problems also involves addressing relationship issues and giving couples education and support regarding sexual matters. If the sexual problems reflect more fundamental relationship problems, it may be that marital issues must take precedence over further infertility treatment. This is especially important if there is evidence of an extramarital affair or sexual behavior that is likely to precipitate a marital crisis, such as homosexuality or sexual behavior for which an individual may be arrested (e.g., victimization, use of prostitutes).

For less serious problems, prevention may simply involve encouraging couples to keep their sexual relationship rewarding, interesting, and enlivened (Table 8). For couples complaining of lost spontaneity, the benefits of planned, special sex 'dates' at nonfertile times may be explored, or they may be given homework in which each partner takes responsibility for planning a sexual 'surprise'. Couples may wish to explore 'nonintercourse' sexual expression, such as massage or sensate-focus exercises (see Table 6) that emphasize physical closeness and nongenital pleasuring. Taking treatment 'holidays' is always a helpful hint, but couples may be encouraged to use the holiday to renew physical intimacy and warmth by spending an evening at a hotel or away from home, renewing their commitment to each other, devoting time in activities that they as a couple find particularly enjoyable, and learning to 'play' with each other again as they did early in their relationship together. For couples who have a difficult time being creative, using books, videotapes, or educational materials may be beneficial, especially those that give ideas on how to be intimate and close. These can, but need not be, actual erotica. For couples complaining of loss of interest or desire

Table 8 Therapeutic recommendations

Ask about sexual functioning and satisfaction; then ask again later

Look for evidence or indications of sexual problems

Watch for signs in spouse or marriage of excessive difficulties coping

Watch for signs of marital conflict and disturbance

Encourage discussion and improved communication between partners about sexual issues

Encourage couple to become educated about normal sexual functioning and sexual activity

Recommend against ritualized, mechanistic, procreation approaches to sex

Suggest planning sexual activities that are not for procreation only

Encourage sexual activities that are playful, enjoyable, or interesting, especially during nontreatment times

Provide educational materials about sexual functioning

Inquire about how stressful patient perceives medical treatments

Be aware of mood disorders that may effect sexual functioning

Make referrals to appropriate sex therapy professional

Encourage patient or couple to discuss the sexual problem with infertility caregiver

(and there is no evidence of depression or other psychological factors), discussions may focus on increasing awareness of sexual cues and what the couple finds erotic or arousing. Homework may involve erotic reading materials, board games, or videotapes that increase the individual's or couple's awareness of what they find exciting.

Although prevention of sexual distress should be a primary goal for all infertility caregivers, it often is not. And worse, it may not be a priority for the infertile couple who is singularly focused on having a baby, after which they believe all their problems will be solved and their sexual relationship will return to its 'preinfertility' level of satisfaction. Of course, this is one of the myths that the infertility counselor must address, helping couples understand that postinfertility (especially when they are parents) will have its own challenges and prevention at this time is worth a pound of cure later on[72].

Ethical Dilemmas

One of the ethical dilemmas of sexual dysfunction in couples undergoing medical treatment for infertility is the patient or couple who requests medical interventions in order to avoid sexual intercourse or treatment of a sexual dysfunction. This may include the patient with primary sexual dysfunction who wishes to have a family or the couple who develops sexual problems secondary to infertility treatment. A couple with unconsummated marriage, sexual aversion, primary impotence, or vaginismus, while acknowledging the dysfunction and refusing appropriate treatment, may present desiring inseminations or even IVF in order to become pregnant. Some couples will develop midcycle impotence or vaginismus, sexual avoidance, inability to produce sperm specimen for IVF or inseminations, or other sexual problems over the course of treatment and request treatments, such as husband insemination, that will accommodate their sexual difficulties. The ethical dilemma is that the sexual problem may mask more severe psychological or marital problems, while at the same time additional medical treatment may further strain individual or couple functioning. Will assisting these couples in achieving pregnancy further impair individual, couple, or family functioning? Should couples be assisted in achieving pregnancy when there is evidence of a disturbance that may impact or impair family or parental adjustment, such as in cases of disturbed gender identity or latent homosexuality? Should medical treatment for infertility proceed unchecked even when patients refuse psychological or sexual treatment, although they have acknowledged the existence of significant problems? What about the well-being of the 'whole' patient or couple and comprehensive care?

These questions often pose very real dilemmas for medical caregivers and for infertile couples, especially if their avoidant coping style and/or their fixation on parenthood clouds their judgment about the health and well-being of their marriage, family, their potential children, and themselves.

It seems that, in accordance with the ethical principle of 'to do no harm', patients with acknowledged primary sexual dysfunction causing infertility should not proceed with medical treatment for infertility, especially as a means of avoiding more appropriate treatment. In addition, although some patients may proceed with infertility treatment in the presence of some sexual dysfunctions, medical treatment should be in conjunction with psychotherapy and/or sex therapy, thereby emphasizing the importance of sexual health and well-being in infertile couples.

Role of the Infertility Counselor

Whether sexual dysfunction is a preexisting condition or an unwelcome side effect of infertility treatment, it can be a devastating and discouraging blow, compounding the disappointment of childlessness and the distress of medical treatment. Although at some point in infertility treatment sex may become regulatory, obligatory, and uninspired, not all infertile couples experience sexual difficulties. Nevertheless, changes in sexual practices or behavior may often occur, such as the initiator of sexual encounters, preferred sexual positions, reduced sexual activity during the luteal phase, or increased midcycle frequency. Adaptation to these changes not only contributes to a couple's self-confidence in managing the crisis and stresses of infertility but can improve communication and marital satisfaction. When infertility results in relationship disturbance or sexual problems, the support and intervention of caregivers is paramount. All too often, the sexual problems of infertile couples are ignored or minimized in a belief that they will dissipate on their own or will have few long-term consequences. Unfortunately, these beliefs are myths. Although some sexual problems may disappear when the pressures of infertility treatment end, sexual difficulties typically linger or become more problematic after treatment ends or parenthood is achieved[73,74].

Most infertility counselors are not certified sex therapists and are therefore not qualified to provide sex therapy as such. However, sexual problems can be integrated into psychotherapy by providing sexual education specific to infertility, brief interventions, and marital counseling (see Table 7). The infertility counselor should, at a minimum, become familiar with the sexual problems relevant to infertility, treatment methods, success rates, and typical as well as atypical psychosexual responses to infertility treatment[72,73]. Also important is an awareness of available resources, organizations, and sex therapists in the area with expertise or special interest in treating infertile couples or willingness to collaborate with a qualified sex therapist with a special interest in reproductive health.

FUTURE IMPLICATIONS

As our understanding of sexual functioning has increased dramatically over the past several decades, so has our understanding of the relation of sexual functioning and infertility. Considerable research has contributed to dispelling long-standing myths and inaccuracies about infertility and sexual functioning (e.g., that failure to orgasm in women or tubal spasms cause infertility or that sperm quality or production is diminished by stress). However, there continues to be a need for well designed research in the area of sexual functioning and infertility. What is the actual incidence of sexual dysfunction among infertile men and women? What is the incidence of sexual dysfunction causing infertility? What is the incidence of specific sexual dysfunctions within the context of infertility and which are more common? Is the incidence of diagnosable sexual dysfunction more common in infertile women or men? Are there specific infertility diagnoses or treatments that are more detrimental to sexual functioning in infertile couples? What are the circumstances that make it easier for patients to bring up sexual problems with their caregivers?

As treatment of infertility involves higher rates of technology use, making sexual intercourse less important, sexual dysfunctions secondary to infertility may become less problematic. And as reproductive technologies become more prevalent and procreation through sexual intercourse less fundamental to the process, it may be that the rates of sexual dysfunction will decline, and sexual intercourse will be valued for the intimacy and relationship rewards that it provides. On the other hand, increased reliance on assisted reproductive technologies may represent the technologizing of our society and interpersonal relationships, allowing more distance, mechanization, and reserve and thereby impeding intimacy, warmth, and connections.

SUMMARY

- The ability to reproduce is intimately tied to sexuality, self-image, and self-esteem. The extent to which this is important varies with cultural expectations, individuals, and the impact of medical conditions and treatment.

- Although sexual problems can occur during infertility, sometimes even causing infertility, sexual difficulties are not universally experienced by infertile couples. The majority of infertile couples do not develop diagnosable sexual problems requiring intensive treatment, although they may experience episodic, transient problems warranting education and support.

- The medical assessment and treatment for infertility may interfere with the infertile couple's sexual pleasure due to performance demand, treatment requirements, or emotional response to treatment or infertility diagnosis.

- A large percentage of sexual problems may be addressed by the infertility counselor educated about the impact of infertility on sexual functioning. Professional attention and education regarding sexual difficulties during infertility can minimize the impact and even prevent many of the sexual difficulties infertile couples encounter.

- Since most couples do not volunteer sexual problems, caregivers must specifically ask questions about sexual behavior as part of a comprehensive medical and social history.

- When sexual dysfunction is the presenting cause of infertility, assessment and therapy for the couple is necessary and should preclude medical treatment for infertility.

REFERENCES

1. Edelmann RJ, Humphrey M, Owens DJ. The meaning of parenthood and couples' reactions to male infertility. *Br J Med Psychol* 1994;67:291–9
2. Fogel CI, Lauver D. *Sexual Health Promotion*. Philadelphia: Saunders, 1990
3. Benedek T. Infertility as a psychosomatic defense. *Fertil Steril* 1952;3:527–41
4. Benedek T, Ham GC, Robbins FP, *et al.* Some emotional factors in infertility. *Psychosom Med* 1953;15:485–98
5. Fischer IC. Psychogenic aspects of sterility. *Fertil Steril* 1953;4:466–71
6. Rubenstein BB. An emotional factor in infertility: A psychosomatic approach. *Fertil Steril* 1951;2:80–6
7. Belonoschkin B. Psychosomatic factors and matrimonial infertility. *Int J Fertil* 1962; 7:29–36
8. de Watteville H. Psychologic factors in the treatment of sterility. *Fertil Steril* 1957;8:12–24
9. Walker HE. Psychiatric aspects of infertility. *Urol Clin North Am* 1978;5:481–8
10. Rutherford RN. Emotional aspects of infertility. *Clin Obstet Gynecol* 1965;8:100–14
11. Cohen HR. The psychosomatic factor in infertility. *Int J Fertil* 1961;6:369–73
12. Eisner BB. Some psychological differences between fertile and infertile women. *J Clin Psychiatry* 1963;19:391–5
13. Riddick DH. Sexual dysfunction: Cause and result of infertility. *Fem Patient* 1982; 7:45–8
14. Elstein M. Effect of infertility on psychosexual function. *Br Med J* 1975;3:296–9
15. Fugate KA, McCluskey MM. The impact of sexually transmitted diseases on fertility: A review of literature and nursing opportunities. *Infertil Reprod Med Clin North Am* 1996;7:521–34
16. World Health Organization. Infections, pregnancies, and infertility: Perspectives on prevention. *Fertil Steril* 1987;47:964–8
17. Kramer DG, Brown ST. Sexually transmitted disease and infertility. *J Gynaecol Obstet* 1984;22:19–27
18. Cook DL, Porth CM. Sexually transmitted diseases. In: Porth CM, ed. *Pathophysiology:*

Concepts of Altered States, 2nd edn. Philadelphia: Lippincott, 1986

19. Infertility and sexually transmitted disease: A public health challenge. *Popul Rep* 1983;11:L113–L51

20. Spector IP, Carey MP. Incidence and prevalence of the sexual dysfunctions: A critical review of the empirical literature. *Arch Sex Beh* 1990;19:389–408

21. Daniluk JC. Infertility: Intrapersonal and interpersonal impact. *Fertil Steril* 1988; 49:982–90

22. van Balen F, Trimbos-Kemper TCM. Long-term infertile couples: A study of their well-being. *J Psychosom Obstet Gynaecol* 1993; 14(suppl):53–60

23. Leader A. Infertility: Clinical and psychological aspects. *Psychiatr Ann* 1984;14:461–7

24. Matthews A, Matthews R. Beyond the mechanics of infertility: Perspectives of the social psychology of infertility and involuntary childlessness. *Fam Rel* 1986;35:479–87

25. Berg BJ, Wilson JF. Psychological functioning across stages of treatment in infertility. *J Behav Med* 1991;14:11–26

26. Carr GD. *A Psychosociological Study of Fertile and Infertile Marriages*. Los Angeles: University of Southern California, 1963. PhD thesis.

27. Andrews FM, Abbey A, Halman J. Stress from infertility, marriage factors, and subjective well-being of wives and husbands. *J Health Soc Behav* 1991;32:238–53

28. Keye WR. The impact of infertility on psychosexual function. *Fertil Steril* 1980;34:308–9

29. van Zyl JA. Sex and infertility, part II: Influence of psychogenic factors and psychosexual problems. *S Afr Med J* 1987; 72:485–7

30. Aribarg S, Aribarg A. Psychosexual factors in infertility. *J Med Assoc Thai* 1985;68:87–90

31. Dubin L, Amelar RD. Sexual causes of male infertility. *Fertil Steril* 1972;23:579–82

32. Mozley P. Emotional parameters of infertility. In: Youngs D, Ehrhardt A, eds. *Psychosomatic Obstetrics and Gynecology*. New York: Appleton-Century-Crofts, 1980

33. Rutledge AL. Psychomarital evaluation and treatment of the infertile couple. *Clin Obstet Gynecol* 1979;22:255–67

34. Rosen R, Leiblum SR. Assessment and treatment of desire disorders. In: Rosen R, Leiblum SR, eds. *Principles and Practice in Sex Therapy: Update for the 1990s*. New York: Guilford Press, 1989:19–47

35. Hamer PM, Bain J. Ejaculatory incompetence and infertility. *Fertil Steril* 1986;45:384–7

36. Pepe MV, Byrne TJ. Women's perceptions of immediate and long-term effects of failed infertility treatment on marital and sexual satisfaction. *Fam Rel* 1991;40:303–9

37. Slade P. Sexual attitudes and social role orientations in infertile women. *J Psychosom Res* 1981;25:183–6

38. Benazon N, Wright J, Sabourin S, et al. Stress, sexual satisfaction and marital adjustment in infertile couples. *J Sex Marital Ther* 1992;18:273–84

39. Keye WR, Deneris A. Female sexual activity, satisfaction and function in infertile women. *Infertility* 1982;5:265–85

40. Hammond KR, Kretzer PA, Blackwell RE, et al. Performance anxiety during infertility treatment: Effect of semen quality. *Fertil Steril* 1990;53:337–40

41. Karahasanoglu A, Barglow P, Growe G. Psychological aspects of infertility. *J Reprod Med* 1972;9:241–7

42. Barraglia AR, Graziano MR, Scafidi MG. Experimental research into the changes in the way sexuality is experienced by the infertile female. *Acta Eur Fertil* 1983;14:67–73

43. Keye WR. Psychosexual responses to infertility. *Clin Obstet Gynecol* 1984;27:760–6

44. Boivin J, Takefman JE, Brender W, et al. The effects of female sexual response in coitus on early reproductive process. *J Behav Med* 1992;15:509–18

45. Berger DM. Impotence following the discovery of azoospermia. *Fertil Steril* 1980;34:154–6

46. Drake T, Grunert G. A cyclic pattern of sexual dysfunction in the infertility investigation. *Fertil Steril* 1979;32:542–5

47. Nachtigall RD, Becker G, Wozny M. The effects of gender-specific diagnosis on men's and women's response to infertility. *Fertil Steril* 1992;57:113–21

48. Kemer P, Mikulincer M, Nathanson YE, et al. Psychological aspects of male infertility. *Br J Med Psychol* 1990;63(pt 10):73–80

49. Baram D, Tourtelot E, Muehler E, et al.

Psychological adjustment following unsuccessful in vitro fertilization. *J Psychosom Obstet Gynaecol* 1988;9:181–90

50. Fagan PJ, Schmidt CW, Rock JA, *et al.* Sexual functioning and psychologic evaluation of in vitro fertilization couples. *Fertil Steril* 1986;46:668–72

51. Laffont I, Edelmann RJ. Psychological aspects of in vitro fertilization: A gender comparison. *J Psychosom Obstet Gynaecol* 1994;15:85–92

52. Masters WH, Johnson VE. *Human Sexual Response*. Boston: Little, Brown, 1966

53. Kaplan HS. *Evaluation of Sexual Disorders: Psychological and Medical Aspects*. New York: Brunner/Mazel, 1983

54. Burns LH. An overview of the psychology of infertility: Comprehensive psychosocial history of infertility. *Infertil Reprod Med Clin North Am* 1993;4:433–54

55. Bernstein J. Psychological evaluation of the infertile couple. In: Seibel MM, Kiessling AA, Bernstein J, *et al.*, eds. *Technology and Infertility: Clinical, Psychosocial, Legal, and Ethical Aspects*. New York: Springer-Verlag, 1993;289–96

56. LoPiccolo L. Low sexual desire. In: Leiblum SR, Pervin LA, eds. *Principles and Practice of Sex Therapy*. New York: Guilford Press, 1980;27–64

57. Schover LR, LoPiccolo J. Treatment effectiveness for dysfunctions of sexual desire. *J Sex Marital Ther* 1982;8:179–97

58. Utian WH, Goldfard JM, Rosenthal MB. Psychological aspects of infertility. In: Dennerstein L, Burrows G, eds. *Handbook of Psychosomatic Obstetrics and Gynecology*. New York: Elsevier Biomedical Press, 1983;231–48

59. Sanderson MO, Maddock JW. Guidelines for assessment and treatment of sexual dysfunction. *Obstet Gynecol* 1989;73:130–5

60. Reading AE. Sexual aspects of infertility and its treatment. *Infertil Reprod Med Clin North Am* 1993;4:559–67

61. LoPiccolo L. Sexual dysfunction. In: Craighead LW, Craighead WE, Kazdin AE, *et al.*, eds. *Cognitive and Behavioral Interventions: An Empirical Approach to Mental*

Health Problems. Boston: Allyn & Bacon, 1994;183–96

62. Bachman GA. Dyspareunia and vaginismus. In: Sexual Dysfunction: Patient Concerns and Practical Strategies, 24th annual postgraduate course of the American Fertility Society, 1991

63. Heiman JR, LoPiccolo L, LoPiccolo J. The treatment of sexual dysfunction. In: Gurman AL, Kniskern D, eds. *Handbook of Family Therapy*. New York: Brunner/Mazel, 1981;592–630

64. Mazor M. Emotional reactions to infertility. In: Mazor MD, Simon HF, eds. *Infertility: Medical, Emotional, and Social Considerations*. New York: Human Sciences Press, 1984;23–35

65. Amelar RD, Dubin L, Walsh PC. *Male Infertility*. Philadelphia: Saunders, 1977

66. Bain J. Sexuality and infertility in the male. *Can J Hum Sex* 1993;2:157–60

67. Ellis A. Treatment of erectile dysfunction. In: Leiblum SR, Pervin LA, eds. *Principles and Practice of Sex Therapy*. New York: Guilford Press, 1980;235–61

68. Masters WH, Johnson VE. *Human Sexual Inadequacy*. Boston: Little, Brown, 1970

69. Bachmann GA, Leiblum SR, Grill J. Brief sexual inquiry in gynecologic practice. *Obstet Gynecol* 1989;73:425–7

70. Annon J, Robinson C. Behavioral treatment of sexual dysfunctions. In: Sha'Ked A, ed. *Human Sexuality and Rehabilitation Medicine: Sexual Functioning Following Spinal Cord Injury*. Baltimore: Williams & Wilkins, 1981;104–18

71. Leiblum SR, Previn LA. The development of sex therapy from a sociocultural perspective. In: Leiblum ST, Previn LA, eds. *Principles and Practice of Sex Therapy*. New York: Guilford Press, 1980;1–26

72. Burns LH. Infertility and the sexual health of the family. *J Sex Educ Ther* 1987;14:30–4

73. Burns LH. An overview of sexual dysfunction in the infertile couple. *J Fam Psychother* 1995;6:25–46

74. Boxer AS. Infertility and sexual dysfunction. *Infertil Reprod Med Clin North Am* 1996;7:565–75

IV.   MEDICAL COUNSELING ISSUES

10

Patients with Medically Complicating Conditions

Donald B. Maier, MD, and Louise U. Maier, PhD

Perfect health, like perfect beauty, is a rare thing;
and so, it seems, is perfect disease.

Peter Mere Latham

HISTORICAL OVERVIEW

Infertility patients with medically complicating conditions often present with complex psychological issues. Medical conditions such as diabetes, hypertension, and endometriosis have always affected some patients seeking infertility services. While these patients with other medical problems have been a relatively small percentage of the infertile population in the past, their numbers are increasing. There are several reasons for this trend. First, due to better medical treatment, there are now more people living with chronic diseases such as diabetes, acquired immunodeficiency syndrome (AIDS), and cancer in remission. Second, the demographic trend of delaying pregnancy has resulted in more older infertility patients, and people are more likely to develop medical problems as they get older. Third, new reproductive treatment options, such as egg donation, intracytoplasmic sperm injection (ICSI), and gestational carrier, make pregnancy and biological parenthood possible for many patients whose medically complicating condition had previously resulted

in untreatable infertility. The purposes of this chapter are:

- to describe the medical conditions that cause infertility or impact infertility treatment
- to discuss the psychological and counseling issues that arise for infertility patients with chronic medical conditions.

MEDICAL OVERVIEW

The first section of this chapter will review the medical conditions that can impact on infertility and its treatment. The impact can be direct, where the medical condition causes infertility, or indirect. In the latter category (indirect) are diseases in which treatment impairs fertility, the desire for fertility alters treatment of the medical condition, genetic traits or the disease itself may be passed to the offspring, or pregnancy outcome is altered by the disease (Table 1). It is important to consider the impact of medical conditions on both the couple's fertility and their subsequent pregnancy.

Table 1 Categories of relationships between medical conditions and infertility

---

1. Medical conditions that may cause infertility
 Endometriosis
 Cancers—testicular, ovarian, Hodgkin's
  disease
 Klinefelter's syndrome
 Turner's syndrome
 Rokitansky-Küster-Hauser syndrome

2. Medical conditions whose treatment may cause infertility
 Male hypertension
 Cancers—testicular, ovarian, cervical, breast,
  Hodgkin's disease
 Endometriosis

3. Medical conditions in which the patient's choice of treatment may be influenced by his or her desire for fertility
 Endometriosis
 Hodgkin's disease
 Breast cancer
 Borderline ovarian cancers

4. Medical conditions in which genetic traits or the disease itself may be passed along to offspring
 Cystic fibrosis
 Severe male infertility
 Breast cancer
 Acquired immunodeficiency syndrome

5. Medical conditions in which the primary impact is on the pregnancy
 Diabetes
 Asthma
 Lupus
 Heart disease

Medical Conditions and Fertility: Categories

It is possible to group the interactions between medical conditions and fertility into five categories (see Table 1). The first category includes diseases or syndromes that cause infertility, and the second involves diseases whose treatment causes infertility. The third category encompasses diseases that have several possible treatments, the choice of which may be influenced by a patient's desire for fertility. The fourth group of medical conditions is one of increasing importance and includes diseases in which genetic traits or the disease itself may be passed along to the offspring. Finally, there are diseases whose main impact is not on conception but on the resultant pregnancy; either the disease process or its treatment may be affected by a pregnancy or the pregnancy may be adversely affected by a medical condition. Some medical conditions will interact with fertility in many ways, and these groupings may be helpful to therapists in categorizing the difficulties faced by some infertile individuals.

Medical Conditions Affecting Males

Male infertility is infrequently caused by medical conditions. Overall, approximately 1% of men referred for urological evaluation because of a low sperm count are found to have a serious medical condition[1]. Diseases impacting male fertility include hypertension (high blood pressure), diabetes, cystic fibrosis, Hodgkin's lymphoma, and testicular cancer. With other medical problems such as AIDS and genetic causes of infertility, transmission of the disease to others is the primary concern.

Hypertension

Hypertension does not cause infertility, but its treatment may. Impotence or difficulty in maintaining an erection are side effects of several antihypertensive medications. Understandably, such difficulties may cause infertility by preventing sexual intercourse. In addition, medications can interfere with a man's ability to ejaculate at specific, stressful times, such as at ovulation or when a semen specimen is needed for in vitro fertilization (IVF). In the latter situation, sperm cryopreservation may be helpful in allowing a man to produce a semen sample under less stressful conditions, with the sample being used later when needed. Alternatively, changing medications may be necessary if there are other medications that can still control the man's blood pressure without these side effects.

One group of antihypertensive medications, calcium channel blockers, can interfere with male fertility more subtly. These medications interfere with the acrosome reaction, a process by which sperm acquire the capacity to fertilize eggs[2]. When men taking these medications are treated with a different medication, their sperm undergo the acrosome reaction at a normal rate. Because this fertilization problem cannot be detected through a routine semen analysis, it is unclear how many men on calcium channels blockers have impaired fertility. Until there is an adequate test for fertilization, it is prudent to have infertile men use another medication. This side effect of these drugs is not commonly known, and a counselor may be the first health care professional to bring this connection to a patient's attention. These medications are also used for prevention of migraine headaches.

Cancer: Hodgkin's Lymphoma and Testicular Cancer

Cancer or its treatment may cause male infertility. This topic has been well reviewed by Meirow and Schenker[3]. Testicular cancer and Hodgkin's lymphoma are two of the more common cancers in young men.

Testicular cancer is a serious cause of male infertility, and male fertility may already be impaired at the time of diagnosis[4]. While the cure rate is high with removal of only one testicle, fertility may be impaired by subsequent chemotherapy. Sperm cryopreservation should be discussed with all men diagnosed with

testicular cancer, even if they have no immediate plans for reproduction. With the advent of ICSI, even a few barely motile sperm may be sufficient to establish a pregnancy. Unfortunately, this option is not always presented to men with testicular cancer prior to chemotherapy. Whether sperm retrieval directly from the testicles would be able to isolate sperm from men with no sperm in their ejaculate after chemotherapy is not presently known. Even if this were possible, it is an invasive procedure that would result in the use of sperm exposed to mutagenic drugs; therefore, cryopreservation of sperm prior to chemotherapy is clearly preferable.

Hodgkin's lymphoma is another cancer that commonly occurs in young individuals. As with testicular cancer, sperm quality may be abnormal at the time the disease is diagnosed and may be decreased by chemotherapy, especially MOPP (mechlorethamine, vincristine [Oncovin], procarbazine, prednisone). However, treatment with ABVD (doxorubicin [Adriamycin], bleomycin, vinblastine, dacarbazine) has much less of an impact on future fertility and has as good a cure rate[5]. Regardless of the type of therapy that is planned, pretreatment sperm cryopreservation should be discussed with these men.

Cystic Fibrosis

It has been known for some time that men with cystic fibrosis commonly have partial absence of the vas deferens (tubes that carry sperm from the testicles)[6]. Recently, physicians have become aware that approximately 50% of apparently healthy men with an absent vas deferens have mutations in the cystic fibrosis gene[7]. With recent advances in microsurgical epididymal sperm aspiration, sperm can now be retrieved from the epididymis and used in IVF. However, there are two important counseling considerations. The first is that some individuals with cystic fibrosis have very minimal pulmonary symptoms and are not diagnosed with cystic fibrosis until they are evaluated for azoospermia. The second is that many individuals with partial absence of the vas deferens are carriers of cystic fibrosis. If their female partners are also carriers, they have a 25% chance of having a child with this typically very serious disease and a 50% chance of having a child who is also a carrier. The counseling issues therefore also involve genetic counseling, as these individuals (and their partners) need to decide between donor insemination and ICSI (see Chapter 11).

AIDS

AIDS does not impair male fertility until the more advanced stages, and its effects may be lessened with antiviral therapy[8]. The primary concern is disease transmission to the partner or child. If the couple has been practicing safe sex, attempts to conceive will put the woman at risk. It is unclear to what extent this risk can be reduced by sperm preparation that may remove the human immunodeficiency virus (HIV). Semprini and colleagues[9] reported a series of 29 HIV-positive men whose sperm was used for intrauterine insemination after having been prepared to eliminate viral contamination. None of the women inseminated became HIV-positive. This technique has not been reported by other investigators, but it may be promising. However, it should be noted that some researchers[10] have observed HIV particles within sperm.

Diabetes

Diabetes can affect male fertility in two ways. Neurological damage may cause difficulties with erection or ejaculation. In addition, sperm counts may be decreased.

Medication Use

In addition to the antihypertensive medications mentioned above, other medic-

ations can affect male fertility, a side effect frequently not recognized as a problem by prescribing physicians. Medications that can reduce sperm counts or motility include sulfasalazine (Azulfidine), used to treat inflammatory bowel disease; cimetidine (Tagamet), an antiulcer medication; nitrofurantoin (Furadantin, Macrobid, Macrodantin, etc.), an antibiotic that is only toxic at high doses; and spironolactone (Aldactone), a diuretic.

Genetic Causes of Male Infertility

Recent advances in the use of ICSI for severely oligospermic males (men with very low sperm counts) has raised a new question. Approximately 13% of these cases appear to be caused by a genetic factor, specifically a deletion in a gene on the Y chromosome called azoospermia factor gene[11]. While these men may now be able to produce children, their sons may be at a high risk for themselves having infertility (or other unknown health problems) because they will inherit this abnormal gene. In the future, genetic testing will be able to assist these men in deciding whether to proceed with ICSI or donor insemination. Mak and Jarvi[12] recently reviewed this rapidly evolving area (see Chapter 11).

Medical Conditions Affecting Females

Medical conditions are more likely to impact females or their treatment. Some of the following diseases are more common in women than in men, affect female but not male fertility, or have effects on the potential pregnancy. These conditions can affect the reproductive system directly, their treatment can damage the ovaries, or they may primarily complicate pregnancies that may already be at high risk because of infertility treatments

Premature Ovarian Failure

Women may have nonfunctioning or absent ovaries for multiple reasons. Turner's syndrome is a common cause of absent ovarian function from birth. Women with this syndrome have only one X chromosome, as opposed to the usual two. They have very early loss of all oocytes, so that at birth the residual ovarian tissue is small (streak ovaries) and nonfunctional. These women also have a characteristic group of physical changes, including significantly short stature and webbing of the neck. However, because the tubes, uterus, cervix, and vagina are formed independently from the ovaries, women with Turner's syndrome can carry a pregnancy as long as donor eggs are used. Other than the potential impact of multiple gestations on women with short stature or on those with certain cardiac conditions that can accompany this syndrome, a woman with Turner's syndrome does not appear to have any special medical considerations differing from those in any woman using donor eggs.

Hodgkin's Disease

As with men, treatment of women with Hodgkin's disease with ABVD is much less likely to cause gonadal failure than treatment with MOPP[13]. Unfortunately, oocyte freezing is not a common technique; typically, a woman cannot have eggs cryopreserved prior to chemotherapy as a man can have his sperm frozen. Therefore, the main hope that women with this disease have for future fertility rests in the development of less toxic chemotherapy regimens. Rarely, it may be possible to perform IVF prior to the initiation of chemotherapy, and then cryopreserve the resultant embryos for implantation after chemotherapy is completed.

Breast Cancer

Breast cancer victims often present with fertility concerns, since 10–20% of breast cancers occur in reproductive-age women[14]. While in most cases breast cancer does not require removal of any reproductive organs, it can profoundly affect fertility. Chemotherapy is commonly used and can result in temporary cessation of menses or permanent ovarian failure. The class of drugs most effective in breast cancer, the alkylating agents, are unfortunately especially toxic to the ovaries. These effects are worse and may be permanent if the dosages are high, the treatment is prolonged, or the woman is older and has fewer oocytes. Even with younger women, rates of ovarian failure are high; it is estimated that 50% of women less than 35 years old will become menopausal after chemotherapy for breast cancer[15]. At the present, there are no good alternatives for a woman facing chemotherapy who would like to increase her chances for subsequent fertility. Unlike the situation with Hodgkin's disease, there are no alternative chemotherapy treatment regimens that have a lesser impact on ovarian function. Use of natural cycle IVF, where the egg or eggs that result from the normal unstimulated menstrual cycle are retrieved, has been reported in one woman with newly diagnosed breast cancer prior to chemotherapy[16]. Her embryos were cryopreserved for future use. This alternative may be helpful for some women, but its use and success are limited. In the future, cryopreservation of ovaries may be a fertility-preserving possibility for these women and others who face imminent loss of ovarian function.

If a woman with a history of breast cancer desires to conceive, it is important for her to consider the possibility that she might have a recurrence of her disease during pregnancy. Breast cancer is more difficult to diagnose and treat in pregnancy. Because most cases of aggressive disease will recur within 2 years of diagnosis, the current recommendation is that women with breast cancer wait at least 2 years before attempting to conceive. It is important to note that there are no reports of any increase in either miscarriages or birth defects in pregnancies conceived by women previously treated with any form of chemotherapy.

Several other issues need to be considered. Besides the initial problem of the effect of disease treatment on fertility, there is also the question of possible effects of pregnancy or fertility treatments on disease recurrence. Many breast cancers are estrogen-sensitive, and it is known that removal of the ovaries or treatment with antiestrogens, such as tamoxifen citrate (Novaldex), will decrease the recurrence risk in these women. Hormonal therapies that enhance conception (superovulation, IVF) and pregnancy itself will result in high estrogen levels. Whether these increased hormone levels would increase the chance for a recurrence is an important question. There are no data that specifically address the issue of fertility treatments and breast cancer recurrence, although the general question of an increased risk of breast cancer from use of clomiphene citrate[17] (Clomid, Serophene) and IVF[18] has been addressed. Rossing and associates[17] found no increased risk of breast cancer in women who had taken clomiphene, compared to the rate in the general population. Similarly, Venn and coworkers[18] found no increase in the incidence of breast cancer in 5564 women who had IVF, compared with 4794 infertile controls who had not. Despite the large number of subjects, this study had a relatively short follow-up period and did not address the question of the recurrence risk faced by a woman who has already had breast cancer.

The data concerning the risk of later recurrence in women who have a pregnancy following breast cancer treatment are more reassuring. There are no studies that show a worsened prognosis in women with a history of breast cancer who conceive compared to those who do not[14]. However, the studies are small and not well designed. Ideally, women whose cancers are estrogen-receptor positive would need to be studied.

Another medical consideration for breast cancer survivors who still have ovarian function is the increased chance that their daughters will have breast cancer. It is apparent that counseling this group of women is a complex task. In the absence of any large, long-term studies, patients, physicians, and counselors are left without data that can help in answering many of their important questions.

Cancer of the Reproductive System

Cervical cancer occurs most commonly in reproductive-age women, and its treatment can be altered if the woman desires fertility. For early-stage cervical cancer, surgery has replaced ovary-damaging radiation therapy. While hysterectomy (removal of the cervix and uterus) may be necessary, the ovaries do not need to be removed. These women can become mothers by having embryos created from their eggs implanted in a gestational carrier.

Ovarian cancer most commonly occurs in women beyond the reproductive years and is therefore an infrequent cause of infertility. When it does occur in younger women, removal of both ovaries is often necessary, as the disease usually is not diagnosed until it has spread. There are some types of borderline tumors of lower malignant potential where removal of one ovary may be curative. It is suggested that these women have the other ovary removed when they are finished with childbearing. Fernandez and Frydman[19] described two women with ovarian cancer who at the time of oophorectomy (removal of the ovaries) had oocytes retrieved for IVF and then had the embryos cryopreserved; however, no similar cases have been reported. If ovarian tissue cryopreservation becomes a reality, treatment options for women with cervical or ovarian cancer who face immediate loss of ovarian function may be dramatically increased.

Endometrial cancer (cancer of the uterine lining) is very uncommon in reproductive-age women. Precancerous lesions can usually be treated medically and subsequent reproduction is not impaired.

Endometriosis

Endometriosis is a common cause of infertility and may create difficult decisions for the woman, her physician, and her counselor. Endometriosis causes both infertility and pain, and the methods to treat one of these symptoms can worsen the other. All medical therapies for pain from endometriosis, except for pain medications, interrupt ovulation and thereby prevent conception. Definitive surgical therapy for pain involves removal of the ovaries. Alternatively, most treatments to enhance fertility in women with endometriosis involve administration of agents such as clomiphene or human menopausal gonadotropins (e.g., Fertinex, Humegon, Metrodin, Pergonal), which stimulate the ovaries and increase estrogen levels. It has not been established whether these treatments accelerate the growth of endometriosis, but they may increase pain levels during the cycles in which they are taken. Therefore, a woman may have to choose between treatment for pain and treatment for infertility. One exception is conservative surgical treatment, commonly using laparoscopic laser therapy. This can relieve pain, while either improving fertility or at least not worsening it.

Many questions still remain about the effects of endometriosis therapy. These include whether treatment of minimal endometriosis, either medically or surgically, improves fertility; whether medical suppression of endometriosis improves fertility; and whether use of medical suppression either pre- or post-operatively improves surgical outcome. For the woman trying to conceive, the lack of definitive information on these subjects can be very frustrating, as she must decide between taking medication and delaying pregnancy for 3–6 months or attempting pregnancy knowing that her long-term outcome may be worsened. The counselor should be aware that endometriosis is a chronic disease of unknown cause with no absolute cure. All available treatments merely suppress or remove existing endometriosis without preventing its recurrence. Patients commonly undergo multiple surgical and medical therapies in the course of their disease and may eventually undergo oophorectomy and hysterectomy.

AIDS

Infertile HIV-positive women present an especially difficult challenge for clinicians and counselors. Perhaps the most difficult issue is the possibility of disease transmission to the offspring. In one study, the rate of transmission from untreated mothers was 25%, and this dropped to 8% in the group in which the women were treated with antiviral therapy during their pregnancy[20]. However, even this rate may be considered unacceptably high, and long-term follow-up on these children is not yet available. Other important issues to consider are the potential effects of pregnancy on the woman's chance for long-term survival, the issue of the amount of parenting that will be available to the child because of the woman's inevitably shortened life expectancy (with the same issue applying to the child's father if he is HIV-positive), and the reluctance of some health care providers to treat these patients if they present with infertilty (see Olaitan and colleagues[21] for a discussion).

185

Diabetes

Prior to the discovery of insulin, it was very uncommon for diabetic women to conceive. With modern diabetic management, these women have a much better chance for conception and normal pregnancy. Diabetes should therefore not be a common cause of infertility in women whose disease is well controlled[22]. Nonetheless, there are several aspects of pregnancy in diabetic women that can affect treatment of infertile women regardless of the cause of infertility. Women with elevated blood sugars who conceive have a higher chance of having a miscarriage or a baby with birth defects. Adequate blood sugar control before conception will reduce these risks. While infertility therapy per se will not alter blood sugar levels or insulin requirements, the additional stress from involved therapies such as IVF may distract the diabetic from closely monitoring herself. Diabetes can also decrease the blood flow to the placenta, potentially resulting in intra-uterine growth retardation, premature delivery, and long-term neurological defects in the baby. Such problems are important for the infertile diabetic woman to consider, especially as treatments such as IVF increase the chance for multiple gestations in which the adverse effects of impaired blood flow are even more harmful.

Other Conditions

Many other medical conditions may coexist with infertility. These conditions may have little impact on fertility or on infertility therapy but can impact the success of pregnancy. These diseases include systemic lupus erythematosus, asthma, and heart or kidney disease. These diseases may increase the chance for miscarriage or may worsen during pregnancy as the increased metabolic demands of pregnancy stress already compromised organs. The more advanced reproductive technologies, such as IVF, which result in an increased rate of miscarriage and multiple births, place the woman at additional risk. In women whose bodies would have difficulty in handling the increased demands from a singleton pregnancy, even twins may create a risk of serious medical complications. These factors must be kept in mind as a patient decides what treatments to pursue. A couple should be encouraged to talk with their infertility specialist or an expert in high-risk pregnancies (perinatologist) to make sure that there will be no interaction between a medical condition and either the conception or the completion of a planned pregnancy.

REVIEW OF LITERATURE

The literature on infertility and medically complicating conditions is primarily concerned with medical treatment issues; little has been written regarding the psychological aspects of these dual-diagnosis patients. In both the medical and psychological literature, patients who are cancer survivors are the primary focus of research.

Male Cancer Patients

The predominant theme in the literature on male cancer patients and infertility has been the importance of sperm banking prior to treatment for testicular cancer or Hodgkin's disease[23-29]. Cella and Najavits[30] found that denial of infertility—that is, unrealistic optimism about being spared treatment-induced infertility—resulted in decisions not to cryobank sperm. Thus, addressing denial may be important in helping men make fully informed decisions and prevent future regret. Several authors[27,28] noted the sensitive issue of discussing sperm banking with adolescent males. Counseling issues include the need for casual but professional discussion of the issues, the provision of accurate information about the differences between infertility and impotence, and the usefulness of having the counselor meet with adolescents alone rather than with their parents present.

Urological cancer survivors reported significant distress and anxiety about infertility and sexual performance[24-26]. Several authors emphasized the ethical and psychosocial importance of discussing treatment alternatives that have a lesser impact on future fertility, and noted that oncologists have become increasingly aware of infertility concerns[24-27,31]. Due to the extremely high cure rates for these early-onset male cancers, quality of life has become a focus of concern in counseling and treatment.

Female Cancer Patients

Literature on female cancer patients and infertility also emphasizes quality-of-life issues[3-33]. Several authors urged discussion regarding the variable impact of different treatment options on ovarian suppression and future fertility, as well as the importance of acknowledging and discussing potential loss of fertility at the time of cancer diagnosis and treatment[28,29,31,33]. Lamb[33] noted that fear of infertility is a common psychological effect of cancer treatment. Lamb[33], Dow and colleagues[32], and Hubner and Glazer[29] discussed the importance of a thorough and responsible case-by-case discussion of options and risks. Dow and associates found that women who had children after breast cancer treatment reported that family issues were an important contributor to postcancer quality of life and that having children contributed to a feeling of being 'cured' and to a sense of reconnection with peers and family. Hubner[31] underscored the importance of the dual 'longing for life'—one's own and that of future

children—expressed by female cancer patients. She recommended the identification and subsequent referral for psychosocial assessment of cancer patients at risk for infertility concerns—those with a history of miscarriage, stillbirth, or abortion, and all premenopausal women without children.

Male and Female Cancer Patients

In their excellent review article, Hubner and Glazer[29] raised five important points for oncology caregivers regarding infertility: (1) Issues of fertility become overshadowed in the face of crisis; (2) significance of fertility must be acknowledged; (3) patients may later experience an 'intolerance of regret;' (4) fertility must be addressed with all patients of reproductive age; and (5) discussion of fertility signifies a belief in the patient's future.

Teeter and associates'[34] large-sample retrospective survey study of decisions about marriage and family among survivors of childhood cancer compared cancer survivors to a control group of siblings without cancer. Although the cancer survivors were not more likely than the controls to have documented fertility problems or offspring with birth defects, they were more likely to have been told by physicians not to attempt to have children. This result suggests that childhood cancer survivors may not be acting on complete or currently accurate information in making childbearing decisions.

CLINICAL ISSUES AND THERAPEUTIC INTERVENTIONS

Taken together, the medical information and psychological literature reviewed here point to several counseling needs and emotional concerns of infertility patients with medical conditions. This section

187

begins with a consideration of the types of decisions faced by patients and the role of mental health professionals in assisting with such decisions. This is followed by a discussion of two types of psychological issues of particular significance to these patients: mortality and loss, and defectiveness and abnormality.

Decision-making

Like other infertility patients, individuals or couples with medically complicating conditions may consult with mental health professionals for assistance with decisions about treatment options. Looked at separately, the decision-making process for either infertility or other medical conditions involves considering treatment options and balancing the potential chances for and benefits of a successful treatment outcome with the risks (physical, emotional, and financial) of the procedures. For these patients, the preferred choice for treating one condition may be detrimental to the other condition, creating a more complex decision process.

Decisions Regarding Treatment of Newly Diagnosed Cancers

A mental health professional may be consulted at the time of cancer diagnosis. If a patient is of childbearing age or an adolescent whose future fertility may be affected by cancer treatment, the oncologist may present treatment options that will differentially affect future fertility. For males with Hodgkin's disease or testicular cancer, the oncologist may recommend cryopreservation of sperm before surgery, chemotherapy, or radiation treatment. In these cases, the mode of psychological treatment is crisis-intervention counseling, in which frightened and highly stressed patients are required to make important life-impacting decisions rapidly, usually

within a few days. The patient and the oncology team will want to treat the cancer rapidly and maximize disease control and life expectancy. At the same time, potentially impaired fertility as a result of cancer treatment is an important counseling consideration.

A mental health professional can assist the patient in expressing fears and feelings of loss and in clarifying the meaning and importance of parenthood in his or her life. The latter task will vary widely, depending on age, marital status, and current parenthood status of the patient. For young single patients, particularly adolescent males, parenthood may have been no more than a remote possibility before the cancer diagnosis, whereas older married patients may have definite family-building plans. The mental health professional should consult with the oncologist to obtain information on treatment choices and their impact on future fertility and cancer control. Such a consultation enables the counselor to assist a distraught patient (whose capacity for memory and concentration is likely to be diminished) with the task of accurately understanding complex information. To avoid confusion, it is also important for the mental health professional to know what the oncologist's views are regarding preferred cancer treatments and what the oncologist has said to the patient in presenting options. With such information, the counselor can optimally assist the patient in a decision-making process that includes accurate risk–benefit factors

Testicular Cancer

When a diagnosis of testicular cancer is made, it is hoped that the urologist will suggest sperm cryopreservation for future inseminations. In such cases, the patient, or patient and his wife, may be referred for discussion of this option. The counselor should ensure that the patient is making an autonomous decision and giving fully informed consent to this choice, especially if it appears that his partner or parents are pressuring him. It is also important to clarify that cryopreservation is a current decision that makes possible but does not guarantee the option of future child-bearing, which will be followed by a separate future decision about whether to utilize that option. This may simplify the complex decision-making process by separating out and postponing the major life decision of whether to become a biological parent. It may also prevent future conflict arising from lack of clarity about the meaning of cryopreservation, in which one member of the couple or family assumes that it means a definite decision has been made to have children, while the other member does not share that assumption. The signed consent forms required by sperm cryobanking centers can promote this process of clarification and support the patient's autonomy if the man alone (and not his partner) signs the forms indicating how long his sperm will remain in storage and what the disposition of the sperm will be if he dies. In the case of a patient who has a partner, the counselor should encourage careful discussion of the issues involved in 'willing' the sperm to the man's surviving partner and the possible utilization of the sperm after the patient's death. These include the child's welfare, each partner's feelings, and attitudes of other family members. The complex ethical and legal issues involved in posthumous reproduction have been discussed elsewhere[35,36] and are beyond the scope of this discussion.

Breast Cancer

Decision-making regarding disease process control and fertility preservation is extremely complex in the case of breast cancer. The most aggressive treatment includes chemotherapy that results in ovarian suppression. However, many women with a strong desire to maintain reproductive capacity will want to choose surgical and radiation treatment without subsequent chemotherapy. The counselor, working in consultation with the oncologist, can help the patient conduct a risk–benefit analysis, address potential denial about cancer or infertility risk, obtain information about pregnancy after breast cancer, and express fears and grief.

Uterine, Cervical, or Ovarian Cancer

The patient with uterine or cervical cancer may be given the options of hysterectomy with or without oophorectomy. Her decision may involve weighing potentially greater cancer prevention through ovary removal against the partial fertility-sparing option of leaving her ovaries intact to use a gestational carrier in the future. Likewise, the patient with early-stage ovarian cancer may be given the option of oophorectomy with or without hysterectomy. Her decision may involve weighing potentially greater cancer prevention against the partial fertility-sparing option of leaving her uterus intact and using donor egg in the future. She also may be experiencing pressure from family members to choose one of the options. Here again, the counselor's role includes advocating for an autonomous informed decision. In cases in which the oncologist recommends hyster-ectomy without oophorectomy, many women currently undergoing cancer treat-ment will be unaware of the gestational-carrier option and will unnecessarily assume that they are losing any chance for future biological parenting. The mental health professional can help patients by educating oncologists about the important psychological consolation such knowledge can provide.

Female Cancer and Cryopreservation of Ovarian Tissue

Cryopreservation of ovarian tissue for potential future childbearing is not currently an approved clinical treatment. Clinicians should be aware of the 1996 American Society for Reproductive Medicine (ASRM) statement on cryopreservation of ovarian tissue, which states that this technique should be used for experimental research purposes only and that it is inappropriate/unethical for patients to be charged fees to cryopreserve tissue for clinical purposes[37]. Cancer patients faced with loss of fertility through surgery, radiation, or chemotherapy could potentially be drawn to ovarian cryopreservation if it is presented as a viable option. The clinician can help such patients by providing accurate information and by helping them accept and grieve the loss of fertility if no fertility-preserving cancer treatment options are available.

Hodgkin's Disease

Because Hodgkin's disease usually strikes men and women in their 20s or early 30s, most of these patients will be of childbearing age. Ideally, the oncology treatment team will discuss the issue of infertility and offer patients the ABVD treatment regimen, which offers a high rate of cure combined with a high rate of future fertility. For men with Hodgkin's disease, the oncologist and mental health professional should be aware that denial of fertility impact may interfere with utilization of sperm-cryobanking procedures[30]. A team approach can help address this denial, so that patients can optimally preserve future fertility and prevent future regret.

Decisions Regarding Treatment of Newly Diagnosed Endometriosis

Use of a common treatment for endometriosis, gonadotropin-releasing hormone agonists (leuprolide acetate [Lupron], nafarelin acetate [Synarel], and goserelin acetate [Zoladex]), results in temporary cessation of menstruation for 3–6 months. Many patients are unconflicted about utilizing this treatment to relieve pain associated with endometriosis. However, other patients feeling an urgency to conceive due to advanced maternal age or other personal factors may find it difficult to choose a treatment that precludes pregnancy for months. Decision-making in this area is complicated by the fact that there is not always a clear-cut link between endometriosis and infertility; many women with endometriosis become pregnant without medical intervention. In cases of endometriosis with severe pain not relieved by medication or surgery, oophorectomy may be recommended to reduce the estrogen levels associated with ovarian function. Women may thus need to decide between preserving their fertility and relieving severe pain. Historically, a hysterectomy was often performed along with oophorectomy, in part because it was thought that this would further reduce pain and in part because fertility was already sacrificed by ovarian removal. However, with the option of donor egg or oocyte cryopreservation, oophorectomy alone allows the possibility of future pregnancy, while potentially relieving much of the pain of endometriosis

Decisions Regarding Infertility Treatment when the Medical Condition has been Previously Diagnosed and Treated

The discussion above has focused on decision-making at the initial time of disease diagnosis. A second major time of decision-making occurs when the patient with a medical condition that has been diagnosed and treated in the past is currently dealing with infertility. If the infertility treatment or pregnancy will potentially make the medical condition worse or create a high risk pregnancy, the patient and her or his caregiver face complex decisions. Once again, the role of the mental health professional is to assist patients in making decisions based on a thorough consideration of the risks and benefits of various choices. The patient may be feeling a sense of urgency about pursuing infertility treatment as soon as possible, or her or his partner may disagree about priorities, with one focused on treating infertility and the other focused on preventing disease recurrence or exacerbation. The therapist's first task may be to help the patient or couple slow down and take time for a carefully considered decision. This does not need to be quick, crisis-intervention counseling.

Male Hypertension

In cases in which calcium channel blockers or other medications for treatment of hypertension result in impotence or reduced fertility, the patient can nearly always be switched to an alternate medication that effectively treats the hypertension without impairing infertility. Informational counseling regarding these options thus precludes the need for more complex either-or decision-making.

Diabetes and Lupus

Interestingly, the desire to reproduce may become a motivator for a patient who has been lax about treating her diabetes to become more vigilant about her care. On the other hand, pregnancy for a diabetic carries the risk of shortened life, kidney damage, and loss of vision. For women with lupus or other autoimmune disorders, pregnancy can shorten life span or have other deleterious effects. The patient may thus need to make decisions that weigh the desire for reproduction against a shorter or less healthy life. In some cases, desire for a

child may lead to denial or minimization of the very real health risks for the patient; such denial should be addressed in counseling.

Breast Cancer

The decision to pursue pregnancy and infertility treatment after breast cancer treatment is complex. Some patients find it difficult to tolerate the recommended 2-year waiting period before attempting pregnancy. Many patients are concerned that pregnancy and use of hormonal therapies will increase their chances for disease recurrence, and they must make their decision in the absence of definitive large-sample longitudinal research studies about these factors. Other patients will be willing to assume the risk associated with pregnancy and use of infertility drugs[38,39]. Patients with complete ovarian suppression whose only options are costly egg donation/IVF or surrogacy may be financially unable to utilize these treatments, exacerbating feelings of anger and frustration about the unfairness of cancer. Some patients desiring infertility treatment encounter opposition from significant others or physicians concerned with pregnancy-caused disease recurrence or maternal death before children reach adulthood. A patient's right to autonomous decision-making and her quality-of-life concerns are important factors to consider as mental health professionals help infertile breast cancer survivors explore these issues.

Decisions Regarding Infertility Treatment when a Genetic or Medical Condition may be Transmitted to Offspring

Patients with cystic fibrosis, severe male-factor problems that are genetically caused, and breast or ovarian cancer may all be concerned with the genetic risks of passing on such conditions to their offspring. Many of these patients will meet with genetic counselors (see Chapter 11), but at times a mental health professional will be consulted about decision-making. Risk factors, alternative treatments such as donor insemination and egg donation, and ethical issues should be included in the discussion.

HIV-positive patients present with concerns about infecting offspring, as well as infecting the female partner in cases in which the male partner is seropositive. Infertility doctors will increasingly see patients who are HIV-positive due to the increased prevalence of HIV infection in women and longer life expectancy from newly developed anti-HIV drugs. With longer survival, HIV-infected patients have broadened the focus from disease management to consideration of quality-of-life issues, including parenthood. Many infertility treatment centers lack clearly defined policies regarding treatment of HIV-positive patients. Olaitan and associates[21] and Rojansky and Schenker[40] pointed to the need for clear ethical guidelines regarding such treatment. The ASRM guidelines on assisted reproduction recommend that risk of transmission, donor insemination, and adoption be discussed with couples seeking infertility services when the male is HIV-positive[41]. Rojansky and Schenker suggested that HIV-positive patients should not be denied treatment and should be counseled regarding five issues: (1) risks of perinatal transmission, (2) possible effects of pregnancy on the maternal condition, (3) available therapy for mother and offspring, (4) preventive measures and safe sex practices, and (5) issues related to infancy and childhood, including orphaned or infected children. Mental health professionals should clarify their own position regarding infertility treatment for HIV-positive patients before counseling such patients, and can advocate for patients by encouraging physicians to develop clear and ethical treatment policies.

Decisions Regarding Infertility Treatment in the Face of Limited Life Expectancy

With diseases such as AIDS, severe early-childhood-onset diabetes, and cancers with low survival rates, patients are faced with the decision of whether to treat infertility and conceive in the face of limited life expectancy. The patient, couple, or infertility doctor may struggle with ethical dilemmas and emotional issues of creating a child whose parent is unlikely to live or to be healthy enough to care for the child until the child has reached adulthood. In this way, some of the counseling issues are identical to those presented by couples where one or both are over the age of 50. The therapist's role may be to assist the patient or couple in facing the realities of limited life expectancy and in making provisions for the care of the child if a parent dies. This process will often include assessment of the supportive role of other family members and friends and evaluation of the family's resources. It is important to recognize and validate the strong 'longing for life'[31] that exists for many patients with life-threatening illnesses, and the ways in which biological parenting may satisfy this longing.

Mortality and Loss Issues

The decision about whether to become pregnant (or to adopt a child) when one's own life expectancy is limited is only one facet of the general psychological issue of loss and mortality faced by infertility patients with a medically complicating condition. Infertility in itself involves multiple potential losses[42]. These include loss of control over reproduction, a healthy sexual sense of self, marital or sexual satisfaction, control over life planning, and an ideal family. The other medical condition can also involve multiple losses. These range from the potential loss of life (from cancer, AIDS, lupus) to the loss of freedom to live an unrestricted life due to daily medical regimens (diabetes, hypertension) or pain (endometriosis).

When patients are facing the dual losses inherent in infertility and their other medical condition, they may respond with depression or anger at the unfairness of life. They may also experience an especially powerful longing for life fueled by the simultaneous threat of loss of life and loss of the ability to create a new life. Overcoming infertility and giving birth are seen as a powerful affirmation of patients' survival of the disease process. If patients are ultimately unable to find a cure for infertility, the grief work involved in the loss of the wished-for child may be compounded with renewed grief for the loss of a full healthy life.

Some patients, faced with these dual losses, may become clinically depressed. The therapist may need to help a patient address previously unresolved grief regarding the medical condition. In some cases, a patient will have grieved at the time of the medical diagnosis, but a future diagnosis of infertility will reopen the grieving process by adding another dimension to the meaning of the illness. In cases in which the depression requires a psychotropic medication that is contraindicated during pregnancy, a patient may need to defer infertility treatment until the depression is alleviated. This postponement, difficult for infertility patients in general, may be particularly difficult for patients with a sense of urgency to reproduce and parent within a potentially shortened life span.

Glazer and Hubner[13] noted that infertility patients with cancer often report feeling a sense of exclusion from the infertile community. They feel that others going through infertility cannot possibly appreciate what it means to face cancer as well, with its additional emotional struggles and losses. Patients may also feel a sense of disconnection from others with their medical condition who are not undergoing infertility treatment. In particular, they may be criticized by others for choosing to have children when the disease itself is life-threatening. Such criticism can increase these patients' sense of isolation.

Defectiveness and Abnormality Issues

Feelings of defectiveness and abnormality are common in infertility patients, as well as those with other medical conditions. A diagnosis of infertility and the process of infertility treatment can compound feelings of defectiveness associated with the other medical condition, causing loss of self-esteem and exacerbating a sense of difference from the 'normal' world. Many of these medical conditions involve problems with sexual functioning, which influence a person's sexual relationships and sexual self-esteem prior to infertility treatment. For instance, males with diabetes or with hypertension often have difficulty maintaining erections or having orgasms. Women with endometriosis may have had unsatisfying sexual relationships due to pain with intercourse. In these patients, the infertility problem can represent an additional experience of feeling sexually abnormal or deficient. Counseling may be needed to assist them in expressing such feelings, to address sexual dysfunction problems that interfere with timed intercourse or the production of semen samples, and to explore general feelings regarding femininity or masculinity. In some cases, the shame associated with feeling sexually abnormal or defective may inhibit one member of the couple from participating actively in the infertility treatment.

More generally, medical diseases can bring up thoughts and feelings of 'my body is defective' and 'I am abnormal', which are exacerbated by infertility. The dual narcissistic injury of infertility and other illness can lead to feelings of being betrayed by one's body. Clinicians should be particularly sensitive to issues of defectiveness in patients whose other medical condition (e.g., testicular cancer, endometriosis, diabetes, Rokitansky-Küster-Hauser syndrome) was first diagnosed in adolescence, a developmental period when difference from peers is particularly challenging to the creation and maintenance of a healthy ego. For such patients, infertility treatment can be threatening to their basic sense of self. The infertility physician can help by being sensitive to these issues and by referring patients or couples for supportive counseling.

Klinefelter's, Turner's, and Rokitansky-Küster-Hauser Syndromes

Patients with these genetic conditions involving sexual abnormalities are particularly vulnerable to experiencing feeling of defectiveness. Women with Turner's syndrome, diagnosis of which usually occurs in infancy, will already have faced issues of looking different throughout life. While egg donation may offer treatment for lack of ovaries, utilizing such treatment can represent another confrontation with a strong sense of difference from the 'normal' world. Likewise, women with Rokitansky-Küster-Hauser syndrome, in which diagnosis often occurs in adolescence, will have already faced feelings of being different from other women. While the option of using a gestational carrier may offer treatment for lack of a uterus, it can also be another painful experience of feeling sexually abnormal. Men with Klinefelter's syndrome are often not diagnosed until they have an infertility problem. At the time of diagnosis, these men often grapple with the feeling of 'not being a complete man' due to the genetic sexual abnormality. This feeling is also common as a result of male

infertility diagnosis in general. Men with Klinefelter's syndrome thus face a double threat to maintaining a healthy sexual ego. Infertility physicians should be sensitive to these issues, and mental health professionals can assist patients in exploring feelings regarding sexuality and masculinity.

FUTURE IMPLICATIONS

The best interests of infertility patients with medically complicating conditions will be served when there is good communication and a teamwork approach among the infertility physician, the mental health professional, and oncologists and other physicians treating the medical condition. By sharing information about the impact on fertility of the disease and its treatment, the impact of fertility on the disease process, and the psychological issues involved, health care providers can assist patients in making decisions that maximize informed consent and peace of mind and minimize the possibility of future regret and distress.

Mental health professionals working in the area of infertility can act as advocates for their patients by educating oncology treatment teams about the options of egg donation for patients who have lost ovarian function and gestational carrier for patients who have had hysterectomies but retain ovarian function. Knowledge of these ways to partially preserve fertility can be extremely comforting to some newly diagnosed cancer patients who otherwise might assume that their cancer means a complete loss of reproductive capacity. Likewise, mental health professionals can act as advocates by encouraging oncologists who treat males with Hodgkin's disease and oncologists/urologists who treat testicular cancer to discuss pretreatment sperm cryobanking with all patients, regardless of age or marital status.

Mental health professionals will increasingly see infertility patients with medically complicating conditions, due to increased survival of patients with cancer and other illnesses combined with improved and expanded infertility treatment techniques such as IVF, ICSI, egg donation, oocyte cryopreservation, and gestational carrier. All of these advanced infertility treatments are very costly, and not all patients will have the financial means to utilize them. Also, none of these treatments is guaranteed to treat the infertility problems. In addition, many of these treatment options carry a risk of multifetal pregnancy, which entails higher costs and greater risks than singleton pregnancies. Thus, health care providers should be thoughtful and realistic in discussing these options to avoid offering false hopes of a simple solution to infertility problems or of a solution that might be financially out of reach.

Issues that need to be clarified in the future include ovarian cryopreservation, treatment of patients with AIDS, and the passing on of genetic problems to children. While ovarian cryopreservation is currently in the early stages of availability, it may become more so in the future. Likewise, techniques for treating sperm of HIV-positive men are not currently widely accepted but may be in the future. Finally, as techniques such as ICSI permit reproduction in men who previously were infertile due to genetic problems, some of these genetic problems will be passed on to the children created through infertility treatment.

SUMMARY

- Infertility counselors can better serve clients by obtaining general medical knowledge about medical conditions affecting infertility.

- Interdisciplinary teamwork among infertility specialists, mental health professionals, oncologists, and other physicians will serve the best interests of dually diagnosed infertility patients with other medical conditions. Counselors can often serve as advocates for patients.
- Mental health professionals can play a vital role in assisting patients with complex decision-making regarding treatment, in which risks and benefits for both disease control and fertility preservation must be considered.
- Cancer treatment decision-making requires rapid crisis-intervention counseling. While addressing primary feelings of fear and grief regarding cancer diagnosis and potential loss of life, counselors can also bring the topic of future fertility into the discussion. Doing so conveys a sense of hopefulness about the future and helps patients avoid future regret.
- The losses faced by infertility patients in general are compounded for patients with other medical conditions. These patients may experience disconnection from the general infertile population who have not confronted personal mortality issues.
- The abnormality and defectiveness issues faced by infertility patients in general are intensified for patients with other medical conditions. Patients whose other medical condition was first diagnosed in adolescence are particularly vulnerable to such feelings.

REFERENCES

1. Honig S, Lipshultz L, Jarow J. Significant medical pathology uncovered by a comprehensive male infertility evaluation. *Fertil Steril* 1994;62:1028–34

2. Benoff S, Cooper G, Hurley I, *et al*. The effect of calcium ion channel blockers on sperm fertilizing potential. *Fertil Steril* 1994;62:606–17

3. Meirow D, Schenker JG. Cancer and male infertility. *Hum Reprod* 1995;10:2017–22

4. Costabile R. The effects of cancer and cancer therapy on male reproductive function. *J Urol* 1993;149:1327–30

5. Ragni G, Perotti L, Viviani S, Santori A, Devizzi L, Della Serra A. Fertility outcome in men with Hodgkin's disease after four different combination chemotherapy regimens. Presented at the 52nd annual meeting of the American Society for Reproductive Medicine, Boston, MA, November 2–6, 1996

6. Mickle J, Milunsky A, Amos J, Oates RD. Congenital unilateral absence of the vas deferens: A heterogeneous disorder with two distinct subpopulations based upon aetiology and mutational status of the cystic fibrosis gene. *Hum Reprod* 1995;10:1728–35

7. van der Ven K, Messer L, van der Ven H, Jeyendran RS, Ober C. Cystic fibrosis mutation screening in healthy men with reduced sperm quality. *Hum Reprod* 1996; 11:513–17

8. Politch JA, Abbott AF, Mayer KH, Anderson DJ. The effects of disease progression and zidovudine therapy on semen quality in human immunodeficiency virus type 1 seropositive men. *Fertil Steril* 1994;61:922–8

9. Semprini AE, Levi-Setti P, Bozzo M, *et al*. Insemination of HIV-negative women with processed semen of HIV-positive men. *Lancet* 1992;340:1317–19

10. Baccetti B, Benedetto A, Burrini AG, Collodel G, Ceccarini EC. HIV particles in spermatozoa of patients with AIDS and their transfer into the oocyte. *J Cell Biol* 1994;127:903–14

11. Reijo R, Alagappan RK, Patrizio P. Severe oligozoospermia resulting from deletions of azoospermia factor gene on Y chromosome. *Lancet* 1996;347:1290–3

12. Mak V, Jarvi K. The genetics of male infertility. *J Urol* 1996;156:1245–57

13. Santoro A, Bonadonna G, Valabussa P, Zucali R, Viviani S, Villani F. Long-term results of combined chemotherapy-radiotherapy approach in Hodgkin's disease: Superiority of ABVD plus radiotherapy versus MOPP plus radiotherapy. *J Clin Oncol* 1987;5:27–37

14. Petrek J. Pregnancy safety after breast cancer. *Cancer* 1994;74:528–31

15. Reichman B, Green K. Breast cancer in young women: Effect of chemotherapy on ovarian function, fertility, and birth defects. *J Natl Cancer Inst Monogr* 1994; 16:125–9

16. Brown JR, Modell E, Obasaju M, Ying YK. Natural cycle in-vitro fertilization with embryo cryopreservation prior to chemotherapy for carcinoma of the breast. *Hum Reprod* 1996;11:197–9

17. Rossing MA, Daling JR, Weiss NS, Moore DE, Self SG. Risk of breast cancer in a cohort of infertile women. *Gynecol Oncol* 1996;60:3–7

18. Venn A, Watson L, Lumley J, Giles G, King C, Healy D. Breast and ovarian cancer incidence after infertility and in vitro fertilisation. *Lancet* 1995;346:995–1000

19. Fernandez H, Frydman R. Cancer and in vitro fertilization. *J In Vitro Fertil Embryo Transf* 1987;4:241–2

20. Connor E, Sperling R, Gelber R, *et al*. Reduction of maternal-infant transmission of human immunodeficiency virus type 1 with zidovudine treatment. *N Engl J Med* 1994;331:1173–80

21. Olaitan A, Reid W, Mocroft A, McCarthy K, Madge S, Johnson M. Infertility among human immunodeficiency virus-positive women: Incidence and treatment dilemmas. *Hum Reprod* 1996;11:2793–6

22. Selby PI, Oakley CE. Women's problems with diabetes. *Diabet Med* 1992;9:290–2

23. Sanger WG, Olson JH, Sherman JK. Semen cryobanking for men with cancer—criteria change. *Fertil Steril* 1992;58:1024–7

24. Schover LR. Sexuality and fertility in urologic cancer patients. *Cancer* 1987; 60: 553–8

25. Rieker PP, Fitzgerald EM, Kalish LA. Adaptive behavioral responses to potential infertility among survivors of testis cancer. *J Clin Oncol* 1990;8:347–55

26. Rieker PP, Fitzgerald EM, Kalish LA, *et al.* Psychosocial factors, curative therapies, and behavioral outcomes: A comparison of testis cancer survivors and a control group of healthy men. *Cancer* 1989;64:2399–407

27. Sweet V, Servy EJ, Karow AM. Reproductive issues for men with cancer: Technology and nursing management. *Oncol Nurs Forum* 1996;23:51–8

28. Kaempfer SH, Wiley FM, Hoffman DJ, Rhodes EA. Fertility considerations and procreative alternatives in cancer care. *Semin Oncol Nurs* 1985;1:25–34

29. Hubner MK, Glazer ES. Now on common ground: Cancer and infertility in the 1990s. *Infertil Reprod Med Clin North Am* 1993;4:581–96

30. Cella DF, Najavits L. Denial of infertility in patients with Hodgkin's disease. *Psychosomatics* 1986;27:71

31. Hubner MK. Cancer and infertility: Longing for life. *J Psychosoc Oncol* 1989;7:1–19

32. Dow KH, Harris JR, Roy C. Pregnancy after breast-conserving surgery and radiation therapy for breast cancer. *J Natl Cancer Inst Monogr* 1994;16:131–7

33. Lamb MA. Effects of cancer on the sexuality and fertility of women. *Semin Oncol Nurs* 1995;11:120–7

34. Teeter MA, Holmes GE, Holmes FF, Baker AB. Decisions about marriage and family among survivors of childhood cancer. *J Psychosoc Oncol* 1987;5:59–68

35. Robertson JA. Posthumous reproduction. *Indiana Law J* 1994;69:1027

36. Ohl DA, Park J, Cohen C, Goodman K, Menge AC. Procreation after death or mental incompetence: Medical advance or technology gone awry? *Fertil Steril* 1996;66:889–95

37. American Society for Reproductive Medicine statement on cryopreservation of ovarian tissue for future reimplantation in women undergoing cancer treatment. *American Society for Reproductive Medicine News* 1996 (Apr)

38. Sauer MV, Paulson RJ, Lobo RA. Successful pre-embryo donation in ovarian failure after treatment for breast carcinoma. *Lancet* 1990;335:723

39. Hussein EE, Tan SL. Successful in vitro fertilization and embryo transfer after treatment of invasive carcinoma of the breast. *Fertil Steril* 1992;58:195–6

40. Rojansky N, Schenker JG. Ethical aspects of assisted reproduction in AIDS patients. *Assist Reprod Genet* 1995;12:537–42

41. American Society for Reproductive Medicine. Ethical considerations of assisted reproductive technologies. Chapter 28: Special considerations regarding HIV and ARTs. *Fertil Steril* 1994;62(suppl 1):85S

42. Menning BE. The emotional aspects of infertility. *Fertil Steril* 1980;34:313–19

43. Glazer ES, Hubner MK. Coping with the double blow: Facing cancer and infertility. RESOLVE Fact Sheet. Boston, MA: RESOLVE Inc, 1992

11

Genetic Counseling and the Infertile Patient

Linda Hammer Burns, PhD, and Bonnie S. LeRoy, MS

We are a spectacular, splendid manifestation of life. We have language ...
We have affection. We have genes for usefulness,
and usefulness is about as close to a 'common goal' of nature as I can guess at.

Lewis Thomas

Genetic counselors and infertility counselors often work together to provide information and supportive care about reproductive medical conditions and treatments. Genetic counselors see infertility patients for two reasons: when a genetic cause is known or suspected, or when it is necessary to assess for genetic risk. Genetic counselors are often the first professionals to respond to the crisis precipitated by the determination that a known or possible genetic factor is the cause of a couple's infertility. As such, it is the responsibility of the genetic counselor to support and assess patient reactions, emotional resources, psychological stability, and ability to understand and 'hear' complicated information, as well to provide appropriate crisis intervention and, when necessary, follow-up referral to a mental health professional. For infertile couples and individuals, appropriate referral is usually to an infertility counselor who is a licensed mental health professional specializing in reproductive medicine, reproductive genetics, and/or perinatology. Alternatively, infertility counselors may encounter patients who present with histories of genetic disorders, confusion

about prenatal or other genetic testing, or genetic causes of infertility in which referral or consultation with a genetic counselor is necessary and appropriate. In addition, couples with a heritable genetic disorder may seek consultation with an infertility counselor to discuss family-building alternatives, such as adoption or assisted reproductive technologies.

In this way, infertility counselors and genetic counselors often provide services that dovetail, working together as integral members of the reproductive medicine team providing comprehensive patient care to infertile couples.

This chapter will:

- address the concepts involved in the applications of reproductive genetic counseling to infertility and infertility counseling
- provide an overview of the applications of genetic medicine to infertility
- outline the basis for testing for the diagnosis of genetic infertility, prenatal genetic testing with applications to infertility, preimplantation genetic diagnosis (genetic testing done during in vitro fertilization (IVF) and before

embryo transfer), and the genetic screening and counseling of gamete and embryo donors

• illustrate how the genetic counselor and the infertility counselor may work together in meeting the complex needs of the infertile patient.

HISTORICAL OVERVIEW

Approximately 3–5% of all live births will have a birth defect, chromosomal anomaly, or genetic disease. To date, more than 8000 diseases are documented as having a genetic basis in McKusick's[1] catalog, a reference text, and also an Internet resource, on single gene disorders that is updated regularly. Moreover, all diseases are suspected of having some genetic involvement, including the susceptibility to infections and common conditions with adult onset such as cancer, heart disease, and mental illnesses. What this means is that we are all at risk for being affected by a condition that has a genetic basis.

Genetic testing and counseling are important to infertile couples for a variety of reasons, including causative factors for infertility, prenatal genetic testing, or genetic inheritance issues with gamete donations. As such, it may be useful to review some basic genetic concepts. The basic units of inheritance are the *genes*, which are the biochemical blueprints from which cells 'read' the instructions needed for normal growth, development, and function. Scientists estimate that there are about 100,000 genes in every cell of the human body, carried in duplicate on the 23 pairs of chromosomes. *Chromosomes* are the 'packaging units' for the genes (i.e., every human cell contains 23 pairs of chromosomes). One chromosome from each of the pairs is inherited from the mother through her egg cell (oocyte or ovum), and the other of the pair is inherited from the father through the sperm cell, for a total of 46 chromosomes. Each of the chromosomes carries hundreds to thousands of genes, and, like the chromosomes, 50% of genes are inherited from the mother, and the other 50% from the father. The first 22 pairs of chromosomes carry genes that every human has in common and that are the same in males and females. The 23rd pair carries the genes that determine the gender of the developing fetus, as well as other information. Females normally have two chromosomes identified as X chromosomes, and males normally have one X chromosome and one Y chromosome. The presence of a Y chromosome with normally functioning genetic material directs the fetus to develop into a male. The absence of a Y chromosome with functioning genetic material, along with the presence of two X chromosomes with normally functioning genetic material, directs the fetus to develop into a female. Changes in the number or the structure of one or more chromosome(s) or changes in the structure and functioning of one or more gene(s) can result in infertility problems and/or the development of a child with a birth defect and/or genetic disease. These changes are the basis of testing that can help diagnose a genetic cause of infertility.

Since the middle 1970s, molecular genetic technologies have evolved to the extent that practitioners can now utilize a variety of methods in the laboratory to analyze hereditary material. Testing is useful in determining the causes of specific diseases that have a genetic basis for diagnostic purposes, in genetic risk assessment identifying carrier status (individuals who are unaffected but carrying genes capable of causing a genetic disease or disorder in their offspring), in predicting an individual's risk of certain adult-onset disorders, and determining genetic causes of infertility[2]. The Human

Genome Project, established during the 1980s in the United States, is an international effort with the overall goal of sequencing the entire complement of human hereditary material. The outcomes of this project will lead to the development of methods that will help scientists locate specific genes responsible for determining particular human traits and causing many diseases. We will also learn more about how genetic factors play a role in human development and behavior. It is hoped that information gained from the Human Genome Project will someday lead to the information needed to treat and cure genetic diseases or disorders, including those related to infertility.

Genetic counseling, as a fully recognized health profession, is relatively new to the health care arena. Genetic counselors are health care professionals with a master's level graduate degree. Formal graduate programs educating genetic counselors are accredited through the American Board of Genetic Counseling and integrate studies in human and molecular genetics, related biological sciences, and psychosocial counseling with clinical application. Graduates must demonstrate clinical skills in a variety of settings with diverse patient populations in order to be eligible to apply for board certification. Genetic counselors work in a variety of settings, such as university medical centers, private hospitals, health maintenance organizations, public health departments, research programs, and laboratory offices. Genetic counselors see patients with issues encompassing preconceptional and prenatal screening and diagnosis, pediatric and adult genetic disease, cancer risk, neurogenetic disease, and a variety of other concerns, including infertility.

The term *genetic counseling* was coined in 1947 by Sheldon C. Reed, PhD, director of the Dight Institute of Human Genetics at the University of Minnesota, who also defined the three requirements of genetic counseling as (1) knowledge of human genetics, (2) respect for sensitivities, attitudes, and reactions of clients, and (3) teaching and providing genetic information to the full extent known[3]. Genetic counseling was originally done by university-based research geneticists involved in research programs. As such, the emphasis was on the provision of genetic information and knowledge-based advice rather than on counseling. With the advent of genetic testing in the early 1970s, genetic counseling moved toward a more medical model of patient care, in which genetic counselors saw their responsibilities as not only providing genetic information but also supportive counseling and clinical services to patients seeking assistance in reproductive and medical care decisions[4].

REVIEW OF LITERATURE

Research on genetic counseling for infertility is sparse, marked by case reports of specific genetic diseases or disorders that feature infertility, with little attention to patient emotional response or psychological adjustment following genetic testing or diagnosis. For the most part, limitations in research are probably due to the fast-paced developments in both genetic and reproductive medicine, as well as the fairly recent recognition of the importance of genetic and infertility counseling in patient care. Recent medical advances have increased awareness and interest in the psychosocial aspects of reproductive genetics: the impact on individuals, couples, and family adjustment; factors influencing reproductive decision-making; and response to diagnosis of infertility due to genetic etiology versus other causal factors. However, research on these aspects has lagged far behind.

A small number of studies have examined psychological factors related to genetic counseling or testing and infertility. These studies have concerned (1) emotional response to genetic diagnosis, (2) patient attitudes regarding prenatal genetic testing or diagnosis, and (3) the personal reproductive and genetic history of the genetic counselor.

Emotional Response to Genetic Diagnosis

Most research on the psychological impact of genetic testing and/or diagnosis has been case reports, group studies, and surveys with outcomes varying from severe depression to improvement in psychological state[5]. This research indicates that women experience greater psychological distress than men, and genetically affected married individuals experience more psychological stress, which is additionally affected by their spouse's reaction. Parents with disabled children experience some measure of guilt about transmitting a disorder (defective gene) to their children. In addition, poorer adjustment is associated with the patient being close to the estimated age of a disorder's onset, at the time of diagnosis.

In a recent study[5] of presymptomatic genetic testing for Huntington's disease, gene positive individuals without children were found to be more hopeless throughout the first year following diagnosis, with peak distress experienced at 6 and 9 months. It was noted that many of the couples had proceeded with genetic testing with the intention of forgoing reproduction if they tested gene positive, so that the positive results highlighted reproductive losses and precipitated contemplation of other family-building decisions. Another follow-up study[6] evaluated the response of men diagnosed with the cystic fibrosis gene resulting in congenital bilateral absence of the vas deferens (CBAVD). It found that 13 of the 14 men did not express high levels of concern about the personal health implications of cystic fibrosis; instead, they viewed the diagnosis primarily in terms of their reproductive potential.

Prenatal Genetic Testing

Several studies have compared patient satisfaction with different forms of prenatal genetic testing. Pergament[7] reported that decision-making by potential candidates for preimplantation genetic diagnosis (PGD) were most influenced by their previous obstetrical experiences. In women who had normal genetic outcomes using standard prenatal testing, only 33% believed that PGD was an improvement, compared with 72% of women who had experienced an abnormal genetic outcome using standard prenatal testing. The three major patient concerns identified in this study were (1) unsatisfactorily high failure rate associated with IVF, (2) high financial cost of IVF/PGD, and (3) possibility of damage to the embryo. In a study comparing respondents' attitudes regarding PGD, Miedzybrodrodzka and colleagues[8] compared five groups of women who had (1) genetic counseling for a single gene disorder, (2) chorionic villus sampling (CVS) for a single gene disorder, (3) CVS for another reason, (4) recently delivered a normal baby, and (5) undergone IVF. Overall, 94% of the women stated they would test a pregnancy if it was at high risk (defined as 25% or 50% chance of 'disease or handicap'), and 68% would terminate an affected pregnancy. With respect to CVS and PGD, 38% of respondents favored PGD, while 42% favored CVS with a subsequent termination of an affected fetus. Religion, family history, opinion of pregnancy termination, and previous CVS outcome did not influence preference for CVS or PGD. However, 40% thought PGD was more morally acceptable, while 34% felt CVS and pregnancy termination were more morally acceptable.

In a rare study comparing the experience of prenatal testing in infertile and fertile couples, Sandelowski and coworkers[9] found that for infertile couples advanced maternal age was the most important determining factor in their decision to proceed with amniocentesis. Prior infertility affected prenatal decision-making in that infertile couples cited a greater variety of reasons for declining amniocentesis, balancing the known premium value of the pregnancy with the value of information obtainable from amniocentesis and the risks associated with the procedure itself. In addition, the authors found that the amniocentesis experience both reprised elements of infertility and interrupted the pregnancy experience. They concluded that because infertile couples were accustomed to failed effort and loss, they were more likely to highly value the pregnancy and baby and, as a result, were more keenly aware of how amniocentesis could both enhance or depreciate it.

Reproductive and Genetic History of the Reproductive Professionals

In an interesting survey study exploring the personal reproductive history of genetic counselors, Martin and Walker[10] found that 36% of survey respondents ($n=522$) identified themselves as personally affected in some way by a genetic disorder or reproductive difficulties. A majority (88%) of the counselors could identify ways in which their personal history was helpful and beneficial in counseling, while fewer (23%) were able to identify ways in which it presented challenges. Interestingly, 49% of the genetic counselors reported disclosing their personal reproductive or genetic history to a client at least once. In a similar survey study of personal reproductive histories of infertility nurses, Marosek and Covington[11] found that 47%

of respondents ($n=70$) had been diagnosed with infertility and 67% received medical treatment for infertility at the same clinic where they were employed. The authors are in the process of a similar study of infertility counselors; however, both studies address the issue of how personal reproductive history and related 'countertransference' may influence the professional's work and patient care in the field of reproductive medicine in both positive and negative ways.

THEORETICAL FRAMEWORK

Genetic counseling uses many of the same principles and theoretical frameworks of psychotherapy, but genetic counseling is *not* psychotherapy. Genetic counseling is based on a definition of counseling as the giving of advice, expert opinion, or instruction in directing the judgment or conduct of another. As such, genetic counseling is not simply the provision of information but the empowering of patients through education, facilitation of information processing, and provision of emotional support. Thus, patients are able to assimilate and integrate the information and, ultimately, to make autonomous decisions. Alternatively, infertility counselors (as licensed mental health professionals) are educated and trained to provide psychotherapy, which is defined as the treatment of personality maladjustment or mental illness by psychological means, usually through personal consultation. While both fields involve providing expert advice and support, only infertility counseling involves the *psychological treatment* of patients.

Client-centered counseling, first described by Carl Rogers, is the fundamental theoretical framework on which genetic counseling is based. Client-centered counseling emphasizes a nondirective approach to counseling, in which a warm, accepting environment and the counselor's

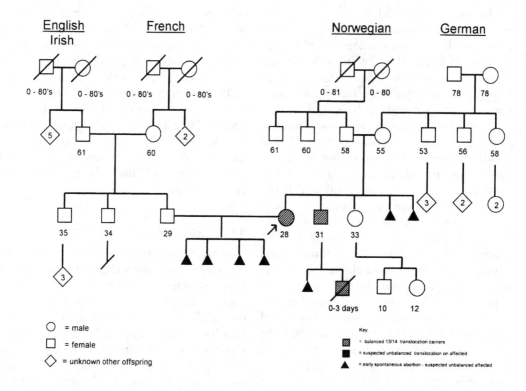

Figure 1 Hypothetical clinical pedigree representing infertility using recommended nomenclature. (Adapted from ref. 66, with permission)

communication of empathy, respect, and unconditional positive regard are thought to facilitate client exploration of feelings, issues, and decisions. The application of respect for autonomy and Rogers' client-centered counseling theory to reproductive decision-making forms the basis for the 'nondirective' tenet in genetic counseling[12]. The Genetic Counselors' Professional Code of Ethics illustrates the basis for this approach by emphasizing the 'respect for client's beliefs, background and culture, and the counselor's duty to enable clients to make autonomous decisions by providing all necessary information'[12].

Kessler[13] characterized the change in emphasis in genetic counseling as a 'paradigm shift', describing the shift in emphasis in genetic counseling from a communication-of-information model of counseling to a preventive medicine model and, finally, the psychosocial medicine approach currently favored[12]. The *psychosocial medicine approach* emphasizes patient self-determination and the genetic counselor's role as a patient advocate, grief counselor, researcher, and health care professional providing supportive care, education, resources, and referrals.

Over time, the application of other theoretical approaches has been suggested, in addition to the client-centered theoretical framework, including a communication/psychological approach and family systems theory. In the *communication/psychological approach* to genetic counseling, the genetic counselor facilitates individual and/or family decision-making by providing unbiased information and assisting exploration of personal views and values regarding medical treatments and available options[12]. The communication model, based on the tenets of nondirectiveness and client self-determination, includes principles from psychotherapy, family therapy, decision-making theory, and cross-cultural counseling. As such, the outcome of genetic counseling is not simply the provision of facts but the processing and integration of information enabling an individual's autonomous decision-making and assimilation of the information.

The application of *family systems theory* to genetic counseling has been suggested because it addresses individual, interactional, and intergenerational issues associated with inherited and genetic disorders[4]. Both genetic counseling and family system therapists use family pedigrees or genograms (see Figure 1) for collecting and organizing information, assessing family patterns of disease and/or behaviors, and developing hypotheses about how family dynamics affect genetic diagnosis, counseling, and even decision-making[4].

Stress theory has also been applied to genetic counseling, providing a framework for conceptualizing the stress-related effects of genetic testing and/or diagnosis[14]. As such, it recognizes the capacity of genetic testing and diagnosis to be either harmful or beneficial, thereby affecting an individual's (and his or her partner's) social support, coping, and psychological resources. It has been suggested that the extent to which genetic testing causes significant distress varies according to (1) test results, (2) characteristics of the disease, (3) uncertainty remaining after testing, (4) degree of uncertainty reduction, (5) availability of coping options, and (6) personal factors such as optimism, perceived risk, or beliefs about disease and disability[14]. This theoretical approach can be particularly helpful in its application to infertile couples who are typically under significant stress related to medical treatment and/or the consideration of family-building alternatives.

CLINICAL ISSUES

Genetic counselors and infertility counselors provide a wide variety of patient care with respect to genetic testing, diagnosis, and issues surrounding infertility, including helping patients consider decisions (1) for or against genetic counseling and testing, (2) genetic counseling and testing for infertility diagnosis, (3) genetic counseling regarding pregnancy losses, (4) prenatal genetic screening and testing, (5) counseling on continuation or termination of a genetically affected pregnancy, (6) the use of assisted reproductive technologies for genetic reasons, (7) PGD during IVF, and (8) genetic screening of potential gamete and/or embryo donors. Genetic screening may be appropriate (Table 1), and there are specific indications for genetic counseling and possible prenatal testing (Table 2).

Deciding For or Against Genetic Counseling and Testing

Decision-making regarding genetic counseling and testing among infertile couples is primarily marked by profound ambivalence. Fundamentally, infertility and genetic diagnoses imply flaw and/or failure, often precipitating feelings of shame, embarrassment, guilt, deficiency, and inadequacy. Inherent in genetic testing is the possibility and potential for narcissistic injury if a genetic disorder, disease, or anomaly is detected either in the individual, the couple, a pregnancy, or potential offspring. The ambivalence and self-protection characterizing an infertile individual's (or couple's) approach to decisions regarding genetic counseling or screening can be understood within the context of additional narcissistic wounds compounding those already inflicted by infertility.

Altered sense of self, stigma, and narcissistic injury as factors influencing decision-making are apparent in a number of aspects of infertility but may be best demonstrated in male-factor infertility. There is considerable evidence that male-factor infertility is more stigmatizing to both men and women than female-factor infertility[15]. This may result in partners' denying or minimizing the male-factor infertility diagnosis or in a couple's colluding by identifying a minor female-factor as causal. This 'protective dance' that couples do around male-factor infertility can have a significant impact on their reproductive decisions and their decision-making process. For example, it is common for wives to proceed with reproductive treatments with which they are uncomfortable in order to protect the relationship and/or the husband's sense of self (see Chapter 1). By the same token, husbands often refuse to consider reproductive technologies that involve nongenetic methods of parenthood or refuse to acknowledge the ramifications of the male infertility diagnosis, often using reassurances such as 'it only takes one sperm'. These issues become even more relevant if responses to genetic diagnosis trigger strong feelings of responsibility, guilt, and defectiveness in the identified patient and blame, shame, and resentment in their spouse.

Western-culture couples often react with grateful enthusiasm in response to reproductive and/or genetic technology and are often reluctant to refuse it when it is offered, despite the costs. They view reproductive and genetic technologies as providing hope and promise and are more aware of the possibility of regret or social criticism if they decide to refuse to use the

Table 1 Questions for screening for genetic risk

Have you or other close relatives had one or more stillbirths or early infant losses?

Did any of your close relatives die at an early age (under the age of 50), and if so, do you know why?

Did you or anyone in your family have more than two miscarriages?

Are you and your spouse related to each other in any way?

Are you and your spouse cousins or do you have relatives with the same last name?

Does anyone in your family have learning problems, or is anyone mentally retarded?

Does anyone in your family have hearing loss, vision loss, or any birth defect?

Does anyone in your family look very different from others in the family (e.g., very tall or very short)?

What country(ies) did your family originally come from?

(Reproduced from ref. 65, with permission)

Table 2 Indications for genetic counseling and possible prenatal testing

Mother over 35 years of age at expected date of confinement

High or low maternal serum AFP screen

Family history of X-linked disorder in male related to mother through female family member

Member of ethnic group in which carrier screening for common disorder is available

Maternal illness

Exposure to medications or substance use

Two or more first-trimester miscarriages

Abnormal finding on ultrasound

Parental anxiety (primarily for reassurance)

(Reproduced from ref. 65, with permission)

technology[16]. By contrast, couples from non-Western cultures are often skeptical of technology and have difficulty recognizing any personal or societal benefit in its use. Their cultural perspective or lack of familiarity may make technological procedures more stressful and frightening, experiences further complicated by language barriers or religious beliefs. In the end, cultural perspectives can influence decisions regarding genetic counseling and testing, as well as acceptable reproductive medical treatments and family-building options (see Chapter 13).

Frequently, couples confuse decisions to pursue prenatal testing as an automatic endorsement of pregnancy termination if a genetic disorder is detected. Although elective termination of an affected pregnancy is a common choice, a certain portion of couples chooses prenatal testing to prepare for the care of a handicapped child. Zuzkar[17] in a review of the psychological impact of prenatal diagnosis of a fetal anomaly found two opposing perspectives in expectant parents: prenatal diagnosis as helping emotional preparation and prenatal diagnosis as prolonging the period of emotional upset. Accordingly, considerations of prenatal testing as preparation for the care of a handicapped child must involve explorations of the expectant parent's personal perspective. Most parents experience a mourning process following prenatal diagnosis or birth of a handicapped child, in which they grieve the loss of the expected healthy child[18]. Advance knowledge of the problem can allow some measure of control over the events surrounding the birth of a handicapped or affected baby, benefiting long-term coping and family adjustment[19]. For couples with a history of infertility, considerations will include issues of parental age, expectations of parenthood, perceived burden versus actual resources, and prior commitments or responsibilities, such as children from previous marriages or elderly parents.

There is considerable evidence that infertile couples' reproductive decisions are less likely to be influenced by statistical probability of generic abnormality and more likely to be influenced by qualitative factors such as a couple's or individual's interpretation or perception of risks[20–22]; desire to have a child[20]; the perceived consequences of having a disabled child, with its impact on marital, family, and the child's quality of life[23]; and the perceived burden of the genetic condition[22]. For many infertile couples, deciding to proceed with genetic testing or counseling is an excruciating decision, usually influenced by past infertility experiences, phase of mourning the losses of infertility, personal identity issues, medical recommendations or indications, and willingness of partners to acknowledge and accept a genetic component to their infertility[24]. The challenges and pressures of infertility may leave couples ill-equipped to cope with potential losses inherent in genetic screening or testing. Already overwhelmed by grief or emotional distress, couples engage in avoidance or have profound ambivalence that may reflect their inability to assimilate or process the implications or ramifications of genetic screening or diagnosis. Acknowledging the need for self-protective measures and the normalcy of ambivalence may reduce anxiety and distress. Alternatively, profound ambivalence, avoidance, and self-protection may also reflect more deep-seated emotional or marital problems warranting psychotherapeutic intervention.

Finally, the experience of prenatal genetic testing alters the experience of pregnancy for previously infertile women, their partners, and even their extended family. Whatever its form, prenatal genetic testing can both validate the existence of a baby (e.g., ultrasound, photos, confirmation of sex) and potentially invalidate the basis for its continued existence (e.g.,

Table 3 Altered adaptation to pregnancy with amniocentesis

Event	*Adaptive response*
First trimester	
1. Confirmation of pregnancy	Acceptance of pregnancy
Early second trimester	
2. Preamniocentesis counseling	Insulation from hurt due to potential subsequent loss leads to delayed acceptance of pregnancy and even anticipatory grief
Awareness of procedure-related miscarriage risk	
Risk of fetal abnormality(ies) assessed	Tentative pregnancy phenomenon
Early to mid second trimester	
3. Sonography performed	Pregnancy suddenly equals baby and becomes a reality, especially for father
Baby 'looks normal'	Enforces dream of healthy baby
Abnormality detected	Point of loss
4. 'The wait' (about 2 weeks)	Continued detachment, delayed acceptance, guarded emotional investment in pregnancy—all in anticipation of potential loss
Mid to late second trimester	
5. The results	
Abnormal	Decision-making
	Grieving process
Normal	Equating normal results on one of two specific tests with normal baby, resulting in greater letdown if baby is born with problems undetectable by amniocentesis
Sex of baby	Reconciliation of fantasies of not 'wished for' sex; naming of baby, elaboration of fantasies, intensified bonding
6. Birth (after abnormal results)	Potentially enhanced coping due to opportunity to prepare for event/loss
7. Birth (after normal results)	
Good outcome	Reconciliation of fantasies regarding idealized child (normal process)
Unexpected outcome	
Death	Grieving process
Birth defect	Grief, adjustment—feeling of 'betrayal' if test results normal

(Reproduced from ref. 47, with permission)

detection of fetal anomaly, absence of fetal heart beat)[25]. The postinfertility pregnancy is a highly valued, purposeful pregnancy achieved after considerable investment of time, money, effort, and emotion. Prenatal testing makes 'tentative pregnancies', in which attachment to the pregnancy and fetus is delayed, the experience of pregnancy is altered, and expectations of parenthood are influenced[26] (Table 3). It is understandable that previously infertile couples often prefer to avoid the whole arena of prenatal testing in an effort to protect against the myriad possible threats, both physical and psychological (see Chapter 24).

Genetic Causes of Infertility

Common genetic factors involved in infertility include chromosomal abnormalities in which the affected individual has a deviation in the amount of chromosomal material. These aberrations can cause a problem in the development of the reproductive system or, with chromosomal structural abnormalities, in the production of gametes with too much or too little genetic information. Single gene disorders can also be a major factor in that the affected individual carries a gene mutation interfering in some way with the development of the reproductive system. There is overwhelming evidence that genetic factors are responsible for failure at all stages of fetal development, accounting for the high rate of most early pregnancy losses[27]. Several studies have shown that at least 50% of clinically recognized pregnancy losses result from chromosomal abnormalities[27,28], while only 7% of all stillbirths are due to chromosomal anomalies[29]. Parental chromosome analysis has shown that one partner in 4–5% of all couples experiencing infertility or multiple pregnancy loss is a carrier of a structural chromosomal anomaly, known as a chromosomal translocation, that affects reproduction. This results in the production of a gamete with too much or too little genetic information, causing early pregnancy loss[27]. In a recent study[30] of the chromosomal structure in discarded oocytes following failed IVF cycles, chromosomal abnormalities were evident in 42.7%.

Genetic causes of infertility have increasingly become an area of investigation, with several important new discoveries regarding male-factor infertility. Pryor and colleagues[31] found that a small proportion (7%) of men with infertility (azoospermia and oligospermia) demonstrated microdeletions of the Y chromosome, although it was noted that deletion did not preclude the presence of viable sperm or the possibility of conception. In a review of the literature on male infertility, Mak and Jarvi[32] noted that the genetic causes of male-factor infertility ranged from gonadotropin-releasing hormone deficiency, to spermatogenic failure, to obstructive azoospermia. Chromosomal abnormalities such as Klinefelter's syndrome can interfere with the development of the male reproductive system and the normal production of necessary hormones.

Azoospermia in men with CBAVD occurs in 1–2% of infertile men and is sometimes referred to as genital cystic fibrosis. Recently, it has been shown that 60–70% of men with CBAVD carry at least one mutation and 10–20% of men with CBAVD carry two mutations for the cystic fibrosis gene, even though these men often have no symptoms of the disorder except for infertility[33]. For men with this type of male-factor infertility, the diagnosis involves learning of not only their infertility/sterility but also the unexpected diagnosis of a genetic disorder with potentially life-threatening medical problems and psychosocial implications for them and even their families. Furthermore, although assisted reproduction using sperm aspiration may facilitate pregnancy for these men, it may also facilitate the transmission of a genetic disorder that was previously undetected and/or untransmittable. For this reason, genetic testing and counseling for men with CBAVD is recommended, as well as cystic fibrosis carrier screening for their female partners. For these couples, it is important to note that if both partners carry a mutation of the cystic fibrosis gene, their risk of having a child with cystic fibrosis is 25%.

Genetic causes of infertility in women usually involve genetic disorders that affect differentiation of the reproductive organs (e.g., testicular feminization, ambiguous genitalia) and chromosomal abnormalities affecting ovarian development and functioning. In addition, women may be carriers of a genetic disorder resulting in pregnancy losses due to a wide spectrum of abnormal processes from fertilization of the ovum, cleavage of the zygote, implantation of the blastocyst, and embryonic development to fetal viability[28]. Turner's syndrome (45, X) is a genetic disorder occurring in about 1 in 2000–5000 women, in which women have a single X chromosome and no other sex chromosome or variation of the sex chromosome structure. In addition, women with this syndrome exhibit webbing of the neck, small stature, and heart and kidney abnormalities. This disorder is typically identified in early childhood or adolescence, as chromosomal ovarian failure affects physical development, resulting in infertility. By contrast, women with mosaic Turner's syndrome (45, X/46, XX) or a chromosomal variation of the disorder are often asymptomatic and normal-appearing and, as such, may present to an infertility clinic seeking services unaware of their genetic disorder. Women with Turner's syndrome may occasionally conceive, although there is a high risk of abnormalities in their offspring. Another genetic disorder of women, typically diagnosed in adolescence, is Rokitansky-Küster-Hauser syndrome, in which women have functioning ovaries together with congenital absence of the vagina and/or uterus, resulting in infertility. With these disorders, psychological issues typically involve personal identity, reproductive choices, and sexual functioning, as well as medical or surgical treatment. Finally, although assisted reproduction may help many women with genetic disorders become biological mothers, the risk of transmission of the disorder to offspring remains an important consideration for them and their partners, especially if they plan to use their own oocytes. Furthermore, it has recently been reported that some women with Turner's syndrome who became pregnant via ovum donation died suddenly in the third trimester of pregnancy due to aortic dissection[34]. This discovery highlights how the avenues of reproduction opened by reproductive technologies may have dramatic and unpredictable consequences.

Genetic Counseling Regarding Pregnancy Losses

A common referral to a genetic counselor involves multiple pregnancy losses. Chromosomal problems causing fetal losses may be in one or both parents (thereby increasing the risk of a subsequent pregnancy loss) or may be due to an error in fertilization or in cell division during egg or sperm cell production ('packaging error'), known as nondisjunction. Genetic causes of miscarriage may be sporadic, chromosomally abnormal, or recurrent due to heritable chromosomal abnormalities. The incidence of sporadic (or isolated incident) miscarriage is 12–15% of all clinically recognized pregnancies. Chromosomal abnormalities account for 50% of sporadic miscarriages, and there is a 25% recurrence risk for miscarriage in the absence of a family history of genetic disorders and/or advanced maternal age[28]. Couples experiencing two or more miscarriages, a miscarriage plus a stillbirth, a malformed fetus, or live-born defective baby should receive a formal genetic evaluation for recurrent pregnancy loss[28]. Genetic evaluation usually involves chromosome studies (karyotyping) of both parents and fetal tissue, detailed family history (see Figure 1), and, when available, photographs of the fetus, radiographic studies, autopsy, laboratory testing, and placenta and cord assessment[35].

Typically, there are both practical and psychological benefits for infertile couples to pursue genetic counseling following a fetal loss, even though information may be provisional or difficult to accept or provide less than 100% accuracy[35]. Often, infertile couples feel that a pregnancy loss is a mixed blessing: The good news is they have achieved a pregnancy; the bad news is the pregnancy was lost. They (and possibly their caregivers) may have difficulty in seeing a pattern in the losses and may respond with alarm when a referral for genetic evaluation is suggested. Alternatively, infertile couples may perceive genetic testing and counseling as an opportunity to reduce ambiguity and gain an explanation or greater understanding of their infertility, even though it carries with it the possibility of a genetic diagnosis. However, the results of genetic testing and even the process of genetic counseling may exacerbate a couple's grieving, reopen wounds, precipitate feelings of defectiveness, touch off a crisis with other family members, and influence future reproductive decisions.

Prenatal Genetic Testing

Men and women undergoing infertility treatment are usually older (past mid-30s) and at an increased risk for having a child with a chromosomal abnormality. At times, they may be unaware of these risks because the focus of their attention has been on getting pregnant, not the challenges and risks of pregnancy itself. Pregnancy after infertility, more often than not, is characterized by ambiguity, isolation, fear, and technological bewilderment[36], and entails a disquieting array of emotions from incredible joy and promise to unanticipated anxiety and ambivalence. The 'technological bewilderment' of these pregnancies refers to the myriad medical technologies that contribute to the creation of the postinfertility pregnancy, as well as its prenatal evaluation and medical management. Adding to this bewilderment are decisions regarding prenatal testing, termination, and the technologies used to accomplish these medical interventions (see Chapter 24).

Prenatal genetic screening and/or testing is usually performed in the second trimester of pregnancy for the purpose of detecting chromosomal abnormalities, single gene disorders, and/or structural fetal anomalies. Recommendations for prenatal genetic testing are usually based on (1) advanced maternal age, (2) family history of a genetic disease or previous child with an anomaly, (3) two or more unexplained miscarriages or prior pregnancies/children with birth defects, (4) exposure to potentially harmful substances, and (5) abnormal ultrasound or alpha-fetoprotein (AFP) or triple test screening.

The most common disorders for which couples seek prenatal genetic testing are chromosomal problems such as Down syndrome and neural tube defects (spina bifida or anencephaly). The chance of having a child with *Down syndrome*, as well as other abnormalities caused by the presence of an extra chromosome, increases with advancing maternal age (Tables 4 and 5). However, it should be noted that what is medically defined as advanced maternal age (older than 35 years at delivery) may not be understood by infertile couples who are typically older. Chromosomal abnormalities may also be due to a parental chromosomal translocation, resulting in an inherited problem in which the fetus is conceived with extra or missing chromosomal material.

Table 4 Risk of having a live baby with any chromosomal problem

Age	Births per 1000
20	1.9
25	2.1
30	2.6
35	5.2
40	15.2
45	47.6

(Reproduced from ref. 64, with permission)

Table 5 Risk of Down syndrome live birth

Age	Risk
20	1/1923
30	1/885
35	1/365
40	1/109
45	1/32
49	1/12

(Reproduced from ref. 64, with permission)

Neural tube defects are malformations of the central nervous system with both a genetic and an environmental component. The risk to the fetus appears to be reduced in some pregnancies by maternal folic acid supplementation (100% of RDA) prior to 28 days of gestation. The highest incidence of neural tube defects is in Northern Ireland, with the lowest incidence in Japan[38]. The incidence of neural tube defects is not related to the age of the mother, although if a couple has had a previous child with a neural tube defect, the risk of recurrence in each subsequent pregnancy is increased to about 1 in 30[38].

Current prenatal screening and testing options include both noninvasive screening measures, such as maternal blood tests or ultrasound, and invasive diagnostic testing (e.g., amniocentesis and CVS) that incur a risk of pregnancy loss. Screening may help assess a risk but are not diagnostic, while testing is more definitive yet still may be inaccurate due to other contributing factors. The currently available prenatal screening involves AFP or triple screen with ultrasound, while diagnostic testing includes CVS, amniocentesis, and in some cases fetal blood sampling (cordocentesis).

Maternal serum AFP is a noninvasive method of obtaining information about fetal development in pregnancy by assessing AFP, a protein produced by the fetus and detectable in the mother's blood. It is helpful in screening for Down

Maternal serum AFP with triple screen, also known as marker assessment of pregnancy (MAP), involves measuring three maternal blood hormones—AFP, human chorionic gonadotropin (hCG), and estriol (Ue3/Ue4)—to provide a more accurate detection of Down syndrome. However, MAP is a limited screening tool, as the results may be influenced by other maternal factors such as age, weight, diabetes, race, other pregnancy elements (bleeding, multiples), and especially the exact gestational time (normal levels at 16 weeks gestation are not normal at 13 weeks). If the AFP or MAP results are abnormal, more extensive (and invasive) prenatal testing is an appropriate option.

Ultrasound (also referred to as sonography) is used as a diagnostic tool for certain structural birth defects and some genetic disorders to determine the sex of the fetus (for situations in which the genetic disorder is sex-linked) and to evaluate fetal growth, well-being, and variations in amniotic fluid. Abnormalities commonly identified on ultrasound include misshapen (club) feet, mild hydronephrosis (fluid on the kidneys), neural tube defects such as anencephaly (absence of skull and brain), hydrocephaly (increased cerebrospinal fluid in the brain), choroid plexus cysts (small pockets of fluid trapped in brain blood cells), facial clefts (e.g., cleft palate), cystic hygromas (cystic swelling in the neck), abnormalities in the heart, diaphragmatic hernia (contents of abdomen outside the chest), limb problems (e.g., dwarfism), and others[39]. Ultrasound can also be used as a screening tool to look for subtle variations that may indicate an increased risk. For instance, fetuses with femur (thigh bone) measurements more than 1 week delayed from the remainder of fetal measurements may indicate an increased risk for Down syndrome.

CVS (occasionally called placental biopsy or placentocentesis), was introduced in the mid-1980s primarily as a method of evaluating fetal chromosomes or testing for single gene disorders. CVS is usually done between 10 and 12 weeks of pregnancy and involves the passage of a needle or cannula into the placenta to withdraw tissue (cells) into a syringe for testing. CVS may be transvaginal or transabdominal, with both methods guided by ultrasound. The risk of miscarriage following CVS in experienced centers is generally reported to be 1%. Results of the chromosome analysis usually takes about 10 days. The use and acceptance of CVS rest almost entirely on the fact that it can be done much sooner than amniocentesis and test results are more quickly available, thereby allowing earlier pregnancy termination if the fetus is determined to have any anomalies. However, the drawbacks of CVS can be significant. For example, while most diseases detectable by amniocentesis can also be detected by CVS, neural tube defects cannot, and ambiguous test results occur in 1 of every 100 tests. In addition, limb damage to the developing fetus has been reported to occur in 1 of every 1000 tests.

Amniocentesis, introduced in the 1930s, initially involved injecting dye into the uterus to outline the fetus on x-ray examination[38]. In the 1950s, it was used to test for Rh factor or fetal blood type when the baby's blood group was incompatible with the mother's. Amniocentesis was first introduced for testing fetuses with

suspected genetic diseases in 1967 and today remains the most common method used for prenatal testing. Amniocentesis was introduced before ultrasound was widely used, but with the benefit of ultrasound, the risk of miscarriage following amniocentesis is currently reported to be 0.6 in 100 pregnancies[38]. Amniocentesis involves the use of ultrasound to guide a needle into the amniotic fluid surrounding the fetus and the withdrawal of fluid containing fetal cells that are used for genetic testing. The most common reasons for undertaking amniocentesis are to evaluate fetal chromosomes and to detect neural tube defects. Amniocentesis is usually performed between 15 and 17 weeks of pregnancy, with chromosome test results available in about 10 days (other testing often taking longer), allowing termination of an affected pregnancy before 21-weeks gestation. However, many women and their partners find the termination of an affected fetus so late in pregnancy a significant drawback of this procedure. Even when the pregnancy is found to be normal, delayed attachment clearly affects a couple's enjoyment of, and attachment to, the pregnancy.

Continuing or Terminating a Genetically Affected Pregnancy

In a review of studies conducted during the past 10 years, it was found that the vast majority of couples chose to terminate pregnancies with severe abnormalities after prenatal genetic testing and usually made the decision to terminate before knowing the results of genetic testing[40]. Sjorgren and Uddenberg[41] found that 62% of respondents had decided to terminate an affected pregnancy prior to having prenatal diagnostic testing. Termination rates ranged from 73% to 90% for prenatal diagnosis of Down syndrome to 100% for prenatal detection of anencephaly or spina bifida[42]. However, for less severe defects, termination rates were as low as 38%[42]. In short, although pregnancy termination for a genetic anomaly is common, a significant number of couples choose to continue their pregnancy after receiving a 'less than normal' diagnosis.

Psychological reactions following the termination of a pregnancy due to fetal anomaly appear to be more similar to psychological responses following spontaneous miscarriage than reactions to elective termination (abortion)[36]. Grief and depression are typical responses to miscarriage, while relief is the most common response to elective abortion. Grief, loss, sadness, depression, and psychological distress were found to be common in couples terminating a pregnancy for genetic reasons[43–47]. Blumberg and colleagues[48] found that depression following termination of a pregnancy for genetic reasons occurred in up to 92% of women and 82% of men, a much greater incidence than that associated with termination of pregnancy for other reasons or following other perinatal losses. However, study participants stated that they felt that terminating an affected pregnancy was preferable to giving birth to an affected child and they would choose the same course of action in another pregnancy. Nevertheless, risk factors for psychological distress following the loss of a wanted pregnancy include prior history of depression, poor social support, ambivalence or coercion about the termination, and disturbed marital relationship[36,49,50].

Infertility counselors may or may not be involved in counseling patients regarding genetic screening or the termination process, although grief issues following pregnancy termination for genetic reasons often become relevant issues in psychotherapy, understandably influencing adjustment and future reproductive decisions.

Psychotherapeutic techniques should help grieving parents distinguish between the healthy child that they had anticipated and the unhealthy child actually lost[35]. Sharing the loss with a few close, nonjudgmental confidants often promotes recovery and reduces shame, as does networking with appropriate support groups. Increasingly, men and women are finding the anonymous support offered by Internet resources helpful. Like other perinatal losses, this loss often reawakens past unresolved losses, disappointments, and/or deprivations, especially those involving elective termination of unwanted pregnancy (see Chapter 12).

Decisions regarding pregnancy termination are always challenging but are even more so when the 'elective' termination involves a *wanted* pregnancy following discovery of a genetic disorder or defect. Even when a couple is certain and confident that termination is the right decision for them, ending a wanted pregnancy is onerous. Adding another dimension to the loss is the variety of decisions that the couple must consider, such as termination techniques, termination facility and/or caregivers, autopsy, genetic testing of fetal tissue, and disposal of fetal remains. Some women prefer procedures that minimize the pregnancy experience and/or physical trauma, while others prefer to experience labor and delivery, recreating as much as possible a 'normal' delivery surrounded by familiar medical caregivers.

The other side of the counseling issue concerns couples who decide to continue a pregnancy despite the genetic diagnosis. The tasks and psychological impact of continuing a pregnancy after an abnormal prenatal diagnosis differ greatly from those associated with termination. For couples who have experienced infertility, the high emotional investment and fear (or actuality) that a future pregnancy may not be possible may strengthen their desire to continue, even after abnormal test results are obtained. When these results indicate a less severe prognosis or only a probability for poor outcome, the option of termination may not even be considered. Further, as medical technology advances, physicians are increasingly able to treat babies, pre- and/or postnatally, for complications of genetic disorders and birth defects. Psychological tasks for these couples often involve attachment to a fetus that is different from what they had anticipated and emotional preparation for parenting an affected (even disabled) child.

Lamentably, prenatal testing procedures have the potential (although minimal) of precipitating a pregnancy loss. This 'preventable' pregnancy loss can be a bitter finale for infertile couples after such extensive and extraordinary efforts to achieve parenthood. These couples may feel angry, guilty, and betrayed by the medical science on which they relied for help, often while personally denying the medical risks of the procedures. However, it is important to note that some of these losses may have been 'natural' miscarriages, perhaps related to the genetic disorder or factors associated with the infertility diagnosis. In a study[51] measuring mood after a pregnancy loss following CVS or amniocentesis, only 20% of the women reported disturbed mood states 6 months later. Women who reported greater mood disturbance at 6 months were more likely to have sought some type of mental health services after the loss, described less support from and congruence with their partners, and reported less support from family and friends. Clearly, a small portion of women (perhaps those with minimal emotional support) may be more emotionally vulnerable and in greater need of emotional assistance and special psychological care.

Use of Assisted Reproductive Technologies for Genetic Reasons

Assisted reproductive technologies are defined as methods of medically assisted conception involving varying levels of technological intervention to retrieve gametes (sperm or oocytes) for fertilization either outside the body (e.g., IVF) or with assistance inside the body (e.g., gamete intrafallopian transfer). Third-party reproduction, sometimes via assisted reproductive technologies, entails the use of donated gametes, donated embryos, surrogacy, or a gestational carrier to facilitate parenthood. In the past, men and women with a chromosomal problem, genetically transmittable heritable disorder, or genetic cause of infertility had few family-building alternatives: childlessness, adoption, donor insemination, or repeated 'trial' pregnancies involving prenatal testing and termination. Today, with the advent of IVF and other forms of assisted reproduction, as well as PGD on their own gametes, the opportunities for achieving parenthood for couples with a detectable genetic disorder have dramatically increased.

Technically, couples affected by a genetic disorder or disease may not be infertile, particularly if their reason for using reproductive technology is to prevent the transmission of a genetic disorder. These couples may be able to conceive or even reproduce, although they may miscarry, give birth to an affected child, or experience repeated pregnancy losses of unknown etiology until a genetic diagnosis is determined. Nevertheless, the psychological experience of infertile couples is similar to that of couples who are childless because of a transmittable genetic disorder. The option of a healthy, unaffected child has been removed, repeated losses often result in profound grief, and the experience of reproductive failure elicits feelings of guilt, shame, and stigma.

An increasing number of men and women with genetic factors affecting fertility are turning to assisted reproduction to have a child. Examples of particular interest are conditions causing sterility such as Klinefelter's syndrome, Turner's syndrome, or Rokitansky-Küster-Hauser syndrome in which assisted reproduction can now facilitate biological parenthood (albeit it with unknown risks). Klinefelter's syndrome (47, XXY) is a chromosomal condition affecting 1 in 1000 men who typically have underdeveloped testes, enlarged breasts, and are infertile as a result of the extra X chromosome. Abnormal testicular development also results in very rare spermatogenesis. While in the past the use of donated sperm was the only reproductive alternative for affected men, now fertilization can be achieved through the use of sperm aspiration from the testes and its injection into the oocyte, enabling previously sterile men to have genetically related children. Retrieval of sperm through aspiration may involve microsurgical epididymal sperm aspiration or testicular sperm extraction, thereby overcoming sperm transport problems, while intracytoplasmic sperm injection overcomes sperm penetration and mobility problems. However, assisted reproduction does not overcome the genetic disorder causing infertility: Affected men still have a chromosomal abnormality, and their child remain at risk of inheriting it or of developing an unknown variation of the disorder[52].

For some women with Turner's syndrome biological motherhood can best be achieved through IVF with donated oocytes, which enables the pregnancy experience but requires the relinquishment of a genetically-shared child. By contrast, women with Rokitansky-Küster-Hauser syndrome may achieve parenthood through the fertilization of their own oocytes using IVF and the assistance of a gestational carrier who bears the pregnancy. While gestational carriers can provide a biological child, this method of third-party reproduction means the relinquishment of the pregnancy experience and involves the risk of genetic transmission of the disorder to the child.

However, the achievement of parenthood through assisted reproduction is not without psychological or social consequences to the rearing parents and even the child (see Chapter 25). In addition, the considerations of these technologies include partner consensus, financial cost, personal well-being, social and familial consequences, and the physical resources of the couple, particularly the woman who must undergo the majority of treatment or may have other health conditions complicating pregnancy. Finally, while assisted reproduction offers hope and opportunity for many, its disadvantages may only discourage and further disappoint others. In a couple's single-minded goal to become parents, one or both partners may minimize the importance of the transmission risk to the child and press on with reproductive solutions that fulfill their psychological need but ignore other concerns, including the physical risks to the mother or the child.

IVF/Preimplanation Genetic Diagnosis

PGD is considered by many a groundbreaking new reproductive technology because it allows individuals or couples with a history of a genetic condition the opportunity to screen for the genetic disorder before pregnancy, thereby decreasing or eliminating the need for prenatal genetic testing and pregnancy termination[53]. In addition, it provides the opportunity for couples to deliver genetically-shared children free of genetic disorders, while avoiding the rigors of 'trial pregnancies' and the moral dilemmas prohibiting abortion as a means of avoiding transmission of genetic disease. PGD involves the integration of three specific medical technologies: IVF, embryo biopsy, and molecular genetic testing[54]. In PGD, one or two cells of an embryo created through IVF are biopsied and tested for a genetic disorder or disease, after which unaffected embryos are transferred to the uterus for gestation. PGD is also known as embryo genetic disorder analysis or blastomere analysis for implantation (BABI). Another method of PGD is polar body analysis and involves analyzing the egg after fertilization for a genetic disorder or disease.

Estimates of success rates or 'take home baby' rates for PGD are generally significantly lower than traditional IVF success rates (10% vs. 35%), probably due mainly to the high rate of embryo wastage involved in PGD. It is estimated that 30–50% of embryos may be lost or damaged as a result of the procedure, posing a potential threat for immediate or long-term risks to those embryos. A few studies have focused on fetal risks due to the manipulation of embryos during PGD. Grifo and colleagues[55] performed biopsies on 122 embryos from patients identified as carriers of a genetic disorder and reported that 28 embryos were diagnosed as unaffected, eight of which implanted, resulting in three deliveries of four babies, three ongoing pregnancies, and one chemical pregnancy. One case of cystic fibrosis was misdiagnosed and was subsequently terminated. Finally, Soussis and colleagues[56] in a comparison of PGD and traditional IVF cycles found that pregnancies resulting from biopsied embryos behaved similarly to control IVF pregnancies, although the preimplantation pregnancies had reduced hCG levels and

smaller ultrasound measurements in early pregnancy.

Criticisms of PGD have focused on its limited accuracy (in comparison to other forms of prenatal genetic testing), its current ability to detect only a limited number of genetic disorders, its invasiveness (e.g., IVF), limited success rates, damage to embryos as a result of embryo manipulation during procedure, the number of embryos lost in the procedure, and the financial cost. Because only a small number of genetic disorders can be detected using PGD, further prenatal genetic testing for other genetic disorders may be necessary and may foreseeably precipitate the discovery of a different genetic or chromosomal disorder warranting pregnancy termination due to fetal anomaly[57]. The financial cost of IVF/PGD is estimated as double that of regular IVF, in part due to its limited availability worldwide. All of these factors have lead some consumers and clinicians to conclude that, at present and for the majority of couples, the disadvantages of IVF/PGD outweigh the advantages. Moreover, these disadvantages are serious enough to mean that IVF/PGD is only applicable to, feasible for, and available to a limited few[58].

Genetic Screening of Potential Gamete/Embryo Donors

Genetic screening of donated gametes and embryos has gained increasing attention and importance by the increasing use and acceptance of 'prenatal adoption' (i.e., pregnancy using donated gametes or embryos), lawsuits and unethical practices regarding donated gametes/embryos, and increasing consumer awareness and demand. Consumers justifiably expect donors of gametes or embryos to have had a complete medical, psychological, and genetic evaluation[54]. As a result, practice guidelines regarding the genetic screening of donors were developed by the American Society for Reproductive Medicine in 1993[59]:

1. The donor should be generally healthy and
    A. Not have a Mendelian disorder or major malformation
    B. Not be a carrier for a known single-gene disorder
    C. Not have or be a carrier for a multifactorial disorder
    D. Not have a major familial disorder
    E. Not have a chromosomal rearrangement
    F. Be young (for males, younger than 50 years; for females, younger than 35 years)
2. First-degree relatives of the donor should be free of
    A. Major malformations
    B. Mendelian disorders
    C. Chromosomal disorders
3. Permanent record keeping

Genetic assessment of potential sperm or oocyte donors typically involves obtaining a family and medical history through a standard questionnaire. Most sperm banks and oocyte donation programs do not engage the services of genetic counselors or involve comprehensive genetic counseling or screening services. Although it has been recommended that genetic testing (karyotyping) be done on all potential sperm and oocyte donors[60], very few sperm banks in the United States offer these services, and it is not typically included in assessments of oocyte donors. Nevertheless, in a recent study of oocyte donors that included genetic counseling and karyotyping, 8.2% of women with normal physical examinations and personal and family histories tested positive for a major genetic abnormality. As a result, it has been suggested that all gamete donor programs use more thorough screening protocols (e.g., karotyping) to minimize transmission or carrier status of genetic abnormalities[60].

Traditionally, sperm donation in the United States has involved varying degrees of physical screening, donor anonymity, and voluntary donation with minimal financial remuneration. Sperm is typically cryopreserved and stored, according to laboratory guidelines, in a commercially operated sperm bank or a bank affiliated with an infertility practice. By contrast, oocyte donation began with known donations, often after the potential donor had been recruited by a family member. Today, oocyte donation also involves medical screening, possible anonymity, and voluntary donations with limited financial remuneration, following recruitment similar to sperm donors. However, currently, oocytes cannot be reliably cryopreserved or banked and thus are usually managed through an infertility practice or a commercial oocyte recruitment program. To date, there are no government regulations of gamete or embryo donor facilities or practices in the United States, although some banks pursue voluntary accreditation of laboratory services.

Embryo donation is usually the result of cryopreserved 'extra' embryos provided by an infertile couple who has undergone IVF. The couple has 'donated' the embryos that they do not intend to use because they do not want them destroyed or used for research. Most embryo donations are available through an infertility practice and are anonymous donations. Most embryo donor couples have not undergone preconception genetic screening, nor have the donated embryos undergone preimplantation genetic screening. Without this screening, donated embryos and the children born as a result of them may very well be affected by a genetic disorder, whether obvious or obscure.

Genetic screening of a recipient couple or individual has not been a major consideration among infertile individuals or their caregivers. However, recipient testing may be important if there is potential for genetic risk due to family medical and pregnancy history, if the recipient and donor ethnic or racial backgrounds are similar, thereby increasing the risk of certain genetic disorders or diseases, or if the recipient couple wishes to screen for a specific genetic disorder (e.g., cystic fibrosis, Tay-Sachs disease)[61,62]. Finally, when considering the genetic issues of donated gametes or embryos, infertile or recipient couples should understand (1) the genetic screening protocols used by the gamete/embryo donation program or bank that they are using, (2) the impossibility of detecting 100% of carrier or genetic disorders, and (3) the possibility of *de novo* genetic disorders (a new gene mutation when there has been no history of one)[54,61,62].

THERAPEUTIC INTERVENTIONS

To aid in patient care and highlight the overlapping roles of genetic and infertility counselors, Shapiro and Djurdjinovic[24] outlined the psychosocial issues of genetic counseling for infertile couples. They pointed out how the emotional vulnerability and reproductive history of infertile couples alters their perspective on genetic and reproductive medicine, often resulting in unrealistic expectations and decisions based on hope versus reality. In fact, research has shown that infertile couples consistently overestimate the success rates of reproductive technologies. In addition, they make decisions influenced more by the perceived burden of a condition than by the actual numerical value of the risk[22]. It is against this backdrop of high expectations, prior narcissistic wounds, long history of medical treatment, and impaired information processing that genetic and infertility counselors provide assistance to individuals

seeking reproductive services who may or may not be infertile.

Genetic counseling typically involves discussions of the medical aspects of a disease or presenting problem, assessment of genetic risk, genetic basis involved in the disease, and appropriate genetic management through available testing. A family history, typically called a 'pedigree', is obtained, and, when appropriate, arrangements are made for obtaining blood samples for chromosome analysis and DNA or metabolic testing (karyotyping) when indicated. The example shown in Figure 1 depicts a couple evaluated for multiple miscarriages, in which it was determined that the wife and her brother were balanced 13/14 translocation carriers, which was the cause of the pregnancy losses. If a genetic disorder is suspected or has been identified, risks for recurrence or transmission, and education regarding the diagnosed disorder are part of the genetic counseling process. Options regarding prenatal testing and diagnosis are also typically explored. In addition, reproductive options are reviewed with the couple, including assisted reproductive technologies, donated gametes, and third-party reproduction, as well as adoption as a family-building alternative. Discussions may also involve exploration of religious or personal ethics, reproductive goals, feasible medical treatments, availability of family support, and acceptability of prenatal genetic testing. Finally, the genetic counselor assesses the emotional response, reactivity, and receptivity of the individuals, their response as a couple and to each other, and their preparedness for pregnancy or assisted reproduction. If problems are noted, an individual or couple may be referred to an infertility counselor or other mental health professional, appropriate support organization, or medical provider, for further assessment and/or psychotherapy.

A diagnosis of a genetic disorder or disease in a partner, the couple, or potential offspring can precipitate a personal crisis and endanger the stability of a marriage. As such, assistance and interventions are directed at helping the couple cope with their acute distress, anxiety, and uncertainty as they struggle with making decisions and deal with the aftermath of the diagnosis[36]. The scarcity of support and understanding for this unique crisis and vulnerability to feelings of stigma, shame, and secrecy highlight the importance of a referral to an appropriate mental health professional and/or support group, patient education materials, and telephone contact from caregivers and support networks[36].

Family factors are often influential in the psychosocial adjustment of infertile couples and are especially relevant if the genetic diagnosis affects other family members or precipitates a family crisis. As such, the emergence of myriad family problems can be expected, such as disclosure of family secrets, dysfunctional communication patterns, inappropriate family reactions to stress and loss (particularly infertility and/or pregnancy loss), boundary violations, divided family loyalties, parental guilt for 'causing' the genetic disorder, and patterns of enmeshment and diffusion. Negative or inaccurate family beliefs regarding heredity, illness, and disability, childbearing expectations, kinship ties, and medical technologies (e.g., genetic testing and/or diagnosis, assisted reproduction) may impair a couple's adjustment by limiting their options and increasing their distress. Alternatively, family values, expectations, and resources may facilitate a couple's adjustment by reinforcing effective coping skills, encouraging adaptability to change, providing emotional warmth and support, and modeling positive mental health habits.

The role, responsibilities, and counseling tasks for both genetic and infertility counselors are influenced by a couple's history of infertility, medical treatments, use of assisted reproductive technologies (especially donated gametes/embryos), infertility diagnosis, and future availability of reproductive options and/or treatments. For this reason, the National Institutes of Health Workshop Statement developed guidelines for the provision of reproductive genetic services[63]:

Reproductive genetic services should not be used to pursue 'eugenic' goals but should be aimed at increasing individuals' control over their own reproductive lives. Therefore, new strategies need to be developed to evaluate the success of such services:

1. Reproductive genetic services should be meticulously voluntary
2. Reproductive genetic services should be value sensitive
3. Standard of care for reproductive genetic services should emphasize genetic information, education, and counseling rather than testing procedures alone
4. Social, legal, and economic constraints on reproductive genetic services should be removed
5. Increasing attention focused on the development and utilization of reproductive genetic testing services may further stigmatize individuals affected by a particular disorder or disability

These guidelines are important not only to genetic counselors but also to infertility counselors, as they emphasize patient autonomy, values, and personal control of reproduction, while recognizing the potential for patient harm and/or discrimination. As providers of patient education, information, counseling, and advocacy, infertility and genetic counselors are in a unique position to facilitate patient decisions regarding reproductive genetics and complicated reproductive technologies.

The role of genetic testing, diagnosis, and treatment in reproductive medicine represents another area about which infertility counselors must be prepared to address complex biopsychosocial issues of childbearing and family building. The couple presenting for infertility services may not know that they have a genetic disorder causing their infertility and may be predictably distressed when confronted with an unexpected *dual* diagnosis: infertility and a genetic disease. Also, increasingly, men and women seeking reproductive medicine and infertility counseling services may not be technically infertile and have other reasons for using assisted reproduction. As such, the psychosocial issues and needs of these individuals are different. The couple with a genetic problem presenting for infertility counseling is more apt to focus on maximizing their opportunities of having a healthy, unaffected infant, exploring their feelings about raising a child affected with a genetic disease or disorder, and addressing their feelings of guilt or anger at transmitting a genetic problem to their offspring. Marital or family-of-origin issues are more likely to focus expectations of 'normalcy' and 'acceptability' in babies or the impact of the diagnosis on other family members. In addition, a couple may have to consider the implications of the genetic disorder on the affected partner's health and longevity, as well as how the disorder may impact childbearing and child-rearing decisions. Alternatively, many of the psychological responses to genetic diagnosis such as feelings of loss, grief, defectiveness, or altered sense of self are similar to those experienced by infertile individuals.

FUTURE IMPLICATIONS

The burgeoning technologies in reproductive medicine and genetics will, no doubt, continue to make available an increasingly complex array of reproductive alternatives and treatments. In actuality, more complicated alternatives cause the decision-making to be more difficult rather than less. As the complexity of alternatives increases, financial costs of reproductive and genetic technologies become more burdensome, the ethical and religious dilemmas more bewildering, and the effects on society will continue to become more profound. Rapidly developing technological choices (e.g., cloning, gene therapy) highlight the conundrums faced by families considering them: Whether what can be done should be done, at what cost, and for whose benefit. Finally, availability of medical technologies does not guarantee that any particular technology is feasible or accessible for the vast majority of individuals or even one couple or that the outcome of assisted reproduction will be the one desired. Given these circumstances, both genetic counselors and infertility counselors may be expected to play an even more important and integral role in reproductive and genetic medicine.

SUMMARY

- Both infertility and genetic counselors, as well as other medical professionals, 'counsel' by advising, supporting, and instructing patients dealing with reproductive health problems. While genetic counselors are trained to provide information and support on genetic issues, infertility counselors are trained mental health professionals who provide psychological treatment with the knowledge of infertility issues. They often work together to counsel

- couples about their reproductive health problems and family-building alternatives.
- Contrary to patient expectations, genetic medicine cannot detect and prevent all birth defects, and reproductive medicine cannot provide everyone with the baby he or she wants.
- Infertile couples (accustomed to failed effort and loss) are more likely to highly value the pregnancy and baby and, as a result, are more keenly aware of how prenatal genetic testing can both enhance or depreciate it[9].
- Emotional reactions to pregnancy termination of a genetically affected fetus appear to be much more similar to reactions following spontaneous miscarriage than to elective abortion[49,50] and are seldom protracted or disturbed[36].
- Prenatal diagnosis of a fetal anomaly may help emotional preparation or prolong the period of emotional upset[17].
- Couples who experience two or more miscarriages or a miscarriage plus a stillbirth, birth of a malformed fetus, live-born baby with genetic anomalies, or have a family history of a genetic disorder should receive a formal genetic evaluation and counseling[27].
- Decisions to proceed with prenatal genetic testing are usually based on (1) advanced maternal age, (2) family history of a genetic disease, (3) two or more unexplained miscarriages or prior pregnancies/children with birth defects, and (4) exposure to potentially harmful substances. The major prenatal testing procedures are: AFP or MAP screening, ultrasound, CVS, and amniocentesis.
- PGD, a ground breaking new reproductive technology, allows individuals with a history of a genetic condition the opportunity to screen for the genetic disorder *before* pregnancy, thereby eliminating or at least decreasing the need for prenatal genetic testing and pregnancy termination[53]. However, the disadvantages of this technology are numerous and need to be fully discussed with the patient.
- Assisted reproduction should not be initiated in men and women with a possible or known genetic cause of infertility without prior genetic counseling and risk assessment[32].
- Genetics is an extremely complicated field that is advancing at the same rapid pace as reproductive medicine. Understanding the new advances and interpreting new testing methods in genetics are of utmost importance to infertility counselors. By the same token, an understanding of advances in reproductive medicine is increasingly important to the work of the competent genetics professional working with infertile patients.

REFERENCES

1. McKusick BA. *Mendelian Inheritance in Man: Catalogues of Human Genes and Genetic Disorders*, 11th edn. Baltimore: Johns Hopkins University Press, 1994

2. Bartels DM, LeRoy BS, Caplan A, eds. *Prescribing Our Future: Ethical Challenges in Genetic Counseling*. New York: Aldine de Gruyter, 1993

3. Reed SC. *Counseling in Medical Genetics*. Philadelphia: Saunders, 1955

4. Eunpu DL. Systemically-based psychotherapeutic techniques in genetic counseling. *J Genet Couns* 1997;6:1–20

5. Codori A, Slavney PR, Young C, *et al.* Predictors of psychological adjustment to genetic testing for Huntington's disease. *Health Psychol* 1997;16:36–50

6. Fitzpatrick JL, Hutton EM, Babul R, *et al.* Counseling and screening for cystic fibrosis in patients with congenital bilateral absence of the vas deferens: Patient perceptions. *J Genet Couns* 1996;5:1–15

7. Pergament E. Preimplantation diagnosis: A patient perspective. *Prenat Diagn* 1991; 11:493–500

8. Miedzybrodrodzka Z, Templeton A, Dean J, *et al.* Preimplantation diagnosis or chorionic villi biopsy? Women's attitudes and preferences. *Hum Reprod* 1993; 8:2192–6

9. Sandelowski M, Harris BG, Holditch-Davis D. Amniocentesis in the context of infertility. *Health Care Women Int* 1991; 12:167–78

10. Martin MS, Walker ME. Exploring the impact on the genetic counseling process when the counselor has a significant genetic or reproductive history. *J Genet Couns* 1995;4:327

11. Marosek KR, Covington SN. Survey results: When you or a colleague is an infertility patient. *Serono Insights Infertil* 1996–7;6–7

12. Fine BA. The evolution of nondirectiveness in genetic counseling and implications of the Human Genome Project. In: Bartels DM, LeRoy BS, Caplan A, eds. *Prescribing Our Future: Ethical Challenges in Genetic Counseling*. New York: Aldine de Gruyter, 1993:101–18

13. Kessler S. The psychological paradigm shift in genetic counseling. *Soc Biol* 1980; 27:167–85

14. Baram A, Friedman AL, Zakowski SG. Stress and genetic testing for disease risk. *Health Psychol* 1997;1:8–19

15. Nachtigall RD, Quiroga SS, Tschann JM, *et al.* Stigma, disclosure, and family functioning among parents of children conceived through donor insemination. *Fertil Steril* 1997;68:1–7

16. Sandelowski M, Harris BG, Holitch-Davis D. Mazing: Infertile couples and the quest for a child. *Image J Nurs Sch* 1989; 21:220–6

17. Zuzkar D. The psychological impact of prenatal diagnosis of fetal abnormality: Strategies for investigation and intervention. *Women's Health Rev* 1987;12:91–103

18. Solnit JA, Stark MH. Mourning and the birth of a defective child. *Psychoanal Study Child* 1961;16:523–7

19. Allen JSF, Mulhauser LC. Genetic counseling after abnormal prenatal diagnosis: Facilitating coping in families who continue their pregnancies. *J Genet Couns* 1995;4:251–65

20. Frets P, Neirmeiher M. Reproductive planning after genetic counseling: A perspective from the last decade. *Clin Genet* 1990;38:295–306

21. Lippman-Hand A, Fraser CF. Genetic counseling—the post-counseling period: 1. Parents' perception of uncertainty. *Am J Med Genet* 1979;4:51–71

22. Leonard CO, Chase GA, Childs B. Genetic counseling: A consumer's view. *N Engl J Med* 1972;287:433–9

23. Beeson D, Goldbus M. Decision-making: Whether or not to have prenatal diagnosis and abortion after detection of fetal abnormality. *Am J Genet* 1984;36(suppl): 122s

24. Shapiro CH, Djurdjinovic L. Understanding our infertile genetic counseling patients. In: Fine BA, Gettig EL, Greendale K, *et al.*, eds. *Strategies in Genetic Counseling: Reproductive Genetics and New Technologies*. White Plains, NY: March of Dimes Defects Foundation, 1990:127–31

25. Sandelowski M. A case of conflicting paradigms: Nursing and reproductive technology. *Adv Nurs Sci* 1988;10:35–45

26. Rothman BK. The tentative pregnancy: Then and now. In: Rothenberg KH, Thomson EJ, eds. *Women and Prenatal Testing: Facing the Challenges of Genetic Technology.* Columbus, OH: Ohio State University Press, 1994:260–70

27. Geraedts JPM. Chromosomal anomalies and recurrent miscarriage. *Infertil Reprod Med Clin North Am* 1996;7:667–88

28. Plouffe L, White EW, Tho SP, *et al.* Etiologic factors of recurrent abortion and subsequent reproductive performance of couples: Have we made any progress in the past 10 years? *Am J Obstet Gynecol* 1992;167:313–20

29. Digman PS. Genetics and pregnancy loss: Value of counseling between pregnancies. In: Woods JR, Esposito JL, eds. *Pregnancy Loss: Medical Therapeutics and Practical Considerations.* Baltimore: Williams & Wilkins, 1987:198–206

30. Ma S, Kalousek DK, Yuen BS, *et al.* Chromosome investigation in vitro fertilization failure. *J Assist Reprod Genet* 1994;11:445–51

31. Pryor JL, Kent-First M, Muallem A, *et al.* Microdeletions in the Y chromosome of infertile men. *N Engl J Med* 1997; 336:534–9

32. Mak V, Jarvi KA. The genetics of male infertility. *J Urol* 1996;156:1245–57

33. Nagel TC, Tesch LG. Art and high risk patients. *Fertil Steril* 1997;68:74–89

34. Reijo R. Diverse spermatogenic defects in humans caused by Y chromosome deletions encompassing a novel RNA-binding protein gene. *Nat Genet* 1995; 10:383

35. Curry CJR. Pregnancy loss, stillbirth, and neonatal death: A guide for the pediatrician. *Pediatr Clin North Am* 1992; 39:157–92

36. Leon IG. Pregnancy termination due to fetal anomaly: Clinical considerations. *Infant Ment Health J* 1995;16:112–26

37. Glaser ES. *The Long-Awaited Stork: A Guide to Parenting After Infertility.* New York: Lexington Books, 1990

38. deCrespigny L, Dredge R. *Which Tests for My Unborn Baby?* New York: Oxford University Press, 1996

39. Romero R, Pilu P, Jeanty A, *et al. Prenatal Diagnosis of Congenital Abnormalities.* Norwalk, CT: Appleton & Lange, 1988

40. Wertz D. How parents of affected children view selective abortion. In: Holmes H, ed. *Issues in Reproductive Technology.* New York: Garland, 1992:161–89

41. Sjogren B, Uddenberg N. Prenatal diagnosis and maternal attachment to the child-to-be. *J Psychosom Obstet Gynaecol* 1988;9:73–87

42. Robinson A, Bender B, Linden M. Decision following the intrauterine diagnosis of sex chromosome aneuploidy. *Am J Med Genet* 1989;34:552–4

43. Magyari PA, Wedehase RD, Callanan NP. A supportive intervention protocol for couples terminating pregnancy for genetic reasons. In: Paul NW, Travers H, Biesecker B, *et al.*, eds. *Strategies in Genetic Counseling: Issues in Perinatal Care.* White Plains, NY: March of Dimes Defects Foundation, 1987:75–83

44. Figa-Talamanca I. Abortion and mental health. In: Hodgson JE, ed. *Abortion and Sterilization: Medical and Social Aspects.* New York: Academic Press, 1981:181–208

45. Nadelson CC. 'Normal' and 'special' aspects of pregnancy: A psychological approach. In: Notman MT, Nadelson CC, eds. *The Woman Patient.* New York: Plenum, 1978;1:73–86

46. White-van Mourik M, Connor J, Ferguson-Smith M. The psychosocial sequelae of a second-trimester termination of pregnancy for fetal abnormality. *Prenat Diagn* 1992:189–204

47. Benkendorf J, Corson V, Allen JF, Ilse S. Perinatal bereavement counseling in genetics. In: Fine BA, Gettig EL, Greendale K, *et al.*, eds. *Strategies in Genetic Counseling: Reproductive Genetics and New Technologies.* White Plains, NY: March of Dimes Defects Foundation, 1990:136–48

48. Blumberg B, Golbus M, Hanson K. Prenatal diagnosis: The experience of families who have children. *Am J Med Genet* 1975;19:729–39

49. Zeanah C, Dailey J, Rosenblatt M, *et al.* Do women grieve after terminating pregnancies because of fetal anomalies? A controlled investigation. *Obstet Gynecol* 1993;82:270–5

50. Lloyd J, Laurence K. Sequelae and support after termination of pregnancy for fetal malformation. *Br Med J* 1985;290:907–9

51. Black RB. A one- and six-month follow-up of prenatal diagnosis patients who lost pregnancies. *Prenat Diagn* 1989;9:795–804

52. Sele B, Cozze J, Chevret E, *et al.* ICSI et syndrome de Klinefelter. *Contracept Fertil Sex* 1996;24:581–4

53. Blatt RJR. Conceiving the future: The impact of the Human Genome Project on gamete donation. In: Seibel MM, Crockin SL, eds. *Family Building Through Egg and Sperm Donation*. Boston: Jones and Barlett, 1996:285–94

54. Jones SL. Advances in human genetics: Implications for infertility nursing practice. *Infertil Reprod Med Clin North Am* 1996;7:577–85

55. Grifo JA, Tang YX, Munne S, *et al.* Healthy deliveries from biopsied human embryos. *Hum Reprod* 1994;9:912–16

56. Soussis I, Harper JC, Kontogianni E, *et al.* Pregnancies resulting from embryos biopsied for preimplantation diagnosis of genetic disease: Biochemical and ultrasonic studies in the first trimester of pregnancy. *J Assist Reprod Genet* 1996; 13:254–65

57. Verlinksy Y. Preimplantation genetic diagnosis. *J Assist Reprod Genet* 1996; 13: 87–9

58. Johnson MD. Practical aspects of preembryo biopsy and diagnosis. *Infertil Reprod Med Clin North Am* 1994;5:213–31

59. American Fertility Society. Guidelines for gamete donation. *Fertil Steril* 1993; 59(suppl 1):1s–9s

60. Licciardi F, Jansen V, Fantini D, *et al.* Strict genetic screening is necessary for oocyte donors. *J Assist Reprod Genet* 1997; 14(suppl):49s

61. Zilberstein M, Verp MS. Genetic issues in gamete donation. In: Seibel MM, Crockin SL. *Family Building Through Egg and Sperm Donation*. Boston, MA: Jones and Bartlett, 1996:94–109

62. Farrell CD. Advances in human genetics: Implications for assisted reproductive technologies in nursing practice. Presented at the Eighth National Conference for IVF Nurse Coordinators and Support Personnel, Boston, MA, May 18–20, 1995

63. National Institutes of Health: Workshop Statements: Reproductive Genetic Testing: Impact on Women. In: Rothenberg KH, Thomson EJ, eds. *Women and Prenatal Testing: Facing the Challenges of Genetic Technology*. Columbus, OH: Ohio State University Press, 1994:295–300

64. Hook EB. Rates of chromosome abnormalities at different maternal ages. *Obstet Gynecol* 1981;58:282

65. Allen JF. A guide to genetic counseling. *J Am Acad Phys Assist* 1991;4:131–41

66. Bennett RL, Steinhaus KA, Ubrich SB, *et al.* Recommendations for standardized human pedigree nomenclature. *J Genet Couns* 1995;4:267–79

12

Pregnancy Loss

Sharon N. Covington, MSW

To contain the whole of death so gently even before life has begun,
and not be angry—this is beyond description.

Rainer Maria Rilke

HISTORICAL OVERVIEW

Pregnancy loss is a broad term used to describe the death of a fetus or baby after conception, during pregnancy, or shortly after birth. Although pregnancy losses have existed since the beginning of mankind, the context has changed dramatically with the advent of reproductive medical technology. For centuries, the death of a baby in pregnancy or shortly after birth was a fact of life—maternal and infant mortality were high and medical intervention almost nonexistent. Some societies and religions protected against this by bestowing 'personhood' only on infants that survived a certain period of time. For example, in China, a child is not recognized as a person until 3 months of age, and in traditional Judaism religious funeral and mourning rituals are not performed before 30 days of life.

However, rapid technological growth in reproductive medicine in the last 50 years has created a picture of medicine-as-god, with the ability to create and continue life. Today, women have more control over their reproductive lives, using a variety of contraceptive devices to avoid pregnancy, advanced reproductive technologies to produce a pregnancy, therapeutic options to terminate or reduce undesired pregnancies, and extensive medical treatment to manage complicated or threatened pregnancies. The consequence has often been an unrealistic expectation that medical intervention can in fact prevent or stop losses in pregnancy.

Just as medical technology has changed, so has the psychological approach to pregnancy loss. Prior to this century, pregnancy and infant losses were a common event and a fact of life in the community, acknowledged, grieved, and mourned in the same manner as other deaths. However, when the treatment of illness, including childbirth, moved from home to hospital, the manner in which death was dealt with changed. Death and dying became sanitized and sterilized. When a baby died, it was handled like a shameful secret, almost as if modern medicine was not suppose to let this happen. The deceased baby was often quietly disposed of without being seen by parents, who were not encouraged to mourn the loss, as it was believed that the whole experience would be too upsetting for them and was better forgotten. 'Out of sight, out of mind' was the emotional approach to a pregnancy loss, and psychological support was minimal.

In the last 20 years, there has been growth in the knowledge and understanding of the psychological ramifications

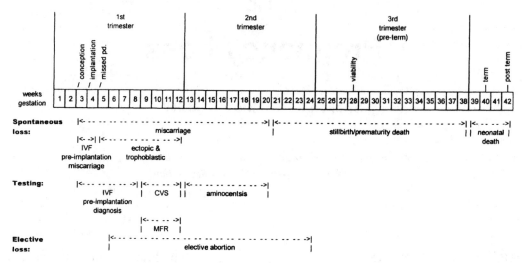

Figure 1 Pregnancy and loss time line

of pregnancy loss, which is frequently a traumatic event in family life.

This chapter will:

- review research in the area
- provide theoretical frameworks that underpin a plan for clinical intervention
- describe psychotherapeutic strategies for counseling couples after a pregnancy loss.

REVIEW OF LITERATURE

Infertility has been defined as the inability to conceive or *carry a pregnancy to a live birth*. This broad definition implies that infertility encompasses both the inability to conceive a pregnancy and the loss of a pregnancy during the perinatal period, that is, before birth. Pregnancy or perinatal loss is a catch-all phrase for the death of a conceptus, fetus, or neonate during the continuum of conception, pregnancy, and birth (Figure 1).

A *miscarriage*, or spontaneous abortion, occurs in the first 20 weeks of pregnancy and is the most common pregnancy loss, estimated to occur in 20–50% of all

conceptions. An *ectopic pregnancy* occurs in 2–3% of pregnancies when the embryo implants and grows in the fallopian tube or anywhere outside the uterus. More rarely, *trophoblastic disease*, or molar pregnancy, happens in 1 out of 2000 pregnancies when the fetus dies but the placenta and/or chorionic villi continue to grow rapidly in a cancer-like way. Both ectopic and molar pregnancies are medical emergencies that may affect future fertility. *Stillbirth* involves the death of a fetus *in utero* after 20-weeks' gestation and before birth, and occurs in 1–2 out of every 100 births. The death of a newborn infant before 28 days of life is termed *neonatal death*, occurring in 1 out of 100 births, and may involve prematurity, birth defects, or sudden infant death syndrome (SIDS). Finally, the term *elective abortion* applies to the voluntary termination of a pregnancy, whether or not the fetus is viable.

Assisted reproductive technologies have further broadened the definition of pregnancy loss. For example, during in vitro fertilization (IVF), conception takes place in the laboratory, and if implantation does not result after transfer of the embryo, it might be called a *preimplantation miscarriage*. Further, the development of genetic testing of fertilized eggs during IVF has resulted in *preimplantation termination* of genetically defective embryos before transfer. Finally, as a consequence of multiple gestation following IVF, *multifetal pregnancy reduction* (MPR), or selective reduction, was developed to terminate a preselected number of fetuses in a multiple pregnancy, usually to maximize the viability of the remaining fetuses or protect the health of the mother.

Early research in the area of pregnancy loss tended to be retrospective, poorly designed, and anecdotal[1-3]. However, it facilitated a growing knowledge-base that pregnancy loss is a significant psychological trauma for parents. A review of the literature covers five areas centering around grief: mourning, gestation, gender, predictors, and interventions.

Grief and Mourning

A significant amount of research has focused on perinatal grief, much of which was based on the early bereavement works of Freud[4], Lindemann[5], Parkes[6], and Bowlby[7]. The grief experience is a universal and predictable process, whereby an individual acknowledges the loss and gradually lets go of the psychological ties to the loved one. Although often used interchangeably, the terms *grief, mourning* and *bereavement* are distinctly different. *Grief* is the emotional response to a loss, manifested by a host of feelings such as shock, numbness, anger, guilt, sadness, and anxiety. *Mourning* is the process, often culturally defined, that one goes through to deal with these emotions. *Bereavement* refers to the time period during which grief is being resolved. Although the mourning process occurs on a continuum of shock, emotional disorganization, and eventual reorganization, the grief experience is like a roller-coaster, where emotional reactions are unpredictable and repetitive. Hence, mourning is a complex process mediated by a wide variety of variables including previous loss, previous childbirth experiences, length of gestation, quality of marital relationship, maternal age, mental health, fertility history, religiosity, physical health, and the likelihood of a subsequent successful pregnancy[8].

The first published study on perinatal loss appeared in 1970 when Kennell and colleagues[9] reported on their interviews with families that had experienced a stillbirth. Subsequent research supports the finding that pregnancy loss involves considerable pain and suffering for parents, with such typical symptoms as sadness, loss of appetite, sleep difficulties, irritability, preoccupation with thoughts of the baby, guilt, shame, and anger[10-14]. Grief is typically intense and begins to decline after the first year of bereavement[15,16]. In addition, there is considerable risk of disordered or pathological grief following a pregnancy loss[16-18]. *Pathological grief* is usually described in terms of psychiatric symptomatology, intense grieving extending beyond the first year, or the absence of grief. Results from these investigations suggests that a substantial number of women, possibly 20–30%, experience significant psychiatric morbidity following a perinatal loss[2].

Grief and Gestation

A common area of interest is the relationship between grief reactions and gestation. There is substantial evidence that the intensity and the duration of grief correspond to the length of gestation[8,14,19,20]. However, other researchers have found no quantitative difference in the grief reactions of mothers who had miscarriages, stillbirths, or neonatal deaths[21]. A more predictive factor in the intensity of grief relates to the sense of psychological attachment to the developing fetus rather than gestational age[8,14]. For example, it has been demonstrated that grief may occur after an unsuccessful IVF cycle, when conception took place in the laboratory but did not result in pregnancy (preimplantation miscarriage)[22].

The kind of loss does not appear to be a determinant in grief and mourning. Grief occurs after ectopic and molar pregnancies, significantly impacting on self- and body image due to the medically intrusive nature of the loss[23,24]. Planned terminations of pregnancies may be distressing and grieved, although not universally and often with no long-term psychological consequences[25,26]. Mothers of a twin who has died experience grief that is quantitatively indistinguishable from mothers who lose a singleton baby[27]. It is also evident that women who terminate a pregnancy because of fetal anomalies experience grief as intense as those who experience spontaneous pregnancy loss and may require similar clinical management[28].

Grief and Gender

Mothers and fathers both mourn a pregnancy loss but will often experience grief in different ways[27,29]. Mothers tend to experience more intense grief, perhaps due to greater prenatal and postnatal attachment[8,14]. However, one study[29] found that 22% of fathers had significantly higher grief scores than mothers. Another study[30] compared grief symptomatology between men and women, with mothers experiencing more emotional and somatic distress, while fathers describing difficulty working, increasing use of alcohol, and social withdrawal. More research on the differing patterns of mourning between mothers and fathers is needed.

Predictors of Complicated Grief

Complicated, disordered, or pathological grief concerns serious psychiatric symptomatology, the absence of grief, or intense grieving beyond the first year that affects the long-term psychological functioning of the individual. The greatest predictor of a pathological grief reaction is a history of poor psychological functioning prior to the loss[8]. One recent study[31] found that women were at five times greater risk of developing depression after a miscarriage than women in the general population. Childless women were also found to be at greater risk of developing a major depression after a perinatal loss. Other risk factors identified in the literature include problematic or lack of social supports, significant life stressors during pregnancy, difficult marital relationship, and poor physical health[8,15,16]. A history of pregnancy or other reproductive loss may also affect the process of grief[20].

Intervention and Grief

Intervention following a pregnancy loss has an impact on grief. There is substantial evidence that family involvement with the deceased baby helps facilitate the grief process[2,9,16,29]. Supportive, reality-enforcing interventions by caregivers to parents, such as seeing, touching, and spending time with the baby, acknowledge the loss and encourage healthy mourning by making it real and tangible. Patients are responsive to open, compassionate, sensitive communication with caregivers and are in need of follow-up care and information, which will facilitate grieving[32]. As important, supportive counseling has been found to significantly shorten bereavement following a perinatal loss[15]. Even a single, follow-up phone call to parents within a few weeks of the loss, in which the grieving process is reviewed and parental concerns are addressed, has been found to significantly reduce guilt and depression several months later[33].

THEORETICAL FRAMEWORKS

Psychology of Pregnancy and Pregnancy Loss

The psychological impact of pregnancy loss is best understood in the context within which it occurs, that is, pregnancy. Pregnancy begins psychologically, long before it occurs physically. From the time girls are little, most play with baby dolls and dream of having children and being mothers. Boys also try on the role of fatherhood in their play. Young couples often carefully plan how their family will grow and talk about their wishes for their children long before they are ready to attempt pregnancy. Thus, men and women lay the psychological and emotional groundwork for adaptation to parenthood and attachment to their child years before the actual event takes place.

Pregnancy is a crisis time when significant changes occur in a short period, and is as much a psychological experience as it is a physical condition. Women experience profound changes in body, sense of self, and in relationship with others. It is a time when psychological defenses are loosened, and unconscious material is apt to emerge. From a psychoanalytic perspective, pregnancy is a regressed state in which early conflicts are revived and repeated[34]. A pregnant woman's identification with her own mother, called maternal identification, is a crucial influence in the psychological course and outcome of pregnancy. Pregnancy is also an intensely narcissistic condition, whereby a man and a woman are recreating themselves. The developing relationship with the baby is based on fantasies, dreams, and images that are reflective of their own psychological issues. There is intense narcissistic involvement, and the pregnancy becomes a source of narcissistic pride or, if problems occur, narcissistic injury. For parents, the psychological challenge in pregnancy is to incorporate and attach to the developing baby, while differentiating the child from one's self[35].

Bonding and attachment, which previously was believed to begin at the time of quickening, have been influenced by the use of new medical technologies[22,36,37]. Women currently have much more control over their reproductive capabilities than ever before through birth control choices, medical treatments, and the option to terminate unwanted pregnancies. Today, blood tests can confirm a pregnancy before a menstrual period is missed. Sonography or ultrasound, much like a window into the uterus, provides an early visual image of the developing baby. Real-time moving pictures of the baby—arms, legs, face, and heartbeat—can be seen before any physical changes have occurred to make others aware of the pregnancy. Genetic testing can be done early in the laboratory during IVF before implantation has occurred, or later with chorionic villus sampling (CVS) and amniocentesis when the genetic makeup and sex of the baby can be learned before a woman is even wearing maternity clothes. Consequently, the information learned from this technology facilitates a very early, intensified psychological involvement with both the pregnancy and the baby, which is seen as a person, not a fetus. (Further discussion of the psychological adaptation to pregnancy can be found in the Chapter 24.)

A pregnancy loss is experienced as an assault on one's psychological foundation. It comes at a time of extreme psychological vulnerability and is in effect a crisis (the loss) within a crisis (the pregnancy). Leon[3] integrated the psychology of pregnancy and pregnancy loss into four areas: a new developmental stage, an instinctual process, object-seeking, and self-enhancement. Pregnancy is a *new phase in life* in which a woman renegotiates the developmental issues of separateness, autonomy, and independence from her mother. If loss occurs, it becomes an obstacle to entering the stage and can result in arrested development and psychological stagnation. Pregnancy is also an *instinctual process*, whereby strong psychological and biological drives come together. A perinatal loss creates an instinctual frustration both by depriving one of the satisfaction of powerful oral drives and by reviving earlier internalized conflicts. For example, mothers often describe a literal 'baby hunger', a profound deprivation of the need to hold, feed, and nurture their baby. Pregnancy is also *object-seeking*, whereby the process of making a person involves internalized interactions that represent both self and others. In addition, pregnancy may be viewed as the pinnacle of both selflessness and self-involvement, a fulfillment of one's most grandiose narcissistic wishes. When a pregnancy loss occurs, there is narcissistic and object loss—the *real* loss of the baby becomes a narcissistic injury and therefore a *symbolic* loss of self. The loss must be understood in terms of the intrapsychic meanings of and the interpersonal responses to perinatal loss.

Unique Aspects of Perinatal Grief

A pregnancy loss occurs at a time of profound developmental change for a couple and may be their first experience with death. However, this death is different from that of a parent, friend, spouse, or even an older child, in which grief is *retrospective* and real memories and experiences are mourned and shared by others. With a perinatal loss, grief is *prospective*: Mourning occurs over the hopes, wishes, and fantasies of the future for a baby known only to the parents and possibly other immediate family. The loss is also *multidimensional* and reflects an individual's unique experiences. For

example, it may reflect a loss of a pregnancy, baby, future relationships, innocence, health, control, reproductive capacity, hopes and dreams, and so on. Further, the narcissistic nature of the loss is different and affects feelings of grief, with mothers often experiencing intense guilt, shame, envy, rage, and self-blame, which are not usually experienced with other losses.

Because the loss is different than other losses and comes at a time of extreme psychological vulnerability, several aspects make grieving particularly difficult[8,34,37]. First, there is little opportunity for anticipatory grieving, as the loss often occurs suddenly and without warning. Second, there is frequently an absence of any visible and publicly acknowledged 'object' to mourn, especially in earlier losses where others may not have even been aware of the pregnancy. Further, there are often few socially acceptable avenues for mourning—no funerals, rituals, or cultural traditions that help to acknowledge loss and facilitate grieving. Fourth, there is a remarkable lack of social support, and the loss is experienced as 'socially unspeakable', often being glossed over or minimized by others. When the loss is not acknowledged or discussed, a deep sense of shame and personal failure is intensified, especially for mothers. Last, and probably most difficult, is the prospective nature of grieving in which fantasies of future interactions must be mourned. When memories of a life are primarily dreams, the grief takes on a new dimension—the pain of not ever knowing. The ability to resolve grief following a perinatal loss often depends on a couple's ability to find avenues to acknowledge the loss and express their emotions.

Although perinatal grief reflects the characteristics of grief identified by a number of authors, mourning is a uniquely personal experience. Each person deals with the feelings in his or her own unique way, based on personality and life experiences. Thus, husbands and wives feel and deal differently with the loss; just as they have bonded differently with the child, they grieve differently. Couples need to be aware that no two people, as close as they may be, experience the loss and deal with the feelings in exactly the same way. They also need to know that different does not mean better or worse, it only means not the same.

Unpredictable Pattern of Perinatal Grief

Feelings of grief are like a tidal wave that sweeps over one, growing and cresting with time. Intense feelings of shock, disbelief, anger, self-blame, rage, guilt, anxiety, and depression occur unpredictably and repetitively. In the author's clinical experience, the feelings seem to peak somewhere between 3–9 months following the loss. This is problematic for parents, as it occurs at a time when social supports, if there were any, may have disappeared. It also may occur within the context of a subsequent pregnancy or other reproductive events, such as infertility. Grieving a perinatal loss takes far longer than most people anticipate, anywhere from a few months to several years.

There are also physical manifestations of grief. Symptoms may include aching breasts and arms, difficulty sleeping, nightmares, lack of appetite, heart palpitations, shortness of breath, difficulty concentrating, forgetfulness, or tiredness. Mothers also may experience their milk coming in and other physical discomforts following delivery, which may enhance the reality of there being no baby. The stress from the loss sometimes brings out physical problems such as headaches, muscle spasms, or a susceptibility to infections, colds, and other viruses. Often, grieving mothers feel as if their bodies have failed

them. The feeling of physical defectiveness is particularly compounded when there are difficulties or complications with physical healing, especially following an ectopic or molar pregnancy. It is also important to recognize that after giving birth, a woman may experience profound hormonal changes that may affect mood and emotions.

As the tidal wave of grief passes, 'swells of grief' remain that are 'triggers' that remind the parents of their loss and rekindle feelings. Peppers and Knapp[38] use the term *shadow grief* to describe this occurrence. It relates to a parent's desire never to forget the baby and also to the general inability to express the feelings to others. Like a shadow, it is always there yet requires no coping mechanisms. Feelings of sadness are often triggered around significant days and events, such as the due date, date of conception, birth date, anniversary of the baby's death. Holidays such as Mother's Day and Father's Day or child-focused celebrations such as Halloween and Christmas or Hanukkah can also be painful. Changes in the season or special places may rekindle memories. However, with time, this sadness becomes a dull ache and not the all-encompassing pain of before.

There are several factors that may adversely affect the grief response—'undercurrents of grief' that may impact the size and duration of the tidal wave. These are circumstances that may complicate the already difficult task of mourning (Table 1). As identified in the research and in this author's clinical experience, the more intense the psychological attachment to the baby, the more significant will be the loss experienced by the parents. Clinicians need to consider the following factors in assessing the risk for complicated bereavement: a history of *poor psychological functioning*, including depression, other psychiatric symptoma-

Table 1 Risk factors for complicated grief

History of poor psychological functioning
History of reproductive loss
Medical history associated with the loss
Medical interventions to achieve or maintain
    pregnancy
Age
Marital instability
Social isolation
Recent crises or losses

tology, and personality disorders; a history of *reproductive loss*, including infertility, prior pregnancy losses, or elective abortions; *medical history*, including risks factors associated with the loss, such as lupus, hypertension, cervical cancer, gestational diabetes, Group B Streptococcus, or overall physical health problems; *medical interventions*, including the use of high-tech infertility treatment to achieve pregnancy, high-risk pregnancy, extended bed rest, and selective reduction or amniocentesis prior to the loss; *age*, including older women facing the biological clock and very young women lacking social support and resources to deal with the loss; *marital instability*; *social isolation*; and *other recent crisis or losses*, such as another death in the family, a move, or job problems. Any of these factors may influence the psychological attachment to the developing baby and intensify the grief reaction. It is important to note, however, that with recurrent pregnancy loss, not every loss will be experienced in the same way or have the same meaning. For example, an early pregnancy loss of an unplanned, unwanted pregnancy may have small emotional significance, while a loss a few years later of a planned, much desired pregnancy may be much more psychologically difficult.

Acceptance or 'resolution' occurs when the loss has been integrated into the person's life and no longer consumes all energy. This point may coincide with a subsequent successful birth, which appears to be an important contribution to resolution of a perinatal loss for some women[39]. For many women, another pregnancy is an opportunity to 're-do' a failed experience and, as such, regain feelings of competency and accomplishment with a successful birth. Although, women often experience a profound 'hole' in their lives following a perinatal loss, some imagine that the way to feel better is to get pregnant quickly, thereby replacing the dead baby. The pregnancy then serves as a means of avoiding grief and may affect the relationship with the subsequent child[2]. Thus, women need encouragement to allow sufficient time to heal physically and emotionally before attempting another pregnancy, understanding that physical healing often occurs long before emotional healing.

CLINICAL ISSUES AND THERAPEUTIC INTERVENTIONS

The goal of all interventions—whether medical or psychological—following a pregnancy loss is to facilitate positive grieving. In addition, it is to restore the patient's narcissistic equilibrium and self-esteem. Because parents mourn regardless of the kind of loss, no distinction will be made in this section between interventions for early versus later gestational losses. However, attention will be given to elected situations of loss, those of multifetal reduction and pregnancy termination due to a genetic defect.

Medical Approaches

Intervention at the time of loss, that is, in the hospital and with medical caregivers, can have a great effect on the course of mourning. Couples often say that the best medicine or the only medicine that helped

Table 2 Interventions after perinatal loss that may facilitate grieving

Medical

Choice of induction/delivery plan

Seeing, touching, spending time with the baby or viewing products of conception

Naming the baby

Taking pictures (if declined by parents, stored in record for later availability)

Providing mementos (e.g., lock of hair, wrist band, foot/hand prints, length/weight certificate, symbolic representations, sonograms)

Planning for disposition of body/tissue

Funeral or memorial service

Choosing room assignment off obstetrics floor or discharge planning

Providing written materials on perinatal grief and support resources

Interim phone call from staff before follow-up office visit

Psychological

Creating a memory box or album (e.g., photographs, sonogram pictures, laboratory reports, IVF petri dish, cards, toy or item of clothing, etc.)

Memorial activities (e.g., planting a tree, selecting a garden statue, donation to special charity, books for support groups, items for neonatal intensive care unit or high-risk unit, etc.)

Self-care activities (e.g., regular exercise, proper diet, avoidance of alcohol/drugs, following a schedule/routine)

Keeping a journal, diary, or audiotape describing the loss and grief

Writing a letter or poem of goodbye to baby

Planning a memorial service, private or with others

Reaching out to a support group or family/friends

following the loss was the compassionate, sensitive care of the medical staff. Conversely, patients' greatest complaints about their medical care often concern feeling traumatized by the lack of sensitivity, responsiveness, communication, and concern by their medical caregivers[32]. This accelerates further narcissistic injury and the projection of rage and blame onto caregivers. It is this author's belief that most medical malpractice following a perinatal loss is *not* due primarily to medical negligence or incompetence but more often to poor and insensitive communication with the grieving couple by the physician and/or medical staff.

Patients need to be presented with reality-enforcing options and allowed to make choices that are right for them (Table 2). These options include the following: choices about induction, delivery, or dilation and curettage (D &C) plan, and whether to wait for the loss to occur naturally or proceed with immediate medical intervention; being able to see, touch, and spend time with the baby or view the products of conception, with careful preparation as to what they will see; having a support person immediately available; taking pictures of the fetus/baby; being provided with mementos such as a lock of hair, wrist band, certificate with length and weight, foot and hand prints, symbolic representation of the fetus/ products of conception, etc.; having a religious/cultural ceremony (e.g., baptism); having a copy of an autopsy or pathology report; burial, cremation, or other disposition of the fetus/tissue; funeral or memorial services; and choice of room assignment or discharge planning. Patients need to be carefully guided as to what to

235

anticipate and expect in considering these options, and need to be given the opportunity to consider and later reconsider if they initially refuse a choice. For example, patients often have fears associated with seeing their dead baby or fetus, yet are embarrassed to express these concerns. However, they need to understand that this will be their only opportunity to see the baby, need to be told what to expect, and advised that other parents have found this useful in making the loss a reality. If they still choose not to see the baby, pictures can be taken and placed in the chart, and the parents informed of access to the pictures later on if they change their mind. Lastly, aftercare needs to be planned, with written materials given at discharge, information provided on support groups and counseling resources, an interim phone call to offer support and understanding, and a scheduled follow-up office visit.

Psychotherapeutic Approaches

A psychodynamic and cognitive-behavioral approach is applicable to perinatal loss therapy. Leon[3] presented a psychodynamic framework in which the intrapsychic meaning of the perinatal death is considered in the context of revived conflicts and identifications occurring in pregnancy. This form of expressive psychotherapy can be used in a short-term or long-term model. Shapiro[40] described a cognitive-behavioral model in which concrete direction and advice are provided by the therapist as a means of improving coping and communication skills to manage the loss. This is a more active counseling approach to therapy that is usually short-term and focused. Both models provide useful tools for psychotherapeutic intervention. This author uses a combination of the two models, based on careful psychological assessment of the patient.

Assessment

Patients presenting for therapy following a perinatal loss are usually in tremendous emotional pain. Leon[3] pointed to the importance of being able to recognize the difference between behavior and affects that in another context would be viewed as pathological. For example, transient hallucinatory descriptions of hearing the baby cry are common. Nonetheless, an awareness of the danger of a pathological outcome is important, which is a matter of degree, affecting the long-range functioning of the individual and his or her relationship with others. History taking must include questions covering the areas mentioned previously regarding the risk factors for complicated bereavement (see Table 1). The assessment phase usually takes from two to four sessions, at the end of which a treatment plan is discussed.

A differential diagnosis needs to be determined between primary perinatal grief and perinatal grief that is secondary to a prior depressive constellation. When there is evidence of preexisting depression, it may be the 'tip of the iceberg' to complicating borderline and narcissistic personality disorders, which cannot be treated in a short-term therapy approach. (However, specific goals that facilitate grief may still be attained.) A complete history of psychological functioning prior to the loss will also assist the therapist in determining true suicidality. Patients often express a wish to be with their dead baby. However, suicidal danger can be ascertained 'by the usual criteria of conscious intent to harm or kill oneself, history of suicidal behavior, reality-testing, impulsivity, and existence of an actual plan'[3].

Two diagnostic codes from the *Diagnostic and Statistical Manual of Mental Disorders*[41] (DSM-IV) that are especially applicable to pregnancy loss are: Adjustment Disorder and Posttraumatic Stress Disorder (PTSD). The most commonly applied is *Adjustment*

Disorder, in which the development of clinically significant emotional or behavioral symptoms is in response to an identifiable psychosocial stressor(s) (i.e., the perinatal loss). Predominant symptoms may be *Depressed Mood* (#309.0), *Anxiety* (#309.24), or *Mixed Features* (#309.28). Further, it is useful to consider how the diagnostic description of *PTSD* (#309.81) also applies to perinatal loss[11]:

> A person has been exposed to a traumatic event in which ... [he/she] experienced a death ... or a threat to the physical integrity of self ... and [the] response involved intense fear, helplessness, or horror. The traumatic event is then persistently re-experienced [with] ... recurrent and intrusive distressing recollections of the event, including images, thoughts, or perceptions; ... recurrent and distressing dreams of the event; [and/or] ... a sense of reliving the experience.

The definition of PTSD accurately describes some of the symptomatology patients experience following a pregnancy loss: flashbacks or, what this author calls, replaying a 'psychological videotape' of the experience; intrusive and distressing thoughts of the event; nightmares; and avoidance of situations (e.g., seeing babies) that trigger the feelings. In recalling the circumstances of learning and experiencing a perinatal loss, patients can often describe in vivid detail what occurred. Women who 30 or 40 years earlier experienced a pregnancy loss can give vivid descriptions of surroundings (who was there, what was said, etc.), almost as if it occurred that very morning[12]. There is often an uncontrollable need and desire to replay the psychological videotape as a means of reliving and working through the traumatic experience. In fact, as with PTSD, it is necessary to be able to repeatedly remember and discuss the experience in order to obtain distance from it.

There are several tools available for therapists to assist in assessment and treatment planning. Porvin and colleagues[43] developed a short version of the Perinatal Grief Scale that is a research measure for assessing response to perinatal loss (see Appendix 6). In addition, Leon[3] developed Clinical Protocols for Perinatal Loss (see Appendix 5), which include background/demographic information; circumstances of loss, such as prior reproductive/medical history, involvement with baby, and future plans; interpersonal reactions of medical caregivers, spouse, family, and friends; intrapsychic responses; and psychotherapy process.

The use of psychotropic medication may need to be considered as an adjunct to perinatal loss therapy. Patients frequently have difficulty sleeping immediately after the loss, and their obstetrician may prescribe sleeping pills or tranquilizers 'to relax'. However, these are short-term solutions to grief symptomatology and need to be carefully monitored so as not to circumvent mourning or precipitate other problems (e.g., history of chemical dependency or abuse). Patients having difficulty with eating, sleeping, anxiety, or depression may be helped with increasing the frequency of therapy, (e.g., from weekly to twice a week), to provide more opportunity to work through feelings. They may also be helped with behavioral techniques, such as regular exercise, deep relaxation, and meditation. If, however, symptomatology does not improve and is adversely affecting daily functioning, a medication referral is warranted. This is particularly important if perinatal grief is secondary to a prior or preexisting depressive constellation. An experienced psychiatrist or psychopharmacologist is the ideal knowledge source for the rapidly expanding options in psychotropic medications (see Chapter 4). Patients may need assistance in understanding that medication is not a 'happy pill' that in effect denies and avoids their grief. Instead, it is a useful tool in alleviating depressive symptomatology, thus giving the patient more energy and cognitive clarity to deal effectively with the problems at hand.

A determination will need to be made about whether the focus of treatment will be individual, couple, or a combination. Sometimes, the decision is made when only one person presents for therapy. However, in the course of obtaining an individual and marital history, it may become apparent that marital instability was a preexisting condition that will need to be addressed. In some relationships, one person will take on the task of grieving for the two, frequently the wife for the husband, in which case both partners may need to be encouraged to participate in the therapy to restore equilibrium and avoid divisiveness. A perinatal loss has the potential of making a good marriage stronger and of destroying a problem marriage. Attention also needs to be given to additional stressors in a couple's life: other children at home; financial problems; job pressures; extended family strains, such as siblings having babies or parents who are ill; health issues, such as continued infertility treatment or the diagnosis of cancer during the pregnancy; sexual dysfunction; or the pregnancy loss representing the end of childbearing and the approach of menopause.

Setting the Stage

Important as it is in treatment to obtain a complete individual and marital history, it cannot take place before the therapist has heard the patient's story of the pregnancy loss. The first session is very important in setting the tone for therapy, and the therapist may want to schedule an extended session (1½ to 2 regular therapy hours) for the initial appointment. The couple needs the opportunity to describe in detail the psychological videotape of the loss—what the circumstances surrounding the pregnancy were; how they learned there was a problem; what happened at the hospital/time of loss; what reality-supporting interventions occurred; what were the availability and reactions of medical caregivers, family, and friends at the time of loss and later; what were the woman or man's emotional reaction at the time and since; and what actions they have taken in response to the loss. If the couple has pictures and/or other mementos of their baby, it is very helpful for them to bring these to a session to share with the therapist. The therapist needs to give sufficient time to go over each item, have the couple talk about what each piece means to them, and offer positive feedback about the specialness of this child. This action communicates the therapist's willingness to emotionally engage in the system and validates the fetus/baby's existence as real and worthy of mourning.

There are two situations in which patients may feel either bolstered or betrayed by medical technology. Infertility patients who lose a pregnancy may feel both success and failure—similar to theatrical masks with one side smiling and the other frowning. These patients often feel bolstered that they have achieved a pregnancy, while experiencing a tremendous sense of loss for the wished-for child in whom they have considerable emotional, physical, and financial investment. With repeated pregnancy loss, there is a recurring cycle of hope and despair that makes it exceedingly more difficult to grieve. On the other hand, patients who have had CVS or amniocentesis genetic testing and shortly thereafter lost a healthy pregnancy often feel betrayed by the medical technology that they thought or were told would be helpful. Understandably, feelings of anger, guilt, and blame may be accentuated and need to be worked through to avoid pathological grief and/or lingering bitterness. While feelings of anger, guilt, self-blame, and blame of caregivers are common, patients may need to be encouraged to dispel hindsight and recognize that they made the best decision at the time with the best of intentions. Often, these patients express complete naiveté about the risks associated with prenatal genetic testing, discounting information that may have been explained to them prior to the procedure. Even patients who understand the risks often cannot believe it happened to them. Consequently, patients need to be prepared for the potential for loss. They will need to recognize that if they would not terminate a problem pregnancy, then the information obtained from the procedure may not be worth the risk.

Patients often present in an emotionally vulnerable and somewhat defenseless manner. Initially, the therapist may need to help them integrate some defenses to deal with the overwhelming feelings. However, if they present in a highly defensive manner, the therapist needs to be very careful about removing any of these defenses until their meaning and purpose for patients are clear. Patients who are defensive believe that there is something that they need to defend against. Further, following a perinatal loss, patients are highly sensitive to perceived criticism and judgment, especially if they think that the pregnancy loss was within their control. Thus, any helping professional must choose words and actions carefully, and appropriately intervene if miscommunication has occurred. The potential for further narcissistic injury is always present because of psychological vulnerability.

The therapist must be able to tolerate the unrestrained, affective outpouring of grief—intense sadness, anger, rage, guilt, self-blame, fear of the future, and remorse—while being ever cognizant of his or her own countertransference to these powerful emotions. If the therapist has experienced a perinatal loss, any self-disclosure should be carefully evaluated as to the appropriateness to the situation at hand and the helpfulness of the content to the patient. Further, if self-disclosure occurs, it is important to process how patients perceive the information, their fantasies and reactions. This is also true of patient education materials, such as personal stories of pregnancy loss or self-help groups in which members recount their loss. These stories may or may not be helpful, so that processing a patient's interpretation of the information is necessary.

One of the difficulties for couples is that there may be no tangible evidence of their baby's existence that can be mourned. With preimplantation losses and early miscarriages, there are few mementos and rituals that validate the loss. At times, patients enter therapy years after the loss, either consciously aware of unresolved grief or unconscious to other events that ultimately relate to unresolved mourning, such as marital problems, depression, problems with subsequent children, or a pregnancy loss of a family member such as a son or daughter. A task of therapy is then to help create mementos and rituals that acknowledge the reality of the lost child.

Therapeutic Goals—Facilitating Grief and Restoring Self-Esteem

Several cognitive-behavioral techniques may be useful in psychotherapy for pregnancy loss and can be presented as options for facilitating grief (see Table 2). Couples may want to put together a 'memory box' or album with small things that represent their wished-for child: a sonogram picture, laboratory report, item of clothing or toy that was for the baby, cards and condolences letters received, positive home pregnancy test, etc. They may also want to consider writing a letter or poem to their baby, in which they name him or her, expressing all their hopes, wishes, and dreams, and then saying good-bye. Keeping a journal of therapy and/or writing a diary of all the events surrounding the loss helps parents find a place to put feelings, so that memories of this special child will never be forgotten. Planning a memorial service, either private or with others, may be helpful even years after the loss. In addition, planting a tree or purchasing a garden statue in their baby's memory helps provide a beautiful, living reflection of their child. Donating money to a special charity, books to a perinatal loss support group, or baby items to a hospital or neonatal intensive care unit may also be a helpful way of recognizing the child. Although these exercises and activities are usually worked on outside the therapy hour, it is often an emotional experience and needs to be processed during the therapy session.

Patients will need assistance in understanding the normalcy of their grief and encouragement for finding ways to express these feelings. Wishes and fantasies will have to be mourned with the realization that the dreams for this special child will never materialize. Where irrational guilt exists, the therapist must carefully explore the origin of the guilt and help patients differentiate between fact and fantasy. At times, patients may need encouragement and assistance in obtaining more medical information to provide the facts. In addition, depression is a common affective response to loss. However, it may be useful to tell patients that depression is often anger turned inward. Thus, a task of therapy becomes helping them express what they are angry or unhappy about and direct the feelings to the source. For example, patients may be feeling very angry at other people, disappointed with their physician, family, or friends who they feel were unsupportive. It can be therapeutic to discuss ways to communicate these feelings to people who have hurt or disappointed them and decide what, if any, action, needs to be taken. Do they want to set up an appointment to talk to the doctor or write a letter expressing their concerns? Do they want to speak with the family or write their feelings in a letter that may or may not be mailed? Role-playing in therapy what the patient would like to say to these people can also help reduce angry feelings and model actions. In addition, it provides the opportunity to determine the reality or justifiability of their anger.

It has been said that a feeling shared is a feeling diminished and that there is strength in numbers. Hence, perinatal loss support groups serve as an important therapeutic resource. These groups prevent parents from becoming isolated with their grief and help connect them to new relationships that will promote healing. For patients with a history of infertility, the group may help them feel more normal and connected to the fertile world. Although a support group may not be for everyone, it is suggested that patients need to go about three times before deciding whether or not it is right for them. For many people, a support group or a group of supportive family and friends is all that is needed to heal the grief. For those who are at risk for complicated grief, a perinatal loss support group may stagnate mourning, unless it is used in conjunction with individual and/or couples therapy.

Patients often need the therapist's encouragement and prompting to take concrete steps for self-care. In short, grieving people often 'forget' how to take care of themselves. Regular exercise is very important in restoring positive body-image, reducing depression and anxiety, and increasing energy. Other activities enhance a more positive self-image, such as massage therapy, facials, manicures, etc. Eating planned, nutritionally balanced meals promotes physical healing. Further, patients may need assistance in instituting a schedule and routine in their life that allows for structure to the boundless experience of grief. They also may need permission to involve themselves in activities that are fun and provide relief from the world of grief. These activities assist in restoring self-esteem.

Elective Termination: Special Considerations

Special consideration needs to be given to situations in which couples choose to reduce a multiple pregnancy or terminate a pregnancy after genetic testing reveals an abnormality. The decision to choose to end a pregnancy is never an easy one for people, especially if they have gone to great lengths to achieve it. It is a decision made in an environment of moral, ethical, and social dilemmas that are conflictual. Further, if spontaneous loss is a socially isolating experience, elected loss is in a complete vacuum. Because the issue of pregnancy termination is politically sensitive and highly emotionally charged, there are few resources available to couples for understanding and acceptance. Thus, there is need for education and emotional support for couples faced with these difficult decisions. The therapist needs to be aware of his or her own moral and ethical feelings about these situations, as it is imperative that patients receive counseling in a neutral environment.

Multifetal Pregnancy Reduction

MPR, an iatrogenic condition, was developed after assisted reproductive technology greatly increased the incidence of pregnancy involving multiple fetuses. Multiple gestation pregnancies pose serious health risks to the mother and children, especially in higher-order pregnancy above twins. The increased risks include loss of the entire pregnancy, premature delivery, preeclampsia, gestational diabetes, and postpartum hemorrhage in the mother, and prematurity, low birth weight, and handicaps in infants. Prematurity can have serious life-long consequences for children and families and may ultimately result in death after extreme medical intervention has failed. MPR is used to terminate a preselected number of fetuses in an effort to increase the likelihood of a successful pregnancy. It is performed at special centers, usually late in the first trimester of pregnancy, and accomplished by means of injection into the cardiac cavities of the selected fetuses, which are eventually absorbed *in utero*.

Since most multiple pregnancies result from infertility treatment, the decision to reduce is a painful irony for couples who so wanted children. There is intense ambivalence—the risk of morbidity and mortality to the babies, while facing the certainty of loss of some of the babies and risk of loss of the entire pregnancy. Despite the concern for psychiatric morbidity, there seem to be few long-term problems for women who resolve their ambivalence and have a successful pregnancy outcome[26,44].

MPR is a distressing and stressful experience that warrants careful counseling both before and after the procedure. Greenfeld and Walther[45] addressed a plan for assisting couples in which they recommended beginning with pretreatment preparation counseling for women undergoing ovulation induction. Couples need to understand (1) that multiple pregnancy is a distinct possibility, (2) that it carries a significant medical risk to fetuses and mothers, and (3) that fetal reduction may be advised. If patients would not consider MPR, they will need to advise the physician before the assisted reproduction procedure and discuss the number of embryos to transfer, or they will need seriously to reconsider participating in this treatment. If a multifetal pregnancy results, couples need psychoeducational materials to facilitate decision-making as well as additional counseling. It is also extremely helpful to have lists of couples who have faced the same decision and are willing to talk to others about their decision to keep the pregnancy or to reduce it. Counseling should help couples anticipate their emotional responses to the stress and be aware of available follow-up.

Pregnancy Termination Due to Genetic Birth Defect

Prenatal testing has become increasingly available and has lead to early detection of genetic defects and fetal anomalies. Preimplantation diagnosis during IVF, CVS during the first trimester of pregnancy, amniocentesis during the second trimester, and high-resolution sonography through-out pregnancy have provided information about a developing baby that a few years ago would not have been known until after birth. However, therapeutic options are limited for many of the problems diagnosed, and parents are faced with the difficult decision: Whether to continue or terminate the pregnancy. A painful dilemma occurs when the pregnancy is very much planned and desired. If termination is decided, the procedure is often intrusive and painful, requiring either a D & C in the first trimester or dilation and evacuation or induction of labor in the second trimester or later.

It seems that women who terminate a pregnancy rarely suffer psychological problems, provided that it occurs in the first trimester and is wanted for genetic or social reasons[25]. However, psychological sequelae following an elective termination are most often experienced by women who have difficulty arriving at a decision to terminate, have the abortion late in the pregnancy, desired the pregnancy[15], and were coerced by their partner or others. Even when couples are firm and clear on their decision to terminate for fetal anomalies, grief can be just as intense as it is for those who experience spontaneous loss, as both grieve for their wished-for baby[28].

Consequently, intervention after a genetic termination involves similar clinical management to that described for spontaneous loss[46]. Patients need to be given the option to participate in all rituals of a perinatal loss as would occur in a normal pregnancy. For example, it is important that they be given the option of seeing and holding the baby, after compassionate preparation of what the baby looks like. Parents' fears and fantasies are often far worse than the reality of any deformities, and spending time with the baby may help bring closure. However, there are several unique issues that need to be recognized in the therapy concerning the *element of choice*, the *perception of loss*, and the *sense of isolation*. First, patients often emotionally struggle with the decision to choose to terminate a pregnancy that was so desired, and yet intellectually know that this is the best for them. They frequently express the wish that the baby had 'just died' versus having to choose to terminate. Second, the narcissistic injury and a perception of defectiveness may be exacerbated due to the fetal anomaly, which may precipitate the discovery of a previously unknown genetic disorder in one or both parents. In addition, people will experience the loss differently: For some, it will be the loss of a pregnancy, while for others it will be the loss of the baby. Finally, these couples often describe feelings of alienation and shame and may not feel free to discuss the experience with others for fear of rejection or condemnation. In fact, it is important for them to be counseled to choose carefully those people with whom they will talk about the termination. This is a time when they need to surround themselves only with people who they know will be supportive. Support groups and resources are now available for this special population, offering acceptance and sustenance. While there is currently no national support organization for this population, a number of local/regional groups have formed, and the physician, genetic counselor, or hospital should be aware of where to locate the support group.

FUTURE IMPLICATIONS

As sophisticated and advanced reproductive technologies have become in creating and sustaining life, there will always be reproductive loss. The continuing challenge will be in providing adequate and available resources for psychological support that encourage the positive resolution of grief. More research needs to be done to understand the differences in the way men and women experience the loss; the effect of reproductive technologies on bonding, attachment, and grieving; and investigation of effective interventions that facilitate grieving, especially for those at risk for pathological mourning. Better designed research and the development of grief assessment tools are needed by clinicians. Further, continuing education of the public about the profound nature of perinatal loss will help change social attitudes toward it.

SUMMARY

- Perinatal death constitutes a major loss for most couples and is a psychically traumatic event.
- Grieving occurs whether the loss is early or late in the pregnancy, and the intensity is more closely related to psychological attachment than length of gestation.
- Couples feel intense emotion, often in virtual isolation because of a lack of social support and societal recognition of this significant experience.
- The narcissistic and object loss occurring at a time of profound developmental change make grieving difficult.
- The goal of intervention is to facilitate grieving and to restore narcissistic equilibrium.
- Actions that acknowledge the loss as real and encourage emotional expression help facilitate grief.
- Situations of elected termination of desired pregnancies require psychoeducation, psychological support, and options to follow mourning rituals as in spontaneous loss.

REFERENCES

1. Kirkley-Best E, Kellner KR. Forgotten grief: A review of the literature on the psychology of stillbirth. *Am J Orthopsychiatry* 1982;52:420–9

2. Zeanah CH. Adaptation following perinatal loss: A critical review. *J Am Acad Child Adolesc Psychiatry* 1989;28:467–80

3. Leon IG. *When A Baby Dies: Psychotherapy for* *Pregnancy and Newborn Loss*. New Haven: Yale University Press, 1990

4. Freud S. *Mourning and Melancholia*. In: Strachey J, ed. and trans. *The Standard Edition of the Complete Psychological Works of Sigmund Freud*, vol 14. London: Hogarth, 1917/1957

5. Lindemann E. Symptomatology and

management of acute grief. *Am J Psychiatry* 1944;101:141–8

6. Parkes CM. *Bereavement: Studies in Grief in Adult Life.* New York: International Universities Press, 1972

7. Bowlby J. *Loss.* New York: Basic Books, 1980

8. Toedter LJ, Lasker JN, Alhadeff JM. The perinatal grief scale: Development and initial validation. *Am J Orthopsychiatry* 1988;58:435–49

9. Kennell JH, Slyter H, Klaus M. The mourning response of parents to the death of a newborn. *N Engl J Med* 1970;283: 344–9

10. Lewis E, Page A. Failure to mourn a stillbirth: An overlooked catastrophe. *Br J Med Psychol* 1978;51:237–41

11. Stack JM. The psychodynamics of spontaneous abortion. *Am J Orthopsychiatry* 1984;54:162–7

12. Bourne S, Lewis E. Pregnancy after stillbirth or neonatal death: Psychological risks and management. *Lancet* 1984;2:31–3

13. Herz E. Psychological repercussions of pregnancy loss. *Psychiatr Ann* 1984;14:454–7

14. Theut SK, Pedersen FA, Zaslow MJ. Perinatal loss and parental bereavement. *Am J Psychiatry* 1989;146:635–9

15. Forrest GC, Standis E, Baum JD. Support after perinatal death: A study of support and counselling after perinatal bereavement. *Br Med J (Clin Res)* 1982;285:1475–9

16. LaRoche C, Lalinec-Michaud M, Engelsmann F, et al. Grief reactions to perinatal death. *Can J Psychiatry* 1984; 29:14–19

17. Cullenberg J. Mental reactions of women to perinatal death. In: Morris N, ed. *Psychosomatic Medicine in Obstetrics and Gynaecology.* London: Karger, 1972;326–9

18. Nicol MT, Tompkins JR, Campbel NA, Syme GJ. Maternal grieving response after perinatal death. *Med J Aust* 1986;144:287–9

19. Kirkley-Best E. Grief in response to prenatal loss: An argument for the earliest maternal attachment. *Dissert Abstr Int* 1981;42(B):2560

20. Janssen H, Cuisinier M, Hoogduin K, deGraauw K. Controlled prospective study on the mental health of women following pregnancy loss. *Am J Psychiatry* 1996; 153:226–30

21. Peppers LG, Knapp RJ. Maternal reactions to involuntary fetal/infant death. *Psychiatry* 1980;43:155–9

22. Greenfeld DA, Diamond MP, DeCherney AH. Grief reactions following in-vitro fertilization treatment. *J Psychosom Obstet Gynaecol* 1988;8:169–74

23. Farhi J, Ben-Rafael Z, Dicker D. Suicide after ectopic pregnancy. *N Engl J Med* 1994;330:714

24. Flam F, Magnusson C, Lundstrom-Lindstedt V, et al. Psychosocial impact of persistent trophoblastic disease. *J Psychosom Obstet Gynaecol* 1993;14:241–8

25. Dagg PKB. The psychological sequelae of therapeutic abortion—denied and completed. *Am J Psychiatry* 1991;148:578–85

26. Schreiner-Engel P, Walther VN, Mindes J, et al. First-trimester multifetal pregnancy reduction: Acute and persistent psychologic reactions. *Am J Obstet Gynecol* 1995;172:541–7

27. Wilson AL, Fenton LF, Stevens DC, Soule DJ. The death of a newborn twin: An analysis of parental bereavement. *Pediatrics* 1982;70:587–91

28. Zeanah CH, Dailey JV, Rosenblatt M, Saller DN. Do women grieve after terminating pregnancies because of fetal anomalies? A controlled investigation. *Obstet Gynecol* 1993;82:270–5

29. Benfield DG, Leib SA, Vollman JH. Grief response of parents to neonatal death and parent participation in deciding care. *Pediatrics* 1978;62:171–7

30. Tudelope DI, Iredell J, Rodgers D, Gunn A. Neonatal death: Grieving families. *Med J Aust* 1986;144:290–2

31. Neugebauer R, Kline J, Shrout P, et al. Major depressive disorder in the 6 months after miscarriage. *JAMA* 1997;277:383–8

32. Covington SN, Theut SK. Reactions to perinatal loss: A qualitative analysis of the National Maternal and Infant Health Survey. *Am J Orthopsychiatry* 1993;63:215–22

33. Schreiner R, Gresham E, Green M. Physician's responsibility to parents after death of an infant. *Am J Dis Child* 1979;133:723–6

34. Leon IG. Psychodynamics of perinatal loss. *Psychiatry* 1986;49:312–24

35. Offerman-Zuckerberg J. Psychological and physical warning signals regarding

pregnancy. In: Blum B, ed. *Psychological Aspects of Pregnancy, Birthing, and Bonding*. New York: Human Sciences Press, 1980;151–73

36. Furlong RM, Hobbins JC. Grief in the perinatal period. *Obstet Gynecol* 1983; 61:497–500

37. Covington SN. Pregnancy loss. In: *Clinical Management of Psychological Issues in Reproductive Health*. Proceedings of the Twenty-second Annual Postgraduate Course of The American Society for Reproductive Medicine; 1989 Nov 11–12; San Francisco, CA. Birmingham, AL: American Society for Reproductive Medicine, 1989;19–36

38. Peppers L, Knapp R. *Motherhood and Mourning: Perinatal Loss*. New York: Praeger, 1980

39. Cuisiner M, Janssen H, de Graauw C, *et al.* Pregnancy following miscarriage: Course of grief and some determining factors. *J Psychosom Obstet Gynaecol* 1996;17:168–74

40. Shapiro CH. *Infertility and Pregnancy Loss*. San Francisco: Jossey-Bass, 1988

41. American Psychiatric Association. *Diagnostic and Statistical Manual of Mental Disorders*, 4th edn. Washington, DC: American Psychiatric Association, 1994

42. Rosenblatt PG, Burns LH. Long-term effects of perinatal loss. *J Fam Issues* 1986; 7:237–53

43. Porvin L, Lasker J, Toedter L. Measuring grief: A short version of the perinatal grief scale. *J Psychopathol Behav Assess* 1989;11:29–45

44. McKinney M, Downey J, Timor-Tritsch I. The psychological effects of multifetal pregnancy reduction. *Fertil Steril* 1995; 64: 51–61

45. Greenfeld DA, Walther VN. Psychological consideration in multifetal pregnancy reduction. *Infertil Reprod Med Clin North Am* 1993;4:533–43

46. Leon IG. Pregnancy termination due to fetal anomaly: Clinical considerations. *Infant Ment Health J* 1995;16:112–26

V. SPECIAL POPULATIONS

13

Racial, Cultural, and Religious Issues in Infertility Counseling

Sherry D. Molock, PhD

If we are to achieve a richer culture, rich in contrasting values, we must recognize the whole gamut of human potentialities, and so weave a less arbitrary social fabric, one in which each diverse human gift will find a fitting place.

Margaret Mead

HISTORICAL OVERVIEW

Infertility represents a violation of cultural norms to parent children. The inability to meet this cultural expectation leaves individuals and couples feeling ostracized, isolated, and alienated. Infertility often represents a crisis not only for the family but for the larger society as well because, understandably, the inability to reproduce would result in the death of society. What is particularly noteworthy is that infertility tends to be perceived as a crisis in most cultures[1-7].

While the perception of infertility as a violation of cultural expectations is fairly uniform, the ways in which different cultural, ethnic, and religious groups perceive infertility have largely been ignored by health care providers and mental health professionals. Yet it is important to consider cultural factors in infertility, for culture shapes our understanding of the world and our behavior. *Culture* is defined as the shared way of life for a group of people and includes knowledge, beliefs, art, morals, laws, customs, and the habits of a group of people[8,9].

The importance of cultural influences on the perception and understanding of infertility cannot be minimized even among people who have been in the United States for generations. There is increasing evidence that ethnic values and identification are retained for many generations after immigration. Second-, third-, and even fourth-generation immigrant Americans differ from the dominant culture in values, life styles, and behaviors. Even when various ethnic groups become acculturated (i.e., make changes in their original cultural patterns as a result of coming in direct contact with another culture)[8], the process of acculturation is uneven. For example, acculturated groups tend to return to their original cultural practices during times of crisis. Because of the stress associated with infertility, clients are more likely to express patterns of beliefs about infertility that reflect their original cultural views rather than a more Westernized notion of infertility, a factor that caregivers must keep in mind.

Infertility cannot be diagnosed or treated without an understanding of the cultural frame of reference of both the client and the health care provider. Cultural groups differ in how they experience pain, what is labeled a symptom, how they communicate about medical and psychological problems, what they believe about the cause of illness, and what their attitudes are toward helpers and about therapeutic techniques and treatment outcomes[10].

This chapter addresses how race, culture, and religion influence:

- beliefs about infertility in culturally diverse clients
- how these viewpoints impact choice of medical interventions, counseling, and treatment outcomes
- suggestions regarding provision of counseling services to culturally diverse infertile clients.

REVIEW OF LITERATURE

Cross-Cultural Research

Most cross-cultural research on infertility has been done outside of the United States. While infertility is universally thought to be undesirable in most cultures, it may be particularly difficult in cultures in which social status and a family's welfare depend on the number of children in the family. This is certainly the case in most African countries, where having children is seen as the supreme reason for marriage. Most traditional African myths of creation point to God's creating man and woman and telling them to go into the world and multiply[7]. In rural areas, children provide a much needed labor force, and having children gives a man social stature.

In most African countries, women bear the responsibility for infertility, even if it is known that male factors are involved. It is hard for African men to admit to any type of disability or illness because this is viewed as a sign of weakness. In South Africa, using assisted reproductive techniques is unacceptable because the child would not be seen as belonging to the husband, even

if the husband's sperm is used in artificial insemination[1]. Infertile women among the Yoruba are often encouraged to 'adopt' a child of a relative in the hope that the spirit of a child who is loved and nurtured will 'attract' a natural child to the infertile woman. The practice of polygyny was also adopted as a way of dealing with female infertility. In this case, the husband is advised by the first wife to marry a younger woman in hope that the spirit of the child of the second wife will 'attract' a child for the first wife[11].

In rural parts of Egypt, *kabsa* is viewed as the principal cause of infertility. *Kabsa* is the unexpected exposure of a vulnerable female to a symbolically polluted individual. Women are thought to be vulnerable when their reproductive genitalia have been recently violated (e.g., abortion, miscarriage, recent birth of a child, female circumcision, etc.). Because of the symbolic 'penetration' of the vulnerable woman's bodily 'boundaries' (i.e., reproductive genitalia) by a polluter (someone who has recently been 'bloodied' by exposure to blood, the dead, or unwashed body fluid), she is thought to be rendered infertile. The vulnerable woman becomes depolluted by being reexposed to the offending polluter or polluting substance[2].

In rural Malaysia, infertile women consult spiritual mediums who enter a trance and speak to the spirits on behalf of them. A combination of classic Chinese medicine, modern Western and Chinese medicine, and magicoreligious healings are used to treat women with infertility[4]. For the Nayars in South India, not only are infertile women social outcasts, but their natal kin are held responsible for their infertility as well. For the Nayars, infertility not only includes procreation but has implications for job opportunities, marriage proposals, and economic concerns as well. When a family member is infertile, the entire kinship group (*taravatu*) becomes involved in a ritual called *pampintullal*, in which they appeal to the family's fertility gods[5].

Cultural Influences and the Infertility Practitioner

While the focus of the discussion thus far has been on the cultural background of possible clients, it is important to understand that infertility treatment is also influenced by the cultural framework of both clients and health care providers. Most health care providers are trained in Western medicine, which is proactive and aggressively tackles medical problems. As new technologies emerge, clients are encouraged or expected to try new procedures, even if the long-term risks involved are not clearly known. This risk-taking occurs in a cultural climate in which using medical interventions is seen as being better than 'doing nothing'. This approach to medical technology reinforces the notion that persistence is good and that the pursuit of the goal will ultimately result in a reward[12]. Thus, a client who decides to wait on God, pray about it, or consult a traditional healer may be interpreted by the health provider as unmotivated, too passive, uncooperative, or, worse, 'strange'.

Practitioners unaware of cultural differences in the understanding of and reaction to infertility may inadvertently dismiss or insult clients. One study[13] looked at how health care providers approached culturally diverse infertile clients and categorized the providers into one of three groups:

- *culturally unaware*: providers who did not recognize cultural differences and treated all clients the same
- *culturally intolerant*: providers who recognized cultural differences but were unwilling or unable to tolerate cultural conflicts in the treatment or were unwilling to change treatment

protocols to be more culturally compatible
- *culturally sensitive*: providers who were aware of cultural differences, acquired information about cultural beliefs, and worked within a client's cultural belief system and adapted assessment techniques and treatments to fit a client's needs.

The study found that culturally unaware providers often perceived their clients as noncompliant or lacking in motivation, and often labeled them as 'difficult', 'unco-operative', and 'uncommitted'. Their clients often terminated treatment. Culturally intolerant providers were aware of cultural conflicts in treatment but were unwilling to change their assessment or treatment techniques. Their clients self-terminated prematurely or were referred to more culturally tolerant providers. Culturally sensitive providers obtained more inform-ation about their clients' cultures and tried to modify techniques when possible to make them more culturally compatible with their clients' belief systems. For example, because Middle Eastern, Asian, and Mexican-American men had more difficulty collecting semen via masturbation, some providers gave the men a special condom that enabled semen collection during intercourse[13].

In summary, cultural factors clearly shape how clients experience and interpret infertility. A review of the literature indicates that infertility is viewed as stressful and stigmatizing across all cultures. Universal across most cultures is the tendency for both men and women to assume that women should take respons-ibility for infertility, even when it is clear that there are male factors involved. Infertility is seen as a crisis in most families, but how this crisis is understood and managed depends in part on cultural factors. Some cultures promote using traditional healers or spiritual inter-ventions. The sexual nature of infertility may result in some clients feeling uncomfortable seeking treatment because of violations of cultural norms and values. Finally, for some cultures, certain medical assessment and treatment techniques are unacceptable, causing cultural conflicts. Infertility treatment providers need to take a culturally sensitive approach in order to enhance the treatment options available to their culturally diverse clients.

THEORETICAL FRAMEWORK

The applicable theoretical framework is the relatively new field of counseling the culturally different, based in part on the American Psychological Association policy statements aimed at increasing the availability and quality of culturally relevant training and provider services[14]. World view is defined as the perception and nature of reality as experienced by individuals sharing a common culture. The world view of culture functions to make sense of life experiences which might otherwise be construed as chaotic, random, and meaningless. The components of world view include group identity, individual identity or self-concept, values, beliefs, and language, all of which play a part in the definition of culture as well as the definition of the individual within a culture[14]. Cultural beliefs, values, and experience are inextricably immersed and intertwined in the concepts of illness and symptoms, and as such infertility counselors must have an awareness and understanding of the health-seeking practices of culturally different patients, particularly their attitudes toward infertility and psychological distress[15]. Beliefs and values regarding medical caregivers and treatment and family-building alternatives and especially relevant, as are cultural beliefs and expectations regarding mental health problems and treatment. These issues must also be considered within the context of cross-cultural marriages, stages of enculturation, individual differences, language barriers, patients from foreign countries, family of origin factors, particular cultural beliefs, cultural or ethnic experiences of cultural racism, as well as the infertility counselor's own cultural background, and sensitivity.

CLINICAL ISSUES

Cultural Groups in the United States

African-Americans

There have been very few studies investigating cultural differences in infertility in the United States. While there are no medical studies examining racial differences in infertility, it is estimated that African-Americans may have a higher risk for infertility than white Americans. African-American families are more likely to live in economically deprived conditions that increase the likelihood of inadequate medical care for conditions that can lead to infertility. Some studies have found that African-American couples have 1.5 times the risk of infertility that white American couples have[9]. African-American women are more likely to have conditions such as pelvic inflammatory disease and ectopic pregnancy that can lead to infertility[16]. Other factors that could contribute to the higher rate of infertility in African-Americans include exposure to occupational hazards that can affect reproduction (e.g., higher concentrations of nuclear waste sites near urban centers) and complications or infections following child birth or abortions[17].

African-Americans are also less likely to seek infertility treatment, compared to white Americans. Many African-Americans think of infertility as a problem that plagues middle-class white Americans. African-American women are stereotypically viewed by the larger society as fertile 'baby machines' who have babies to increase their welfare check. African-

American men are often negatively viewed as highly sexed 'studs' who are more interested in making babies than in parenting them.

There are clear economic barriers to infertility treatment for African-Americans as well. African-Americans are more likely to live below the poverty line and have inadequate health insurance. They often cannot afford expensive infertility treatments. Some researchers view the cost of these procedures as racially and economically divisive. As assisted reproductive technologies become more sophisticated and hence more expensive, they become an elite form of medical care that only a few can afford[12]. As a result, low-income minority families rarely receive information about the treatment options available to them when they do experience infertility[17-19].

In addition, African-Americans also tend to have a holistic approach to health care in general, and many feel that assisted reproductive technologies are unnatural and devoid of anything spiritual. Spirituality is a very important cultural value for African-Americans[20]. Some African-Americans feel that assisted reproductive techniques remove the spiritual or divine nature of creation from the process of conception, and as a result, may turn to spiritual rather than medical solutions. This is surprising to many health care and social service providers, who assume that middle-class, educated African-Americans are not concerned about the spiritual realm of creation. However, the centrality of spirituality in the African-American community cuts across all economic groups. Some African-American couples question whether assisted reproduction is immoral; since most African-American denominations have not formally addressed this issue, infertile couples are deprived of spiritual guidance on this critical issue.

African-Americans may be uncomfortable with some assisted reproductive techniques because they are relatively new, are considered to be experimental, and can impact on reproductive capacities. Past abuses by the medical profession have resulted in the involuntary sterilization of African-American women in the South and in an experiment conducted in Tuskegee, Alabama, in which African-American men with syphilis were left untreated for over 40 years. African-Americans also have lingering doubts about cultural genocide, so they are particularly distrustful of techniques involving assisted reproduction.

Because adopting healthy infants may be a more viable option for African-American families (relative to white Americans), many may feel that this is a more feasible alternative to family building. This may be particularly true because it has been a culturally condoned practice: African-Americans have informally adopted children for centuries. Although there is a common perception that African-Americans do not adopt, when informal adoptions are taken into account, they adopt at a rate higher than any other ethnic group[21].

Hispanic Americans

There have been very few studies examining infertility in the Hispanic community. One study[3] looked at the psychosocial impact of infertility on Hispanic women and found that they expressed feelings of anxiousness, loneliness, and isolation. They often held themselves responsible for the infertility and protected their male partners from dealing with it even when it was evident that male factors were involved. The study also found that the spouses or male partners of the women had little interest in attending infertility workshops.

Understanding Hispanic culture, especially the importance of family in Hispanic communities, can help health care and mental health practitioners provide infertility services to Hispanic clients. It is important to note that the Hispanic community is not homogeneous. For example, Mexican-Americans hail from a culture that is a mixture of Spanish and Indian influence; Cuban-Americans have more of a Spanish, African-influence. These differences have influenced the cultural mores of these groups. While there are differences among the various Hispanic groups, there are some commonalties as well. Most Hispanics share a common language (Spanish) and are largely Roman Catholic. There is an emphasis on spiritual values and a belief that the spiritual world is inhabited by good and evil forces that influence behavior. Family relationships tend to be emotionally intense and openly affectionate, with an emphasis on the group, not the individual. The family is patriarchal, and respect for one's elders and for males in particular is very important. The family is embedded in an extended family network, and family ties are close. Families are typically large, and children are felt to validate the marriage[22,23].

Machismo is an important concept in Hispanic families. The male figure in the family is often described as aggressive and dominant, and wives are described as humble, virtuous, and submissive. While this pattern is displayed in public, in private, there are many variations, particularly in younger families and in third-generation families. Nevertheless, mothers wield considerable power at home through their children, and motherly love is felt to be stronger than wifely love[22,23].

Like their African-American counterparts, many Hispanic families may have difficulty with access to medical treatment for infertility because of economic barriers. Hispanic families are more likely to be underemployed or unemployed and to have inadequate health insurance. Hispanic families may be more comfortable turning to a traditional healer in the community or a priest to deal with infertility. The traditional healer or priest is someone that the family knows and trusts and is often located in close proximity to where the family lives. In contrast, the infertility clinic is typically located far from the community, offers services only in English, and is impersonal[24].

Some of the procedures used during the assessment phase of treatment are culturally incompatible with Hispanic cultures. For example, Mexican-American men do not feel comfortable collecting semen specimens via masturbation. It is also more difficult to get Hispanic males in general to come in for infertility work-ups because their sense of masculinity is threatened. When Hispanic families go to a traditional healer, there is not a lot of discussion about the 'treatment;' instead, the family expects to be reassured and the healer should 'fix' the problem quickly. This contrasts with infertility treatment, which can take months or years[25].

Hispanic families may also conceptualize infertility very differently from mainstream American culture. Because it is common for emotional feelings to be experienced as somatic complaints (e.g., anxiety = *aigre*: 'bad air'), Hispanic family members might not seek medical intervention for certain somatic problems. The strong emphasis on spirituality also leads some Hispanic Americans to believe that infertility is 'God's will' or a test of faith. As such, people are expected to persevere, accept their fate, or pray, but not necessarily seek medical intervention[24].

Asian-Americans

In spite of the stereotype that Asian-American families are the 'ideal' ethnic group that is successful and upwardly mobile, they are also a heterogeneous group with different ethnic identities. Chinese-American and Japanese-Americans have a longer history of immigration in this country, and many Chinese- and Japanese-Americans who are third- and fourth-generation may be quite acculturated. Individuals from Vietnam, Cambodia, and Laos are more likely to be more recent arrivals to this country, to come from lower socioeconomic status backgrounds, and to continue to struggle with acculturation and assimilation.

In Asian-American families, the concept of time and family extends forward and backward; personal actions reflect on the nuclear and extended family, and all preceding generations and behaviors impact on future generations. The father is the head of the nuclear family, and he enforces family rules and is responsible for providing for the family. Women have a much lower status in the family. In traditional families, women are absorbed into their husbands' family, where their status is lower than that of their spouse and their in-laws, particularly their mother-in-law. The focus in the family is on a mother's relationship to her children, particularly her oldest son, who may help elevate her status. Sons are more valued than daughters[25].

Asian-Americans also have a different communication style from that of Westerners. Apart from the obvious language barriers, what is communicated between persons depends on the age, sex, education, occupation, and social status of the speakers. For example, Asian-American clients may not establish eye contact with a clinician as a sign of respect for the clinician's authority. This is important to remember when treatment information is conveyed. Direct confrontation is to be avoided, and questions or concerns tend to be communicated indirectly[25]. Thus, if a client disagrees or has questions about the information given during infertility assessment or treatment, Asian-Americans are less likely to voice their opinion because of fear of insulting the physician, who has high status because of his or her educational background.

Asian-Americans are more likely to turn to family members first to resolve a problem. Infertility is viewed as a family problem that should not be discussed with strangers. One study[13] noted that Asian women tend to be very modest and feel uncomfortable with pelvic examinations, as well as discussions of sexual matters with strangers. Because they find many surgical procedures (e.g., laparoscopy) intrusive, many feel more comfortable with herbal medicines and acupuncture.

Native Americans

Because of the heterogeneity of the Native American community, it is hard to generalize how infertility is viewed within it. There are many Native American tribes in the United States, and perceptions of infertility, views on traditional versus Western medical interventions, family structure, and views on assimilation into mainstream white culture vary from tribe to tribe. However, most tribes view the extended family as the basic family unit. There is an emphasis on the community rather than individuals, and behavior is evaluated in the context of how the individual benefits the tribe. Most Native American tribes emphasize cooperative behavior and have a time orientation that moves from the present to the past. The tribe promotes people's living in harmony with nature and achieving balance in their life[24].

Native Americans are the only ethnic minority group in the United States that is not immigrant, and they are the only minority group that must define its ethnicity using federal guidelines. The active attempt to destroy native culture and communities in the expansion of the

United States has resulted in many Native Americans living in economically impoverished, psychologically distressed communities where the unemployment rate, suicide rates, and rates for substance abuse are very high. Access to marginal health care is poor, with long waits, language barriers, and impersonal, unfriendly care delivery often being the rule rather than the exception. In this context of medical care, infertility treatment on many reservations is minimal at best. While there are no data that examine infertility in the Native American community, the limited access to good medical care, the high rate of substance abuse, and the practice of having multiple sexual partners suggest that the rate of infertility of Native Americans might be higher than that of white Americans.

Even if infertility treatment were available, Native Americans would be less likely to avail themselves of it because of the emphasis on balance with nature and spirituality within this community. Thus, Native Americans would be more likely to go to a spiritual healer or use traditional medicine for infertility. Many Native American practices for infertility cures involve the use of the earth or soil because of curative powers in the earth[26]. Infertility is viewed as being out of balance with nature, possibly affected by some evil spirit. Infertility treatment is not strongly supported within this community because it is seen as unnatural. Since strong emotions are not publicly expressed, it would be very unusual for a Native American couple to seek infertility counseling outside their community. The tribe often emphasizes accepting rather than modifying difficult situations, so accepting childlessness is viewed as a more culturally accepted option than infertility counseling or treatment. Adoption also is more culturally sanctioned and often occurs informally within extended families.

Religious Factors

It is somewhat artificial to separate cultural and religious factors regarding infertility because there is some overlap between the two: cultural factors are influenced by religious issues. For example, since many Hispanic Americans are at least nominally Roman Catholic, many issues pertaining to Roman Catholicism apply to this cultural group as well. Judaism is both a religion and a culture, but there are different forms of Judaism. Some Jews may be Orthodox, while others may consider themselves Jewish in terms of their cultural heritage but not religiously. However, for clarity, cultural and religious factors are discussed separately.

Certain aspects of infertility automatically bring up religious issues. The first commandment in both the Christian Bible and in the Torah, the Jewish holy book, commands humans to 'be fruitful and multiply'. This commandment is found in most major religions and in the creation myths of most cultures as well. What follows is an overview of how infertility and infertility treatment are viewed from different religious perspectives. This discussion is largely taken from Schenker's[27] excellent review of religious views on infertility.

Judaism

In Jewish culture and religion, the centrality of family is crucial. The first commandment in the Torah is to 'be fruitful and multiply'. Thus, procreation is felt to be an obligation and a responsibility. Among Orthodox Jews, the ultimate goal of sex is procreation; children are seen as a blessing and an extension of the worth of the parents[27]. The Talmud allows a man to divorce his wife if she is barren: 'Any man who had no children is considered as a dead man'. Clearly, even among many non-Orthodox Jews, having children is a central function of the family[27].

Hebrew law suggests that infertile couples should be diagnosed and treated as a single unit. Intrauterine insemination (IUI), in vitro fertilization (IVF), embryo transfer (ET) without a donor, and corrective surgical techniques (e.g., tubal repair) are considered to be appropriate methods to treat infertility. Gamete donation (i.e., donor insemination [DI] or ovum donation [OD]) is considered inappropriate because of issues with adultery, inheritance, and the legitimacy of the child. Some interpret Jewish law to hold that a child conceived by DI is the product of an adulterous relationship because the husband's sperm was not used, while others differ with this interpretation. Problems of inheritance stem from the lack of genetic link between the father and the child when DI is used. In the case of OD, a problem arises in the interpretation of who the child's mother is: the donor or the woman who carried and delivered the child[27,29].

Some treatment protocols or options may not be sanctioned. Some researchers have noted that Orthodox Jews do not openly discuss sexual matters, making it difficult to obtain a good medical history[29]. Orthodox Jewish women are particularly concerned that test procedures will result in bleeding because they would have to refrain from sexual intercourse for 8 days and undergo a ritualistic purification[13]. Orthodox Jews may also have restrictions regarding sexual intercourse during certain periods of the woman's menstrual cycle or may have restrictions on the Sabbath, thereby interfering with treatment protocols.

Islam

Islamic law is called *Sharia* and is based primarily on the Quran (the Islamic Holy book) and the Hadith, the authentic traditions and sayings of the prophet Mohammed. Islam also views sexual relations within the context of procreation and family building. Because procreation is considered a duty in marriage, Islam encourages the treatment of infertility, so IUI, IVF, and ET are deemed appropriate interventions, as long as they do not involve gamete donation. DI, OD, embryo donation, surrogacy, and adoption are forbidden because they are viewed as either adulterous or violations against legal inheritance. If the sanctioned assisted reproductive technologies are unsuccessful, Islam promotes acceptance by the couple that the marriage will remain childless[27].

Roman Catholicism

The Roman Catholic Church has some of the most restrictive views on the use of assisted reproductive technologies to treat infertile couples. In 1987, the Congregation for the Doctrine of the Faith clearly stated that for assisted reproduction to be sanctioned by the Church, human life must be protected, respected, and treated with dignity from conception. Procreation cannot be separated from the relationship between the parents. Children must be a product of a physical union between the husband and wife and must be conceived through an act of love and sexual intercourse. Thus, procreation cannot be performed by a physician, although physicians can assist a couple in conceiving by using corrective techniques that do not involve procreation (e.g., ovulation-induction medications, etc.)[30].

As such, the Roman Catholic Church views IUI, IVF, DI, OD, embryo donation, zygote intrafallopian transfer, gestational carrier and surrogacy as impermissible because the procedures separate human procreation from sexual intercourse and/or do not protect human life (e.g., in the case of IVF, there is concern that the zygotes may be damaged or destroyed during the procedure). Gamete intrafallopian transfer is allowed because the sperm can be removed from the vagina after normal intercourse and implanted into the fallopian tube[27]. It is interesting to note that the Roman Catholic Church is the only denomination that the American Society for Reproductive Medicine (ASRM) has directly responded to regarding the denomination's views on assisted reproductive technologies. In 1988, the ASRM wrote a direct response to the Congregation for the Doctrine of the Faith, vehemently disagreeing with the Church's interpretation that the separation of the unitive and procreative aspects of sexual relations interferes with sexual intimacy and, hence, with the emotional relationship in marriage[31].

Protestantism

There are a number of Protestant denominations with varying degrees of acceptance of assisted reproductive technologies both across and within denominations. Many denominations do not have 'official' policies regarding these techniques, so the interpretation of their use is often decided by the local pastor or the parishioner him- or herself. Most Protestant denominations view the Bible as the only religious authority, and while the Bible does not say much about assisted reproduction, it says quite a bit about infertility.

There are seven well known cases of women in the Bible who were barren and who received an annunciation from God promising an end to their barrenness: Sarah, wife of Abraham (Genesis 18:9–15); Rebecca, wife of Isaac (Genesis 25:19–26); Rachel, wife of Jacob (Genesis 30:1–8, 22–24); the unnamed wife of Manoah and mother of Samson (Judges 13:1–24); Hannah, wife of Elkanah and mother of Samuel (I Samuel 1:1–28); an unnamed Shunammite woman (2 Kings 4:8–17); and Elizabeth, wife of Zacharias, and mother of John the Baptist (Luke 1:7–25, 39–80). Of these seven women, only Elizabeth is found in the New Testament[32]. It is also interesting to note that the author could not find one example of barren men in the Bible, with the exception of eunuchs (men who were castrated, often to protect the harem of a prominent male).

However, the curse and stigma associated with infertility for the women in the Bible is very dramatic and clear. When Rachel was unable to have children and envied her sister Leah's ability to have several children by Jacob, she told Jacob to 'Give me children, or else I die' (Genesis 30:1–3)[32]. When Rachel became pregnant, she thanked God, saying 'God has taken away my disgrace' (Genesis 30:23)[32]. In the New Testament, when Elizabeth became pregnant, she proclaimed: 'In these days he has shown his favor and taken away my disgrace among the people' (Luke 1:24–25)[32].

The theological motif of these stories is that the child is born to a previously barren woman and that the child is special and is a gift from God. These children are all extraordinary, they all face dangers, and in some cases they lose their lives. Theologically, if God gave the child to the woman in the first place, then he has a right to ask for the life of the child (i.e., a sacrifice)[33]. This motif is important because it helps explain why many Protestant couples view infertility as a punishment from God: If children are gifts from God and we cannot have children, then what have we done to be undeserving of the gift?

Infertility can represent a crisis of faith in the lives of individuals and couples. It places an individual or couple in touch with mortality because children are often an important link to the future. It also impacts on their notion of God as provider and divine healer[34]. Not only do infertile individuals feel that they are being punished (e.g., for an earlier abortion, delaying childbearing for educational or career goals), but they wonder why, if they are not going to have a child, God does not take away the desire to have one[35]?

Many religious couples will approach their pastor (who may or may not be familiar with infertility and assisted reproductive technologies) for spiritual advice or counsel. Some Protestant pastors feel that assisted reproduction is an appropriate mode of treatment, as long as it involves the married couple and if only the gametes of the couple are used. Others strongly prohibit gamete donation and have concerns about the damage that can occur to preembryos and embryos[28]. Some fundamentalist groups object to the practice of masturbation in the collection of semen, and some religious men may feel uncomfortable with the use of visual aids in semen collection rooms[29].

Unfortunately for some couples, the very place where they go to for support may inadvertently provide the least support because of the minister's own discomfort with talking about infertility. Some pastoral counselors suggest that ministers refrain from offering infertile parishioners religious platitudes such as 'God can work miracles', 'God knows best', 'It's God's will' and treat infertility like any other chronic medical condition[35]. Others suggest helping individuals and couples struggle with the meaning of suffering, the use of prayer, and dealing with anger at God[34]. Pastors can also help couples grieve and can be more sensitive on special holidays such as Mother's Day, Father's Day, and Christmas[35].

Churches can also support other options such as child-free living and adoption. Some pastors have become advocates of adoption, noting that Moses and Jesus were adopted[36]. Some also note that Jesus advocated adoption during his crucifixion when he told his mother Mary and his disciple John: ' "Dear woman, here is your son;' and to the disciple, 'Here is your mother" ' (John 19:26–27)[32]. Many African-American churches are involved in the national One Church One Child program, which advocates adopting African-American children.

In summary, the religious background of infertile clients is also an important influence on how they adjust to infertility and its treatment. For Roman Catholic and Orthodox Jewish couples, many of the procedures may be prohibited, limiting treatment options or creating conflict for those who choose to participate in treatment protocols that violate religious beliefs. Infertility may precipitate a spiritual crisis. Clearly, religious and cultural factors have to be considered in the provision of psychotherapeutic interventions for couples and individuals experiencing infertility.

THERAPEUTIC INTERVENTIONS

In providing infertility counseling for culturally and religiously diverse individuals and couples, it is important to have a good understanding of how their cultural or religious background shapes their understanding of infertility, how infertility impacts on them psychologically, and how it shapes their perception of the available treatment options. Infertility counselors must have a working knowledge of an individual's cultural and/or spiritual values. This may feel overwhelming to therapists, who cannot possibly have a cultural anthropologist's understanding of all the various ethnic, cultural, and religious groups that one might encounter in counseling infertile clients. However, a great place to start is an awareness that culture and religion can influence how infertility impacts the psychological adjustment of a client. Having a general understanding of how the major cultural and religious groups in this country *traditionally* view family building, fertility, and infertility is also helpful.

While it is important to recognize cultural differences, it is also important not to stereotype clients based on their cultural or religious backgrounds. During the initial stages of counseling, it is important to note how salient cultural practices are in a client's life. Some of this information can be obtained while gathering general background information from clients. Clients who have more education, live in middle-class communities, and have professional occupations have more contact with mainstream culture and thus may be more acculturated. It is also important to asks clients about their understanding of infertility, not just from a medical standpoint but on a 'personal level'. For example, this author often ask clients to explain what they thought about infertility before they began their diagnostic work-up. Many African-American clients have shared that they never knew any black people who were infertile; they thought it was mostly 'a middle-class white women's disease'. It can also be enlightening to ask clients how 'elders' (e.g., parents, grandparents, fictive kin, etc.) in their community conceptualize infertility, because this also gives both a familial and a cultural perspective of what infertility means to the clients.

It is important to be sensitive to the fact that some cultural groups may feel uncomfortable seeking counseling for infertility because (1) they are uncomfortable discussing issues concerning sexual behavior, (2) they are uncomfortable seeking counseling in general, and (3) counseling is not a culturally approved activity. Women from Asian-American, Hispanic, Middle Eastern, or Orthodox Jewish communities may feel uncomfortable discussing infertility because of the close association between infertility and sexuality. Infertility counselors can acknowledge this discomfort and, if appropriate, acknowledge the cultural differences in discussing such topics in an open manner with strangers. This helps validate clients' feelings and gives them permission to discuss infertility when, and if, they feel comfortable doing so. It is also important for infertility counselors to recognize and respect that some behaviors that create cultural barriers for clients and counselors will never be overcome (e.g., discussing sexual behavior).

Counselors also need to be sensitive to the fact that many persons from minority groups are uncomfortable venturing into counseling because they prefer to resolve 'emotional' problems with the help of family, friends, neighbors, and members of the clergy in their own community. There is a tendency to distrust disclosing personal information to 'strangers', and there may be strong feelings about airing 'family business' in public. There is also a stigma attached to seeking professional mental health services, which many members of ethnic groups view as being designed for 'crazy' people or for 'rich white people'. Their level of discomfort may be heightened by the fact that a counselor is culturally different from them[37]. Because of their discomfort with using mental health professionals, the individuals or couples experiencing infertility may not come in for counseling until the situation has reached a crisis. For some, a culturally different counselor may be an advantage in that he or she is not connected to their community, and therefore it is easier to disclose personal information.

In acknowledging cultural differences in perceptions of infertility, it is also important not to interpret differences as being 'deficient'. Some counselors view a reluctance to use certain techniques as 'ignorance' or 'noncompliance' on the part of clients and become impatient waiting for these clients to 'catch up' to other, mainstream clients. Such attitudes are condescending and are not respectful of cultural *differences* in views on infertility. For example, this author had several African-American clients resist doing a sperm penetration assay test (see Chapter 2). While this may seem straightforward to many health care providers, to some African-American clients, it feels 'unnatural' and 'experimental'. Given the history of medical abuses of African-American men, it is understandable that they may be uncomfortable with tests involving reproductive processes, particularly when the test involves the use of *nonhumans*. Acknowledging a client's ambivalence and explaining *why* a procedure is being used often is helpful in alleviating distrust and anxiety.

Infertility counselors must also respect a client's decision to terminate infertility treatment, even if they think that other treatment options could prove to be successful, particularly if the reasons for termination are culturally based. Counseling techniques may also have to be modified to be more culturally compatible with a client. For example, while many therapists prefer to treat infertility in marital or couples therapy, African-American and Mexican-American men may be particularly reluctant to engage in counseling. If this is the case, a counselor may want to begin counseling with the female partner only, with the understanding that the male partner may join subsequent sessions. Inviting the male partner to a time-limited, problem-focused session may be more helpful and less threatening.

Counselors who work with low-income families have to be sensitive to a family's environment and broader community. It is important to do the counseling within a client's community and, if possible, in his or her native language. This will ease some of the barriers to the therapeutic process by providing the counseling in a familiar language and environmental setting. Sensitivity to the large number of stressors that often impinge on these families is also imperative, as is recognition that infertility

may not be the most pressing concern each week when a person comes in for counseling. Concerns with employment, housing, and household finances may understandably take precedence over infertility. Counselors must be careful not to interpret this behavior as 'defensive' or 'resistant'. Therapists who work with low-income clients need to know the social service system well and be willing to make contacts with various service providers when necessary[37].

Even when clients come to counseling, their cultural background will influence their expectations regarding the therapeutic process. For example, Asian-American clients may expect the therapist to be more directive, because the therapist is seen as an authority figure. If the therapist uses a model in which he or she takes a more passive role in the session, this may be viewed as an indication of lack of knowledge and skill. The therapist might need to take a more directive approach in the initial stages of counseling. Respect for traditional roles in the family is also important, even when gender role behaviors are incongruent with a counselor's beliefs about gender roles in families. In more traditional Hispanic and Asian-American families, the male is the authority figure in the home. Thus, it might be helpful to address initial inquiries and requests for information to the husband first[25]. It may also be difficult for a client to disagree with the counselor or ask questions for clarification because of cultural views with respect to authority figures. Here, the therapist should pay close attention to nonverbal cues to discern when a client is uncomfortable.

Counselors must also explore their own values and belief systems about working with clients of different religions or cultures. One of the difficulties that therapists may have in dealing with culturally diverse clients is having to come to terms with the fact that they may unconsciously harbor prejudiced views of different cultural groups. Even when therapists feel that they genuinely believe in a 'color-blind society', they must appreciate that this is not the experience of most of their clients. Thus, while cultural differences may not matter to a therapist, they may be very important to a client. Also, denying a client's cultural or religious differentness is denying a central part of who he or she is.

In addressing religious issues with clients, counselors must address how they feel about their own spirituality. This can be particularly difficult for therapists, because most have been trained to avoid religious issues in counseling. However, it is important for infertility counselors to appreciate that infertility represents a spiritual crisis to many clients. Infertile individuals often have to reevaluate their view of and relationship with God. Other clients will have to wrestle with deciding to pursue treatment options that are not sanctioned by their religion, creating another source of stress and cutting off a valued avenue of support. For example, this author has several Catholic clients who have vigorously pursued IVF, although they recognize that this goes against the teachings of their church. What was particularly agonizing for one couple was that they no longer felt comfortable going to their priest for support during this stressful period in their lives.

Therapists who feel comfortable doing so can help clients explore what their spirituality means in the face on infertility. It is particularly helpful to explore with clients how their spirituality helps and impedes their ability to cope with infertility. It is important to respect clients' religious views on infertility and not interpret decisions to use only certain procedures as 'defensive' or ambivalent. If a therapist is uncomfortable discussing spiritual issues,

he or she should offer a referral to a pastoral counselor who has been trained to address both spiritual and psychotherapeutic issues.

Therapists can also encourage the development of support groups within particular cultural and religious communities. The advantage of support groups is that they minimize the stigma attached to using mental health services and help clients see that they are not alone in their infertility experience. This may be a particularly important treatment option for minority groups who have a level of mistrust for mainstream mental health services.

While many national organizations report that support group attendance is low among ethnic minority groups, there are several ways for counselors to enhance participation. First, it is best when support groups are initiated by persons *within* a client's cultural or religious community. Clients may feel more comfortable with counselors and group members who have a similar cultural or religious background, particularly when their native language is not English. This may be particularly important for members of fundamentalist and orthodox religious groups who may be uncomfortable receiving services from groups outside of their religious community for fear that the information will be contrary to their group's doctrine. Church-based support groups also give religious clients 'permission' to deal with the emotional distress associated with infertility without having to worry that seeking counseling means that they are having a spiritual crisis or that they lack faith in God's healing powers.

Second, locating the support group within the cultural or religious community makes services more easily accessible. One reason that support groups tend to have such low participation from minority groups is that they are often located in predominantly white, middle-class communities. Support services located outside the community also send the message that they are not designed for people within the community. It is important for counselors and group leaders to recognize that members of different cultural groups may use support groups in a manner different from white middle-class clients. Because many ethnic minority members tend to rely on family and friends for emotional support, they may only use support groups during times of crisis. Support groups can also be developed in sororities, fraternities, other religious and cultural organizations, and in community-based health clinics, where are easily accessible.

FUTURE IMPLICATIONS

While white middle- and upper-class couples have historically been the primary consumers of infertility treatments, that may be changing. Through education, insurance access, and more user-friendly clinics, an increasing number of minority or culturally diverse couples are seeking medical assistance to treat infertility. As this phenomenon increases it is incumbent upon medical caregivers in the field to be culturally sensitive and adaptive. They must be prepared to tailor treatment procedures and alternatives to patients' cultural or religious restrictions or expectations.

An additional cultural phenomenon impacting medical caregivers is the increasing number of foreign patients seeking medical treatment for infertility in the United States[38]. Patients from around the world are known to seek treatment in the United States because particular medical treatments for infertility are unavailable in their own country or the laws

governing a preferred treatment are restrictive. As such, an increasing number of clinicians, particularly those offering assisted reproductive technologies or third-party reproduction, will encounter cross-cultural issues involving the religious beliefs, cultural norms, and even different language of patients pursuing family-building through infertility treatments.

SUMMARY

- Cultural and religious factors can impact the understanding and treatment of infertility.
- In infertility counseling, examination of a client's cultural and religious background and the infertility practitioner's cultural and religious framework is important.
- Certain assessment and treatment techniques may present cultural and/or religious conflicts for clients from other cultures.
- Insensitivity to cultural and spiritual barriers can result in premature termination or inadequate treatment of infertility.
- Understanding that infertility can also represent a spiritual crisis for individuals and couples can clarify some of the barriers to treatment and help individuals and couples work through the stress associated with infertility.
- Diagnostic work-ups, treatment procedures, and infertility counseling can be provided in a culturally sensitive context, which can enhance the treatment and therapeutic outcomes for infertile clients.

REFERENCES

1. Bornman MS, Schulenburg GW, Boomker D, *et al.* Observations in infertile African males at an andrology clinic in South Africa. *Arch Androl* 1994; 33:101–4

2. Inborn MC. Kabsa and threatened fertility in Egypt. *Soc Sci Med* 1994;39:487–505

3. Miranda C, Larrazabal F, Laban P. Family counseling in infertility couples. *Rev Chil Obstet Ginecol* 1995;60:75–8

4. Mo B. Black magic and illness in a Malaysian Chinese community. *Soc Sci Med* 1984;18:147–57

5. Neff DL. The social construction of infertility: The case of the matrilineal Nayars in South India. *Soc Sci Med* 1994;39:475–85

6. Rosenblatt PC, Peterson P, Portner J. A cross-cultural study of responses to childlessness. *Behav Sci Notes* 1973;8:221–31

7. Uka EM. The African family and issues of woman's infertility. *Afr Theol J* 1991; 20:190–200

8. Berry JW, Poortnga Y, Segall MH, Dasen PR. *Cross-Cultural Psychology: Research and Application.* Cambridge: Cambridge University Press, 1992

9. Tseng W, McDermott JF. *Culture, Mind, and Therapy.* New York: Brunner/Mazel, 1981

10. McGoldrick M. Ethnicity and family therapy: An overview. In: McGoldrick M, Pearce JK, Giordano J, eds. *Ethnicity and Family Therapy.* New York: Guilford Press, 1982;3–30

11. Gbadegesin S. Bioethics and culture: An African perspective. *Bioethics* 1993;7:256–62

12. Becker G, Nachtigall RD. Born to be a mother: The cultural construction of risk in infertility treatment in the United States. *Soc Sci Med* 1994;39:507–18

13. Blenner JL. Health care providers' treatment approaches to culturally diverse infertile clients. *J Trans Nurs* 1991;2:24–31

14. Dana RH. *Multicultural Assessment Perspectives for Professional Psychology.* Boston Allyn & Bacon, 1993

15. Comas-Diaz L, Griffith EEH. *Clinical Guidelines in Cross-Cultural Mental Health.* New York: John Wiley & Sons, 1988

16. Cannon EO. Religiosity and the outcome of pregnancy. *Society for the Study of Social Problems* 1990;1–9

17. Calica J. Infertility: An unacknowledged health problem. *Adopt Me* 1995;4:1,7

18. Molock SD. Impact of infertility on African Americans. Unpublished manuscript, 1994

19. Molock SD. Religious and culture aspects of infertility in the African American community. Presented at the national One Church One Child annual conference, Chicago, IL, 1995

20. Jones J. TRIOS. In: Boykins AW, Yates F, Franklin AJ, eds. *Research Directions of Black Psychologists.* New York: Russell Sage, 1980; 340–65

21. Molock SD. Barriers to adoption in the African American community. *Adopt Fam Am* 1995;28:14–16

22. Falicov CJ. Mexican families. In: McGoldrick M, Pearce JK, Giordano J, eds. *Ethnicity and Family Therapy.* New York: Guilford Press, 1982;134–63

23. Garcia-Preto N. Puerto Rican families. In: McGoldrick M, Pearce JK, Giordano J, eds. *Ethnicity and Family Therapy.* New York: Guilford Press, 1982;164–86

24. Bornstein J. Multicultural variables in infertility. Unpublished manuscript, 1995

25. Shon SP, Ja DY. Asian families. In: McGoldrick M, Pearce JK, Giordano J, eds. *Ethnicity and Family Therapy.* New York: Guilford Press, 1982;208–28

26. Sha JL. *Mothers of Thyme: Customs and Rituals of Infertility and Miscarriage.* Minneapolis, MN: Lida Rose Press, 1990

27. Schenker JG. Religious views regarding gamete donation. In: Seibel MM, Crockin SL, eds. *Family Building Through Egg and Sperm Donation.* Boston: Jones and Bartlett, 1996;238–50

28. Herz FM, Rosen EJ. Jewish families. In: McGoldrick M, Pearce JK, Giordano J, eds. *Ethnicity and Family Therapy.* New York: Guilford Press, 1982;364–92

29. Nutting SC. Potential cultural and religious implications faced by an ART couple. *Sereno Symposium USA Newsletter* 1995:4–5

30. Congregation for the Doctrine of the Faith. *Instruction on Respect for Human Life in Its Origin and on the Dignity of Procreation: Replies to Certain Questions of the Day.* Libreria Editrice Vaticanna, Vatican City, 1987

31. Ethical considerations of the new reproductive technologies: Ethics committee (1986–87) of the American Fertility Society in light of instruction on the respect for human life in its origin and on the dignity of procreation issued by the Congregation for the Doctrine of the Faith. *Fertil Steril* 1988;49(suppl):1s–7s

32. *The Layman's Parallel Bible*, New International Version. Grand Rapids, MI: The Zondervan Corporation, 1991

33. Ackerman S. Child sacrifice: Returning God's gift: Barren women give birth to exceptional children. *Bible Rev* 1993;9:20–9

34. Devor N. Pastoral care for infertile couples. *J Pastoral Care* 1994;48:355–60

35. Spring R. Ministry to the infertile. *Leadership* 1988;9:95–7

36. Guoth-Gumberger M. Buried under a mango tree: Infertility and faith. *Daughters of Sarah* 1992;18:12–13

37. Boyd-Franklin N. *Black Families in Therapy: A Multisystems Approach*. New York: Guilford Press, 1989

38. Kolata G. Infertile foreigners see opportunity in US. *New York Times*, Jan. 4, 1998

14

Lesbian Couples and Single Women

Mary Casey Jacob, PhD

The reality is that society brings home to us its most painful contradictions, not only through our internal experience of parenting, but through the experience of our children.

Jan Clausen

What do lesbian couples and single women have in common? Why write about them in the same chapter? They are linked by two key issues: (1) While they need the assistance of medical professionals (once they decide not to conceive via intercourse or self-insemination with a known donor), they generally are not infertile or known to be infertile; and (2) many people think that they should not become parents. Thus, we generally see that infertility programs decide to treat both groups or to exclude both groups from treatment; it is rare that a program will treat only one group or the other.

An additional possible area of overlap, of course, is that single women may be lesbian, and thus some of the issues discussed in this chapter regarding lesbian couples may apply equally to some single women. For example, Leiblum and colleagues[1] reported that 4 of 14 lesbian donor insemination (DI) patients were not living with lovers, and other studies[2,3] have shown similar proportions of single lesbians. At the University of Connecticut Health Center program, there has been only one instance of a single woman self-identifying as lesbian.

This chapter:

- contains some of the background that can be helpful in preparing to work with these populations
- addresses counseling issues unique to these groups.

It should be read in conjunction with the chapters on psychosocial evaluation of the infertile patient (see Chapter 3), recipient counseling for donor egg and donor sperm (see Chapters 18 and 19), and parenting after infertility (see Chapter 25). Those chapters cover many topics also applicable to single women and lesbian couples, such as donor and disclosure issues.

In this discussion, the term *single woman* should be taken to mean an unmarried, unattached woman. Unmarried heterosexual couples needing donor sperm or donor eggs are nowadays generally able to secure treatment and are not the subject of this chapter.

HISTORICAL OVERVIEW

Historically, it has been assumed that lesbian couples were not, and single women should not be, mothers. Tables 1 and 2

Table 1 Objections to lesbian parenthood

Lesbians are emotionally and sexually maladjusted[4,13,77].

Lesbian mothers are more focused on their relationships than on the children[8].

Lesbians are not maternal[1,8,54,77].

Lesbians will teach the children to be homosexual either consciously or through role-modeling[4,8,10,11,13,14,16,26,74,77–82].

Lesbians will molest their girl children[4,10,13,14,79].

Preference for girl children leads to rejection of boys[3,10].

The children will have disturbed gender role development[4,8,11,13,14,16,44,48,74,77,80,83,84].

The children will be socially stigmatized[4,8,10,13,14,16,35,44,72,74,77,79,82].

Lesbian parents will have an impact on children's mental well-being[8,11,16,77].

Lesbian parenthood lacks male role models[77,83].

Note: The citations given are both pro and con the concern specified.

Table 2 Criticisms of single women becoming parents

Children should have two parents, a mother and a father[2,20].

Absence of a father can impact a child's psychosexual development[20,35,60].

Because a single mother needs to work, the reduced time with a child will impact cognitive and social development[20,35,60].

Becoming a single parent is just a selfish act[2].

Parenthood is too stressful for one parent to manage[2,60].

A single-woman parent may have an impact on a child's mental well-being[2,85].

Women who want to be single mothers are emotionally abnormal[2].

Women who have not been sexually active may not be acceptable candidates for donor insemination[60,86,87].

There are financial stressors in single parenting[35,60].

Note: The citations given are both pro and con the concern specified.

delineate the arguments that have been made in this regard. The issues in these tables that can be scientifically operationalized have been studied.

Published reports suggest that as many as five million lesbians have children conceived in heterosexual relationships[4–8]. Reviews of lesbian parenthood[5,8–16] have summarized the literature on a range of variables 'including gender role development and sexual identity, separation-individuation, psychiatric evaluations, assessments of social adjustment and behavior problems, personality, self-concept and self-esteem, locus of control, development of moral judgment, and intelligence'[9]. The results do not show that children of lesbians are disadvantaged in any unique way. They do show of course the effects of marital distress and divorce on the children.

The effects of family break-ups are also apparent in studies of families headed by single mothers, showing that the children may have less educational, occupational, and economic success, are more likely to begin their own families at a younger age, and are more likely to become separated or divorced themselves[17]. Probably, these disadvantages are more the result of a loss of socioeconomic status when a family breaks up than the lack of a second residential parent per se[18,19]. Other studies[20] have suggested that children of female-headed families are similar in cognitive abilities to those of two-parent families, are likely to be independent and achievement-oriented, and have good self-esteem.

Studies of nontraditional families have also identified some variables that predict good adjustment and some unique strengths. For example, not only does the literature support the notion that children of lesbians are normal and healthy, but it also suggests that they tolerate and value diversity to a greater extent than children in intact heterosexual families and may feel more able to challenge traditional sex-role stereotypes[21]. The quality of parent–child communication, social support, and socioeconomic status have been linked to success in single-parent families, both for their own intrinsic value and for how they contribute to the mental and physical well-being of individuals[22].

There is so little literature on families headed by single-mothers-by-choice that a special issue of *Family Relations*[23] on the topic of single parents did not have a single chapter on this subgroup. Mechaneck and associates[24] did report on this group, however, following interviews with 20 women who elected to become single mothers either proactively or after conceiving an unplanned pregnancy. The women in this study were all white, with an average age of 39 and average annual income of $39,000 (in the mid-1980s). One was a high school graduate, four had bachelor's degrees, six had master's degrees, three had doctorates, two were lawyers, and one was a medical doctor. Nineteen were heterosexual; 18 hoped to marry in the future. The decision to become a single mother took an average of 4 years. Four women used DI, six adopted, and 10 used intercourse. One mother had two children; others wanted second children but did not proceed for financial reasons. Overall, the women reported being happy with their decisions, and single motherhood for these goal-directed women seemed a viable choice. Frank and Brackley[25] reported two case studies from a nursing perspective. The women were 38 and 44 years of age. Each had made the decision to have a baby over 5 or more years. Desire for a child and a sense of being ready were important factors in the decision, and the women seemed goal-oriented and independent in general. Both planned to include men in their support system, so the children would have male role models. Both understood the enormity of their decisions. In each of these reports, the women did not fit the societal stereotypes of single mothers. They were mature, independent, deliberate women who understood that they would need the help of family and friends to care well for the child.

This brief historical overview documents the existence of lesbian and planned single motherhood. Even so, professionals who work with lesbian couples have generally assumed that all children of lesbians were the issue of previous heterosexual marriages. The degree to which this was true can be seen, for example, in a large study[26] of homosexual and heterosexual men and women in which the homosexuals were asked about children only in the context of marriage. In the past, even lesbians themselves assumed parenting was not an option. One woman, in explaining why she felt restricted by her lesbian status stated, 'The person I love and live with might someday want a child, and I could never give it to her, nor could she to me'[26]. Single women have not been categorized as unable to have children in this way. Instead, it has generally been assumed that single mothers conceived by accident or carelessness, not design. For both groups of women, the notion of motherhood by choice has only recently been more widely recognized by doctors and other health professionals.

REVIEW OF LITERATURE

Even after recognizing that children might be desired by lesbian couples and single women, and in spite of the data supporting their fitness as parents, practitioners and the public have continued to expressed the concerns listed in Tables 1 and 2[27-31]. The expression of these concerns and the reluctance to treat these women are consistent with Melton's[32] observation that public policy regarding children and families is often based on myths of what ought to be rather than on the facts of what they are and what they do. Others[33-35] cite uncertainty regarding the legality of treating single women or lesbian couples. For several decades now, however, feminist and lesbian literature[36-43] has argued for the rights of these women and has given information about how they might conceive without the assistance of the medical establishment. Most recently, a body of literature has appeared in which arguments are made that there are no a priori reasons to exclude single women and lesbian couples from assisted reproduction programs. These discussions stem from both medical ethics[9,12,35,44-46] and legal[33,34,47] perspectives. Some articles also attempt to give guidance to physicians regarding how to incorporate single and lesbian women into existing treatment programs[35,44,46]. Additionally, several practitioners have published retrospective reports describing their program's DI patients, and these reports show that single women and lesbian couples are being treated in some programs.

McCartney's[2] report showed that 2 of 12 single DI candidates were lesbian. In Leiblum's and coworkers[1] report of 45 unmarried women who underwent DI, 28 were heterosexual, 14 lesbian, two bisexual, and one celibate. There were few differences between the groups, except that heterosexual women tended to be older. In the combined sample, over 70% of the women reported four factors that prompted them to begin DI treatment: (1) They felt secure in their employment; (2) they had 'worked through' parenting issues for themselves; (3) they felt that time was passing; and (4) they felt that they had sufficient social support. All the women planned to disclose to the children the facts of their conception but were not always sure how and when to do so.

A recent report by Wendland and colleagues[3] showed that of 115 DI recipients treated over 4 years, 65% were married, 17%

single, 14% lesbian couples, and 4% unmarried heterosexual couples. The married women and those who identified themselves as single did not state their sexual orientation. The report gave demographic information for the different groups and compared them on factors related to deciding to use DI versus alternatives, undergoing the DI procedure, preparing for a child, disclosure and social support, the impact of the use of DI on the relationship, and the use of counseling in DI. The groups did not differ significantly on demographic variables, except that lesbian recipients were less likely to belong to a mainstream religious group. For all groups, recipient age and emotional readiness to have a child were key factors in deciding when to proceed. Lesbian couples reported that they decided which partner would try to conceive by weighing desire to experience pregnancy and childbirth more heavily than age or insurance issues. Of lesbian couples, 38% reported that the other partner would attempt conception later, and two of the partners already had biological children. Lesbian women were more likely than single or heterosexual-coupled women to consider intercourse with a fertile and consenting man, and 13% had attempted this. Major reasons for not attempting this were concerns over the donor's parental rights and involvement, and moral objections. Only 12% of married couples discussed custody issues prior to initiating DI, but 97% of lesbian couples had done so. Among lesbian couples, 29% had drawn up legal documents regarding custody. One-third of all subjects indicated a gender preference (mostly for girls), and the percentages did not vary among groups.

Lesbian Couples

Seligmann[7] has reported that 5000–10,000 planned lesbian families exist. Patterson[48] referred to this as a 'lesbian baby boom'. Steckel[49] was one of the first authors to report on planned lesbian families. She compared separation and individuation in children of lesbian couples to those of heterosexual couples. There were 11 children in each group of 3- and 4-year-old children. She found the two groups to be very similar in that neither group had more pathology or difficulties than the other.

McCandlish[50] reported interviews with five lesbian two-parent families with 7 DI-conceived children between them ranging in age from 18 months to 7 years. All children old enough to talk demonstrated a healthy gender identity and knowledge of gender differences, normal development, and no evidence of behavior problems. The mothers expressed some difficulties with the transition to parenthood, particularly that the biological mother felt uncomfortable when the co-mother was called and treated as 'mom' by the child or children.

In 1989, Brewaeys and colleagues[51] may have been the first team to report that their practice was treating lesbian couples. They described the approach their team used to screen the 27 applicant couples and gave information about the 21 couples accepted into the program. The mean age of the women was 30 years, 6 months. All had completed secondary education, and 40 of the women worked, while two were homemakers. The relationships varied in length from 3 years to 10 years, with a mean of 6 years. All were in regular contact with their own families. Most (40/42) were open with friends about being lesbian, while half were open at work. Jacob and associates[52] found similar results in 1994 with the first 14 lesbian couples to enter a longitudinal study of DI recipients. In a comparison of the couples with single women and heterosexual couples using DI following a vasectomy, few differences were found in demographics or motivations for using DI compared with adoption. The lesbian couples (and the single women) were more likely to have disclosed to numerous others and to intend to tell the child, and the partners of lesbian women were more likely to attend the inseminations.

Patterson[48] reported a study of 37 families headed by either single lesbian parents or lesbian couples. While she did not state specifically that the women used DI to conceive, all conceived after coming out as lesbians. The 37 children studied were all between the ages of 4 and 9 years. They were examined on social competence, behavior problems, self-concept, and sexual identity. The first three variables were evaluated with standardized measures and compared to published norms for non-clinical samples. The scores for social competence and behavior problems were also compared to clinical norms. In each case, the scores of the children were higher than those of the clinical samples (where applicable) and did not differ from the normal samples, with one exception. Children of lesbian mothers reported greater stress reactions than children of heterosexual mothers, but they also had a higher overall sense of well-being. Because all the children tested were prepubertal, consideration of sexual identity focused on sex-role behavior. Most children reported preferences for sex-role behaviors considered normative for their age. All children reported that their friends were mainly or entirely of their own sex. Only one child reported favorite toys that were typed as opposite-gender, and only two reported favorite characters that were opposite-gender-typed.

In this study[48], 26 families were headed by lesbian couples. These families were also studied in terms of division of labor, relationship satisfaction, and the psycho-social adjustment of the 26 children as it related to the first two variables[53]. The rationale for this study was based on the accumulated evidence that heterosexual transition to parenthood has been associated with increasing role specialization. Given that lesbian couples without children tend to divide household tasks equally and to see this as an important thing to do, what happens when children are added to the household? Patterson[48] found that couples with children continued to divide most household tasks evenly but that biological mothers ended up with more responsibility for child care and non-biological mothers ended up working more hours for pay. Further, the children's psychosocial adjustment (which in general was very good) was better in households where this unequal division of labor did not occur. Relationship satisfaction was not related to either the division of labor or the adjustment of the children.

Flaks and colleagues[54] compared 15 lesbian couples who became parents via therapeutic donor insemination (DI) to 15 matched heterosexual families. Each family had at least one child between the ages of 3 and 9 years. The children's cognitive functioning and behavioral adjustment, as well as the parents' relationship and parenting skills, were studied. All measures were standardized and included a report completed by the children's teachers. No significant differences were found between the two groups of children or parents, except that lesbian parents exhibited more parenting-awareness skills.

Gartrell and associates[55] recently published preliminary data from an ongoing longitudinal study of 84 DI lesbian families, 70 of which had two parents. Families were recruited and first interviewed during the insemination process or the pregnancy. The authors reported on parental relationships (or desire for a relationship, if single), plans regarding the sharing of parenting tasks, social supports, making the decision to have a child, preferences for the sex of the child, issues of known versus anonymous donors, concerns about stigmatization, and plans regarding being open about their lesbianism. Variables were

chosen with an eye to information to which these women might have liked access as they considered becoming mothers. Couples had been together for a mean of 6.1 years, and they listed shared values and communication skills as the most important strengths of their relationships. Unlike in McCandlish's[50] study, these women did not have different rates of concern about bonding between co-mothers and the children. Gartrell and coworkers'[55] subjects did, however, report concerns about ways in which they and their children might be stigmatized. They recognized they were a nontraditional family in a sexist and homophobic world. Further, the children were conceived unconventionally, and some were nonwhite or non-Christian. All of these variables provided opportunities for others to discriminate against the families. The preliminary data suggested that the families were thoughtfully conceived by women with good relationships with friends and extended family. They were knowledgeable about the difficulties that they may encounter and had access to support groups. The authors hope to follow this cohort for 25 years.

As one hopeful lesbian mother-to-be put it, lesbian families offer 'not a "traditional" family structure, but a family with traditional values—integrity, compassion, honesty, spirituality and morality'[56]. This applies equally to what single mothers by choice offer.

Single Women

Published discussions of the possibility that single women might request DI date back to the 1940s, and evidence 'great concern and distaste'[33]. Potter and Knaub[57] took the debate a big step forward when they made an important distinction and argued the need to begin separating the data regarding families of 'single mothers by choice' from families of women who became single mothers 'by accident' via rape, divorce, widowhood, or accidental conception.

Reports of single women requesting DI from fertility clinics began appearing periodically in the 1980s and triggered a still ongoing controversy about the appropriateness of offering the service[1,35,57,58]. Strong and Schinfeld[35] described the approach that their clinic was taking and gave case reports of some single women accepted for DI treatment. McCartney[2] reported the findings of a psychiatric evaluation of 12 unmarried women requesting DI. The psychiatrist's task was to give an opinion about each woman's mental health, rationality, and preparation for the stresses of single parenting. She found that one woman's statement represented a summary for the group: 'Nothing is missing from my life, I just want to expand it'. All had discussed their plans with parents, and all parents accepted their daughters' plans. All the women had male friendships, and the 10 heterosexual women were hoping eventually to have committed relationships. The two lesbian women had long-term partners. Seven of the women had reason to believe that they would have trouble conceiving. All were financially stable, with good social support in the family and from friends. These women were goal-oriented and independent. Of this group, two women were counseled to delay conception; the authors did not say why.

Klock and coworkers[59] compared single and married DI candidates and found that they did not differ in reported psychiatric symptoms, self-esteem, or attitudes and concerns regarding DI. Single women did take longer to decide to proceed with DI and were more likely to be planning to disclose to the child the facts of his or her conception.

In perhaps one of the most negative reports available, Baetens and colleagues[60] reported on 94 single women who requested DI and the 41 who were accepted for treatment. The authors were very clear that, in their view, choosing to become a single parent is very different from choosing to become a parent with another person (male or female): The financial challenges, the social isolation, and the kinds of reasons given for making this choice are more often problematic with single women. The primary reasons for refusals were a lack of autonomy, ongoing problems with relationships, current financial or psychiatric instability or legal uncertainties (e.g. illegal immigrants), and available social supports. The authors noted that these problems were much less prevalent in the lesbian population applying for treatment in the same setting[51].

THEORETICAL FRAMEWORKS

Lesbian Couples

Loulan[61] proposed that there are five general stages that lesbians pass through in choosing to be mothers:

- It is possible; some lesbians are mothers.
- It is attractive but may not be for me; maybe I'm not competent (internalized homophobia).
- I can do it, but I am not ready.
- I am ready and can begin planning.
- I've made a plan and am acting on it.

She also made suggestions about how therapists can be of assistance at the different stages, such as working with a client to bolster self-esteem or to deal with ambivalence about one's sexual orientation, exploration of reasons for wanting to be a mother, investigating or establishing good support systems, referrals to support groups of other lesbians working toward motherhood, medical referrals, and practical information about issues such as finding child care.

Slater and Mencher[62] noted that while family theory has begun to account for the ways in which some kinds of diversity are demonstrated in families, little has been written of diversity in terms of sexual orientation. They first reviewed the structural elements of family theory as presented by Carter and McGoldrick[63]. These elements include (1) predictable stages of family life, including mate selection, bearing or adoption of children, raising of children, and having grown children leave home and begin the next generation; (2) a consistent context of social supports; (3) the use of *public* ritual to negotiate transitions between stages; and (4) the use of public ritual to validate the existence of the family. Slater and Mencher[62] then showed that this model is difficult to apply directly to lesbian families. First, there is no road map in terms of stages as there is for the heterosexual culture. Second, the model assumes the presence of family support because in the heterosexual culture a lack of these supports is deviant; in the lesbian culture, however, it may be the norm. Third, the model is child-centered, and it has not been the norm for lesbian families to have children. This last point is especially complicated because it correctly identifies a conflict for lesbians: The heterosexual world does not expect them to have children, but neither does their lesbian world. Finally, the model assumes social validation of the family unit, but this validation is generally not available to lesbian families. 'There is no act, commitment, or length of time spent together that moves such a couple into a sanctioned social status. The couple must fight both active and passive disregard throughout life'[62].

In addition to reviewing the applicability of traditional family theory to lesbian families, Slater and Mencher[62] took a brief look at relationship theory as well.

They noted that fusion, or a sort of psychic melding, has been noted to be present in a significant number of lesbian relationships and has generally been thought to be maladaptive. This argument was made after a comparison of lesbian relationships to heterosexual ones. In view of contemporary theory about the development of girls and women[64], however, it may be the norm for women to demonstrate fusion in their relationships with one another, and this may be particularly functional in lesbian relationships if it is not taken to an extreme[62]. Other authors[65] have made similar arguments.

Single Women

Baetens and colleagues[60], in describing their method of evaluating the DI requests of single women, reported using the guidance of Satir's family systems theory. This theory centers on the family as a working system, not just a group of people. It recognizes the importance of all family members, both in the family of origin and the present constellation. Psychological health is a function of positive self-esteem in family members, good communication, open relations with the environment, and well balanced and clear family roles. Single candidates for DI are therefore, in this setting, questioned about many aspects of family history to see whether they meet the basic criteria for healthy functioning à la Satir.

CLINICAL ISSUES AND THERAPEUTIC INTERVENTIONS

For pretreatment counseling, many of the issues discussed with single women and lesbian couples need not differ from those discussed with heterosexual couples. These issues have been outlined elsewhere in this book and also by Klock and Maier[66]. There are, however, a number of additional issues to raise with these nontraditional applicants for DI.

Deciding to Parent and How to Parent

For many people, the desire for children is hard to explain. The motivations for parenting given by single women and lesbian couples do not differ from those of married women: Many say that they always wanted to be mothers and looked forward to the experience; some hope to combat loneliness; and some hope to fulfill the expectations of family. Lesbians and single women should not be required to articulate their desire for children more clearly than married women do .

The evidence suggests that most of these women have been thoughtful and deliberate in deciding to conceive[1,24,25,67,68]. Occasionally, however, a woman will make a hasty decision, not having discussed the matter with family or friends. She may need to be encouraged to take more time and seek the support of others.

How does a woman know when she is ready to proceed? Reasons given include being financially stable, having dealt with ambivalence, having social supports in place, and feeling that if she waits too long, it will be too late biologically. Lesbian couples and single women are a part of the larger society and, as such, may well carry some of the prejudices of the culture, including the belief that children should have two parents, a male and a female. Counselors should encourage clients to express any uncertainties that they have about whether they are doing the right thing. Lesbians also state that completing the coming out process with family and friends is an important step in preparation. Sometimes, lesbians have not come out with parents, at work, or with neighbors and have not given thought to what it might be like for a child to have to bear the burden of this secret. It is important that they be challenged to think this through, and it could be argued that the coming-out process should be completed or well underway before the insemination procedure.

Having decided to parent, women must decide how to proceed: to get pregnant or to adopt? Those who decide to adopt generally do not come to an assisted reproduction program. For those who have decided on anonymous DI, it is important to ask a few questions: Why DI? Why not a known donor? Why an infertility program and not their private gynecologist? Sometimes, in the course of this discussion, the women or couples learn about a new avenue that they had not considered. Mostly, however, women choose DI through a sperm bank for some of the following reasons: greater medical safety, greater legal protection, less chance that the donor/father will interfere or have a role, absence of a male friend who is willing to donate without being a father in the child's life, reluctance to have sex with a man purely for conception, or belief that it is wrong to use a man for conception only or that doing so is breaking a vow of fidelity.

Lesbian couples have the additional task of deciding who will carry the baby. In this author's experience, the most common reasons given for the choice that they have made is that one woman always wanted to be pregnant and the other has no desire, that one is too old or known to be infertile, that one has already borne a child, or that the eldest will go first and the younger will have a second child later. When both women want to carry the baby, this is a very difficult decision. By the time the couple presents to the DI program, this decision is generally made. Some couples will have gone to counseling for help in deciding. In these more challenging cases, additional factors may come into play. For example, a couple may recognize that one set of grandparents will be more likely to accept the child as family if their daughter carries it or that one woman has excellent maternity and medical benefits and the other does not. Regardless of how the decision was made, if the DI program counselor is alert to this issue, he or she can help the couple know what to expect as they go through the process. For example, the co-mother may have to struggle with feelings of envy and being left out.

Legal Issues

It is important to advise all lesbian couples and single women to consult a lawyer and have documents prepared outlining what their intentions are regarding parenting and what they want to happen in the event of death or, for couples, separation. Lesbian couples should document their intention and desire to parent together with equal rights and responsibilities and, in the event of the death of one or the other, to have the surviving partner be the parent. They should investigate the options in their state for the co-mother to adopt the child; in Vermont and Massachusetts, for example, this is allowed[69]. While published reports[3] and this author's experience suggest that almost all lesbian couples have considered these issues, few consult lawyers prior to the birth of a child.

Relationships

The literature suggests that most single women who choose to have a child hope to have a life partner later in their lives. It is important for these women to understand how difficult it can be to find time to make new relationships, while being a single parent. It is difficult on a practical (time) and financial (baby-sitters) level, as well as emotionally. If a woman is already working full-time and away from her child most of the day, it can be very difficult to leave the child for an evening out, especially when the child is quite young. It is important, however, for all parents to have some time

to themselves and to recognize that when they do nurture themselves, they do a better job of caring for their children.

Most single women and lesbian couples using DI expect to conceive rapidly. Not only do few of them have any reason to doubt their own fertility, but few understand that even quite fertile women may require a number of cycles before conception occurs. (In this, they are not different from married women who employ DI because of a partner's known sterility, and thus they have not yet experienced failed attempts at conception.) The chance of conception in any one month using frozen donor sperm is about 10–12%. Most are probably also ignorant about the prevalence of early miscarriage or age-related genetic issues.

All partnerships can be strained by attempts to conceive and by parenting, but lesbian relationships have some unique risks in this regard. Because a couple may be undergoing stressors that their friends are not, support may be in short supply. Wendland and associates[3] reported that 56% of lesbian couples reported stress from DI treatments, compared to only 26% of married couples. If it takes a while to conceive, a woman attempting pregnancy may become more and more focused on her own body and her sadness, while her partner may be bewildered or angry or may wonder whether the desired child is more important to her partner's happiness than she is. This is very much the dynamic seen in heterosexual couples, and the interventions used for infertile heterosexual couples are very appropriate to use here (see Chapters 6 and 8).

Lesbian couples also need to be encouraged to read about co-mothering. The nonbiological mother will be in a constant struggle not to be invisible to the child's school, doctor, and the biological mother's family. Even the co-mother's family may not look on the child as 'theirs' and may need education and encouragement to feel a part of the family.

Disclosure

Lesbian parents have two sets of disclosure issues to consider: disclosure of the facts of conception and disclosure of their lesbianism. In this author's practice, disclosure about sexual orientation is an area few lesbian couples have considered. They seem to expect that because they will be living together and will both be parents, the child will 'just know'. Couples need to be educated on this subject and to be reminded of something that they already know: Children do not want to be different. It has been reported that when children are told of their mothers' lesbianism in childhood or as older teens, they cope with the information better and have higher self-esteem, compared to those informed as young teens[6,70,71]. In one study[72] of 164 children with at least one homosexual parent, the parents reported that by age 6 the children could understand the concept of homosexuality. Berzon[73] has written a thoughtful article meant to help lesbians prepare for speaking openly with their children.

The fact that their mothers are lesbian is almost sure to be an issue, and one that the child will need to be able to talk about not just with his or her mother but with others. The literature suggests that children do hide and disclose this information selectively[72–75] and that they wish they had peers in similar situations to talk to[70,72,75]. Sometimes, the local gay and lesbian community center has organized groups for this purpose. In this author's practice, a list of first names and telephone numbers of lesbian couples who would like contact with others is kept. Patients new to the practice can have the list if they are willing to be part of it. Not only does this allow couples to develop support for themselves in the

present but, hopefully, for their children in the future.

The published literature suggests that virtually 100% of single women and lesbian couples plan to disclose to the children their use of DI to conceive[3,76]. The ongoing longitudinal study by Gartrell and colleagues[55] is an exception to this, with only 91% stating an intention to be fully open.

FUTURE IMPLICATIONS

In the last few years, it has become apparent that many programs are beginning to treat single women and lesbian couples as a matter of course. It is this author's recommendation that they be treated as much like heterosexual couples as possible. For example, if pretreatment counseling is required, it should be required of all patients wanting to use a donor to conceive, regardless of social circumstances or sexual orientation. The topics may differ a bit, but the goals of the pretreatment counseling are the same: to attempt to ensure psychological and relationship stability and to go through an informed consent process.

What does the future hold? There are legislative initiatives in a number of states regarding same-sex marriage, parenting, and guardianship of children. There are a number of longitudinal studies in place now that will provide prospective information about these planned nontraditional families[52,55]. Since most of these families plan full disclosure to the children, the longitudinal studies will also allow an evaluation of the impact of disclosure on children. This information in turn can be shared with patients who use DI and are inclined toward privacy or secrecy.

SUMMARY

- The published literature would suggest that children in lesbian and single-mother families are not uniquely disadvantaged. Many of the difficulties that these children experience are due to the breakup of their biological family and to financial circumstances. In planned families, there does not appear to be significant drawbacks for children.

- The reasons to offer or require pre-treatment psychoeducational counseling for single women and lesbian couples are the same as those for heterosexual couples: individual and relationship stability and informed consent; only the details may vary.

- Doctors' offices that offer infertility treatments to lesbian couples and single women should prepare paperwork and resource materials that are not worded for heterosexual married couples only.

- Doctors' offices that offer infertility treatments to lesbian couples and single women should offer educational materials and resources and referrals to support groups.

REFERENCES

1. Leiblum SR, Palmer MG, Spector IP. Non-traditional mothers: Single heterosexual/lesbian women and lesbian couples electing motherhood via donor insemination. *J Psychosom Obstet Gynaecol* 1995;16:11–20

2. McCartney CF. Decision by single women to conceive by artificial donor insemination. *J Psychosom Obstet Gynaecol* 1985; 4:321–8

3. Wendland CL, Byrn F, Hill C. Donor insemination: A comparison of lesbian couples, heterosexual couples and single women. *Fertil Steril* 1996;65:764–70

4. Falk PJ. Lesbian mothers: Psychosocial assumptions in family law. *Am Psychol* 1989; 44:941–7

5. Gottman JS. Children of gay and lesbian parents. In: Bozett FW, Sussman MB, eds. *Homosexuality and Family Relations*. New York: Haworth Press, 1990;177–96

6. Pennington SB. Children of lesbian mothers. In: Bozett FW, ed. *Gay and Lesbian Parents*. New York: Praeger, 1987;58–74

7. Seligmann J. Variations on a theme. *Newsweek* 1990;Winter/Spring Special Issue: 38–46

8. Patterson CJ. Children of gay and lesbian parents. *Child Dev* 1992;63:1025–42

9. Jacob MC. Lesbian couples and therapeutic donor insemination. *Assist Reprod Rev* 1995; 5:214–21

10. Cramer D. Gay parents and their children: A review of research and practical implications. *J Couns Dev* 1986;64:504–7

11. Gibbs ED. Psychosocial development of children raised by lesbian mothers: A review of research. *Women Ther* 1988;8:65–75

12. Golombok S, Tasker F. Donor insemination for single heterosexual and lesbian women: Issues concerning the welfare of the child. *Hum Reprod* 1994;9:1972–6

13. Hutchens DJ, Kirkpatrick MJ. Lesbian mothers/gay fathers. In: Schetky DH, Benedek EP, eds. *Emerging Issues in Child Psychiatry and the Law*. New York: Brunner/Mazel, 1985;115–26

14. Moses AE, Hawkins RO Jr. *Counseling Lesbian Women and Gay Men: A Life Issues Approach*. St. Louis, MO: Mosby, 1982

15. Sears JT. Challenges for educators: Lesbian, gay, and bisexual families. *High School J* 1994;77:138–56

16. Tasker FL, Golombok S. Children raised by lesbian mothers: The empirical evidence. *Fam Law* 1991;21:184–7

17. Mueller DP, Cooper PW. Children of single parent families: How they fare as young adults. *Fam Rel* 1986;35:169–76

18. Golombok S, Rust J. The Warnock Report and single women: What about the children? *J Med Ethics* 1986;12:182–6

19. Adams PL, Milner JR, Schrepf NA. *Fatherless Children*. New York: Wiley, 1984

20. McGuire M, Alexander NJ. Artificial insemination of single women. *Fertil Steril* 1985;43:182–4

21. Riddle DI. Relating to children: Gays as role models. *J Soc Issues* 1978;34:38–58

22. Hanson SMH. Healthy single-parent families. *Fam Rel* 1986;35:125–32

23. The single-parent family. *Fam Rel* 1986;35(special issue)

24. Mechaneck R, Klein E, Kuppersmith J. Single mothers by choice: A family alternative. In: Braude M, ed. *Women, Power, and Therapy: Issues for Women.* New York: Haworth Press, 1988;263–81

25. Frank DI, Brackley MH. The health experience of single women who have children through artificial donor insemination. *Clin Nurse Spec* 1989;3:156–60

26. Bell AP, Weinberg MS. *Homosexualities: A Study of Diversity Among Men and Women.* New York: Simon and Schuster, 1978

27. Kerr MG, Rogers C. Donor insemination. *J Med Ethics* 1975;1:30–3

28. Dunstan GR. Ethical aspects of donor insemination. *J Med Ethics* 1975;1:42–4

29. Sauer MV, Gorrill MJ, Zeffer KB, *et al.* Attitudinal survey of sperm donors to an artificial insemination clinic. *J Reprod Med* 1989;34:362–4

30. Leiblum SR, Barbrack C. Artificial insemination by donor: A survey of attitudes and knowledge in medical students and infertile couples. *J Biosoc Sci* 1983;15:165–72

31. Shenfield F. Particular requests in donor insemination: Comments on the medical duty of care and the welfare of the child. *Hum Reprod* 1994;9:1976–7

32. Melton GB. The clashing of symbols: Prelude to child and family policy. *Am Psychol* 1987;42:345–54

33. Kritchevsky B. The unmarried woman's right to artificial insemination: A call for an expanded definition of family. *Harvard Women's Law J* 1981;4:1–42

34. Harvard Law Review. Reproductive technology and the procreation rights of the unmarried. *Harvard Law Rev* 1985; 98:669–85

35. Strong C, Schinfeld JS. The single woman and artificial insemination by donor. *J Reprod Med* 1984;29:293–9

36. Wikler D, Wikler NJ. Turkey-baster babies. The demedicalization of artificial insemination. *Milbank Q* 1991;69:5–40

37. Robinson S, Pizer HF. *Having a Baby Without a Man: The Woman's Guide to Alternative Insemination.* New York: Fireside/Simon and Schuster, 1985

38. Pies C. *Considering Parenthood.* San Francisco: Spinsters/Aunt Lute, 1988

39. Lane FE. Artificial insemination at home. *Fertil Steril* 1954;5:372–3

40. Klein RD. Doing it ourselves: Self-insemination. In: Arditti R, Klein RD, Minden S, eds. *Test-Tube Women: What Future for Motherhood?* London: Pandora Press, 1984;382–90

41. Hornstein F. Children by donor insemination: A new choice for lesbians. In: Arditti R, Klein RD, Minden S, eds. *Test-Tube Women: What Future for Motherhood?* London: Pandora Press, 1984;373–81

42. Wolf DG. Lesbian childbirth and woman-controlled conception. In: Darty T, Potter S, eds. *Women-Identified Women.* Palo Alto, CA: Mayfield Publishing, 1984;185–93

43. Hanscombe G. The right to lesbian parenthood. *J Med Ethics* 1983;9;133–5

44. Barwin BN. Therapeutic donor insemination (TDI) for women without partners and lesbian couples: Considerations for physicians. *Can J Hum Sex* 1993;2:175–8

45. Jacob MC. Concerns of single women and lesbian couples considering conception through assisted reproduction. In: Leiblum SR, ed. *Infertility: Psychological Issues and Counseling Strategies.* New York: Wiley, 1997;189–206

46. Englert Y. Artificial insemination with donor semen: Particular requests. *Hum Reprod* 1994;9:1969–71

47. Kern PA, Ridolfi KM. The fourteenth amendment's protection of a woman's right to be a single parent through artificial insemination by donor. *Women's Rights Law Rep* 1982;7:251–84

48. Patterson CJ. Children of the lesbian baby boom: Behavioral adjustment, self-concepts, and sex role identity. In: Greene B, Herek GM, eds. *Lesbian and Gay Psychology: Theory, Research, and Clinical Applications.* Thousand Oaks, CA: Russell Sage, 1994;156–75

49. Steckel A. Separation-individuation in children of lesbian and heterosexual couples. Berkeley, CA: Wright Institute Graduate School, 1985. Doctoral dissertation

50. McCandlish B. Against all odds: Lesbian mother family dynamics. In: Bozett FW, ed.

Gay and Lesbian Parents. New York: Praeger, 1987;23–36

51. Brewaeys A, Olbrechts H, Devroey P, *et al.* Counselling and selection of homosexual couples in fertility treatment. *Hum Reprod* 1989;4:850–3

52. Jacob MC, Klock SC, Maier D. Lesbian couples as therapeutic donor insemination recipients: Descriptive and psychological factors. Presented at the 50th annual meeting of the American Fertility Society, 1994

53. Patterson CJ. Families of the lesbian baby boom: Parents' division of labor and children's adjustment. *Dev Psychol* 1995; 31:115–23

54. Flaks DK, Ficher I, Masterpasqua F, *et al.* Lesbians choosing motherhood: A comparative study of lesbian and heterosexual parents and their children. *Dev Psychol* 1995;31:105–14

55. Gartrell N, Hamilton J, Banks A, *et al.* The national lesbian family study. 1. Interviews with prospective mothers. *Am J Orthopsychiatry* 1996;66:272–81

56. Anonymous. Family options (a personal story). *Insights Infertil* 1996;Winter/Spring special issue:3–4

57. Potter AE, Knaub PK. Single motherhood by choice: A parenting alternative. *Lifestyles: Fam Econ Issues* 1988;9:240–9

58. Pakizegi B. Emerging family forms: Single mothers by choice—demographic and psychosocial variables. *Mat Child Nurs J* 1990;19:1–19

59. Klock SC, Jacob MC, Maier D. A comparison of single and married recipients of donor insemination. *Hum Reprod* 1996;11:101–4

60. Baetens P, Ponjaert-Kristoffersen I, Devroey P, *et al.* Artificial insemination by donor: An alternative for single women. *Hum Reprod* 1995;10:1537–42

61. Loulan J. Psychotherapy with lesbian mothers. In: Stein TS, Cohen CJ, eds. *Contemporary Perspectives on Psychotherapy with Lesbians and Gay Men*. New York: Plenum, 1986;181–208

62. Slater S, Mencher J. The lesbian family life cycle: A contextual approach. *Am J Orthopsychiatry* 1991;61:372–82

63. Carter B, McGoldrick M. *The Changing Family Life Cycle: A Framework for Family*

Therapy. Needham Heights, MA: Allyn & Bacon, 1989

64. Jordan JV, Kaplan AG, Miller JB, *et al. Women's Growth in Connection: Writings from the Stone Center*. New York: Guilford Press, 1991

65. Rohrbaugh JB. Lesbian families: Clinical issues and theoretical implications. *Prof Psychol Res Pract* 1992;23:467–73

66. Klock SC, Maier D. Guidelines for the provision of psychological evaluations for infertile patients at the University of Connecticut Health Center. *Fertil Steril* 1991;56:680–5

67. Engelstein P, Antell-Buckely M, Urman-Klein P. Single women who elect to bear a child. In: Blum BL, ed. *Psychological Aspects of Pregnancy, Birthing, and Bonding*. New York: Human Sciences Press, 1980;103–19

68. Martin A. *The Lesbian and Gay Parenting Handbook: Creating and Raising our Families*. New York: HarperPerennial, 1993

69. Crockin SL. *Beyond Tammy: Co-Parent Adoptions in Massachusetts*. Boston Bar J 1994; Sept/Oct:7–8,18–21

70. Paul JP. Growing up with a gay, lesbian, or bisexual parent: An exploratory study of experiences and perceptions. Berkeley, CA: University of California at Berkeley, 1986. Doctoral dissertation

71. Huggins SL. A comparative study of self-esteem of adolescent children of divorced lesbian mothers and divorced heterosexual mothers. *J Homosex* 1989;18:123–35

72. Riddle DI, Arguelles MD. Children of gay parents: Homophobia's victims. In: Stuart IR, Abt LE, eds. *Children of Separation and Divorce: Management and Treatment*. New York: Van Nostrand Reinhold, 1981;174–97

73. Berzon B. Sharing your lesbian identity with your children: A case for openness. In: Vida G, ed. *Our Right to Love: A Lesbian Resource Book*. Englewood Cliffs, NJ: Prentice-Hall, 1978;69–77

74. Javaid GA. The children of homosexual and heterosexual single mothers. *Child Psychiatry Hum Dev* 1993;23:235–48

75. Lewis KG. Children of lesbians: Their point of view. *Soc Work* 1980;25:198–203

76. Brewaeys A, Ponjaert-Kristoffersen I, Van Steirteghem AC, *et al.* Children from anonymous donors: An inquiry into homosexual and heterosexual parents'

attitudes. *J Psychosom Obstet Gynaecol* 1993;14:23–35

77. Kirkpatrick M, Smith C, Roy R. Lesbian mothers and their children: A comparative survey. *Am J Orthopsychiatry* 1981;51:545–51

78. Green R. The best interests of the child with a lesbian mother. *Bull American Academy of Psychiatry and the Law* 1982;10:7–15

79. Hall M. Lesbian families: Cultural and clinical issues. *Soc Work* 1978;23:380–5

80. Green R. Sexual identity of 37 children raised by homosexual or transsexual parents. *Am J Psychiatry* 1979;135:692–7

81. Golombok S, Spencer A, Rutter M. Children in lesbian and single-parent households: Psychosexual and psychiatric appraisal. *J Child Psychol Psychiatry* 1983;24:551–72

82. Tasker F, Golombok S. Adults raised as children in lesbian families. *Am J Orthopsychiatry* 1995;65:203–15

83. Harris MB, Turner PH. Gay and lesbian parents. *J Homosex* 1985;12:101–13

84. Hoeffer B. Children's acquisition of sex-role behavior in lesbian-mother families. *Am J Orthopsychiatry* 1981;51:536–44

85. Pinkerton CR. Artificial insemination for the single woman [letter]. *Lancet* 1982;i:968

86. Jennings S. Virgin birth syndrome. *Lancet* 1991;337:559–60

87. Heywood A. Immaculate conception? *Nurs Times* 1991;87:62–3

15

The Older Infertile Patient

Miriam B. Rosenthal, MD and Sheryl A. Kingsberg, PhD

Sarah became pregnant and bore Abraham a son in his old age ... Abraham was 100 years old when his son Isaac was born. Sarah said, 'God has given me cause to laugh and all who hear of it will laugh with me. Who would have told Abraham that Sarah would nurse a child! Yet I have borne him a son in his old age.'

Genesis 21:1

HISTORICAL OVERVIEW

In the Book of Genesis, Sarah, the wife of Abraham gave birth to her first child, a son, Isaac when she was 90 years old. Her husband was 100 at the time. Perhaps this Biblical tale foreshadowed what was to come in the days, thousands of years later, when not only has the life expectancy of women markedly increased, but reproductive technology has enabled many women and men past traditional reproductive age to conceive and in many instances carry a pregnancy to term. The *Guinness Book of World Records* reports that the oldest spontaneous pregnancy occurred in a woman 57 years and 120 days old. A Scottish woman was reported to have given birth to her sixth child at age 62 years[1]. Most recently, Paulson and colleagues[2] reported that a 63-year-old woman using anonymous ovum donation gave birth to a healthy baby girl.

Despite these very unusual accounts, it is well known that fertility in women, and less so in men, declines with age. Some of the earliest research on age and fertility was done on the Hutterites, a religious sect in North America in which contraception was not used, family size was not limited, and mostly intact healthy families continued to have children as long as they were able to do so[3]. Researchers found that while overall fertility rates were very high, they declined for women at around age 35 with 33% of women infertile by age 40 and 87% infertile by age 45. A large study[4] of reproductively healthy women who had artificial insemination by donor because their husbands were azoospermic also demonstrated a gradual decline in pregnancy rates with increased age. The pregnancy rate in women less than 31 years of age was 74% and fell to 54% in women over 35 years of age. In addition, the majority of older women who did conceive required more treatment cycles to do so[4,5]. Since the 1960s the percentage of women under 30 who are childless has doubled from 12 to 25%[6]. About 20% of American women are having their first child at ages 35 and older. This represents a 50% increase from the last decade[7].

A significant factor in older parenthood is that couples are marrying later and delaying childbearing. More than half of women aged 20–24 years, and one-quarter of women aged 25–30 had not married in 1992. Women today have their children an average of 3 years later than women 20 years ago[6]. Mothers over 30 years of age had 1 in 3 births in 1992, which was more than four times as many as teenage births in the United States that same year.

Furthermore, many unmarried women in their late 20s and 30s are choosing to have children without a partner. Unmarried women aged 25 and older account for more nonmarital births (35%) than do women younger than 18 (13%) or younger than 20 (30%)[8]. Perhaps, this increase in single women and lesbian couples having children is related to an increase in societal acceptance of children born to women without husbands, as well as to the availability of medically assisted donor insemination (see Chapter 14).

Older fatherhood is a more complicated statistic to determine. The National Center for Health Statistics reported in 1980 only 48,000 babies (or 1.5% of births) were born to fathers aged 45 or older. In 1991, this figure was 67,000 or almost 2% of births[9]. Some older fathers are first-time fathers who (like women) have postponed parenthood until later in life. Other older fathers are 'repeat parents': they had children earlier in their lives but now, with a younger partner (who perhaps does not have children) have decided to become parents again in a new relationship (see Chapter 16). For the older man, infertility is as likely to be due to prior sterilization (e.g., vasectomy) as it is to be the result of medical factors. Barriers to proper care in the older infertile man are often myths or misconceptions such as that vasectomies can always be successfully reversed or that if a man already has children he cannot have a fertility problem.

Although statistics indicate that in the last quarter of the 20th century an increasing number of men and women are becoming first time and repeat parents at older ages, often facilitated by the use of assisted reproductive technologies, despite these increases, older or 'elderly' parents are still in the minority and, as such, present with a variety of unique psychosocial issues.

This chapter will:

- outline the incidence and characteristics of age-related infertility in men and women
- provide an overview of medical evaluation of infertility in the older patient
- define the complex psychosocial issues of older parenthood, differences between older infertile men and women, and pregnancy in the older woman
- address the bioethical issues of older parenthood, its impact on children, and its context within society.

REVIEW OF LITERATURE
Fertility in Older Women

Fertility rates for women decline steadily with age, with a significant drop from age 35 onward. It is estimated that about one-third of women who delay their first pregnancy until age 35 or older will have difficulty with conception. About half of those women who wait until age 40 or older will have problems with conception, carrying a fetus to term, or increased fetal anomalies[10]. The primary reason for the decline in fertility for older women is the decline in the quality of their oocytes resulting in increases in follicular atresia, chromosomal abnormalities, menstrual abnormalities, and follicular-stimulating hormone (FSH) levels. The uterus may become less receptive to pregnancy maintenance as well, although this is not always the case[7,11].

There are controversial data about the outcome of pregnancy in women 35-40 years of age and older, but the overall conclusion in the United States seems to be that in healthy women who receive good prenatal obstetrical care and good care during labor and delivery, a good outcome can be anticipated[5,12]. However, while there has been a decrease in rates of fetal death in women of all ages since the 1960s, 'older women' have an increased risk of poor embryo viability and fetal demise[13].

Fertility in Older Men

Age also affects male fertility, although anecdotes and media accounts about very elderly men fathering babies perpetuate the myth that male fertility is endless. There is some evidence that sperm quality declines with age, particularly in men with urological disorders (e.g., prostate cancer) or other health problems. The older father is a risk factor for trisomies[5] and some genetic disorders are thought to be due to male gene mutations that increase in men over the age of 50 (see Chapter 11). Older men have been found to be at risk of increased incidence of autosomal dominant mutations (e.g., dwarfism) in offspring[19]. In addition, aging males have lower androgen levels resulting in decreased sexual interest and sexual activity, decreased frequency of ejaculation, and decreased sperm production and motility.

Despite these statistics and the reality of fertility problems in older men and women, the incidence of infertility in the older couple may be more an issue of *delayed* conception than failed conception. It has been estimated that one-third of infertile couples may conceive within 2-7 years of stopping infertility treatments. In addition, because older couples feel a great deal of pressure to conceive within a short time, they often seek therapy in fertility clinics earlier than younger couples and are often encouraged to do so by medical caregivers[7,14].

THEORETICAL FRAMEWORK

The application of developmental theory to infertility in the older individual makes some sense, although it also highlights how later parenthood is out of synch with traditional developmental tasks (see Chapter 1). Levinson[15], in his interviews of men, found that middle adulthood was often the fullest and most creative era in the adult lifecycle marked by the individual being more deeply attached to others and yet more separate and centered in the self. Levinson also reported that during early adulthood men were more focused on their careers while in middle age the focus often returned to their families. Men who had become fathers early in life often found that their renewed interest in family came at time when their children had left or were leaving home and were least interested in their attention. This finding may support the perception that older parents may be less distracted by the interest or necessity of career establishment and, as such, more readily available to enjoy their children and give them the attention and time they need.

Feminist theory provides an interesting perspective on older parenthood, especially older motherhood facilitated by assisted reproduction and oocyte donation. Within this context the reproductive playing field between men and women has become more even: Men *and* *women* may become biological parents whenever they choose without regard to age or 'biological clocks'. Historically, feminist criticism of reproductive medicine has contended that the male-dominated character of Western medicine and male-domination of the medical system reinforces a subordinate role for women[16]. In addition, Western science and technology embody stereotypically male values such as control, distance, power, objectivity, and domination which promote invasive solutions to problems—often at the expense of women. However, for the older woman, reproductive medicine (e.g., donated sperm, donated oocytes) may actually enhance a woman's control, distance, objectivity, and power over her reproductive life by enabling her to have children when she chooses to, and without a partner.

These technologies have not only provided women more opportunities, but increased the pressure (external or internal) to use them. And while these treatments offer opportunities for parenthood, they do not always provide opportunities for genetic motherhood. Furthermore, medical treatments for infertility and reproductive technologies remain inequitable: Women continue to endure the lion's share of medical treatment and more invasive procedures. Nevertheless, it is often women consumers (especially older financially independent women) who have demanded the opportunities for parenthood that assisted reproduction can provide.

CLINICAL ISSUES

Evaluation of the Older Infertile Couple

For women 35 years and older, referral to an infertility specialist should be sought under the following circumstances[6]:

- after 6 months or more of adequate sexual intercourse without the use of contraception at ovulation times (as opposed to 12 months for women less than 35 years)
- irregular menstrual periods
- two or more miscarriages
- prior use of an intrauterine device for birth control
- male with a prostate infection
- history of a sexually transmitted infection in either partner
- in utero exposure to diethylstilbestrol (DES)
- infection in genital or pelvic area
- prior abdominal surgery in either partner or prior reversal of sterilization procedures in either partner
- single women (heterosexual or lesbian)

who want to become pregnant by donor insemination.

Given the significant drop in fertility rates for women over 35, evaluation of an older couple or a couple with one older partner, should typically proceed quickly, particularly if the woman partner is over the age of 40 or the male partner over the age of 55. In the female partner, assessment of ovulation should include menstrual cycle regularity and length, as menstrual cycle lengths tend to get shorter in women over the age of 40. Cycle lengths of less than 25 days or more than 36 days as well as increased cycle irregularity may suggest ovulatory problems. Measurement of FSH levels in women over 35 years of age may indicate decreased ovarian response and is measured by blood levels along with estradiol on the second or third day following onset of menses. The response of the ovaries may decrease as FSH levels increase, but there is marked cycle-to-cycle variation in basal levels of gonadotropins. Clomiphene citrate challenge test, also used to determine ovarian response, is a more sensitive indicator of ovarian response. 'When patients with the same basal FSH levels are compared, pregnancy rates are lower in older women'[7]. There is some controversy surrounding the occurrence of shortened luteal phases in older women, but some studies suggest that it occurs more often in women over 45 who still cycle. Infertility treatments should probably not be continued in women with early follicular-phase FSH levels greater than 15 mU/mL unless using donated oocytes.

It is important to check thyroid function and evaluate endocrine or hormonal changes. Symptoms such as hirsutism, galactorrhea, hot flushes, weight loss, and obesity are important markers for potential endocrine problems. Older women with type I or type II diabetes and with autoimmune disorders (e.g., lupus, arthritis) also need particularly careful evaluation (see Chapter 10). Psychiatric disturbances, depressive illnesses, or use of psychotropic drugs also warrant consideration as potentially impacting fertility (see Chapter 4).

Evaluation of infertility in the older male includes a complete semen analysis as age-related infertility is often due to diminished sperm motility, sperm morphology, and semen volume[17]. In men who have had a vasectomy reversal, semen analysis should include assessment for sperm antibodies. A complete physical examination is warranted as lower testosterone levels have been found in older men with health problems resulting in diminished fertility either from the illness or the medications used to treat it[18]. Prostate cancer, hypertension, diabetes, heart disease, peripheral vascular disease, depression, and general ill-health affect fertility in men both directly and indirectly by affecting quality of life and sexual functioning. Evaluation of the older man should also include an assessment of depression and other psychiatric disorders, history of sexually transmitted diseases, sexual history including past and current frequency of sexual intercourse and masturbation, evidence of sexual dysfunction, history of urological disorders including exposure to DES, and prior reproductive problems. Finally, although the association between advanced paternal age and serious birth defects has received less attention than the effect of advanced maternal age, there is increasing evidence of increased risk of serious birth defects in older men, particularly over the age of 50[19].

The Menopausal Woman

Natural menopause is defined as the occurrence of the final menstrual period with a uterus and at least one ovary intact. This is defined retrospectively if there has been no menses for a year and no pregnancy or lactation. It represents ovarian failure and, subsequently, the inability of the woman to conceive. Surgical menopause occurs when the uterus or both ovaries have been removed, causing cessation of menses. The average age for natural menopause is 50.5 years, with a typical range of 45–55 years.

Menopause, whether natural or surgical, tended to provide clear boundaries and closure to the issue of whether a woman can reproduce. For some women, menopause arrives prematurely (e.g., before the age of 35) or before they are psychologically prepared to give up the idea of having a first child or more children. In these cases, third-party reproduction may reopen a door too quickly shut, by providing opportunities for parenthood, or may provide a means for denying the realities of aging. For other women, menopause is a welcome marker of closure on reproductive ability. Regardless of whether the closure of menopause is experienced as a loss, a relief, or a little of both, it is usually perceived as final. The fact that technologies now may extend women's reproductive life past menopause may cause significant distress, confusion, ambivalence, or joy.

Management Issues with Older Infertile Patients

Infertility treatments for older women are typically the same as for younger women. Usually, ovulation induction with intrauterine insemination for women over 40 years of age involves an increase in the dosage of menopausal gonadotropins and the days of treatments, just as the number of mature follicles and preovulatory estradiol levels decrease[20]. In addition, progesterone supplementation or supplemental human chorionic gonadotropin

(HCG) may be used to increase receptivity, with progesterone given after embryo transfer[21]. Finally, more aggressive treatments are usually offered to women more than 39 years of age, especially if they are using their own oocytes.

In vitro fertilization (IVF) can be used in women over 40, although with poorer results at every step: Fewer oocytes are retrieved and embryos transferred, implantation and pregnancy rates are lower, and miscarriage rates are higher[22,23]. IVF data from 1993 show that about 15% of all stimulation cycles were done on women aged over 40, although success rates were lower[7]. Even with ovulation induction, response is typically not encouraging in older patients using reproductive technologies without oocyte donation (OD)[24] as very few pregnancies occur in women aged over 43. Therefore, OD has offered the older woman much better chances for successful pregnancy and parenthood[25-27]. It may be unkind or worse to continue treatment cycles if there is no chance for success using her own oocytes. As such, older couples should receive counseling which includes discussion of alternative options such as the use of donated oocytes, a surrogate, adoption, or living without children[28].

As noted previously, infertility in the older male may be due to a prior vasectomy or may be the result of age-related fertility problems (e.g., decreased sperm motility or semen volume) or may be due to other medical conditions. If the older man's fertility problem is related to a prior vasectomy (e.g., sperm antibodies), treatment, or age-related sperm quality, parenthood may be achieved through the use of sperm aspiration techniques (e.g., MESA, TESA) or with ICSI. However, if these techniques are not successful or feasible for a couple, the use of donor sperm may be the most viable or preferable option to successful parenthood (see Chapter 18).

Pregnancy in Older Women

There is not a considerable amount of data on pregnancy outcome in women over 45 years of age. Despite the reality that fertility is compromised in older women, pregnancies obviously occur—and with reproductive technologies are occurring with greater frequency. Therefore, a discussion of older women and infertility would not be complete without discussing pregnancy. As with fertility, pregnancy after age 35 may be accompanied by more frequent problems than pregnancy in the younger women. For example, Paulson and Sauer[29] reported pregnancy-induced hypertension, gestational diabetes, stillbirths, and babies of small size for gestational age in older women. However, many of these complications may be typically dependent upon the general health of the woman before pregnancy.

Maternal mortality rates are about 58.3 per 100,000 live births for women over 35. The maternal death rate for women over age 45 is 71.5 per 100,000 for white women and 602.4 for black women. While overall maternal mortality rates are falling due to improved prenatal care and medical care during labor and delivery, women with cardiovascular disease, pulmonary hypertension, or myocardial infarctions probably should not undertake pregnancy at any age[12,30,31]. Furthermore, risks of pregnancy related to assisted reproductive technologies such as multiple gestations and preterm labor, must also be carefully considered by the older woman. It has been suggested that older women are willing to endure considerable personal health risks (even endangerment) if the well-being of their babies can be ensured—an approach that often contributes to ill-considered decisions and inappropriate risk-taking[32].

An additional concern for the older pregnant woman is the increased incidence of fetal problems including retarded fetal

Table 1 Positive and negative factors for biological parenthood in older people

Positive	Negative
Procreative liberty: the moral right of everyone to reproduce	Risk of parental death or age-related disability
Parenting skills: more experience, patience, time, desire	Less physical stamina/energy for parenting
Financial security	Social stigma for offspring
Medically safe for postmenopausal women in good health	Use of limited resources for less than optimal candidates
Clearly motivated to have a child	Limited financial resources
	Medical risks for older women
	Questionable motivations for reproducing at an older age

growth, stillbirths, chromosomal abnormalities, and perinatal mortality. While the use of donated oocytes from younger women can prevent chromosomal anomalies which correlate with the age of the oocyte donor, increased risks to the baby may be the result of assisted reproduction, multiple gestation, and/or prematurity due to medical conditions in the mother. For the older woman pregnant with her own oocytes, blood tests, chorionic villus sampling (CVS), amniocenteses, and/or ultrasound can aid in the detection of chromosomal anomalies (see Chapters 11, 12, 24). However, women and their partners are then presented with choices about continuation or termination of the pregnancy if abnormalities are detected.

THERAPEUTIC INTERVENTIONS

Counseling Issues

The stresses of infertility and infertility treatments put anyone at risk to experience some psychological difficulties or distress and can impair one's ability to make rational, well-informed decisions regarding treatment options. However, there are a number of issues that are unique to older men and women and relevant for the counseling of this group of patients (Table 1).

One important area for counseling of older women that is frequently overlooked or addressed too late is basic fertility education. Increasingly successful reproductive technologies have led women to believe that their ability to procreate may not be limited to their 20s and 30s, giving many a false sense of security regarding their ability to procreate at will without regard to age. Regardless of age, all women should be informed about the decline in fertility with aging, as well as all the other possible factors that might affect their ability to conceive, cause repeated fetal loss, or the birth of a child with problems. Even for young women who do not want children immediately, education about fertility and reproduction should be readily available. By contrast, men and women considering sterilization should be carefully counseled that it is a permanent and not temporary medical procedure. This is not only necessary for understanding options but may influence reproductive choices[33,34].

For older infertile men and women, counseling should address motivations for wanting a child. Motivation is a particularly important issue for the older individual because reasons for wanting a child may change considerably over the life cycle. What was considered important or a primary motivator to a person in their 20s, may be quite different from what motivates them in their 30s or 40s. Some men and women may not be aware that they are currently making choices based on old motivations that are no longer relevant but that continue to drive their current behavior. Distinguishing past and current priorities and goals may help clarify issues related to infertility and decision-making regarding treatment. This may be particularly helpful for couples who have been trying to conceive for many years and may have lost sight of their original motivations or have confused them with their present ones. Counseling issues should also help individuals and couples distinguish their personal motivations from that of others such as past or current partners, children from previous relationships, or other family members.

Many older infertile individuals may have delayed having children for a variety of reasons, such as continuing education, building a career, taking care of parents, not finding a suitable partner, not wanting children, or having a partner who did not want children. As the biological clock ticks away, many men and women who at one time decided not to have children may change their minds with the realization that they might lose the opportunity to experience pregnancy or raise and nurture a child. Some women or couples may develop a desire to have children as they observe their friends who have children, or they feel left out, as the majority of their peer group has chosen this option and lifestyle. In addition, there may be family, religious or cultural pressures to have children as the expected default behavior in most societies is for heterosexual couples to have children. Childless couples are typically asked to explain or justify why they do not have children, and there is often an underlying negative judgment or suspiciousness that accompanies such

questions. The death of parents is sometimes a stimulus and a motivation for women (or men) to want to become parents themselves, as they identify with their mothers (or fathers) or mourn their loss. Remarriages in middle age (sometimes to much older or much younger partners) may cause some individuals to reevaluate their decisions regarding childbearing, for example, women who are now married to men who want children or would make great fathers. An older woman may be in the same relationship for many years but may have developed secondary infertility, may have changed her mind about having children, or may be considering new options that were not available years earlier. In this regard, newer medical treatments may inadvertently be coercive: Because they are available, some individuals or couples feel pressured to use them.

In addition to understanding their general reasons for wanting children, counseling may help women understand their desire for pregnancy and the pursuit of fertility treatments. This insight, in conjunction with psychotherapy, can be very useful in processing the loss and subsequent grief if fertility treatments are unsuccessful. Furthermore, having an accurate assessment of motivations to parent and the form of parenting (i.e., having a genetic child, using donor gametes, or adopting) is essential for maximizing psychological adjustment and for making appropriate decisions regarding what treatment options to pursue and when to terminate treatment.

More specifically, the older individual needs to try to understand what is most important to them in their pursuit of infertility treatment. There are typically three distinct goals which often inextricably overlap: (1) the desire to have one's genetic child, (2) the desire to experience a pregnancy, and (3) the desire to parent. Counseling can help couples differentiate goals regarding fertility and parenting. Insight into which of these goals (one or more) is most important may help to evaluate treatment options and determine treatment decisions. For example, if the desire to experience a pregnancy is a pressing goal, then the option for an older woman to use OD may be suggested. Similarly, if having a genetic child is critical (and is still physiologically possible), then IVF with or without a gestational carrier may be considered. If parenting appears to be the most important goal, then alternatives to reproductive technologies may also be explored, such as adopting, being a foster parent, or working with children in other roles.

For individuals who use gamete donation or a gestational carrier (surrogate) there may be grief over the loss of the ability to have a genetic child, the pregnancy experience, or over the need to have another woman carry their child. Many individuals need to work through these losses regardless of their choices. It is important for mental health professionals to normalize the grief response and dispel unnecessary fears, such as that grieving is an indication the couple will not be able to accept another parenting solution or will not be acceptable to an agency. By contrast, there is concern about an older couple's unresolved grief acting as a primary motivator in their pursuit of infertility treatment—that they are in pursuit of a baby as a replacement for a previous child who died. Counseling is essential to address the psychological needs and stability of the individuals as well as to address marital issues affecting the couple's adjustment.

In the counseling of the older infertile individual or couple it is important to bear in mind that psychological reactions to infertility are influenced by many factors: each individual's age and stage of development, personality style and defense mechanisms used to deal with the stressors of life, coping mechanisms, lifestyle, financial status, causes of infertility, length of infertility, medical problems, support systems, and past history in regard to parenting opportunities and responsibilities. In addition, individual differences in psychological reactions to infertility may be a source of conflict and distress for couples, especially if one partner is more motivated toward parenthood, has been a parent earlier in life, or has financial obligations to children from previous relationships. Many couples experience relationship conflicts when considering pregnancy or child-rearing. Another remarried man who has adult children may not wish to start a new family for a variety of reasons. He may feel it is morally wrong to be an elderly parent or may resent the additional financial demands necessitating the postponement of retirement. He may not have enjoyed parenthood earlier in life and, therefore, does not wish to repeat the experience. He may feel that he is at a stage in life in which he prefers a lifestyle that is more self-indulgent, or he may have remarried with the expectation that the new relationship would be child-free and feel that his spouse's desire to have children is a breaking of the marital contract. By the same token, his younger wife may feel entitled to experience parenthood for the first time or she may want to ensure her place in the family constellation of step-children and ex-wives. By contrast, an older woman married to a younger man, may feel pressured to have a child 'for him' or to stabilize the relationship, and may agree to medical treatments that are in opposition to her personal moral code or wishes. Men or women may feel parenthood achieved through the use of their own gametes or minor medical treatment to be acceptable, but that the use of 'extreme measures' involving a third person such as a donor or surrogate carrier entering the dyad may be far less acceptable. Brief marital counseling prior to or during active pursuit of infertility treatment can often preempt the development of problems and is certainly recommended should such conflicts arise.

In addition to the relationship conflicts that often develop over procreative options, couples may also experience sexual problems. The increased pressure for older couples to have intercourse to become pregnant may cause sexual problems. Treatment side-effects, the stress of being infertile, and the potential relationship conflicts can also lead to sexual problems, including loss of desire, erectile dysfunction, dyspareunia, or vaginismus. Furthermore, age-related sexual problems such as decreased frequency and sexual dysfunction secondary to health problems may have a detrimental effect on sexual functioning and thereby fertility (see Chapter 9).

If an older woman is able to achieve a pregnancy, she may experience significant distress. There is a certain amount of stigma attached to pregnancy in older women. Peers may have older children or even be grandparents and may not be able to relate to their experience. Older women may receive less social support during infertility and pregnancy than their younger counterparts from friends, co-workers, or family members, and often experience less empathy from others who believe she is too old anyway. She may have more difficulty when she is trying to arrange time off for doctor appointments in the infertility clinic or obstetrician's office, or fewer offers of help in general. Older women often cannot rely on family members as much as can younger women. Many may have already lost their parents or may actually be caring for them, while also trying to have a child or raise one. Ironically, our society may be as judgmental about older women having children as it is about adolescents having children, and

although older men may experience some stigma as older fathers, just as often they are praised or complimented on their achievement of parenthood—an achievement that is often viewed as a measure of their masculinity. Nevertheless, the stigma experienced by the older infertile individual and older parent reinforces the importance of providing good mental health care for these couples, which should be an integral part of any infertility program.

Bioethical Issues

A number of ethical issues have been raised about using reproductive technologies in older men and women. The primary ethical issue is that of procreative liberty[29,35]. If one believes that everyone has the moral right to reproduce, then the other issues related to age are rendered moot. Procreative liberty is not dependent on age. However, if one believes that there are exceptions to procreative liberty, then issues around age can be raised. The most frequently raised issue tends to be whether older women and men are being irresponsible or too selfish by having children. That is, would their offspring be at too much risk to be orphaned/abandoned because their older parents might die before they reach adulthood, or would they be left to care for disabled elderly parents? Thus, in contrast to procreative liberty, older parenting raises questions about the rights of offspring or the greater society, which may end up being the financial or social support of a group of children who are orphaned by older parents or elderly parents dependent on social security[7]. Another ethical problem is: What is considered 'older', or, maybe more to the point, what is considered 'too old?' Certainly, one cannot equate a 40-year-old with a 60-year-old, or can one? If there is such an age that would be 'too old', who determines that age? The American Society for Reproductive Medicine? Each individual fertility program? The government? Would age as the exclusion category be modified by one's medical condition? With reports[2] of women in their 60s successfully giving birth to and breast-feeding a baby, medical risk for women may not be a major factor in setting age limits for pregnancy. Similarly, with OD becoming increasingly more common, menopause no longer limits a woman's ability to reproduce. If procreative liberty for all is considered one end of a spectrum, and an absolute age limit (e.g., 55 years of age) the other end, would the establishment of guidelines be a more moderate position or completely unacceptable to everyone?

Another question related to older parents is whether their age, above and beyond death and major infirmity, would impair their ability to adequately parent (relative to younger parents). Will they have enough energy or the physical stamina to appropriately interact with and stimulate young children? This position is greatly weakened by numerous examples of wonderful parenting by older foster parents and grandparents who have adopted their grandchildren. In addition, there may be a number of benefits to being an older parent, including the possibility that older parents may have more patience, time to spend, experience, and financial security.

The motivation of older women and men to have a child has been raised as an ethical issue. Having children in midlife and beyond may be considered such a marked change from our established developmental markers that some may question the motives of those who challenge these norms. For example, is the person or couple trying to retain their youth or trying to replace a child that has died? In such cases, is it the fertility program's or mental health professional's ethical responsibility to evaluate

motivations, when determining whether to provide reproductive technology services.

As discussed earlier, many consider the questioning of older people as parents to be blatant ageism. Similarly, since this issue has only become popularized with the increase in older women reproducing, many also consider it to be sexism as well. Society has not had as dramatic a reaction to older men becoming fathers as it has had with older women becoming mothers.

A final ethical issue to consider is that of the consumption of limited resources. In many cases of older women or couples seeking to reproduce, there will be the need for donor oocytes and the medical technology for IVF. Given that, to date, donor oocytes are still in very limited supply, there is concern over using these resources for older women for whom success rates may be lower.

FUTURE IMPLICATIONS

The lightning speed of advances being made in reproductive technologies indicates that there will continue to be increasingly more 'unusual' ways to reproduce. This forced those of us involved in considering the related ethical and psychosocial issues to look beyond what we consider hard and fast boundaries of possibility and to try to keep up with the science driving our thinking. It is obvious that reproductive technologies will only continue to make it easier for older women to reproduce, thus making it essential that some resolution be reached regarding the related issues of older reproduction and parenting.

Yet, as each issue is resolved, others will most likely appear, some of which we cannot even contemplate in the 20th century. Even today, we are already having to address unusual cases that our technologies have made possible. Without age or reproductive organs as barriers to having children, we anticipate an interesting future for parenting in the 21st century and beyond.

SUMMARY

- Fertility in women declines with age, with a significant drop from age 35. Fertility also declines in men, although age of onset and causal factors are not as defined as they are for women.
- One-third of women who delay their first pregnancy until age 35 or older will have difficulty with conception.
- Infertility treatments for older women are typically the same as for younger women, but are associated with decreased chances of success and should be started earlier.

- Reproductive technologies, including OD, may now extend women's reproductive life past menopause.
- Counseling older men and women or couples must address specific issues, including motivations for wanting a child, distinguishing past and current priorities, societal versus personal values, relationship stability, and goals of genetic parenting versus raising a child.
- A number of ethical issues are raised about using reproductive technologies in older men and women, including procreative liberty, what is considered 'older', the pros and cons of older parents, and the use of limited resources with less than optimal candidates.

REFERENCES

1. Speroff L. The effect of aging on fertility. *Curr Opin Obstet Gynecol* 1994;6:115-20
2. Paulson RJ, Thornton MM, Salvador HS. Successful pregnancy in a 63 year old woman. *Fertil Steril* 1997;67:949-51
3. Tietze C. Reproductive span and rate of reproduction among Hutterite women. *Fertil Steril* 1957;8:89–97
4. Federation CECOS, Schwartz D, Mayaux JM. Female fecundity as a function of age: Results of artificial insemination in 2193 nulliparous women with azoospermic husbands. *New Eng J Med* 1982; 306:404–6
5. Speroff L, Glass RH, Kase HG. *Clinical Gynecology Endocrinology and Infertility* , 5th edn. Baltimore, MD: Williams and Wilkins, 1994:811–15
6. Berger J, Goldstein M, Fuerst M. *The Couples Guide to Fertility*. New York: Doubleday, 1995
7. Ethics Committee of The American Society for Reproductive Medicine. Ethical considerations of assisted reproductive technologies. *Fertil Steril* 1997;67(Suppl): 25-35
8. Foster EM, Hoffman SD. Nonmarital childbearing in the 1980s: Addressing the importance of women 25 and older. *Fam Plann Perspect* 1996;28:117–19
9. Carnoy M, Carnoy D. *Fathers of a Certain Age: The Joys and Problems of Middle-aged Fatherhood*. Minneapolis, MN: Fairview Press, 1997
10. Stovall DW, Tomah SK, Hammond LM, Talbert LM. The effect of age on female fecundity. *Obstet Gynecol* 1991; 77:33–36
11. Navot D, Drews MR, Bergh PA, Guzman I, *et al*. Age-related decline in female fertility is not due to diminished capacity of the uterus to sustain embryo implantation. *Fertil Steril* 1994; 61:97–101
12. Wolff KM, MacMahon MJ, Kuller JA, Walmer DK, Myer WR. Advanced maternal age and perinatal outcome: Oocyte recipiency versus natural conception. *Obstet Gynecol* 1997; 89:519–23
13. Fretts RC, Usher RH. Causes of fetal death in women of advanced maternal age. *Obstet Gynecol* 1997;89:40-5
14. Jones HW, Toner JP. The infertile couple. *New Eng J Med* 1993;23:1710–15
15. Levinson D. *Seasons of a Man's Life*. New York: Alfred A. Knopf, 1978

16. Ratcliff KS. Healing technologies for women: Whose health? Whose technologies? In: Ratcliff KS, ed. *Healing Technology: Feminist Perspectives.* Ann Arbor, MI: University of Michigan Press, 1992:173–98

17. Schwartz D, Mayaux MJ, Spira A, *et al.* Semen characteristics as a function of age in 833 fertile men. *Fertil Steril* 1983;39: 530

18. Meacham RB, Murray MJ. Reproductive function in the aging male. *Urol Clin North Am* 1994; 21:549–56

19. Martin RH, Raemaker AW. The effect of age on the frequency of sperm chromosomal abnormalities in normal men. *Am J Hum Genet* 1987; 41:484–92

20. Jacobs SL, Metzger DA, Dodson WC, Haney FF. Effect of age on response to human menopausal gonadotropin stimulation. *J Clin Endocrinol Metab* 1990; 71:1525–30

21. Meldrum DR. Female reproductive aging; ovarian and uterine factors. *Fertil Steril* 1993; 59:1–5

22. Romeu A, Muasher SJ, Acosta AA, *et al.* Results of in vitro fertilization attempts in women 40 years of age and older: The Norfolk experience. *Fertil Steril* 1987:47: 130-6.

23. Check JH, Lurie D, Callan C, Baker A, Benfer K. Comparison of cumulative probability of pregnancy after in vitro fertilization embryo transfer by infertility factor and age. *Fertil Steril* 1994; 61:257–61

24. Society for Assisted Reproductive Technology, American Society for Reproductive Medicine. Assisted reproductive technology in the United States and Canada: 1993 results generated from the American Society for Reproductive Medicine/Society for Assisted Reproductive Technology Registry. *Fertil Steril* 1995; 64:13–21

25. Sauer MV, Paulson RJ, Lobo RA. Reversing the natural decline in human infertility: An extended trial of oocyte donation to women of advanced reproductive age. *JAMA* 1992; 268:1270–5

26. Sauer MV, Paulson RJ, Lobo RA. Pregnancy after 50: Application of oocyte donation to women after natural menopause. *Lancet* 1993;341:321–32

27. Sauer MV, Avy BR, Paulson RJ. The demographic characterization of women participating in oocyte donation: A review of 300 consecutively performed cycles. *Int J Gynaecol Obstet* 1994;45:147–51

28. Rosenthal J. The desire for childbearing in women of advanced reproductive age. Presented at the North American Society of Psychosomatic Obstetrics and Gynecology, Chicago, IL, February 14, 1997

29. Paulson RJ, Sauer MV. Regulation of oocyte donation to women over the age of 50: A question of reproductive choice. *J Asst Reprod Genetics* 1994; 4:177–182

30. Hansen JP. Older maternal age and pregnancy outcome. A review of the literature. *Obstet Gynecol Surv* 1986; 41:726–42

31. Hollander D, Breen JL. Pregnancy in the older gravida: How old is old? *Obstet Gynecol Surv* 1990; 45:106–12

32. James CA. Female fertility over 40. *Inf Rep Clin North Am* 1996:467–82

33. Maranto G. Delayed childbearing. *Atlantic Monthly.* June 1995:55–66

34. Callahan D. Babies in late life? Choices we make, prices we pay. *Washington Post Health.* Nov. 27, 1990

35. Robertson JA. *Children of Choice: Freedom and the New Reproductive Technologies.* Princeton, NJ: Princeton University Press, 1994:22–42

16

The Remarried Family and Infertility

Nancy Hafkin, PhD, and Sharon N. Covington, MSW

One never knows how much a family may grow; and when a hive is too full, and it is necessary to form a new swarm, each one thinks of carrying away his own honey.

George Sand

HISTORICAL OVERVIEW

Over generations and throughout history, remarriage, the stepfamily, and infertility have been linked. Prior to the last half of the 20th century, mortality was the almost universal reason for remarriage. Wars, illness, famine, shorter life spans, maternal death during childbirth, and sterility were all factors influencing the incidence and necessity of remarriage. For men and women widowed at relatively young ages, remarriage served important societal functions: financial security (particularly for women and children), housekeeping and child care for surviving children (particularly for men), sexual release, and the opportunity for further childbearing[1]. Remarriage for reasons of divorce was rare or nonexistent, except in cultures in which divorce was allowed when a marriage was childless or without an acceptable heir. The most famous historical example is King Henry VIII of England, who changed the religion of a nation and the destiny of an empire to remarry. There are Biblical accounts and cultures where divorce, remarriage, and even the taking of multiple wives occurred when a marriage was childless. And in all these situations, it was usually the wife who was blamed for being 'barren'. In short, history is filled with accounts of infertility, death, divorce, and remarriage, all influenced by societal norms, circumstances, and acceptable 'solutions' to these events.

The second half of the 20th century has been marked by significant social changes, especially regarding remarriage. During the last 25 years in the United States, divorce rather than death has been the primary reason for remarriage: 50% of all first marriages and as many as 70% of all remarriages end in divorce. Today, remarriage after divorce outnumbers remarriage after the death of a spouse by 10 to 1[2,3]. As in the past, age differences between spouses in subsequent marriages continue, with a remarried male likely to be as much as 6 years older than his wife[3]. However, there is a changing trend today, with older women marrying younger men either in a first or subsequent marriage, posing unique reproductive challenges for this couple. While a male's age may effect his motivation for having children, it is usually not an issue in his fertility, unless he is sterilized. Since infertility rises with maternal age, it may be a factor for a remarried woman. Finally, approximately half of all remarried women of child-bearing age give birth during a subsequent marriage: the majority within the first 2 years of the second marriage[4]. If the first marriage was ended by death, women in their childbearing years are 44% more likely to have a child in their second marriage than women whose first marriage was ended by divorce[4].

In the general population, infertility effects 1 of every 8 couples and is generally attributed to delayed childbearing, non-barrier methods of contraception, and sexually transmitted diseases. While no statistics are available on remarriage infertility, women in second marriages tend to have lower fertility than women in first marriages, probably because they are generally older in remarriages[1,3]. In addition, infertility in subsequent marriages is more likely to be due to surgical sterilization (vasectomy and tubal ligation) during first marriages. Thus, it appears that while a significant number of remarried couples experience infertility, the majority who present for treatment involve remarriages in which one partner has children and the other partner is childless.

Remarriage not only involves the union of adults but may also involve the *blending* or *reconstituting* of their families of procreation. *Stepfamily* is generally defined as a family in which children from previous relationships either live with or visit their parent, his or her subsequent spouse, and perhaps the spouse's children. As in the past, children from previous marriages are a significant factor in remarriages: At least 7 million American children, or 11% of all children under the age of 18, currently live in a reconstituted family[3]. Remarriages and reconstituted families face a number of challenges, including new definitions of the meaning of *family*, forming new and reconstructing previous kinship relationships, redefining family roles and responsibilities, reorganizing family boundaries, and creating a new family identity. Not surprisingly, these challenges are often daunting, fraught with difficulties and obstacles for adults and children alike. The normal transitions and adaptations of new relationships are influenced by a myriad of factors in the individuals and the new family system, such as family history before remarriage and individual expectations of the new family. Therefore, additional stressors such as infertility can be particularly traumatizing and distressing, not only for the new husband and wife in the reconstituted family but for any children already in the stepfamily.

A couple faces significant challenges when struggling with the crisis of re-marriage and infertility, including differing reproductive agendas, negotiating the developmental tasks of the reconstituted family, and revisiting past reproductive decisions or experiences. The therapist must understand not only the complicated and stressful intricacies of infertility but also the conflicts and struggles of step-family living.

This chapter will:

- apply current theoretical frameworks to remarriage infertility
- explore clinical issues regarding infertility in the remarried family
- identify therapeutic techniques for assisting families dealing with the tandem emotional process of infertility treatment and stepfamily integration.

REVIEW OF LITERATURE

Although the number of remarried couples presenting at infertility clinics for medical treatment is increasing, there remains a marked dearth of research on the impact of infertility in this population. Available research focuses on the separate issues of stepfamily adjustment and on the emotional crisis of infertility (see Chapter 1).

Research on stepfamilies has virtually exploded in the past 30 years as attention has turned from the effects of divorce on families to what happens when divorced people remarry and their families are reconstituted. The first study appeared in 1966 with Fast and Cain's[5] pivotal article that offered insights into the role of the stepparent and the working of the remarried family. They believed that role confusion doomed a stepfamily—since there was no definitive, set behavior for steprelationships, people assumed stepparents would behave as biological parents would. Their work supported a new idea that the stepfamily needs to be considered a unique and structurally different unit for childrearing. Duberman[6], another early researcher, paid attention to the ways in which social and demographic factors affected relationships between stepparents and stepchildren. She found that stepfathers were more likely to achieve better relationships with stepchildren than were stepmothers. Stepmothers' relationships were better with children younger than 13 than with teenagers, while younger stepmothers had better relationships with children of all ages. Other factors highly correlated with good stepfamily relationships were less education in stepfathers, a new baby, and two sets of children sharing a house. Duberman also found that stepmothers without biological children have a more difficult time than stepmothers with biological children, fathers, or stepfathers. Bohannon[7] focused on the role of stepfathers and found that they viewed themselves and their children as less successful and happy, a view not shared by the children and their mothers.

Other studies found that families were inadequately prepared for remarriage and reconstitution. Messinger and colleagues[8] studied couples' reactions to the upheaval involved in forming stepfamilies. As a result of finding inadequate preparation for remarriage, they developed group techniques to clarify steproles, offer support, and educate about the structural differences between biological and stepfamilies. They found that the combination of support, factual information, and opportunity to interact around emotions was reassuring to couples and assisted them in feeling less alone and better able to cope. Similarly, Cherlin[9] emphasized the confusing and murky path for stepparents as they attempt to create a workable relationship with stepchildren. He contended that stepparents often feel they have little assistance in forming a working stepfamily out of an association of biologically and legally related persons. Finally, Visher and Visher[10] examined discipline of children in a stepfamily and the ambivalence of the biological parent. They concluded that the presence of parental guilt had the potential to cripple stepfamily formation. They also concluded that there is an absence of guidance for stepparents from mental health professionals. Consequently, resources regarding the counseling process were generated and the field of stepfamily counseling was born[11-13].

THEORETICAL FRAMEWORKS

A theoretical framework for understanding remarriage infertility must be developed by applying models from both stepfamily and infertility psychology. While stepfamilies go through a developmental process founded on loss, the emotional process of infertility follows a parallel course.

Stepfamily Developmental Model

Theoretical frameworks of the stepfamily have been influenced by the groundbreaking work of Papernow[14], who developed a life-cycle model describing the normative changes in the formation of a

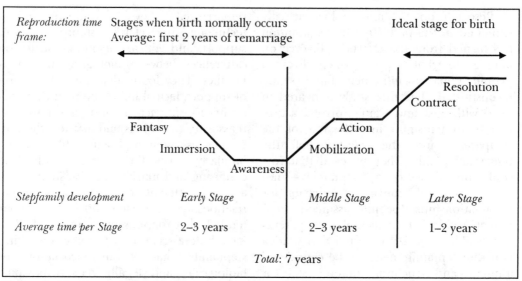

Figure 1 Developmental stages in remarried families and fertility. (Adapted from ref. 14, with permission)

well functioning stepfamily unit, a process taking 4–7 years (Figure 1). Papernow divided stepfamily development into: early stages (fantasy, immersion, and awareness), middle stages (mobilization and action), and later stages (contact and resolution).

Early Stages

The early stage of stepfamily development takes 2–3 years to evolve, while the family structure remains biologically oriented. This is characteristically a tumultuous time for families and yet is the time when most births occur[4]. During the first phase, *fantasy*, the task of the stepfamily is to become aware of and articulate the fantasies and dreams that each member has for the new family. Unrealistic hopes must be grieved and abandoned. The *immersion* phase is characterized by frustration and distress as the stepfamily members confront their differences amid intense feelings. The goal of this phase is to endure the emotional intensity, struggle through uncomfortable feelings, and continue to connect with each other. During the

awareness phase, members become curious and empathic about their own role in the stepfamily and about the roles of others. Goals become clearer and mutual understanding forms the foundation necessary to move on to the middle stage.

Middle Stages

While early phases are marked by biological organization within the family, as the family matures major reconstruction takes place. The middle stage, averaging 2–3 years, entails the family's changing from a collection of biologically organized mini-families to a working stepfamily unit. In the *mobilization* phase, the stepfamily airs its differences openly and discusses step-issues with sophistication. Differences between previous families, adults, and children—insiders and outsiders—are reviewed, and the new stepfamily begins to form a new identity. By the time a family reaches the *action* phase, it is ready to loosen biological ties and establish new boundaries around step-relationships. New traditions, new family rituals, and new customs become the norm. Still, some of the old family structure must be in place so that all members can feel comfortable.

Later Stages

By the later stage, biological ties loosen, while firm, new boundaries are established to define step-relations. The *contact* phase is characterized by intimate, authentic step-relationships—the stepfamily is working and enjoying the connections that it has forged with each other. By the time the *resolution* stage is established, the stepfamily is a fully functioning unit. Boundaries are permeable: Children are secure members of two households and move back and forth with little stress. The important task of this stage of development is retaining the new family ties across life-cycle events, such as graduations and weddings. These occasions also provide opportunities to work again on old issues which may threaten the functioning of the stepfamily.

Stepfamily and Infertility Loss Theory

Pioneering work on stepfamily counseling developed by Visher and Visher[15] provides a theoretical perspective that has important implications for counseling the remarried family facing infertility. According to these investigators, the stepfamily is born of loss and created over the grave of a previous marriage. Grief feelings of anger, hurt, loss, and guilt are common. Whether the prior marriage was ended by divorce or death, feelings of loss and grief affect all members of the original family unit. Further, the step-family experiences a sense of disequilibrium as the old family system reorganizes and the new family system is defined. For people who prefer order and are uncomfortable with ambiguity, being a stepparent (or an infertility patient) can be very difficult.

While the stepfamily goes through a developmental process founded on losses

that must be grieved, infertility often involves a parallel process. For example, infertility is frequently described as an 'emotional roller coaster', similar to the early tumultuous stages of stepfamily development. Around the same time when stepfamily theory was first being published, theory about infertility was changing: The psychological sequelae associated with infertility were likely the *consequence*, not the *cause*, of infertility, as earlier believed. The first work in this area was done by Menning[16], who wrote about the life crisis of infertility as a developmental block affecting future plans, self-esteem, and self-image that must be grieved. Mahlstedt[17] described infertility as fraught with losses affecting multiple aspects of a person's being and a couple's life. The myriad losses—control, health, self-worth, sexual well-being, hopes, dreams, relationships, and so on—are experienced as a grief reaction with normal feelings: shock, anger, guilt, blame, anxiety, depression, and despair. However, the grief is more chronic in nature: the losses emerge slowly over time as the couple identifies infertility as a problem, seeks medical treatment, and looks for solutions[18]. Furthermore, infertility is stressful and played in the high-stakes world of rapidly advancing reproductive technology, which presents complex choices and physical, emotional, and financial demands for couples.

Feelings of anger, hurt, guilt, and disbelief common to infertility can be exacerbated by the losses and ambiguity of the stepfamily experience. If the first marriage ended by death, infertility in the remarriage may revive past losses, enhancing the cumulative effect and exacerbating feelings of vulnerability by denying the life-long, life-affirming connection of a child. A further complication, common to both infertility and the reconstituted family, is the *lack of a shared-loss experience*. It is difficult for the losses of a previous marriage to be shared or grieved by the new spouse, just as the losses of infertility are often individual for each spouse. Further, if only one of the partners has children, infertility will not be a shared loss. This may mean that the level of investment in rectifying the condition of childlessness may differ within the couple. The inequitable level of investment may contribute to feelings of anger, betrayal, loss, and guilt. For remarried couples facing infertility, the lack of a shared loss can contribute to increased marital divisiveness and instability. Finally, as in other infertility situations, the ability to procreate is seen by society as completion of a developmental process of attaining adult status[4,16] and completing one's family[19]. Remarried individuals or couples also may feel that a baby is required to 'validate' a new marriage in the eyes of society or as a solution to the myriad struggles of the reconstituted family[4]. Thus, the inability to have a mutual child may be experienced as a block to the process of development both as an individual and as a stepfamily.

CLINICAL ISSUES

The two emotional minefields of stepfamily adjustment and infertility pose unique clinical challenges for infertility counselors. The differences in first and subsequent marriages, including the differences in the experience of infertility, need to be addressed to discern the unique aspects of remarriage infertility. In addition, therapists must understand the meaning and implications of infertility for all members of the stepfamily: the biological parent, the children, and the stepparent.

Differences Between Initial and Subsequent Marriages

Remarriage is different from, and more complicated than, an initial marriage for a number of reasons[20]. First, an initial marriage and subsequent marriages take

place at different points in an individual's life and within different social and historical contexts. Age, life experience, social status, and maturity are factors that cause individuals to see similar events in strikingly different ways. This seems particularly relevant in terms of infertility, in that the failure to conceive at age 25 may not have the magnitude or urgency as it does at 35 or 45 years of age.

Second, a current marriage bears the continuing imprint of previous marriages, in that the prior marriage is an experience that can be compared and contrasted with subsequent relationships, often contributing to unhealthy comparisons and unfair expectations. Although couples usually make an effort to differentiate marital styles, it is not always possible, as each partner may bring 'remarriage baggage' to the new relationship. Remarriage baggage may involve a belief that one's previous partner was completely to blame for the disintegration of the first marriage, freeing the individual from painful self-examination and contributing to the 'same marriage, different partner' phenomenon. The imprint of this first marriage experience has the potential for creating havoc in the second marriage, especially if infertility is used by a spouse as the 'cause' of marital problems, and therefore a defense against self-examination or addressing marital issues.

Third, when a previous marriage involves children, there is a constant psychological presence in the remarriage of the 'other' biological parent, whether that parent is dead or alive[11]. It is a common myth that it is easier to reconstitute a family when a parent has died because an idealized deceased parent is impossible for a stepparent to compete with. In addition, it is a fact (often difficult for subsequent partners to accept) that formerly married partners with children continue to have some sort of relationship with each other, linking their previous and present partners together in a 'remarriage chain'[7,21]. The challenges and demands of this remarriage chain can be considerable for the infertile remarried couple. The infertile partner may feel envious of the ex-spouse who was able to have a child or may disapprove of the ex-spouse's parenting style, magnifying a sense of loss. Further, the infertile partner may resent a spouse's relationship with their children, highlighting issues of loyalty, commitment, and love.

Differences of Remarriage Infertility

The etiology of and emotional response to infertility in remarriage usually differ from those of a first marriage. Often, infertility in a stepfamily is due to *prior elective sterilization*, which is usually a decision made after careful thought and consideration. Most individuals decided on sterilization at a point in their lives when parenthood or their desired family size had been achieved. However, if the marriage ends and the sterilized person marries a partner who longs for children, a dilemma results. There may be the wish to make a new partner happy by having another child, while feeling ambivalent about starting a family all over again. Assisted reproductive technologies may be an option to having a child together, albeit at great financial and emotional costs, and may create conflict over how far to pursue treatment. For example, if tubal reversal is not possible or successful, in vitro fertilization (IVF) can be considered. However, if a vasectomy reversal is not successful, male fertility can be affected and render a man sterile. Under these circumstances, artificial insemination by a donor or adoption may be the only solution for childlessness. The husband may have been reluctant to have a genetic child but is even more resistant to parenting a nongenetic child. If the wife is older and uses a donated oocyte, pregnancy can still be experienced, although issues still remain in raising a child that is not genetically related to both parents. Hence, there would not be a mutual child in this stepfamily who was related to everyone as the couple, no doubt, originally intended.

Age-related infertility may be a significant factor in the reconstituted family because at least one of the partners in subsequent marriages is usually older and potentially less fertile. While age is usually a more significant factor for women than men, it contributes to pressured feelings to proceed with infertility treatment before a stepfamily has emotionally adjusted. Finally, *preexisting infertility* may be a factor in the breakup of a first marriage, and thus a pivotal influence in reproductive decisions and childbearing time-lines in a remarriage. Sometimes, a partner may leave an infertile marriage in an impulsive attempt to prove his or her own fertility, to punish either oneself or a former spouse for being infertile, or because reproduction is so highly valued. While there may be no surprise that infertility is a factor with which to contend, the history of preexisting infertility can be a heavy legacy to bring into a new marriage.

Infertility in the Stepfamily

Infertility treatment in a stepfamily is similar to a movie production on a busy set. The co-stars act out their drama in the midst of directors, technicians, and bit players. The couple feels exposed in front of a cast of characters that includes an ex-spouse without fertility problems, stepchildren, in-laws, friends, and neighbors. The drama is public, chaotic, lonely, misunderstood, and expensive. The substantial needs of children do not cease because a stepparent is undergoing treatment; their lives and demands continue, and resentments may build. Stepparents and biological parents may also become resentful as their needs are thwarted by the experience of infertility.

The subject of money is an emotionally charged issue in stepfamilies, with or without infertility. The emotional overtones begin long before a stepfamily is formed, and the bitterness can endure into adulthood. There may be alimony payments to a former spouse, child-support payments to children living outside the home, and child-support payments coming in. Sometimes, no payments exist, which means that the new couple provide all support. The exchange of money—or lack of it—binds the former spouses together and fuels feelings of guilt and anger[11]. To complicate matters, the cost of infertility treatment is anxiety-laden and can be extraordinarily expensive. Decisions about the investment of financial resources may become a minefield: A childless partner may wish to use financial resources in the pursuit of parenthood, while a spouse with children feels obligated to use the money on current, not future, children. Further, a charged similarity between these two— stepfamilies and infertility—may create a dual battleground: the former spouse and the insurance company.

Issues for Biological Parents

Parents in an infertile remarriage may have markedly different levels of investment and motivation in having a *mutual child*. A parent may feel ambivalent or even opposed to 'repeat parenthood', while at the same time wishing to please or fearing the loss of the new partner if she or he does not agree to having more children. Ambivalence or reluctance may involve the biological parent's personal goals: a return to diapers and preschool is less appealing than launching young adults and considering the joys of an empty nest, not wanting to share their partner

with a new baby, or, if older, feeling it irresponsible to have a child later in life. At other times, ambivalence and reluctance to be a 'repeat parent' involves concerns about their current children and their needs: regret or guilt about neglecting their needs, lingering conflicts in their relationship related to the divorce, and an overwhelming sense of financial and emotional responsibility to their children in general.

In addition, investment and motivation for a mutual child may change dramatically if it becomes clear that it will not be a genetically related mutual child. A remarried parent's age or prior sterilization may result in sterility, and donated gametes or adoption are the only solutions to childlessness in the current marriage. These parents may be resistant to consider alternative family building when the opportunity for the genetically-shared mutual child to 'solidify' the stepfamily is eliminated.

The *unshared loss of infertility*, when one partner has children and the other does not, presents other issues. Often, a new set of guilt feelings emerges: an infertile spouse desperately needs emotional support, and the parent may not have it to give. The guilt may be due to ambivalence and inequitable motivation for having a mutual child or to the emotional demands of their children that leave little energy for their partner. Also, children from a previous marriage represent one partner's reproductive ability, a fact that may distress an infertile partner. Infertile partners may resent these children who symbolize what they are unable to achieve or feel jealous or bitter of their partner's fertility, or they may feel angry and resentful if their inability to have a child is due to their partner's sterilization during the previous marriage.

Issues for Children

The challenges for an infertile remarried couple are even greater when children from a previous marriage are involved.

Undeniably, children from previous marriages involve a constant psychological bond, financial obligation, and emotional presence, as well as a continuing relationship with the other biological parent. Whatever the age of children, a host of emotional responses may occur: dependent children with physical, emotional, and financial demands, and adult children with emotional reactions to their parent's starting another family.

Children of all ages typically have feelings about their parents trying to have a baby and recreating a new family. Older children may resent the financial costs or energy spent on infertility treatment or, more primitively, be offended by their parent's obvious sexual activity. In fact, infertility and the motivation for parenthood can become a decisive roadblock in the development of rewarding relationships in the reconstituted family. Children from previous marriages may feel (or actually are) ignored or unappreciated, and normal parent–child conflicts may be exacerbated by infertility issues. Children ready to dislike a stepparent for his or her part in destroying the fantasy of a 'nuclear family reunion' may resent the potential mutual child as a further threat to this fantasy and the exclusivity of their relationship with their biological parent.

A unique issue for an infertile remarried couple is the consideration of family-building alternatives in terms of the needs and demands of the stepchildren. Frequently, these children live with the infertile remarried couple on a part-time or full-time basis and are aware, in varying degrees, of infertility issues. Often, children have thoughts or feelings about the issues that may precipitate a variety of responses from the infertile couple. As in all family communication, parents who ignore their children's feelings or opinions, dismiss them as irrelevant, or avoid dialogues risk a disturbed relationship with their children.

Further, the infertile remarried couple must consider the ages, circumstances, and their relationship with current children, when exploring medical alternatives, especially those involving donated gametes. For example, is a decision not to disclose the circumstances of the child's donor-conception realistic and feasible if children from a previous marriage are aware or may be told by an angry ex-spouse of the parent's prior sterilization? Although all infertile couples must explore the issues of raising a child who is not genetically linked to both parents, these issues are more complex when children from previous marriages are part of the equation.

Issues for Stepparents

The primary task of a new spouse in a remarriage is establishing a relationship with stepchildren that is workable, rewarding, and positive. However, this task can be exceedingly challenging and usually involves a number of unique stressors[22-24]. Common problems include feelings of exclusion from original parent–child relationships, difficult relations with stepchildren, struggles over discipline of stepchildren, life-cycle disequilibrium with their spouse, and financial problems. Cherlin[22] argued that stepparents face role ambiguity and have no socially approved means to establish a system of behavior that allows a satisfactory reconciliation of roles or provides a clear role definition. Frustrations with role ambiguity (operating as a responsible parent without being acknowledged as one) and the desire for social acceptance as a parental figure may become motivating factors in the pursuit of a biological or mutual child for the reconstituted family. This is an important issue for stepmothers who tend to assume greater responsibility for childrearing than stepfathers in reconstituted families.

Expectations of the steprelationships can be an additional significant issue in the reconstituted family. Stepparents who believe that a good stepparent feels 'instant intimacy' with a stepchild become disappointed and believe that they have failed when the fantasy is not realized[24]. Further, women often work very hard to dispel the image of the 'wicked stepmother' and find themselves feeling disappointed, angry, hurt, rejected, and guilty when the instant intimacy does not occur. These feelings may exacerbate the longing for a mutual child who will heal the pain and provide the intimacy the stepchild does not. By contrast, some stepparents enter a reconstituted family not wanting or expecting intimacy from stepchildren and are ill-prepared for the parenting needs and demands. Other stepparents enter the remarriage situation with a belief, either explicit or implicit, that stepparenting will meet their needs to regenerate and parent. Months or years later, when the dynamics of the situation or the longing for one's own child becomes paramount, the entire reconstituted family can be thrown into turmoil. A biological parent may feel betrayed that the stepparent wants to change the original agreement, while a stepparent feels cheated and manipulated that he or she agreed to something that goes against one's primal needs. It may seem that there can be no 'win–win' solution to rewriting the marital contract. Making the struggle over having a mutual child can be difficult to resolve[25].

Successful stepparenting appears to involve consistent change and adaptation to behavior and role performance over time. Initially, during the first year, a position of interested and invested 'friend' seems to promote good functioning. Over time, the role of stepparent involves more active parenting, including discipline and decision-making[26,27]. Stepparents who attempt to hurry the process are often disappointed and fail to be integrated into the family unit.

It is important to point out that a reconstituted family does offer an excellent opportunity for stepparents to experience the joys and rewards of parenting, as well as participating in the lives of children. Although these relationships may not be the same as those of biological parenthood, they can be exceedingly warm and rewarding, especially when the children have experienced parental relationships that were disappointing, painful, or disturbed. In these cases, the affection and emotional investment of a caring step-parent can be a child's saving grace, mutually rewarding and healing for both parties, and a welcome substitute for what 'might have been'. The rewards of these relationships are often difficult for stepparents to see or accept, especially if they are focused on relationships with children that are defined only in biological or genetic terms. While adoption may not be feasible for an infertile remarried couple, investing in stepchildren is a source of relationship rewards that can last a lifetime.

THERAPEUTIC INTERVENTIONS

Helping individuals who previously belonged to another nuclear family carries the potential for complex family dynamics. New roles are assumed, new territory is defined and new relationships are formed. A systems framework is helpful, and traditional techniques are not always sufficient, given the many intimacy issues in stepfamilies[13].

Helping infertile couples and individuals in a stepfamily requires a thorough understanding of infertility, as well as familiarity and knowledge of stepfamily dynamics. The diversity of stepfamily needs and the emotionally laden quality of these needs requires a therapist who is active, resourceful, flexible, and capable of directing emotionally volatile sessions, utilizing different modalities[28,29]. Problems in the reconstituted family frequently stem from the wish to view or experience the stepfamily as a reworking of the nuclear family[30]. Families need assistance in avoiding the longing for instant unity and intimacy, which stems from the desire to avoid pain, vulnerability, and the fear of another failure. Losses need to be grieved and fantasies examined so that more realistic goals and expectations of normal adjustment can be adopted by all family members.

Tandem Processes of Infertility and Stepfamily Integration

Since most births in remarriage occur within the first 2 years of the marriage, it is reasonable to assume that this is the most likely time period of infertility. In Papernow's[14] stepfamily cycle (see Figure 1), this stage is also the most volatile, conflicted, and unstable period, marked by the greatest risk for marital breakup and the greatest likelihood of more children entering the family. Thus, couples need assistance in understanding that they are coping with two highly stressful situations replicating similar feelings.

Loss of control, anger, guilt, ambiguity, and a cycle of disappointment are but a few of these 'simultaneous' feelings. Stepparents often feel a lack of control over stepchildren and issues related to their spouse's or ex-spouse's involvement with these children. Similarly, a common feeling expressed by infertile couples is the loss of control over how infertility treatment has taken over their lives. Anger is very much a part of the divorce, stepfamily, and the infertility experience. Anger may be directed at people close to the situation or at intangibles, such as the unfairness of the experience. Guilt may be experienced on many different layers: guilt at the way one is dealing with others; guilt over ambivalent, conflicted feelings toward having another child; lack of positive feelings toward innocent stepchildren; and guilt over past deeds (e.g., sterilization, abortion). Further, these feelings facilitate an ongoing cycle of disappointment and sense of loss for the fantasized stepfamily and wished-for mutual child. It may be difficult at times to distinguish the origin of these feelings—is it infertility or the stepfamily?—resulting in emotions that are ambiguous and projected onto each situation. Infertile remarried couples need assistance in identifying the origin of their feelings and channeling them in appropriate ways.

Both stepfamily members and infertile couples report that validation and normalization of their feelings and experiences are essential for effective adjustment[14,18,30]. Additionally, clarifying issues and insights, understanding of self and others, and depathologizing the stepfamily experience are helpful[28]. Intense emotions—anger, guilt, grief, and a sense of being out of control—are critical to acceptance, understanding, and integration of the experience. Often, these feelings run parallel in a family: to integrate a stepfamily and resolve infertility, couples must run an emotional gauntlet that is intense and similar.

Grief work is necessary to let go of fantasies and accept losses[12,16,17]. Families must be able to identify the dreams, acknowledge the feelings, and communicate the experience to be able to mourn the loss of the nuclear family and the mutual child. It is only through the communication of these feelings, shared in an effective manner that is received and validated, that resolution will occur.

Communication, Conflict Resolution, and Decision-Making Skills

Effective communication, decision-making, and conflict resolution are essential family-living skills that may be taught by the therapist and modeled in therapy. Clients learn to safely express their thoughts and feelings, be acknowledged and validated, and receive feedback on their behavior[31]. For effective communication to take place, three sequential components must occur:

- Each person must know how she or he feels.
- The person must be willing to share the feelings.
- Each person must feel that she or he has the ability to share feelings effectively.

For individuals who are unable to distinguish or do not know how they feel, individual or group therapy and personal exploration strategies such as journal writing may be useful for learning how to identify feelings. A reluctance to share feelings or thoughts requires exploration as to the meaning of the unwillingness or inability to communicate. Often, the barrier relates to trust and safety issues in the relationship where the person feels it is too risky to share. The ability to communicate effectively is a matter of experience and can be addressed through communication-training exercises in therapy or as 'homework'. Difficult situations are better understood and resolved by learning these communications skills.

At times, infertile stepfamily couples reach an impasse or stalemate, especially when dealing with how far to pursue infertility treatment and family-building alternatives. They may not be able to reach a compromise or agree on a win–win solution that is satisfactory or acceptable to all parties. One useful technique is to persuade each partner to 'walk in the other's shoes'. In this situation, a dialogue occurs in which each person assumes his or her partner's position and role-plays what he or she knows and understands the partner to feel. The therapist may ask them to change seats as they change identities and talk about the problem. The process is then discussed after the content dialogue takes place, exploring how it feels to be in the other partner's position, what they heard, and what they learned from the exercise. To facilitate the process, the therapist may assign the couple homework to continue the role reversal outside the session. During this period, each partner pursues learning more about the other's position: reading books or articles on the subject, attending information meetings or support groups, or just being open to think about the positive associated with their partner's viewpoint. For example, one partner may want to pursue donor conception, while the other partner is resistant to more children and has only been amenable to a genetically-shared pregnancy in this marriage. The task will be for the 'resistant' partner to learn all that he or she can about the issues of donor conception, while the 'donor' partner pursues an understanding of the benefits of remaining childless in this marriage and investing in stepparenthood. This technique is often helpful in facilitating the process of conflict resolution and decision-making.

Another helpful technique in facilitating conflict resolution is educating couples on the important elements of good decisions and the consequences of unilateral, default, and mutual decisions. Unilateral decisions, in which one partner makes a decision affecting the couple, are authoritarian decisions that may seem effective in the short-run but will result in the non-participating partner's becoming angry and resentful, potentially undermining the decision so that it becomes ineffective. Passive or default decisions occur when one or both partners relinquish participation in the decision-making process, frequently to avoid conflict. While short-term consensus may have been achieved by inaction, it often results in later regret and guilt by the failure to invest in the decision-making process or allowing a unilateral decision. Compromises or mutual decisions, in which each party gets something of what he or she wants or needs, are the most effective decisions with the highest long-term compliance.

For infertile remarried couples who have polarized their positions, finding a win–win situation can be exceedingly difficult, especially if the partners have difficulty addressing 'bottom lines'. In some situations, a compromise may be that the couple reaches an agreement to reevaluate the decision in a given period of time (e.g., 3–6 months). For example, it is common to find couples polarized when one partner has children and the other does not, the *lack of a shared loss* situation. Here, the infertile remarried couple may decide not to pursue further treatment at this time and to realign priorities so that the stepparent feels more a part of the reconstituted family and is given more time or attention by the parent. The couple may then set a date for reviewing this arrangement to assess its success, as well as the stepparent's satisfaction or comfort with remaining childless. At that time, it may be that the noninfertile partner has not realigned priorities or that the infertile partner believes that she or he cannot live without a biological child, and the decision-making process is begun again.

Genograms

A family systems approach that can be useful in assisting people in understanding the complexities of stepfamily life involves the construction of *genograms*, diagrams indicating relationships between current or former family members[1]. In addition, genograms can be helpful in visualizing complex family relationships and assist the therapist in organizing large amounts of data from complicated histories. The genogram also allows the therapist to shift attention from the individuals and the presenting problem to thinking of the larger family system. It usually takes only a few minutes of the therapy hour, and if the therapist allows the clients to see the developing genogram, their participation may elicit more information. While creating the genogram, the therapist can ask questions such as: 'And how did this (remarried) relationship begin? 'Can you tell me about the individuals in the family group who experienced any problems with alcohol, drug abuse, legal difficulties, mental or physical health?' 'Can you give me a "Reader's Digest" version of why this marriage ended (whether it is the client's prior marriage or their parents')?' This additional information provides not only useful family history but a glimpse of the family's overall functioning and stability.

An example of a typical genogram of remarriage infertility involves an older husband, divorced, with children and a younger, childless wife (Figure 2). This genogram can assist in exploring issues of shame and guilt and the circumstances under which original families were created and dissolved and new relationships begun. It can also be useful in exploring the fantasies and beliefs about what a new baby will bring to the relationship. It is a common fantasy that the wished-for child will cement the relationship and be the glue that binds the new family together[32]. However, the likelihood of a new baby's increasing or decreasing the glue in a stepfamily depends very much on the developmental stage of the family when the baby is born, ongoing family relationships, and relationship expectations in the reconstituted family. It can be helpful to

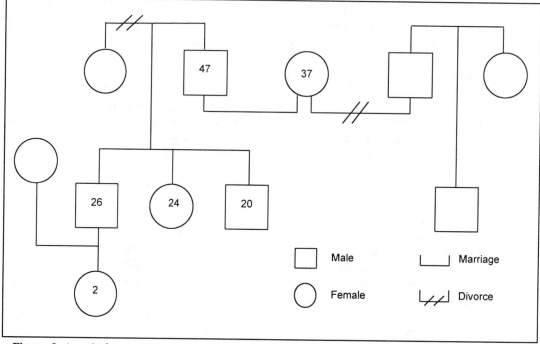

Figure 2 A typical genogram of remarriage infertility

have couples describe how they see their own family picture or genogram with a new child. Often, each member of the step-family has a different image of what the new family will or should look like: the stepparent may see it as 'you, me, and our new baby', while the biological parent may see it as 'you, me, our new baby, and my children'[14].

Finally, for some infertile remarried couples, the reality may be that the rewards of the marriage cannot outweigh the costs of childlessness or the demands of the stepfamily. In these cases, the best that the therapist may be able to do is assist the couple in ending the relationship in a respectful and nondestructive fashion that protects the well-being of both partners and the stepchildren. The considerable demands of the reconstructed family and the emotionally damaging effects of infer-tility can leave remarried couples at risk during a particularly vulnerable point in a stepfamily's life cycle. Understanding these circumstances can diminish blame and enhance understanding for both partners. Ultimately, infertile remarried couples, like other couples experiencing infertility, may have to accept the unacceptable: there may be no desirable alternative, and their course in therapy will be to resolve the losses of the wished-for child and family.

Infertile remarried couples are under extraordinary stress as they become a stepfamily, while dealing with infertility. The tandem process of stepfamily develop-ment and infertility experience is compli-cated by the duality of feelings on both issues—loss, anger, guilt, grief, blame, lack of control, ambiguity, and hurt. These families must develop skills to deal with these negative feelings and develop a clear understanding of the process and dynamics of their situation. Without this knowledge, they are at risk of a continuing cycle of despair and failure—another failed marriage and thwarted reproduction.

FUTURE ISSUES

Given the high incidence of remarriage and infertility in the general population, it is reasonable to expect that infertility counselors will encounter a significant number of remarried couples and reconstituted families in which infertility is an issue. There is a void of research on this population and an enormous need to examine the implications of the dual experiences of infertility and remarriage for couples and their children or stepchildren. Complicating the picture further is advancing medical technology that makes family building and thus family dynamics and kinship ties increasingly more complex. The issues of donor conception, surrogacy, gestational carrier, conception from deceased spouses, and possibly cloning add new meaning to the words 'reconstituted families'. Infertility counselors must be prepared to assist these families with the complex task of integration and adaptation to a new, healthy family unit.

SUMMARY

- Research on stepfamilies and infertility has exploded in the last 30 years, providing information on counseling and assisting these populations. However, no research is presently available on the impact on stepfamilies of the combined issues of infertility and remarriage.
- Initial marriages differ from remarriages in that they (1) take place at different points in an individual's life and involve (2) the 'continuing imprint' of previous marriages and (3) the presence of a 'remarriage chain', of former spouse, children, and remarried parent and stepparent.
- The etiology of infertility in remarriages is more often the result of (1) prior elective sterilization, (2) age-related infertility, and (3) preexisting infertility.
- Stepfamily integration takes from 4–7 years, the most difficult time being the first 2–4 years of the remarriage. The majority of new births take place within the first 2 years (when infertility would typically be experienced) during a period of considerable transition and disequilibrium.
- Parallel feelings occur during the process of stepfamily development and infertility that may confuse and hinder healthy progress, including feelings of anger, loss of control, guilt, hurt, blame, grief, ambiguity, and disappointment.
- Dual issues exist between stepfamily integration and infertility, which are often weathered in tandem and are experiences born of loss that must be grieved. Stepfamilies require assistance in understanding and managing the duality of these emotional challenges.
- Infertile remarried couples need to develop skills in effective communication, conflict resolution, and decision-making.
- Geograms can be useful in history taking and providing a visual representation of the complexities of stepfamily life.
- Infertility counselors must have a thorough understanding of infertility as well as knowledge of stepfamily family dynamics to effectively counsel infertile remarried couples.

REFERENCES

1. Spanier GB, Furstenberg FF. Remarriage and reconstituted families. In: Sussman MB, Steinmetz SK, eds. *Handbook of Marriage and the Family*. New York: Plenum, 1987:419–34

2. National Center for Health Statistics. *National Estimates of Marriage Dissolution and Survivorship*. Hyattsville, MD: US Department of Health and Human Services, Public Health Service, Office of Health Research, Statistics, and Technology, National Center for Health Statistics, 1980. United States, Series 3, No 19

3. Glick PC. Remarriage: Some recent changes and variations. *J Fam Issues* 1980; 4:455–78

4. Wineberg H. Childbearing after remarriage. *J Mar Fam* 1990;52:31–8

5. Fast I, Cain AC. The stepparent role: Potential for disturbance in family functioning. *Am J Orthopsychiatry* 1966;36:435–91

6. Duberman L. The reconstituted family: A study of remarried couples and their children. Chicago: Nelson-Hall, 1975

7. Bohannon P, ed. *Divorce and After*. New York: Doubleday, 1971

8. Messinger L, Walker KN, Freeman SJ. Preparation for remarriage following divorce: The use of group techniques. *Am J Orthopsychiatry* 1978;48:263–72

9. Cherlin A. *Marriage, Divorce and Remarriage*. Cambridge, MA: Harvard University Press, 1981

10. Visher EB, Visher JS. Common problems of stepparents and their spouses. *Am J Orthopsychiatry* 1978;48:252–62

11. Visher EB, Visher JS. *Stepfamilies: A Guide to Working with Stepfamilies and Stepchildren*. New York: Bruner/Mazel, 1979

12. Sager CJ, Brown HS, Crohn H, *et al. Treating the Remarried Family*. New York: Brunner/Mazel, 1983

13. Martin D, Martin M. *Stepfamilies in Therapy*. San Francisco: Jossey-Bass, 1992

14. Papernow PL. *Becoming a Stepfamily*. San Francisco: Jossey-Bass, 1993

15. Visher EB, Visher JS. *Stepfamily Workshop Manual*. Palo Alto, CA, 1980

16. Menning BE. *Infertility*. Englewood Cliffs, NJ: Prentice-Hall, 1977

17. Mahlstedt PP. The psychological component of infertility. *Fertil Steril* 1985; 43:335–46

18. Covington SN. Psychosocial evaluation of the infertile couple: Implications for social work practice. In: Valentine D, ed. *Infertility and Adoption: A Guide for Social Work Practice*. New York: Haworth Press, 1988:21–36

19. Blake J. Is zero preferred? American attitudes toward childlessness in the 1970s. *J Mar Fam* 1979;41:245–57

20. Furstenberg FF. Conjugal succession: Reentering marriage after divorce. In: Baltes BB, Brim OG, eds. *Life Span Development and Behavior*. New York: Academic Press, 1982:4

21. Furstenberg FF. Reflections on remarriage. *J Fam Issues* 1980;1:443–53

22. Cherlin A. Remarriage as an incomplete institution. *Am J Sociol* 1978;84:634–50

23. Furstenberg FF. The new extended family: The experience of parents and children after remarriage. In: Pasley K, Inhinger-Tallman M, eds. *Remarriage and Stepparenting Today: Current Research and Theory*. New York: Guilford Press, 1987;42–64

24. Visher EB, Visher JS. *Old Loyalties, New Ties: Therapeutic Strategies with Stepfamilies*. New York: Brunner/Mazel, 1988

25. Bernstein AC. *Yours, Mine, and Ours*. New York: Scribner's, 1989

26. Bray J. Children's development during early remarriage. In: Hetherington EM, Arastek J, eds. *The Impact of Divorce, Single-Parenting and Stepparenting on Children*. Hillsdale, NJ: Lawrence Erlbaum, 1988;279–98

27. Hetherington EM, Cox M, Cox R. Long-term effects of divorce and remarriage on the adjustment of children. *J Am Acad Child Psychiatry* 1985;24:518–30

28. Pasley K, Rhoden L, Visher EB, Visher JS. Successful stepfamily therapy: Clients' perspective. *J Mar Fam* 1996;22:343–57

29. McGoldrick M, Carter B. Forming a remarried family. In: Carter B, McGoldrick M, eds. *The Changing Family Life Cycle*. New York: Gardner, 1988;399–429

30. Walsh W. Twenty major issues in remarriage families. *J Couns Dev* 1992; 70:709–15

31. Ganong L, Coleman M. Do mutual children cement bonds in stepfamilies? *J Mar Fam* 1988;50:687–98

32. Mandell D, Birenzweig E. Step families: A model for group work with remarried couples and their children. *J Divorce Remarriage* 1990;14:29–41

17

Secondary Infertility

Harriet Fishman Simons, PhD

Secondary infertility hurts ... because these couples are not childless, they are often ashamed of their sorrow. They are so lucky ... Who are they to complain? But the pain is real and no less legitimate that anyone else's ... our pain is our pain and it really does hurt.

Judith Calica[1]

HISTORICAL OVERVIEW

Secondary infertility is medically defined as the inability to become pregnant or carry a pregnancy to term following the birth of one or more biological children to the same couple. Some doctors consider a couple to be experiencing secondary infertility when they have conceived together and then experience a pregnancy loss or stillbirth. However, psychosocially, the overriding factor is the experience of being parents rather than the diagnostic potential of having conceived. Therefore, involuntary childless couples regardless of pregnancy or childbearing history are best treated as experiencing *primary* infertility. On the other hand, many women have given birth in a previous relationship only to experience infertility with a subsequent partner. While medically they would not meet the criteria for secondary infertility, their identity as mothers having difficulty conceiving again would categorize them psychologically as secondarily infertile.

Secondary infertility is statistically more common than primary infertility; however, only half of those with secondary infertility

seek medical help[2]. This appears to be changing as more and more couples conceive their first child as a result of assisted reproductive technologies, such as in vitro fertilization (IVF), or adopt, and then return to treatment in the hopes of having additional children. In addition, these couples may be more aware of available treatment options.

The issues to be addressed in this chapter are:

- the impact of secondary infertility on couples, families, and children
- how secondary infertility effects treatment decisions
- the impact of secondary infertility on children already in the family
- therapeutic interventions for helping couples with secondary infertility move on.

REVIEW OF LITERATURE

What surprises many people, including even infertility clinicians, is how much secondary infertility hurts. While secondary infertility shares much of the pain of primary infertility, Simons' study[3] of 60

313

women with secondary infertility reveals additional complications as well. Women who had experienced both primary and secondary infertility reported that they received less social support once they had a child. An additional complication was that couples frequently felt less united in their desire for another child than for a first child.

Individuals suffering from secondary infertility are more apt to be criticized and feel guilty for having normal feelings of grief. The pervasiveness of the depression that often accompanies secondary infertility is underestimated not only by the general public but also by those experiencing it, who question why they aren't coping 'better'[3]. Parents are also concerned about the potential impact of this distress on their existing child or children. Although no formal research has been done on children in families experiencing infertility per se (although there are anecdotal accounts of distress), a follow-up study was done on families in which stillbirth occurred[4]. This research confirmed that even if pre-schoolers do not understand intellectually, they will pick up on the emotions of the event knowing that it is a sad moment.

Understandably, for women having given birth before, the inability to give birth to additional children represents a very tangible loss. Many have a desire not only to have another child, but also to reexperience pregnancy, childbirth, and breastfeeding. These may have been peak emotional experiences, a time during which they felt special, and they are eager to recapture those feelings. Many parents question whether or not the positive experiences of parenting their biological children would make it difficult to parent a child whom they adopted. A survey of over 1000 mothers[5] (biological, adoptive, and both biological and adoptive) compared adoptive and biological mothers and found virtually no difference in the quality of the mother–child relationships. Nor, as many couples feared, did bioadoptive mothers feel closer to their biological children. About one-third of the adoptive mothers in this study had both biological and adopted children. The mother-child relationships were just as close with their adopted children as with their biological offspring: 'Not all wonderful relationships, but no better or worse than biological.' In fact, those women who also had biological children were reported to have 'a psychological edge' over mothers who had adopted children only. With such firsthand experience of parenting both adopted and biological children, there seemed to come a feeling of security and confidence that they were as real a mother to their adopted children as to their biological children.

THEORETICAL FRAMEWORK

Theoretical approaches to secondary infertility primarily involve developmental theory, particularly family life cycle theory and the idealized family size. A comprehensive family life cycle model was developed by Carter and McGoldrick[6] who divided the family life cycle into six distinct stages: (1) the launching of the single young adult, (2) the joining of families through marriage, (3) families with young children, (4) families with adolescents, (5) launching children and moving on, and (6) families in later life. Secondary infertility occurs during the family growth phases: during the expansion phase the addition of new family members is an expected and desired developmental task and a strong boundary is established around the nuclear family. However, during secondary infertility the family boundary is ambiguous as it remains uncertain when, how, and if additional new members will actually enter the family. Further, according to family system theory ambiguous boundaries increase individual and family stress, particularly if it is prolonged as is the case in secondary infertility.

An additional theoretical application is the concept of family definitions, which in terms of infertility is often a romantic image definition of the family[7]. Within this context, public and private definitions of the ideal family size work to increase psychological pressure to have a certain sized family. Most people base their image of family either on a replication of or reaction to the family in which they grew up. Often, family relationships which are viewed realistically as less than ideal still determine the script for what a family should be, (e.g., a 'big, happy family'). Often, couples strive to create the 'ideal' family for their child, one they lacked in their own childhood. Mazor[8] theorized that unresolved issues with siblings become reactivated during infertility. Often, those who have been disappointed in their relationship with their own brothers and sisters are more motivated to provide their children with the ideal relationship that they themselves lacked. In short, personal family experience affects one's definition or perception of the idealized family as much as social circumstances or ideological abstraction[7].

Secondary infertility affects definitions in terms of latent feelings about the family of origin and siblings, as well as what constitutes a real or ideal family. While on one level couples know that they and a single child are a family, it may not always feel like what a *real family* should be. It is difficult for some to reconcile fantasy and existing families. While others may define their family as complete, there is a gap between expectation and reality, leading some to describe this hole in their lives in images of, for example, an empty chair at the table or an empty seat in the car. Within this context, the actual family is less than ideal and consequently does not meet the romanticized definition of the family, thereby affecting psychological response and family adjustment.

An additional theoretical approach is grief and loss. While primary infertility is often described as an invisible loss grieved in isolation, secondary infertility represents an even more socially isolating grief. The lack of understanding of the enormity of the loss may cause patients to feel guilty about grieving and prevent some from receiving needed support to cope with this life crisis. Guilt may be exacerbated for those with recurring infertility who may have 'bargained' that just one child would make them happy, or for those who already have more than one child. Infertility counselors need to validate the real losses that accompany secondary infertility and give parents permission to take the necessary time and emotional space needed to deal with their emotions.

CLINICAL ISSUES

Throughout time, couples have been unable to complete their families and could be diagnosed as being secondarily infertile. However, the lack of knowledge of such a condition and the assumption that 'once fertile, always fertile' have caused many couples and even doctors to fail to recognize this problem. Because these couples are not childless, secondary infertility has been largely invisible and remains an even more hidden form of infertility. Confusion about the nature and even the existence of the problem is rampant and affects doctors and patients alike. Many couples delay seeking treatment by rationalizing that they obviously are not infertile; after all, they live with a daily proof of their fertility. It is very tempting to take a wait-and-see approach, as some doctors suggest, rather than to enter into extensive infertility treatment. However, many patients later regret that they did not proceed with treatment sooner because they were presumed to be 'fertile'.

It is hard for parents to accept that past fertility is no guarantee of future fertility.

When a problem is finally acknowledged, couples frequently react with shock and often blame themselves or one another for not having had additional children earlier while everything was 'working'. If couples have previously experienced primary infertility, they may experience a painful sense of *déjà vu* and disappointment that the infertility was not cured and that they must go through extensive medical treatment with no guarantee of another success.

The lack of recognition that secondary infertility is problematic often results in parents' enduring even more than their share of insensitive remarks. While there may be some recognition that couples may not be childless by choice, there is very little understanding about those who have 'proven' fertility. Unknowing, others pry and make assumptions that are unfounded and hurtful. Those who hide their infertility may have to defend against stereotypes that do not apply to parents of single children. Even when the infertility is shared with others, these infertile couples often find themselves receiving little or no validation of this loss. In fact, many reactions are insensitive and actually 'blame the victim' for wanting another child, with the admonishment to be grateful for the child(ren) they have.

Parents experiencing infertility are uniquely isolated, belonging neither to the world of the fertile nor of the childless. Many parents of one child report casting around for others in the same situation, studying school directories, eyeballing crowds for families that look like their own. Ironically, those who may have been their greatest support in parenting their first child may now become the greatest source of distress as they go on to repeat the previously shared parenting experience with subsequent children. Feeling left behind is exacerbated when peers or family members go on to have not only second children, but third or more. The enjoyable

activities of parenthood such as participating in a parent/toddler class, attending child-oriented parties, or religious ceremonies (e.g., baptism) may not be enjoyable at all, but rather acts of courage. Further, some parents, typically mothers, may have foregone career advancement or taken part-time work or time-out to parent, cutting off other potential sources of personal gratification and support.

For mothers experiencing infertility, and fathers perhaps to a lesser extent, infertility represents not only the loss of the longed-for child but also the inability to perpetuate the parenting role, which may have been central to their identity and daily existence. In some cases, parents have a desire to build on their parenting experience. Normal regrets are intensified for some parents who fear that this may have been their only chance at parenting. The desire to excel as parents and to have their child validate their parenting can be strong, or they may simply wish to experience the joys of parenting more than once. For other women, parenthood provides a welcome or needed shelter from ambivalence or confusion about other career plans, so that failure to achieve parenthood enhances feelings of anxiety, confusion, and distress about future roles or career goals.

Infertile parents often experience additional guilt and sorrow at being unable to provide a sibling for their child. For some, the sense of failing their child is the most difficult part of secondary infertility, often exacerbated when the child pleads for a sibling. It is difficult to cope not only with their own reactions and their spouse's but with their child's as well. In some cases, parents project their own longing for a baby onto their child. One of the challenges of secondary infertility is not to impose their own feelings onto the existing child and to allow the prospective sibling normal feelings of ambivalence about a new arrival. It is also important to recognize that a smaller or single-child family may not be a deprivation but may even be advantageous to their child(ren) (see Chapter 25).

Ironically, the very joy of parenting can also underscore the pain of infertility. The paradox is that the positive feelings about their existing child underscore their pain if they are unable to have another. Unfortunately, some parents find that their mixed emotions make it hard for them to enjoy the children that they do have. The existing child can become a constant and bittersweet reminder of the longed-for children. Some parents, distressed by their infertility, temporarily experience a loss of interest in the existing child; this has the potential to compound their loss. Berkeley[8] cautioned that the child who is there will never be any younger and that parents who cannot enjoy their child(ren) as they mature may experience regrets later.

A smaller family than expected can raise unexpected issues of boundaries between parent and child, and challenge their sense of completeness and legitimacy, causing feelings of failure and even acute distress. The inability to achieve the desired family can cause couples to mourn for their intended children, who may have been visualized in great detail, and for the desired 'family personality'[3]. Many lack a model for parenting a single child, which may be very different from the way in which they were raised and, as such, they may need help in identifying the positives of parenting a smaller or single-child family.

THERAPEUTIC INTERVENTIONS

Facilitating Decision-making

Decisions about treatment and alternate ways of family building are also considered through clients' lens as parents. Time, emotional energy, and financial constraints characterize secondary infertility decision-making. Some couples who feel that they might have been able to be 'child free' feel unable to parent a single child. Ideas about the spacing of siblings sometimes increase the sense of urgency and distress in reaching a decision. The needs of the existing child are often paramount in consideration of the financial, physical, and emotional costs of adoption and/or expensive medical treatment.

Parents are often torn between their desire for another successful pregnancy and child, and their feelings of responsibility to the existing child. It is hard to divide their resources, both emotional and financial, between the child they have and the child they long for. Some parents decide to stop treatment because they need to be more accessible to their child, while others feel they cannot justify the expense and/or fear managing multiples. Often parents feel that decisions about family resources must take into consideration the well-being of all current family members. They feel it morally or sensibly wrong to 'spend' or invest inordinate amounts of the family resources (time, energy, financial, emotional well-being) on a potential family member at the expense of actual and current family members.

A common theme expressed by mothers is the difficulty in remaining a good parent while undergoing the stress of medical treatment for infertility and medications. The awareness that treatment is compromising their ability to parent causes some parents to discontinue treatment[3]. While parents lament the fact that they may not have any additional children, their children definitely will not have any other parents, and their performance in the parenting role is vital.

While the vast majority of women say that they would have considered adopting if they were childless[5], the decision is less automatic when a couple already has a child. Many people feel they could easily parent in a family formed by adoption have concerns about their ability to parent if their children enter the family in different ways. This is a fear that is not supported by research (see Chapters 22, 25).

Having conceived and given birth to at least one child together, couples are shocked to learn that this is no longer possible and that any future pregnancy will be the result of using donated gametes. When considering whether or not to achieve a pregnancy via donor sperm, donor ovum, or surrogacy, couples must consider the investment of time and money, as well as their ability to accept a child who is biologically a half-sibling of their existing child. Some couples attach a great deal of importance to equity, feeling that it is crucial for both parents to have the same biological relationship to the child and for the children to have the same biological relationship with the family members. Others feel that the genetic input and the chance to experience another pregnancy are overriding positives. They believe their parenting will not be adversely affected by the different ways in which the children joined their family[9] (see Chapters 18 and 19).

Reassessing a desired family size requires confronting the fantasy of the ideal family, mourning its loss, and reevaluating whether or not the couple can make a positive decision to accept the status quo. This process is markedly different from that of abandoning treatment and feeling defeated by the process. Affirming the family as it is requires making a conscious decision with positive motivations. Usually, it takes grieving for what might have been and acknowledging the benefits of what is. It is accepting what may not occur, acknowledging the benefits of other options, and defining life according to what the couple has and the family is[10].

Helping Families with the Impact on Children

One of the hardest parts of experiencing infertility as a parent is the worry about its effect on the existing child or children. Just as infertility, regardless of diagnosis, is considered a 'couple problem', secondary infertility must be considered a family problem (see Chapter 25).

Parents must determine whether and how much to tell their children about infertility. Children can sense when parents are preoccupied and not emotionally accessible. Young children become quite adept at reading their parents' moods; after all, both their physical and emotional survival depend upon them. This vulnerability causes them to become particularly attuned to their parents' well-being. Although most parents feel badly or even guilty about exposing their children to sadness, this experience can actually be a good preparation for life. Appropriate expressions of emotions by parents can give their children a model to follow. Crying in front of their child might actually be a positive act reassuring the child that life continues in spite of pain[11]. The important dynamic is that the child sees that the parents are coping with the crisis and seeking the support of other adults to help them resolve their feelings.

If not given an explanation for the sadness, children might rely on their own egocentric perspective and conclude that somehow whatever is wrong is their fault. Magical thinking is common; however, children need to realize that they are not so powerful that their thoughts will prevent conception or cause a loss to occur. Neither will their 'being good' make everything all right.

Even quite young children with whom infertility has never been overtly discussed may experience dreams about 'the baby' or talk about 'my brothers and sisters'. Johnston[12] agreed that children often know more than they have been told and advised parents to respond to questions with simple and age-appropriate information.

Some parents are quite open about their longing for another child, while others prefer to share as little as possible. They wish to protect their children and maintain privacy around such a personal issue. Johnston[12] felt that technical information about reproductive technologies such as IVF or gamete intrafallopian transfer is the parents' information and too sophisticated for children to process. She believed that even young children can understand the need for boundaries and that some information is simply the private business of parents.

The fear of something happening to the parents, common at a young age, may be heightened by the knowledge that the mother or, in some cases, both parents are undergoing medical intervention. In this case, fantasy and reality converge. Children, as do most adults, equate doctors and hospitals with illness and need to be reassured that their parents are not sick. Children who have seen their mothers experience a pregnancy loss may become especially fearful, particularly if they have been told that their brother or sister died. Many children refuse to believe that children can die; the idea is just too threatening. Or they may fear that their own life is in danger. Children need to have as much continuity and consistency in their lives as possible. They need to hear that they did nothing wrong, are loved, and will be taken care of; to be reassured that the parents are not sick; to understand enough so that they can maintain trust; and to be given permission to verbalize their feelings.

Parenting during infertility has its own distinct emotional sequelae and challenges. There are common reports of being overprotective or fearful about the existing child, as well as feeling ambivalent about developmental advances which might otherwise be occasions for joy. For those who have been unable to have other children, every developmental step is particularly poignant, greeted with pride but also with the realization that this stage will not come again. A normal desire for a child to separate and gain autonomy can be particularly painful if the parents are experiencing the 'empty lap' syndrome[3]. Being unable to have another child can make it harder to let go of the existing child who may be needed to fill a void.

The knowledge that things can and do go wrong, coupled with the negative mind set resulting from repeated treatment failures, can lead to intense fears about the safety of the existing child, creating the potential for hypervigilant parenting. Just as overprotectiveness has been observed in those parenting after infertility, it occurs in those parenting during infertility. Mothers report having nightmares about harm to their existing children and struggle to avoid psychologically smothering them (3).

Facilitating Coping

Families coping with secondary infertility are particularly motivated to resolve their crisis. They realize the effects of their struggle on their existing children and want to be able to enjoy them completely. They feel the passage of time as they see their child mature. They are not inclined to drift but rather often spend a time-limited period intensely exploring all alternatives. At some point, many feel the desire to reclaim their lives is stronger than their desire for another child. Some specific suggestions for these families include:

- facilitate the grieving process
- normalize single-child family constellation
- encourage self-education and other active coping techniques
- help couples explore additional treatment options and/or family building alternatives.

Couples should be validated about the normalcy and legitimacy of their feelings of grief, anger, and loss. There is no hierarchy of suffering; even though they have had a child, they are still lacking their future children and their desired family. Infertility counselors may encourage couples to explore what having another child means to each of them, and normalize the fact that couples experiencing secondary infertility often differ in their desire for additional children. While it is not necessary for one partner to mirror the other's feelings, it is necessary for each partner to understand and respect their partner's feelings and perspective. It may be important to introduce techniques for improving communication and/or problem-solving, especially if the couple has very divergent opinions. Additionally, sharing memories of their child's birth and infancy, or looking at pictures of their child, may help identify the particular losses of secondary infertility for each partner as well as for the couple and family. Support groups, especially those that address secondary infertility, are helpful in countering feelings of isolation, expanding support networks, and providing education and information.

Couples should be empowered to take control and be more active in their coping. This may mean setting limits in difficult situations or on the amount of medical treatment, developing coping strategies that increase self-esteem, or developing more coping strategies that involve the support of others. Infertility counselors should make available to couples recommended reading about both the medical and emotional aspects of infertility. In addition, couples should be encouraged to learn as much as possible about their options in treatment and family building. It is important that neither they nor their medical providers make treatment decisions or assumptions based on their past fertility. Finally, other family building options should be addressed with the couple. This may include helping them to reality-test any concerns about adoptions, including familiarizing themselves with families in which the children came into the

family both through birth and adoption, and with the research on such families.

Parenthood and parenting are important facets of secondary infertility. For this reason, couples should be given permission and guidance on how to communicate with their children in age-appropriate terms. They should be offered concrete suggestions for parenting under stress while being fundamentally reassured that they and their children will survive the crisis of infertility. The infertility counselor must allow parents to confront any fears about parenting an 'only child' in order to reality-test them; some parents actively research this topic and are reassured by what they learn, some appreciate having a chance to meet other families like their own.

Parents should also explore strategies for parenting a single child which will address both their immediate and long-range concerns: for instance, the infertility counselor may recommend joint child care or play groups, and discussions about financial planning and long-term care insurance for older parents, to allay fears of burdening their child.

FUTURE IMPLICATIONS

Secondary infertility can be expected to be a growing issue as parents have their first child later in life and experience difficulty having additional children. Also, as more couples are successful in having a first child through assisted reproductive technologies, they will return to treatment in an attempt to repeat that success.

The stigma traditionally surrounding an 'only child' may be lessened by the fact that more and more couples are opting for a one-child family. In fact, this has been described as the most rapidly increasing family form. However, the fact that couples are voluntarily limiting their family size can mask the existence of those families with secondary infertility. While the one-child family is certainly a viable option for some, that should not obscure the pain caused when others who choose to have more than one cannot achieve their desired family size.

Increasingly, couples experiencing secondary infertility will consider family building alternatives that involve third-party reproduction and various forms of prenatal adoption (e.g., donor insemination, embryo donation). For these couples the complex issues of family definition may involve parenting children that are not genetically related to each other or to each parent in the same way. Family kinship may be 'genealogically bewildering' and complicate the individual and family adjustment to secondary infertility.

SUMMARY

- Secondary infertility is statistically the most common form of infertility.
- Secondary infertility is an even more hidden form of infertility.
- Guilt over grieving their loss and social invalidation of that loss are part of the emotional sequelae of secondary infertility.
- The diagnosis of secondary infertility initially causes shock and denial, causing couples to reassess their self-image.

- The couple may be uniquely isolated because their support network may have centered around parenting activities.
- The infertility is experienced by parents as the loss of a child.
- Parents often feel guilty about not providing a sibling for the existing child.
- Parents often experience both logistical and emotional difficulty in combining treatment with parenting.
- Parenting can become a bittersweet experience as their delight in the existing child exacerbates the feelings of loss at not having additional children.
- Decision-making is complicated by concerns about the existing child and fears about parenting children who come into the family by birth or adoption.
- Issues arise over how much to share with the child and how to process the feelings around the infertility of both parents and child.
- Letting go of the existing child can be problematic for parents who desperately want another child.
- Parents experiencing infertility are highly motivated to resolve this crisis and get on with their lives.

REFERENCES

1. Calica J. Secondary infertility: An unexpected disappointment. *Chicago Parent* Oct. 1987:8
2. Beck M, Quade V. Baby blues: The sequel. *Newsweek* July 3, 1989:62
3. Simons, HF. *Wanting Another Child: Coping with Secondary Infertility.* New York: Lexington Books, 1995
4. Defrain J, Martens L, Stork J, Stork W. *Stillborn: The Invisible Death.* New York: Lexington Books, 1986
5. Genevie L, Margolies E. *The Motherhood Report: How Women Feel about Being Mothers.* New York: Macmillan, 1987
6. Carter EA, McGoldrick M. Overview: The Changing Family Life Cycle. A Framework for Family Therapy. In: Carter EA, McGoldrick M, eds. *A Framework for Family Therapy.* New York: Gardner Press, 1988:3–28
7. Settles BH. A perspective on tomorrow's families. In: Sussman MB, Steinmetz SK, eds. *Handbook of Marriage and the Family.* New York: Plenum Press, 1987:157–80
8. Simons HF. Secondary infertility. *Conceive.* May/June 1990:12–15
9. Cooper S, Glazer E. *Beyond Infertility: The New Paths to Parenthood.* New York: Lexington Books, 1994
10. Carter J, Carter M. *Sweet Grapes.* Indianapolis, IN: Perspectives Press, 1989
11. Grollman E. *Talking about Death.* Boston MA: Beacon Press, 1990
12. Johnston P. *Taking Charge of Infertility.* Indianapolis, IN: Perspectives Press, 1994

VI. THIRD-PARTY REPRODUCTION

18

Recipient Counseling for Donor Insemination

Aline P. Zoldbrod, PhD, and Sharon N. Covington, MSW

... children are a bridge joining this earth to a heavenly paradise ...
Blessed indeed is the man who hears many gentle voices call him father!

Lydia M. Child

For couples with severe male-factor infertility, donor insemination (DI) has been shrouded in myths, misinformation, and misperceptions, as well as by psychological factors including stigma, shame, and secrecy. It was usually offered as a medical treatment option rather than a family-building alternative without full acknowledgment of the man's feelings about his infertility or education of the couple about the psychosocial issues of DI. Historically, women have been the primary focus of medical investigation and treatment for infertility, often out of a misplaced belief that men could not be infertile. As a result, some infertile couples were not fully informed or cognizant that their infertility was attributable to male factors. Myths, such as 'it only takes one sperm' or 'infertility is a female trouble', often prevented couples from acknowledging the husband's less-than-ideal sperm parameters and thereby infertility.

Given the dramatic increase in the practice of DI and the number of children conceived and born as a result of donated sperm, it is not surprising that an increasing number of mental health professionals recommend pretreatment counseling to address:

- the man's psychosocial adjustment to male-factor infertility
- his comfort with societal attitudes regarding this method of achieving fatherhood
- marital and sexual adjustment of the couple considering DI
- issues of secrecy and DI[1-3].

This chapter will explore these areas, with special attention to patient screening and preparation regarding the use of donated sperm following a diagnosis of male-factor infertility.

HISTORICAL OVERVIEW

The first recorded births resulting from insemination were reported in the United States and France almost simultaneously in 1884, while the first use of *donor* sperm for insemination was reported in 1909. However, it was not until after World War II that DI became more popular; between 1950 and 1960 an estimated 1000–7000 DIs were performed yearly in the United States. Until recent decades, artificial insemination by donor involved the almost exclusive use of fresh sperm, donor anonymity, and the counseling of couples to keep the child's donor conception secret. Cryopreservation became more common during the 1950s, enabling the establishment of sperm banks with paid, recruited sperm donors. Sperm banks were usually part of a university medical center, commercial business, or private operation catering to special populations. Today, there are more than 400 sperm banks in the United States, and it is estimated that 23,000–30,000 children are born each year in the United States as a result of donated sperm[1].

The practice of DI changed dramatically in the 1980s as a result of two important social events. First, several women in different countries became infected with human immunodeficiency virus (HIV) after being inseminated with donated *fresh* sperm; this resulted in the banning of the use of sperm worldwide. Globally, the laws, practice guidelines, and government policies changed so that only cryopreserved sperm is now used. Further, exclusive anonymity regarding donated sperm was no longer the rule. In the United States, practice guidelines developed by the American Society for Reproductive Medicine (formerly the American Fertility Society) and the American Association of Tissue Banks recommended the exclusive use of cyropreserved sperm and the continued practice of donor anonymity. By contrast, Sweden and New Zealand required that all donors be willing to be identified, resulting in a drastic decline in sperm donors. Second, during the 1980s, the use of donated oocytes became feasible and was originally almost exclusively sister-to-sister identified donations, a practice that influenced sperm donation procedures. Some countries, such as states in Australia, developed laws establishing a central donor registry and required that the birth certificate of every child conceived via donor gametes indicate donor conception, so that the child may obtain information

about the donor from the central donor registry after the age of 18.

REVIEW OF LITERATURE

Research on DI has focused on three areas: men's feelings about their infertility, research on DI, and research regarding the issue of disclosure. The amount and quality of research on the psychological response of men with male-factor infertility have been limited and afflicted by a number of problems, including an underrepresentation of infertile men, male face-saving explanations that presented the infertility diagnosis as unexplained, or couple's providing public explanations of infertility as a lessor female diagnosis rather than the actual male-factor diagnosis. Research on men who with their wives pursue DI as a family-building alternative has been plagued by small sample sizes and concentration on the limited time period during or soon after DI treatment (e.g., studies ranging from pretreatment to 12 years).

Psychological Response in Men to Male-Factor Infertility

Recent studies have addressed how men feel about their own infertility. Kedem and colleagues[5] compared the psychological functioning of 107 infertile men to 30 fertile men and found that infertile men suffered more from psychological distress, including decreased self-esteem, higher anxiety, and more somatic symptoms. Nachtigall and associates[6] also found that men experienced a sense of stigma, loss of potency, role failure, and diminished self-esteem in response to male-factor infertility. Mason[7] interviewed 22 men diagnosed with male-factor infertility and found all of them to be disturbed by their diagnosis. Some men were most concerned about the impact of the diagnosis on their marital relationship, while others were most affected by a decreased sense of self-esteem. In sum, although there is evidence that infertility is psychologically more distressing to women than men, men with male-factor infertility appear to experience significant distress especially around issues of self-esteem.

Donor Insemination Research

Researchers have explored the reasons why DI was a preferred alternative[8] and the length of time couples took to make the decision to proceed with DI[9]. In addition, early investigations of DI focused on obstetrical outcomes, normal infant development, and satisfaction with DI as an alternative. These studies reported no increased risk of obstetrical complications, no evidence of increased risk of abnormal infant development or congenital anomalies, high satisfaction with DI as an alternative, and, interestingly, very low divorce rates[10–13]. Most research has indicated that DI parents and children fall within normal range on indicators of family and psychological functioning[9,14–16]. Amuzu and colleagues[12] reported in a follow-up of 427 families who had conceived a pregnancy by DI over a 12-year period that the children were normal and the divorce rate significantly lower than in the normal population. Klock and colleagues[14] in a prospective study of 42 couples undergoing DI found participants to be within normal limits in terms of marital and psychological adjustment. Schover and coworkers'[16] results were similar in their evaluation of 52 couples, reporting psychological, marital, and sexual adjustments within the normal range.

Research on the practice of DI found that patients prefer having the husband present during insemination, fewer medical caregivers involved in treatment, planning a ritual on or around the time of insemination, and having intercourse after insemination[8,9,14,17]. Mechanick-Braverman and Corson[18] investigated patient pref-erences for known versus anonymous donors and found that there was a wider acceptance of the use of known donors than had previously been seen.

Research on Disclosure

The issue of disclosure—telling the child the truth about his or her donor origins—and secrecy has received increased attention and been the focus of con-siderable research. Despite changing attitudes and policies, the evidence con-sistently indicates that although a majority of parents have told someone (friend or family member) about the donor conception, they do not plan to tell their child the truth about it. There is ongoing debate among professionals about whether or not parents have an obligation to their donor children to disclose their origins. However, there is no reputable, large-scale body of retrospective or prospective data that indicate whether openness or secrecy is the best option for the child or the family. In a review of the research on the issue of privacy and disclosure among couples using donor sperm to conceive, Klock[19] developed a summary of research findings on parental attitudes about disclosure that showed that rates of disclosure are consistent across treatment, countries, and sex, with only a minority of individuals (range, 12–44%) stating that they would tell others. Equally stable have been stated disclosure rates (donor recipient stated plans to tell child): in the United States, 14–29%[14,16,20]; Canada, 30%[21]; Great Britain, 20%[22]; and New Zealand, 22%[2].

Manuel and associates[23] in a study in France investigated plans regarding disclosure in 72 couples and found that 61% did not plan to tell, while 39% reported that they plan eventually to tell the child. Reasons for nondisclosure included: (1) The child 'belongs' more to the couple if he or she does not know; (2)

the parents believed the child would be socially stigmatized if others knew of the child's donor origins; (3) the parents feared a negative reaction from the child; and (4) the parents wished to protect the husband's self-esteem. Interestingly, 41% of the parents felt that donated sperm was preferable to adoption, in that it allowed male-factor infertility to remain confidential. Similarly, in an Australian study[24] in which 56% of couples did not plan to tell, 9% planned to tell, and 35% were uncertain. The three most common reasons for not disclosing the child's origins were: (1) the couple wanted to protect the man's self-esteem; (2) they feared social stigma of the child; and (3) the couple wanted to feel more 'ownership' of the child.

In an ongoing longitudinal study of DI families, following them from their initial infertility diagnosis to the present, Klock and colleagues[14] found that the majority of parents (56–86%) did not plan to tell the child of his or her donor origin. This was in spite of the fact that many couples had told family and friends before or during the pregnancy. Further, as time went on, the researchers found that parents became less inclined to disclosure, with those who had been truthful regretting their prior openness. Amuzu and associates[12], studying 427 couples who conceived by DI, found that many (47%) did not plan to tell, or thought they would not tell (14%), their children about their conception. In Schover and coworkers'[16] study of 52 couples, 74% of the women and 80% of the men reported that they did not think that children conceived by DI should be told about the method of conception. Sewall and Mason[25] found that although 87% of couples thought that their child had the right to know about his or her donor origins, only 58% planned to tell.

In a recent study by Nachtigall and colleagues[20], 184 couples who had become parents by DI completed questionnaires assessing disclosure and stigma. They found that the disclosure decision was not linked to parental bonding with the child or the quality of the interparental relationship. Disclosure decisions were affected by the male-factor infertility diagnosis (azoospermia, post-vasectomy, oligospermia) in that couples with azoospermia were more likely to have disclosed to others, while wives of oligospermic men were less likely to disclose. Increased likelihood of disclosure by couples was found to be related to younger age, azoospermia, lower stigma scores, and having more than one child by DI. Fathers who reported higher scores on stigma indicated less parental warmth and less fostering of independence in their child.

Agreement between husbands and wives regarding disclosure is another focus of research. Disagreement between spouses is fairly common. Klock and colleagues[14] found that 16% of couples disagreed on whether or not to tell others about DI. Schover and associates[16] found a higher percentage of women than men supported disclosure (26% vs. 20%). In their study, wives worried about husbands' attachment to the child, but husbands reported very little concern about loving their donor-conceived child.

THEORETICAL FRAMEWORKS

No single theoretical framework is universally applicable to male-factor infertility and the use of donated sperm to facilitate parenthood. However, several theoretical frameworks have been applied to male-factor infertility, including Freudian theory, pertaining to oedipal jealousy and family-of-origin issues; Goffman's stigma theory; Kohut's self-psychology theory, relating to narcissistic impact on male sense of self; and grief and loss theory. Each theory offers insights into different aspects of male-factor infertility that are relevant to how men consider and feel about DI as an alternative to child-lessness.

Freudian Theory

Freudian theory originally focused on family-of-origin issues and competitiveness with one's father. This perspective lead some early psychoanalysts to assert, as Gerstel[26] did, that 'a decision to participate in artificial insemination, in itself, is indicative of an emotional disturbance'. It was her belief that the diagnosis of male-factor infertility, compounded with the revival of the oedipal conflict inherent in the process, would necessarily lead to severe psychopathology in the couple and the resulting child. Although this approach has fallen into disfavor, more recent approaches continue to consider the importance of family-of-origin issues and the ways in which men were parented as factors in how they manage the crisis of infertility. For some men, particularly those who did not have a close relationship with their father, the essence of the masculine role is reproduction, and therefore the ability to impregnate their wife is the measure of their masculinity[27]. These men mistake fertility for virility and believe that loss of reproductive ability necessarily means the loss of sexual function, self-esteem, and diminished manhood. Under-standably, for these men, considerations of DI are often met with reactive refusal, for to do so would be only further emasculation by acknowledgment of the loss of manhood.

Stigma Theory

The concept of *stigma* has been applied to infertility but is particularly relevant to male infertility because many infertile men feel that infertility is a handicapping defect and makes them different from other men. Goffman[28] explained, 'Given that the stigmatized individual in our society acquires identity standards which he applies to himself in spite of failing to conform to them, it is inevitable that he will feel some ambivalence about his own self.' It is common for infertile men to have feelings of being damaged, defective, and worthless, as well as strong feelings of guilt, despair, loneliness, isolation, and stress. They struggle with stigmatized feelings that make them feel like less than a man, powerless and diminished.

Self-Psychology Theory

Kohut's[29] psychology of self established the centrality of a stable and sustainable sense of self to happiness and well-being. The self is viewed as the organizing force of personality that guides how an individual lives life, which can be disrupted by a disappointment or frustration of a person's innermost hopes and expectations. When the loss is significant or fundamental to the individual's sense of who he or she is, there can be a perceived deficit in the self with concomitant loss of hopefulness and depression. The primary effect of a deficient or faulty sense of self is shame.

Guilt and shame are common responses to male-identified infertility. Infertile men often feel like 'losers', 'duds'[6], 'damaged goods'[30], or powerless because they have 'no balls' or are 'shooting blanks'. Many interpret their infertility as punishment for wrong-doing[31], such as masturbation, adolescent sexual experimentation, promiscuity, homosexual activity, or illicit drug use, or simply as punishment from God[32]. Predictably, altered self-concept and self-image is a significant factor in male infertility and impact a man's perspective or decisions regarding DI, particularly initially: feeling shameful and defective, he may oppose donor parenthood because it may publicize his defect; he may acquiesce to his wife's wishes because he feels powerless and impotent; or he may insist on secrecy about donor conception because his damaged and fragile sense of self cannot acknowledge or integrate his loss of fertility. To illustrate, one study[33] reported that 80% of the men expressed feelings of guilt about their infertility that prevented them from acting like real fathers, as it provided proof of their loss of manhood.

Grief and Loss Theory

The grief and loss model was initially applied to infertility by Menning[32] as a useful explanation for the typical feelings and psychological response to infertility in both men and women (see Chapter 1). Nevertheless, grieving the numerous and complex losses of male infertility presents different issues for men and women. For example, a common reaction to grief in men is to offer their wife a divorce, especially among working class men who may have been socialized in more traditional gender roles[33]. Men who have been socialized more traditionally may conceal rather than reveal their emotions and feelings of grief and loss[34], having been taught not to have or show vulnerable feelings. For some men, feelings of grief and loss are so unacceptable that they have difficulty identifying and expressing these feelings[35]. As a result, many react to losses with separation, distraction, and disengagement, rather than sharing or expressing[36]. Men from families with specific talents in which blood ties are highly valued or men viewed as the 'crown prince' (being the last male with the family name) feel devastated and guilty at not carrying forward their father's line or not living up to family expectations. Focus on the narcissistic loss of genetic connection for the man often obscures the loss for the wife, who longs to carry her husband's child. A wife may grieve at length for the child who would have been the image of her husband or shared his personal characteristics. Menning[37] noted the importance for a couple of grieving the lost genetic connection to a child and, as important, to each other.

It has also been suggested that in response to grief and loss, men are the forgotten mourners. This phenomenon has also been described as the *keening syndrome* in reference to the Irish custom of mourning, in which the women, weeping and wailing, prepared the dead body, while the men sat soberly around the edges of the room watching. The keening syndrome refers to the way in which many couples grieve the losses of infertility: women weep and men watch—resulting in the husband becoming the 'forgotten mourner' because he is not as verbal and outward in his grief as wife is. Ultimately, failure to acknowledge and appropriately grieve the losses of male-factor infertility impacts a man's long-term adjustment to infertility, as well as his perspective and decisions regarding parenthood and DI as a family-building option.

CLINICAL ISSUES

DI is not a treatment for infertility. It does not provide a 'cure' or medical treatment for male-factor infertility. As such, even if parenthood is achieved via the use of donated sperm, the diagnosis and etiology of male-factor infertility remains unchanged. DI is an effective and positive method for building a family, enabling involuntarily childless men and women to become parents. Couples choose DI as a family-building alternative over adoption because it is expeditious, less expensive, and allows for control of the prenatal environment and the experience of pregnancy, as well as providing a genetic link to one marital partner. For many men, DI is a positive choice because it allows them to support their wife's pregnancy in the traditional manner and gives them a feeling of control and contribution toward the couple's desired goal: parenthood. By contrast, a couple may choose adoptive parenthood over DI because it provides an equitable connection to the child for each partner in the relationship, because it is consonant with personal or a couple's values (e.g., believing that it is better to give a home to an existing child rather than create another), because pregnancy is unimportant to both partners, because DI is inconsistent with religious beliefs (e.g., believing that it is unethical or immoral to use donor gametes or procreate without sexual intercourse), or because one or both partners has a special connection or investment in adoption.

Couples considering DI may be referred to an infertility counselor or decide on their own to seek counseling prior to treatment. Increasingly, infertile couples are required to receive educational counseling as part of medical treatment before undergoing DI. In such cases, counseling is generally a unique combination of educational, therapeutic, and evaluative components. As in all psychotherapy, reasons for presenting to counseling are instrumental in determining treatment agendas and goals.

Infertility counselors working with medical practices must make the treatment goals and agendas clear to couples at the outset. This may be done through a standard informed psychological consent form and, if the infertility counselor is independent of the medical practice, a signed authorization for release of information to the referring physician or clinic (see Appendix 11). In some cases, the medical practice expects an evaluation that is instrumental in determining whether or not the couple proceeds with further medical treatment. However, in most cases, the medical practice expects the infertility counselor to assess the couple's readiness, outline any special circumstances or issues that contraindicate the couple's proceeding with medical treatment, and, foremost, educate the couple about the psychosocial issues and implications of sperm donation and about special parenting tasks. Although infertility counselors are sometimes expected to provide a 'screening opinion', in most practices decisions about patients' or couples' proceeding with treatment are not their sole prerogative. In the majority of infertility practices, these are treatment team decisions or, ultimately, the treating physician's prerogative.

Sometimes a couple is referred for educational counseling, and it becomes clear that they are not ready to proceed with medical treatment and/or are unprepared for parenthood via donated gametes. Clearly in need of additional counseling, the couple may decide on therapy with the infertility counselor with a new set of therapeutic goals, or they may prefer to be referred to another infertility counselor in preparation for DI later. Although it is probably ideal for the couple to be referred to a separate infertility counselor for psychotherapy, this is not always logistically feasible or preferable to the couple who do not want to start over with someone new.

When a couple is self-referred for DI counseling, the goals and agenda of counseling are explicitly therapeutic. In these cases, the couple presents for counseling with the mindful purpose of addressing marital conflict, especially regarding the decision to pursue DI; exploring the implications of the husband's infertility; grieving the actual or potential loss of the genetically-shared child they had dreamed of; and examining DI as a family-building alternative, including sperm bank choices, known versus anonymous donor, treatment preferences, and the issue of disclosure. In addition, the infertility counselor guides the couple in their

Table 1 Deciding between donor insemination (DI) and adoption

Pros of DI

Wife genetically connected to child

Able to have more genetic information about the child than adoption

Husband and wife able to share pregnancy experience

Able to control the prenatal environment

Typically more expeditious than adoption

Typically less expensive than adoption

More 'normal' or typical means of family building, therefore less stigma for whole family

Cons of DI

Inequity of husband and wife's genetic relationship to the child

Inability of parent to accept child who is not biologically related to father

Legal concerns in some states

Religious, ethical, or moral objections to this means of family building

Pressures of unique method of parenthood: secrecy, lack of genetic information

exploration of the myriad choices regarding the implications of medical treatment, family-building options, and childlessness. Support groups for couples considering or undergoing DI may be particularly helpful in assisting in the understanding, acceptance, and decision-making about donor issues (see Chapter 7).

It is important that infertility counselors maintain a neutral position and support the couple's process of exploration of all of the issues and consequences of choosing DI as a means of family building. Although they may have their personal bias about such issues as secrecy and disclosure, therapists must present the pros and cons of each position in a balanced and unbiased manner. It may also be helpful for therapeutic goal-setting to provide patients with a short list of the relevant issues of DI so that they understand the process of therapy (Tables 1 and 2).

THERAPEUTIC INTERVENTIONS

Therapeutic interventions in DI counseling may cover three areas:

- exploring the implications (both medical and emotional) of male-factor infertility
- grieving the loss of the genetically-shared pregnancy or child
- examining DI as a family-building alternative, including assessing readiness, providing support, and addressing disclosure issues.

Exploring the Implications of Male-Factor Infertility

Exploring the implications of male-factor infertility involves inquiring about a man's understanding of his infertility diagnosis, as well as his feelings about it.

Implications of the Medical Condition

Contrary to many myths and misconceptions, infertility affects men as often as it does women: 40% of infertility is caused by a male factor and 40% by a female factor. The most frequent causes of male-factor infertility are problems with sperm production, sperm transport, and fertilization. Sperm production or transport may be affected by genetic disorders, illness, injury, or ingestion or exposure to toxic agents. Mumps orchitis and testicular cancer, for example, destroy the ability to produce sperm. Other causes of male-factor infertility are inherited or genetic disorders such Klinefelter's syndrome and congenital bilateral absence of the vas deferens (CBAVD). Although there has been some awareness of the effect of toxic agents on male-factor infertility, it is only recently that men have become more educated about protecting their reproductive health by not smoking tobacco, abusing alcohol, or using recreational drugs (particularly

Table 2 Considerations regarding openness versus secrecy

Pros for openness

Avoids burden of deceiving child (and others) over a lifetime

Avoids burden of others' deceiving child over a lifetime

Avoids chance disclosure by others or discovery of secret by child

Acknowledges ethical right of child to know circumstances of his/her conception

Allows child to integrate truth of conception into his/her identity in normative fashion

Information about child's genetic parentage available for later circumstances

Pros of secrecy

Father's infertility to remain secret, protected

Avoids stigma of unique conception for child

Avoids potential stigma for other family members or family as a whole

Avoids potential legal problems

Extended family or friends unable to respect boundaries, have potential for destructive or retaliative behavior, or believe choice is sinful and will, as a result, treat child badly

Current practice of donor anonymity means child unlikely to have information or access to donor

marijuana); wearing boxer underwear; avoiding overheating of the testicles (e.g., hot tubs); and watching their general health habits.

Historically, it was thought that most male-factor infertility was idiopathic, caused by idiosyncratic problems that could not be treated and were thus of little import to couple decision-making. There were few treatment options for male-factor infertility (especially azoospermia), the most common being insemination with the husband's sperm after it was spun and 'washed'. If this failed, it was not long before couples with male-factor infertility were considering DI. Making these considerations more difficult was the reality that the infertility was inexplicable: often, there was no identi-

fiable causative factor that could help the man and his spouse adjust to the diagnosis. By contrast, today, an increasing number of male-factor infertility problems can be diagnosed and treated with increasingly sophisticated and successful procedures. In addition, an increasing number of patients are men who have had a vasectomy and, due to changed life circumstances, wish to pursue reproduction again (see Chapter 16).

In recent years, several treatment options have become available, including intracytoplasmic sperm injection (ICSI), microsurgical epididymal sperm aspiration (MESA), and testicular sperm extraction (TESE). Treatments such as MESA and TESE help to overcome sperm transport problems, while ICSI helps overcome sperm penetration and mobility problems. However, as in the majority of male-factor infertility therapies, the lion's share of treatment is still experienced by the woman, who undergoes ovulation induction and in vitro fertilization (IVF) to maximize the potential for conception and the chance of having a genetically-shared child, even though her fertility may not be impaired in any way.

Recent advances in genetics indicate that a significant portion of severe male-infertility (azoospermia and oligospermia) may be due to genetic disorders involving CBAVD, microdeletions on the Y chromosome, and/or subtle abnormalities in other genes that are often not detectable on a gross karyotype[38]. This discovery has altered the significance of male-factor infertility for many men: instead of an idiopathic problem, these men have a genetic disorder that may have significant ramifications for their health, as well as their reproductive ability. For example, azoospermic men with CBAVD have been found to be at increased risk for cystic fibrosis but have often been asymptomatic. With the discovery of the infertility problem, they also discover the presence of a genetic disorder and potentially life-threatening or life-altering medical problem (see Chapter 11).

These discoveries have also impacted men's reproductive choices. While ICSI now allows men with severe defects in spermatogenesis to reproduce, MESA and TESE allow the transmission of genetic mutations, the consequences of which are not yet understood. For this reason, some European countries, including the Health Council of the Netherlands, issued an immediate moratorium on MESA and TESE, until further research is completed on the rate of transmission of chromosomal aberrations and abnormalities, as well as a call for additional counseling for couples considering the use of ICSI, MESA, and TESE[39].

For many couples with male-factor infertility, ICSI, MESA, and TESE represent treatment choices that make a genetically-shared pregnancy more feasible than ever before, but not without significant demands and drawbacks. Increasingly, couples with male-factor infertility are being offered these options as a medical treatment alternative or as a diagnostic tool. A growing concern for infertility counselors is that this option is often presented with the possibility of 'donor backup', if fertilization fails. While ICSI, MESA, or TESE allows a couple to pursue a genetically-shared pregnancy, 'donor backup' does not do so, and this distinction is not always implicitly clear to couples, who are often anxious and driven in their desire to conceive. Making treatment decisions much more complicated is the potential of passing on genetic anomalies, having children with chromosomal disorders, having a donor child or, worse, twins who have different genetic fathers, without adequate consideration or preparation. In short, many infertile men and women are ill-prepared for the complexities and challenges of these treatments or potential outcomes. They have not been properly counseled or equipped to handle the potential distress that conception via assisted reproductive technologies impose on a couple.

For these reasons, couples considering ICSI, MESA, and TESE must be informed about the possibilities and range of risks: that more is unknown than known at this time and that the potential impact on a man's future health, as well as on genetic children or subsequent generations, is unclear. Thus, these couples may not simply be making a decisions for the most expeditious means of genetically-shared parenthood. More important, they may be making decisions about their child's well-being, genetic makeup, and even, unknowingly, inherited genetic disorders, with unknown health consequences that may have been prevented (see Chapter 11).

Implications of the Emotional Response

Some men, like some women, find integrating medical information about themselves both difficult and detestable. Refusing to accept the reality of male-factor infertility and its implications, some men may use inappropriate means of handling their feelings; these include sexual acting out such as affairs or seeing prostitutes; bullying, controlling, or blaming their wife or medical caregivers; or trying to escape their feelings through alcohol, drugs, or gambling. In addition, male-factor infertility may precipitate disturbing, intrusive changes in a man's body image and sexual functioning; flashbacks of sexual vulnerability unresolved from adolescence; or spontaneous, negative visual imagery of a defective body[40].

Many men encounter difficulty maintaining positive self-esteem and self-image, especially if they have preexisting shame about their body, heightened guilt feelings, or misperceptions about bad behavior causing infertility. There is clinical evidence that men who have significant difficulty and are more devastated by a diagnosis of male-infertility are (1) men who were emotionally close to their fathers, while growing up, and/or have positive internalized images of fatherhood; (2) men who highly value their genetic lineage or bloodlines; (3) men with preexisting narcissistic wounds about body image and masculinity; and (4) men with preexisting sexual problems[27]. Intense feelings of defectiveness need to be processed before proceeding to DI, for the well-being of the man, the family, and the child conceived by DI, whom the man may later view as a mark of his impairment instead of the joy of his life.

Men are socialized to take responsibility for the well-being of others, especially their family. Consequently, infertile men believe their role is to take care of their wife, whom they perceive as more upset or more entitled to distress. As a result, men may agree to DI as an alternative to make their wife happy, not because it is their choice. Although it can be difficult to get men to express these vulnerable feelings, becoming a DI father before such emotions are worked through may pose some hazards to the father–child bond.

Exploring the implications of male-factor infertility also means that the husband is able to acknowledge and accept his wife's painful feelings of loss without feeling responsible, blamed, or shamed. In fact, her losses may trigger some of his losses (e.g., she will not carry his baby). While the husband's losses are fundamental, the wife's losses are as important, warranting equal recognition and validation. A couple's relationship can become closer and stronger by each partner's recognizing, confirming, and sharing their pain and grieving the losses of male-factor infertility together. Acknowledgment and acceptance of male infertility means giving it a personal meaning, improving decision-making skills, prompting a closer marital relationship, reevaluating the meaning of masculinity and parenthood, and becoming aware of inner resources.

Finally, cultural issues may be a factor and are especially relevant in the matter of male-factor infertility. There may be strong, culturally defined attitudes regarding masculinity, fertility, virility, and male roles that influence a man's emotional response to infertility and consideration of DI. Cultural values and fundamental beliefs are not always apparent, especially if the man and his partner do not present with obvious cultural differences (see Chapter 13).

Grieving the Genetically-shared Pregnancy

It is probably self-evident that every couple pursuing parenthood, plan, wish, and hope for a genetically-shared pregnancy, a child that is a genetic link to both parents. The genetically-shared pregnancy and child represent all the things that the couple had hoped and dreamed for in their child. Letting go and saying goodbye to this child is a painful process and represents the most significant loss to be grieved in the genetically-shared pregnancy. Grieving the loss of the genetically-shared pregnancy also entails mourning the husband's biological connection to the child, the marital equity of each parent's connection to the child, and the couple's reproductive plans and choices.

Grieving the genetically-shared pregnancy involves deciding to end treatment in which the genetically-shared, biological pregnancy is the goal and addressing the myriad issues of 'when enough is enough'. It may begin with a medical opinion that the prognosis does not warrant continued medical treatment with the couple's gametes, or with the couple's realization that their financial and/or emotional resources are seriously diminished. One or both partners, in shock and disbelief, may have difficulty accepting the prognosis, insist on second and third opinions, or continue treatment despite poor predictions of success. Furthermore, evaluating their resources—time, money, energy, hope, courage, and commitment—couples may have difficulty in accepting that further investment will not produce successful results. Either partner may react with anger and protest at how unfair infertility is, how uncontrollable the future has become, how things are not as they should be, or how this is not what either partner wants or deserves.

The anger of grief may be the most comfortable emotion for many men with male-factor infertility. As a result, the targets of their far-reaching and all-encompassing anger may be to direct it at their wife, medical caregivers, insurance companies, coworkers, siblings, and ultimately themselves. Further, men who place considerable faith and optimism in science and technology, may feel shocked and betrayed when assisted reproductive technologies are not successful. Their anger is as much about the failure as it is about the loss of a predictable and understandable world. Alternatively, wives' anger may be toward their partner, whom they perceive as unable to give them what they most want. Although angry, women may also feel guilt, remorse, and shame about these feelings and yet are unable to relinquish or reconcile them. As a result, many women attempt to protect themselves and their husband from their anger, in that preventing the expression of his anger will avoid triggering her own.

Couples' conflict is a frequent response to grieving the genetically-shared pregnancy. The wife may feel that she can no longer continue treatment, while her husband still holds hope for success. By the same token, couples' conflict may erupt around family-building options. Couples may experience, in isolation or together, a multitude of feelings: depression, guilt, shame, defensiveness, and anger. Unfortunately, grief can complicate conflict resolution, making shared perceptions and easy communication difficult and conflict resolution very challenging.

At times, couples may want to proceed quickly to DI as a means of avoiding painful feelings and grief. Hence, it is helpful to have a protocol time period, for example, 3–6 months, between receiving the diagnosis and being apprised of the option of DI, and undergoing treatment. Grieving the loss of a shared child must occur before decisions on alternative family-building can be made. Ideally, a level of reorganization and transcendence regarding infertility will have been reached before couples attempt to examine the myriad issues of DI as a family-building alternative. They will have been able to integrate the experience and not be overwhelmed by distress, sadness, and emotional reactivity triggered by grief and loss.

Examining Donor Insemination as a Family-Building Alternative

The three important issues of DI counseling to be addressed include assessing readiness, providing support, and addressing disclosure issues.

Assessing Readiness

Fundamental to assessing a couple's readiness for DI is an exploration of their reasons (individually and as a couple) for actively choosing the use of donated sperm to build their family. First, it is paramount that both partners have a thorough understanding of what the use of donated gametes entails, and have considered the pros and cons of DI (Table 3). Second, the couple should show positive marital and sexual functioning, healthy communication, and good problem-solving skills. Third, both partners have grieved the loss of the genetically-shared child that they had hoped to have and consider the use of donated sperm as a positive option. Fourth, the couple understands the implications of secrecy versus disclosure and the responsibilities of their choice, and are comfortable with them. Finally, the couple has agreed on a plan regarding their choice. Many couples find it helpful to make a plan 'for now' regarding their choice, which they agree to reevaluate later, either at a set date or as situations develop. In this way, the couple does not have to agree on a 'decision to last a lifetime'.

Neither partner should acquiesce to DI because it has been medically recommended and is the next step in the infertility treatment plan, nor should they do so if it has been suggested as 'donor backup' for other medical treatments because, as such, it is a decision by default without careful consideration. Further, neither partner should be coerced, bullied, or pressured into proceeding with DI as a means of parenthood or before they are prepared. Assessing readiness often entails exploring or investigating subtle and overt pressures regarding DI; for example, a husband who had a vasectomy during a previous marriage and is ambivalent about repeat parenthood, or a wife for whom pregnancy is a paramount requirement of motherhood. For this reason, it is imperative that the couple agree on the decision to proceed with the use of donated sperm and consider it a positive alternative.

Although a screening process is often in place, it is ultimately better when couples 'screen themselves out' by recognizing either that the choice is not for them, that they are not in agreement, or that one or both partners are not prepared. Often, screening means postponing proceeding with treatment and allowing couples the opportunity to address their problems in therapy in preparation for proceeding at a later date. However, there are instances in which screening may result in denial of treatment; these include evidence of relationship instability, overt psychopathology, nonacceptance of the procedure by one partner, or evidence of coercion[19].

Providing Support

A primary role of infertility counselors is to provide education and support while a couple addresses DI as an option for family building. This includes providing both partners a professional, unbiased environment for the free expression of feelings and the safe exploration of beliefs and attitudes about the use of donated gametes. In addition, it involves provision of various education materials regarding the psychosocial aspects of male-factor infertility, DI, the use of donated gametes, and medical treatment of male-factor infertility. Couples are interested in information that provides a fair presentation of the different aspects of DI, as well as access to information that is not readily available through their own resources, for example, the opportunity to page through available storybooks for children on DI (see Resources at the end of the volume).

When considering DI, couples must consider the special circumstances of their own lives, cultures, and personalities, and recognize the genetic inequity of the choice. The infertility counselor can support both partners as they explore their feelings about the fact that DI will make the father's genetic relationship to the child (and that of his genetic relatives) uneven and inequitable to the child's relationship with the mother (and her genetic relatives). For many couples, this is one of the primary negative aspects of DI, while for other couples genetic and biological linkages are unimportant.

Table 3 Pros and cons proceeding with donor insemination (DI)

Indications	Contraindications
Husband	*Husband*
• Able to put his feelings into words about his inability to be a genetic father	• Would see the donor child as a symbol of his failure as a man
• Supportive, with positive feelings about the alternative	• Feels intensely guilty about the infertility diagnosis
• Not being coerced, assuaging his guilt about his infertility, avoiding his grief, or using DI to prevent dissolution of the marriage	
• Addressed his feelings about his relationship with his parents, defined fatherhood for himself, and has positive feelings about his own role as a father	
• Shows evidence of good self-esteem, which he feels will be further enhanced by choosing fatherhood through DI	
• Has intact body image and integrated the infertility diagnosis into a sense of self	
• Able to picture himself in the future with his donor child, without minimizing the complexities of the choice	
Wife	*Wife*
• Sorted out her own feelings of loss about not having her husband's child	• Coercing husband to pursue DI and/or parenthood, and would retaliate or leave the marriage if he does not acquiesce
• Continues to hold her husband in positive regard despite the infertility diagnosis and does not denigrate him regarding his reproductive ability or sexuality	
• Sensitive to the issues posed by having a genetic bond with the child that her husband will not	
• Able to picture herself in the future with his donor child, without minimizing the complexities of the choice	
Couple	*Couple*
• Positive marital and couple functioning evidenced by good communication and problem-solving	• Intense marital instability or conflict, especially about infertility, treatment, and/or DI
• Have grieved the loss of the genetically-shared child that they had hoped to have	• Objection to DI by either partner for any reasons
• Have thoroughly considered the pros and cons of DI	• Presence of significant psychopathology in either partner
• Have thoroughly considered the implications of secrecy versus disclosure, agreed on a plan for the present and future regarding their choice, and understand the implications and responsibilities of their choice	• Current alcohol or drug abuse
	• Impaired cognitive functioning or mental incompetence so that either partner is unable to provide an informed consent or understand the short- and long-term implications of choice
	• History in relationship of violence or emotional, physical, or sexual abuse in either partner
	• History of child abuse, neglect, or abandonment in either partner
	• History of legal problems, especially involving criminal activity, in either partner

Some couples, having decided on DI, seek counseling for support as they consider their beliefs and preferences about the donor: do they wish to use a known (identified) sperm donor (e.g., father, brother, cousin, or friend) or an anonymous donor? How much information do they want about the donor? Do they want the child to be able to contact the donor at a later date? Or as they consider their preferences regarding the sperm bank: how much information is provided about the donor? What are the bank's policies about anonymity, donor profiles, donor availability, and/or agreeability to contact from adult offspring? Again, the infertility counselor can be helpful in providing additional information or resources for couples during their decision-making process.

Once these decisions have been agreed on, Vercollone and associates[41] suggest that a couple determine whom they will include in their 'inner circle of confidantes', that is, with whom they as a couple or as individuals will discuss DI. Whatever the couple has decided regarding secrecy (privacy) and disclosure, they must agree on a few close intimates (friends or family) who will be privy to the information. Some couples may decide to tell no one, in which case the infertility counselor and/or medical staff becomes their primary support network regarding DI. Other couples elect certain close family and friends, while others are eager and willing to make their decision very public (e.g., newspaper articles, television appearances). In these considerations, the couple should contemplate their unborn child's privacy, realizing that once the information is shared, it is no longer the child's information to share about him- or herself. Furthermore, decisions on the 'inner circle of confidants' may reflect clashing beliefs or even unhealthy attitudes about boundaries: boundaries that are too permeable versus boundaries that are too rigid.

Finally, couples must be reassured again and again that this is *their* decision and only theirs. Infertility counselors can be helpful sources of support and information, providing an unbiased perspective and acting as a sounding board for ideas or a mediator for disagreements, but in the end it is the couple who must decide when, where, and how they will proceed with the use of donated gametes to build their family.

Addressing Disclosure Issues

Historically and traditionally, the practice of using donated sperm has been strongly influenced by secrecy and donor anonymity for several reasons: to bond the child emotionally to the recipient father, to keep the father's infertility secret, to protect the father's self esteem, to enhance parental feelings of 'ownership' or 'entitlement' to the child, to avoid any potential negative psychological effects on the child, to deter any social stigmatization for any of the family members, to maintain privacy for the family, and to avoid any legal issues[42,43]. In addition, parents state that they do not want to tell their child because they do not have adequate information on how and when to tell the child, and because there is only limited information available on an anonymous donor.

An increasing number of mental health professionals and consumers have advocated against secrecy and deception, and for a greater degree of openness, suggesting that not only do donor children have a *right* to know but they *need* to know the truth about their conception[44-47]. They argue that truthful information about a child's conception and access to information about the donor (e.g., diagnosis of a genetic medical disorder) is fundamental to a child's identity formation. Furthermore, the burden of long-term deception, the corrosive effects of secrets, and the perpetuation of a delusion regarding parentage may contribute to adjustment problems in parents, children, and the family. Many professionals also believe that donor children will intuitively figure out that something is going on in the family, and that their suspicions (e.g., mother had an affair) or fantasies (e.g., a virgin birth) are more destructive than the truth[48]. Finally, openness is often encouraged because it enables parents to control the process of revelation (as opposed to unintended disclosure).

Today, few mental health professionals rigidly advocate secrecy or disclosure, preferring a 'client self-determination' or 'modified disclosure' approach[19,41]. This moderate, social work perspective advocates the right of clients to self-determination regarding decisions about disclosure and nondisclosure. The client self-determination approach recognizes the positives of openness, as well as the fact that some families have good reasons for maintaining secrecy or a certain level of privacy. For some families, reasons for nondisclosure, secrecy, or measured privacy include family-of-origin issues, the inability of family and friends to respect boundaries, concern that the information would be used in a destructive or retaliatory manner or that it would increase stigma for the child or family within the family's social network, or evidence of family dysfunction or individual psychopathology. The client-determination approach takes into consideration the family's special circumstances, the stage of the family's development, the environment or community in which the family lives, and the child's personality, stability, and age.

According to research studies and our clinical experience, the primary desire of couples considering DI and parents who have not yet disclosed to their child is for more detailed information. Parents would like specific guidance on how and when to tell, delivered in a nondogmatic, nonbiased fashion. Parents also want respect for their doubts and fears and acknowledgment of their ability to eventually discern and choose what is best for their children. In addition, parents want accounts from other parents who have moved slowly toward openness in a way that maintained as much privacy as possible in the wider world. Finally, parents want educational materials including books on DI, storybooks for children, and more personal accounts of donor offspring. Several recent books and articles are helpful to parents understanding the experience of parents and children in donor-formed families[41,49,50] (see Resources).

It is important to note that since the 1950s at least a million DI children have been born in the United States during the practice of secrecy/privacy and anonymity. However, there has not been a spontaneous eruption of vast numbers of donor families seeking or needing psychological assistance or searching for donor 'fathers'. Although there have been popular press reports of disturbed parent–child relationships following DI, these are not the majority of accounts or clinical evidence. Furthermore, there has been some research on adult offspring discovering their donor conception later on in life, indicating that the offspring were not traumatized or rejecting of their psychosocial father[51].

FUTURE IMPLICATIONS

In spite of recent advances in the treatment of male-factor infertility, DI will continue to provide a viable option for family-building. While male-factor infertility has been shrouded in secrecy, infertile men have been isolated from emotional support and information regarding the frequency or occurrence of this condition. These men need more first-person accounts of the reactions of other men to their involuntary childlessness. In addition, they need to learn more of the experiences of men who have chosen different pathways: parenthood by DI, adoption, generativity through relationships with others' children, and child-free living. In general, more open communication about these issues within society will help diminish the shame and stigma that surround male-factor infertilty and DI.

Infertility counselors must be advocates with reluctant caregivers for a more balanced and informed approach to educating patients about DI, especially about disclosure. They need to advocate for clinics to use sperm banks, which may allow more specific information on the donor, or the possibility of some form of contact between adult donor children and their genetic fathers. This may take the form of a central donor registry. Also, mental health professionals need to continue to advocate for counseling services for all patients considering DI, especially when it is offered as a 'backup' for ICSI, MESA, and TESE. Medical teams must be prepared to offer parents and donor offspring supportive services or referral, not only at the time that services are provided but long into the future.

Although there has been considerable research on DI, there are a number of areas where information is sorely limited. Research is needed addressing more diverse populations, including nonwhite, non-middle-class fathers who have achieved parenthood through DI; comparison and longitudinal studies of different infertile populations; investigation of long-term family adjustment, comparing families who have chosen openness versus families who have chosen to be private/secretive about their child's donor conception; and evaluating the impact of class, race, culture, and religion on men's feelings about their infertility; as well as how infertile men's feelings have changed over time. Because of shame and stigma, selection bias and small sample sizes have been problems with the existing research on families created by DI. In addition, medical teams should begin to ask patients who pursue DI whether or not they would be willing to be contacted in the future.

Prospective parents need more descriptive literature that helps them understand the experience of growing up knowing that one was conceived through DI. Patient education materials, including children's books that assist parents in understanding the issues and implications of raising a donor-conceived child, need to be more readily available.

SUMMARY

- Although DI has been occurring for almost 100 years, the recognition of the need for patient counseling regarding the implications of treatment has been recent but well established.
- Infertility counseling for couples pursing DI includes exploring the medical and emotional implications of male-factor infertility, grieving the genetically-shared pregnancy, and thoroughly examining DI as a family-building option.
- Infertility counselors must be prepared to assess for readiness, identify any issues or circumstances that contra-indicate proceeding with treatment, and provide ongoing education and support to DI couples.
- It is important that infertility counselors actively help couples process their infertility experience and assist them in making an informed decision about whether or not to use DI to create a family. This involves knowing about the common advantages and disadvantages of using donor sperm and being knowledgeable about community resources.
- Although there has been an increasing

push for openness in DI families, the vast majority of couples choose *not* to disclose to their child the truth about his or her donor conception.

- Reasons for openness include feeling that the child has a right and/or need to know the truth about conception and birth, a belief that keeping the secret would be destructive or impossible, a belief that it would be bad for the family as a whole to have a secret, and increasing social and emotional support through resources, groups, and educational materials.

- Reasons for nondisclosure are a desire to keep the man's infertility private, fears that the child will not love the psychosocial father once the secret is out, fears that the child will be stigmatized by others, and a belief that being truthful about the child's genetic origins is pointless because there is little opportunity for contact or additional information on the donor/ genetic father.

- Infertility counselors must be aware of their personal biases regarding disclosure and nondisclosure and remain neutral in counseling to allow couples to determine what is best for them.

Acknowledgment

The authors wish to thank Carol Frost Vercollone for her substantial contribution to this chapter.

REFERENCES

1. Klock SC. Psychological aspects of donor insemination. *Infertil Reprod Med Clin North Am* 1993;4:455–69

2. Daniels KR. Artificial insemination using donor semen and the issue of secrecy: The views of donors and recipient couples. *Soc Sci Med* 1988;27:377–83

3. MacNab RT. Psychological issues associated with donor insemination. In: Seibel MM, Crockin SL, eds. *Family Building Through Egg and Sperm Donation: Medical, Legal, and Ethical Issues*. Boston: Jones and Bartlett, 1996;53–60

4. Orenstein P. Looking for a donor to call dad. *New York Times Magazine* June 18, 1995:28–51

5. Kedem P, Mulincer M, Nathanson Y, Bartoov B. Psychological aspects of male infertility. *Br J Med Psychol* 1990;63:73–80

6. Nachtigall R, Becker G, Wozny M. The effects of gender-specific diagnosis on men's and women's response to infertility. *Fertil Steril* 1992;57:113–21

7. Mason M. *Male Infertility: Men Talking*. New York: Routledge, 1993

8. Wendland CL, Byrn F, Hill C. Donor insemination: A comparison of lesbian couples, heterosexual couples, and single women. *Fert Steril* 1996;65:764–70

9. Klock SC, Maier D. Psychological factors related to donor insemination. *Fertil Steril* 1991;56:489–95

10. Milson I, Bergman P. A study of parental attitudes after donor insemination (AID). *Acta Obstet Gynecol Scand* 1982;61:125–8

11. Clayton CE, Kovacs CT. AID offspring: Initial follow-up of 50 couples. *Med J Aust* 1982;1:338–9

12. Amuzu B, Laxova R, Shapiro SS. Pregnancy outcome, health of children, and family adjustment after donor insemination. *Obstet Gyencol* 1990;75:899–905

13. Bendvold E, Skjaeraasen J, Moe N, *et al.* Marital break-up among couples raising families by artificial insemination by donor. *Fertil Steril* 1989;51:980–3

14. Klock S, Jacob M, Maier D. A prospective study of donor insemination recipients: Secrecy, privacy and disclosure. *Fertil Steril* 1994;62:477–84

15. Golombok S, Cook R, Bish A, Murray C. Families created by the new reproductive technologies: Quality of parenting and social and emotional development of the children. *Child Dev* 1995;66:285–98

16. Schover LR, Collins R, Richards S . Psycho-

logical aspects of donor insemination: Evaluation and follow-up of recipient couples. *Fertil Steril* 1992;584–9

17. Zoldbrod AP. The emotional distress of the artificial insemination patient. *Med Psychother* 1988;1:161–72

18. Mechanick-Braverman A, Corson S. Factors related to preferences in gamete donor sources. *Fertil Steril* 1995:6;543–9

19. Klock SC. To tell or not to tell: The issue of privacy and disclosure in infertility treatment. In: Lieblum SR, ed. *Infertility: Psychological Issues and Counseling Strategies*. New York: Wiley, 1997;167–88

20. Nachtigall RD, Quiroga SS, Tschann JM, *et al*. Stigma, disclosure, and family functioning among parents of children conceived through donor insemination. *Fertil Steril* 1997;68:1–7

21. Berger DM, Eisen A, Suber J, *et al*. Psychological patterns in donor insemination couples. *Can J Psychiatry* 1986;31:818–23

22. Cook R, Golombok F, Bish A, *et al*. Disclosure of donor insemination: Parental attitudes. *Am J Orthopsychiatry* 1995;65:549–59

23. Manuel C, Chevret M, Cyzba J. Handling the secrecy by AID couples. In: David G, Price E, eds. *Human Artificial Insemination and Semen Preservation*. New York: Plenum, 1980;419–30

24. Rowland R. The social and psychological consequences of secrecy in artificial insemination by donor (AID) programmes. *Soc Sci Med* 1985;21:391–6

25. Sewall G, Mason L. Parental acceptance, disclosure, and decision making amongst recipients in an anonymous donor oocyte program. In: Program and Abstracts of the American Society for Reproductive Medicine, 1995 Annual Meeting, Seattle, WA. Birmingham, AL: American Society for Reproduction Medicine, 1995;S252–3

26. Gerstel G. A psychoanalytic view of artificial donor insemination. *Am J Psychother* 1963;17:64–77

27. Zoldbrod A. *Men, Women and Infertility: Intervention and Treatment Strategies*. New York: Lexington Books, 1993

28. Goffman E. *Stigma: Notes on the Management of Spoiled Identity*. Englewood Cliffs, NJ: Prentice-Hall, 1963

29. Kohut H. *The Restoration of the Self*. New York: International Universities Press, 1977

30. Mazor M. Emotional reactions to infertility. In: Mazor M, Simons H, eds. *Infertlity: Medical, Emotional and Social Considerations*. New York: Human Sciences Press, 1984; 23–35

31. Fisher S. *Sexual Images of the Self: The Psychology of Erotic Sensations and Illusion*. Hillsdale, NJ: Erlbaum, 1989

32. Menning B. *Infertility: A Guide for the Childless Couple*, 2nd edn. New York: Prentice-Hall Press, 1988

33. Owens D. The desire to father: Reproductive ideologies and involuntarily childless men. In: McKee L, O'Brien M, eds. *The Father Figure*. London: Tavistock, 1982

34. Pleck J, Sawyer J, eds. *Men and Masculinity*. Englewood Cliffs, NJ: Prentice-Hall, 1974

35. Levant R, Kopecky G. *Masculinity Reconstructed: Changing the Rules of Manhood*. New York: Dutton, 1995

36. Snarey J, Son L, Kuehne U, Valliant G. The role of parenting in men's psychosocial development: A longitudinal study of early adulthood infertility and mid-life generativity. *Dev Psychol* 1987;23:593–603

37. Menning BE. Donor insemination: The psychosocial issues. *Contemp Obstet Gynecol* 1981;10:155–72

38. Reijo R. Diverse spermatogenic defects in humans caused by Y chromosome deletions encompassing a novel RNA-binding protein gene. *Nature Genet* 1995;10:383

39. How to resolve ICSI genetic dilemmas. *IVF News* 1996;7:3

40. Zoldbrod A. *Getting Around the Boulder in the Road: Using Imagery to Cope with Fertility Problems*. Lexington, MA: The Center for Reproductive Problems, 1990

41. Vercollone C, Moss R, Moss H. *Helping the Stork: The Choices and Challenges of Donor Insemination*. New York: Macmillan, 1997

42. Marsh M, Ronner W. *The Empty Cradle: Infertility in America from Colonial Times to the Present*. Baltimore: Johns Hopkins University Press, 1996

43. May ET. *Barren in the Promised Land: Childless Americans and the Pursuit of Happiness*. New York: Basic Books, 1995

44. McWhinnie A. A study of parenting of IVF and DI children. *Medicine Law* 1995;14(7–8): 501–8

45. Gordon ER. Blended families: Adopted, ART, and natural children. In: Postgraduate course XII: ART parents and children. American Society for Reproductive Medicine, Seatttle, WA, October 7–8, 1995;78–83

46. Lieber-Wilkins C. Talking to children about their conception: A parent's perspective. In: Postgraduate course XII: ART parents and children. American Society for Reproductive Medicine, Seattle, WA, October 7–8, 1995;163–73

47. Barran A, Pannor R. *Lethal Secrets*. New York: Amistad Press, 1993

48. Snowden R, Mitchell GD. *The Artificial Family: A Consideration of Artificial Insemination by Donor*. London: Unwin Books, 1981

49. Sherry SN, Sherry M. Explaining gamete donation to children. In: Seibel MM, Crockin SL, ed. *Family Building Through Egg and Sperm Donation: Medical, Legal, and Ethical Issues*. Boston: Jones and Barlett, 1996;274–7

50. Topp K. Personal perspective: Positive reflections: Growing up as a D.I. child. *Can J Hum Sex* 1993;2:149–51

51. Snowden R, Mitchell GD, Snowden B. *Artificial Reproduction: A Social Investigation*. Winchester, MA: International Publishers, 1983

19

Recipient Counseling for Oocyte Donation

Dorothy A. Greenfeld, MSW

there is only one image in this culture of the 'good mother' ...
She loves her children completely and unambivalently.

Jane Lazarre

HISTORICAL OVERVIEW

The first pregnancy achieved as a result of oocyte donation (OD) was reported in 1984 by a group from Monash University in Australia[1]. A 25-year-old woman with premature ovarian failure was the recipient of a single oocyte donated by a 29-year-old woman undergoing an in vitro fertilization (IVF) cycle. Since that initial success, OD has become increasingly acceptable and integral part of assisted reproductive technology programs around the world[2–4]. On this continent, for example, a 1993 registry of births from assisted reproductive technologies reported that in that 1 year alone there were 135 OD programs in the United States and Canada, resulting in 227 live-born infants[5].

This successful technique is a reproductive advance that allows the retrieval of eggs from one woman, their fertilization through the process of IVF, and their transfer to the uterus of another woman; it extends the potential for pregnancy to an entirely new cohort of women heretofore unable to conceive. Typical candidates for this treatment are women with premature ovarian failure or surgically removed ovaries, carriers of genetic disease, and those with diminished ovarian function due to treatment for cancer with chemotherapy and/or radiation[6]. Moreover, since substantial evidence suggests that much of female infertility is due to poor-quality embryos rather than poor-quality endometrium (egg quality may become diminished, but the uterus carries on), a rapidly expanding group of patients is participating in OD[7–9]. This group includes women who have a history of failed IVF treatment or of repeated pregnancy loss as well as those who are postmenopausal or of advanced reproductive age[10]

The success of OD, in which the pregnancy rates are double those of standard IVF[5], is somewhat diminished by the complexity of ethical and psychological concerns surrounding the treatment. These concerns include increasing numbers of women well past reproductive age who are becoming mothers; sisters or other relatives donating ova within a family, thereby creating wholly unique bonds within families; and the payment of substantial fees to women for the donation of their eggs, with the potential for the exploitation of needy women as donors for the more affluent. Because of these concerns, infertility counselors from the outset have been active members of OD teams, and there has been a consistent emphasis on the importance of psychological preparation, evaluation, and support for participants in this treatments[11-13].

This chapter describes the psychological aspects of OD, with the focus on recipients of this treatment. Crucial clinical issues for this population include:

- assessing appropriate candidates for OD treatment
- implications of lost fertility and genetic connection to the pregnancy the recipient will carry
- donor considerations such as anonymous versus known, and the nature of the relationship (if any) with the donor
- disclosures issues regarding OD
- patient preparation for OD.

REVIEW OF LITERATURE

Despite the fact that OD is entering its second decade of success, there are relatively few studies in the literature that specifically address the psychological issues for recipients of donated oocytes. Studies on the psychological aspects of infertility and assisted reproductive technologies have a general applicability to this population in some ways, but in many respects they do not address the issues particular to the donor-egg population. For example, not all recipients of donated egg are technically infertile: they may have had children earlier in their lives and are now past reproductive age. Furthermore, the addition of a third party—the donor—is a crucial ancillary factor that has an important impact on families created through this technology and although a parallel may be drawn with male-factor infertility and donor sperm (see Chapter 18), women who become mothers via donated oocytes still have the biological connection to the child through pregnancy and childbirth.

Studies are just beginning to appear in the literature that consider the psychological experience of OD for recipients of the treatment. In a program in which recipients recruit their own donors and anonymous donors are excluded, Barlett[14] studied the psychological experience and attitudes of 14 oocyte recipients over a 2-year period. In terms of psychiatric symptomatology, all were within normal range. Although all gave the primary motivating factor for participation as the desire to have a child, a number of recipients chose their sisters as donors and agreed that a genetic link was an important motivating factor for doing this.

In a program in which recipients may choose between an anonymous donor recruited by the program or a donor recruited by themselves, Greenfeld and associates[15] studied the first 90 recipients in their program: 64 subjects using anonymous donors and 26 using their own donors. The authors reported no significant differences between groups on social and demographic variables, but the groups differed significantly on the issue of disclosure. Recipients using a known donor were more likely to have told others about their participation in an OD program and were more likely to indicate that they intended to inform the child about the nature of his or her conception. It should also be noted, however, that the participants chose anonymous donors over their own donors in the ratio 2:1.

In France, where donor anonymity is the law and payment of donors is illegal, one program has come up with a unique solution termed *personalized anonymity*. This procedure involves a recipient couple's recruiting a donor (usually a sister or close friend) who then is matched to another recipient in the program, and vice versa. Studies from this program report that recipients are pleased with this arrangement. In terms of psychological symptomatology, the authors found that women with premature ovarian failure had a higher degree of depressive symptoms and were more inclined to have 'relationship problems' than recipients with other diagnosis[16].

THEORETICAL FRAMEWORK

Just as there is no clear psychological profile of recipients of OD, there is also no clear theoretical model universally applicable to all candidates for this treatment. However, theoretical models that explore motivations for parenthood and embody a woman's identity and sense of self are applicable to female-identified infertility and have been well described in other chapters: these include psychoanalytic self-psychology, feminist theory, and grief and loss theory (see Chapter 1). Each theoretical perspective offers insights into different aspects of female-identified infertility and family-building through the use of donated oocytes.

Early psychoanalytic views of the psychology of women was based on the psychology of self which Horney[17] described in terms of the actual self, the real self, and the idealized self. According to Horney, a woman's efforts to achieve independence and/or a career were insignificant because her interests should focus 'exclusively upon the male or upon motherhood'. From this perspective, the loss of fertility may be viewed as the loss of real and actual selves as well as the idealized self: mother. Although OD may provide the opportunity to recapture motherhood, it is within the context of a deep narcissistic wound to the idealized self.

Feminist theory has been critical of infertility treatments, particularly assisted reproductive technologies that may be perceived as victimizing women or a certain segment of women (e.g., lower economic status). However, Sandelowski[18] has suggested that questioning the motherhood motives of infertile women shatters sisterhood and alienates women who may already feel alienated from their fertile friends and relatives. Furthermore, assisted reproductive technology, especially oocyte donation, provides women opportunities to become mothers later in life, as men always have. In this respect, feminist advocacy of equality between men and women may be interpreted as an endorsement of assisted reproduction and the opportunities for reproductive equity it provides.

Family systems theory is applicable to oocyte donation when the donation is within the family (e.g., sister to sister donation). The concept of family boundaries is especially important in that research and theory contends that ambiguous and blurred boundaries create stress within family systems. Within this context oocyte donation may be consider a family stressor to which the family must adapt and realign, redefining family boundaries, relationships, and kinship ties. Family systems theory also becomes relevant in terms of the long-term adjustment of the family and the impact of the circumstances of conception on the child. Of importance are the family's relationship dynamics, values and beliefs (particularly about children), and rules about loyalty and obligation. These issues are particularly useful for the infertility counselor in evaluating recipients and donors considering intrafamily oocyte donation. Many have found the genogram a useful tool in facilitating this assessment.

The theoretical model of grief and loss is probably most applicable to candidates entering OD treatment. Nonetheless, it is important to remember that women considering OD vary widely in their degree of psychological adaptation to their loss at the time they enter treatment. Mahlstedt's[19] description of specific losses common to infertility provides a theoretical framework for consideration of the grief and loss experienced by women unable to be genetically related to their (potential) offspring:

- loss of a (potential) relationship
- loss of health
- loss of status or prestige
- loss of self-esteem
- loss of self-confidence
- loss of security
- loss of fantasy or hope of fulfilling an important fantasy
- loss of something or someone of great symbolic value.

A theoretical concept more directly applicable to recipients of OD was put forth by Mahlstedt and Greenfeld[11], who suggested that patient preparation and education are fundamental to all candidates considering participation in OD. Pre-treatment preparation that emphasizes time for consideration of this treatment as crucial to decision-making should focus on two aspects of the process: (1) identifying and resolving the specific ways in which infertility and infertility treatment have affected patients individually and as couples, and (2) discussing the specific issues involved in the treatment and developing ways of coping with them.

CLINICAL ISSUES

The psychological experience of participation in egg donation as a recipient requires consideration of several issues: mourning the loss of one's fertility and the inability to use one's own gametes for reproduction, making the decision to incorporate a donor into one's reproductive life, and thinking about the choice of an anonymous donor or, alternatively, a known donor such as a sister, close relative, or friend. Finally, the recipient must consider the inequity implications of giving birth to a child genetically related to her partner but not to her self.

There is no clear psychological portrait of the recipient in egg donation. After all, the first recipient of this treatment was a 25-year-old with premature ovarian failure, while at the other end of the spectrum are the well known reports of the 60-year-old postmenopausal Italian woman who gave birth to a donor-egg baby following the death of her only (grown) child[20] or the 63-year-old postmenopausal American woman who gave birth to a donor-egg baby (her first child) after she had reportedly deceived the clinic about her age[21]. These cases illustrate how diffuse the entire range of incentives (and ages) may be in this population. Thus, to appreciate the clinical consequences and impact of participation in an OD recipient program, we must have some appreciation of the recipient's motivation and incentives for participation. For example, is the recipient's participation in this program an extension of earlier treatment? Is there a history of failed IVF treatment? Did she lose ovarian function at a young age or is she a cancer survivor?

Formerly IVF was regarded as the so-called 'end of the line' in medical treatment, the last stage in what usually was a long, painful quest for a successful pregnancy. For some, OD has extended the treatment possibilities. Hence, donor-egg programs have become an extension of the 'end of the line', so that those women who have failed cycles of IVF are now given the opportunity to enter egg-donation treatment. In fact, only a small proportion actually go on to become egg recipients. For those women, it is appropriate to extend our knowledge about the psychological aspects of infertility to their experience as oocyte recipients.

A number of women participating in donor-egg programs are not patients who have failed other infertility treatment programs. Many are women who have had children before, perhaps in previous relationships. Some are women who lost ovarian function at a young age, or were born without it, and it is apparent that they need to have a donated ovum to achieve a pregnancy. Others may be in a second marriage and, having diminished ovarian reserve or lost ovarian function (for whatever reason, including menopause or age), seek an OD program because they want to have a child with their current spouse. Others are women who are known carriers of a genetic disorder and do not want to transmit it to potential children For these patients, OD is a 'miracle', offering a new and dramatic possibility to give birth. Consequently, these women usually experience different psychological issues than women who have endured long and unsuccessful prior infertility treatments only to discover that advanced maternal age has become the barrier to having a child. What all women entering into an OD program have in common, however, is their reliance on the participation of a 'third party'—a donor—to become a biological, if not genetic, mother.

Clinicians working with recipients of donated oocytes and their partners can take heart from studies on recipients of donated gametes. Research literature indicates that, for the most part, participants appear to be psychologically sound, and using donor gametes does not appear to adversely affect their marital or sexual relationships. Nevertheless, participants entering into this treatment have a myriad of psychological issues to consider. Thus, intake assessment and pretreatment preparation with a mental health professional trained in assisted reproduction is recommended[13,22,23]. Infertility counselors can help patients make the determination about whether or not the treatment is one that they could tolerate and understand and whether or not they could comfortably accept a donor into the parenthood equation. Infertility counselors can also help them understand the psychological stresses that are inevitable consequences of the treatment, whatever the outcome. Thus, infertility counselors serve as counselor, educator, and guide as recipients of donated oocytes go through this process.

The quality of the donor-recipient experience depends in part on how the process is conducted and managed. While helping couples learn about what they are going to have to deal with, infertility counselors can facilitate discussions of issues as they come up, and in many instances can help a couple make many of these decisions as the interview unfolds. Clinicians working with this population need to consider that recipients of OD—whether they intend to utilize an anonymous donor or a designated or known donor (e.g., a relative or a friend)—face complex questions and concerns. Recipients must deal with the knowledge that this treatment may not work, that there are advantages and disadvantages to using either a known or anonymous donor, that there are crucial decisions to make about issues of privacy and disclosure of the procedure to relatives and others, and finally that there is the ultimate issue of whether, when, and what to tell the child conceived in this manner.

THERAPEUTIC INTERVENTIONS
The Clinical Interview

Although this chapter has placed emphasis on the experience of the women who are recipients of egg donation, the clinical interview, informational and evaluative, needs to include the couple. In addition to the normal content of any psychological evaluation, this process, which may take more than one meeting, offers couples the opportunity to work through common concerns of participating in OD, such as mourning the loss of the potential child genetically related to both partners, addressing coercion and/or ambivalence about the treatment option, discussing the pros and cons of using a known versus an anonymous donor, and addressing the issues of who should know and who should not know about their participation in egg donation, including the potential child resulting from this treatment.

The purpose of the clinical interview is to determine whether the participants are psychologically prepared to undertake such decisions, are able to give informed consent, and do not have complicating psychiatric, marital, social, or legal problems that would interfere with their ability to participate in treatment or to become parents. The interview should include reproductive history, history of infertility, marital and sexual history, social stability, and available resources including financial stability, social support, physical health and well-being, and coping style and strategies. A good basis for the interview is *The Comprehensive Psychosocial History of Infertility* (CPHI) (see Appendix 2) which provides an outline of issues relevant to infertility although does not address assisted reproduction or third-party reproduction. During the clinical interview a couple is encouraged to address the issues fundamental to this unique form of family-building. It is important that all of these issues be addressed up-front, even though definitive answers to many issues may not come until considerably later:

- Has the couple considered the possibility of treatment failure?
- How has the couple or the individual partners adapted to the loss of the woman's fertility: is there any anger, resentment, or blaming?
- Has the couple considered other options such as adoption, and why is adoption less acceptable or donor oocyte more acceptable?

- Have they considered the possibility and consequences of multiple pregnancy and/or multifetal pregnancy reduction?
- Are they clear about their chances of pregnancy with this process?
- What thoughts do they have about distribution of extra embryos resulting from treatment?
- Do they plan to use a known donor or an anonymous donor?
- If they have chosen a known unrelated donor does there appear to be excess attention to donor characteristics (e.g., interest in creating the 'perfect baby')?
- Have they told others about their participation in an OD program?
- Do they plan to tell the child?
- What are their reasons for their disclosure decision?

While the clinical interview is typically both informative and evaluative, it is important to inform the couple up-front whether the interview may ultimately exclude them from participation. Klock and colleagues[24] described the difference between evaluation and counseling in the following way:

> The goal of the evaluation is to gather information to determine whether the couple can psychologically and socially cope with gamete donation treatment. The goal of counseling the gamete recipient couple is to provide an empathic environment for working through and resolving issues related to the gamete donation procedure and its consequences.

Obviously, the skilled infertility counselor can, and typically does, address both goals, but couples need to be clear about these goals at the outset. They need to be given documentation such as authorization for release of information or informed consents for mental health counseling (see Appendices 10–11). Patients need to be informed about any summaries or reports the infertility counselor must provide the treatment team, and the amount and kind of information that is typically included in the report. If psychological testing is performed as part of the evaluation, tests results should be reviewed with the individuals., although they should be informed that they will not receive the actual test report or raw data.

In the event that the psychological evaluation results in treatment being deferred (but not refused), it is typically the infertility counselor's responsibility to clearly state the criteria to be met before the couple proceeds with treatment. In addition, the infertility counselor usually tracks the couple's compliance and progress toward meeting the criteria. Alternatively, if the couple does not meet the criteria for participation, it is usually the infertility counselor's responsibility to inform them and to ensure that they experience no undue harm as a result. In such instances, referral to another mental health professional for supportive care may be warranted.

Positive indications for participation suggest that the couple is well informed, well prepared, and socially and psychologically stable enough to tolerate the demands of treatment, pregnancy, and parenthood. Contraindications for proceeding include evidence that:

- the couple may not be appropriate candidates for treatment
- the couple may need more time before pursuing egg donation
- the couple or individuals may need psychotherapeutic interventions before pursuing treatment.

Factors that may contraindicate participation in egg donation include:

- marital instability including overt or covert partner coercion
- legal problems including family violence, bankruptcy, and/or criminal activity

- psychiatric illness (past or present) that includes significant symptomatology
- current chemical dependency problem that includes drug-seeking behavior or marital conflict
- significant physical illness that may impact pregnancy and/or longevity
- chaotic social or familial functioning including significant life stressors
- impaired cognitive functioning
- conflicted gender identity or homo/bisexuality that impacts marital functioning
- sexual trauma that impacts personal or marital functioning

Finally, although an important function of the clinical interview is information gathering, a great deal of decision-making often takes place during the interview process as couples address issues of third-party reproduction they had not previously considered, examined, or discussed at length. Frequently, the infertility counselor becomes a facilitator when couples encounter challenging or conflictual issues that they cannot discuss, or reach an agreement on, on their own. These discussions can are helpful for patient preparation, informed consent, and shared decision-making so that the infertility counselor must be prepared to provide additional counseling sessions if necessary. It is this factor of additional discussions and/or time that patients and caregivers often underestimate in their rush to proceed with OD as a treatment option. Failure to allow sufficient time for further sessions and/or to thoughtfully process the decision may result in patients who are ill-prepared and who experience significant post-treatment regret.

Making the Decision Between Anonymous and Known Donors

Rules and regulations regarding donor anonymity, the use of friends and family members as donors, and donor compensation vary greatly around the world. In the United States, the experience regarding these same factors fluctuates greatly from program to program and from one part of the country to another. Thus, some patients make the decision to use an anonymous donor because they do not know anyone who would be a good candidate, or they may choose a known or identified donor because the treatment program that they are using does not have an anonymous donor program. Other patients may work with a program in which they are given the option of recruiting their own previously anonymous donor who becomes known to them. Some programs provide a list of donors, including a superficial description of each donor's characteristics such as height, weight, eye color, hair color, blood type, and level of education. Other programs provide more extensive information including a photograph or intelligence testing of the potential anonymous donor.

For many couples, the process of deciding whether or not to participate in egg donation is the more critical decision: the decision-making and the psychological work revolve around the issue of saying goodbye to the idea of having a child that is biologically related to both partners. Often, this more crucial work takes place with a mental health professional (usually an infertility counselor), making the decision of whether or not to use a donor known to them or anonymous easier. In the ideal scenario, a couple has given the process a great deal of thought and they have had sufficient time to process their feelings. They have worked through any ambivalence regarding the procedure, the choice of donor, and the boundaries and limitations of what information they may or may not have or want regarding the donor. Finally, they have considered what information is available for them to pass on to any

potential child resulting from this treatment. Obviously, decisions about choosing between anonymous and known, as well as other important factors about the donor, are precisely the issues to discuss in the meeting with the mental health professional.

Anonymous Donor

In the use of an anonymous donor, couples may or may not have selection issues. Some programs make the donor choices for the couples and only provide brief information if the procedure is successful. Other anonymous donor programs provide more of an array of choices in which case couples need to consider what characteristics are important to them in the selection of an anonymous donor. Typical concerns are that the donor resemble the recipient in height, weight, eye color, and/or ethnic background. Others are more concerned about the donor's level of education or intelligence, health, personality type, family history of health or genetic problems, and/or intelligence. Questions to be considered during the clinical interview regarding the use of an anonymous donor include:

- How important is it to the couple that the donor physically resemble the recipient?
- Is the couple satisfied with the amount and type of information provided?
- Should they consider going to a program in which they can learn more about the donor, or even meet her?
- How do they feel about the adequacy of the information provided to pass on to a child resulting from this technology?

Too much emphasis or high expectations of an anonymous donor may reflect a failure to accept the necessity of donor reproduction and/or a need to replicate the recipient. In addition, high expectations may represent inaccurate expectations of genetics (e.g., able to accurately predict a child's qualities) or a desire to create a perfect or 'designer' child.

Known Donor

Although some programs will introduce anonymous donors to recipients, for the most part, recipients have no direct relationship with donors. However, when couples utilize eggs from their close friends, sisters, or other relations, the relationship with the donor is an important part of the interview. Ideally, the interview extends to the recipient couple and the known donor and her partner (if applicable). The quality and the history of the relationships between the couple and the potential donor need careful consideration. Furthermore, the relationship of the donor with the potential child needs to be considered and clearly defined for all parties. Should the relationship between the donor and recipient turn hostile at some time in the future, there is potential for trauma to the child caught in the middle of this complex set of relationships. It is important to evaluate the quality of the relationship boundaries and investigate any history of boundary violations (e.g., incest) which may contraindicate participation. Questions to be included in the clinical interviews with recipients and their known donors are:

- Is the known donor being coerced or pressured (overtly or covertly) to participate?
- Is the recipient feeling coerced or pressured by family or friends to use a (or this) known donor rather than an anonymous donor?
- What is the compensation arrangement?
- How will participation affect their future relationship with each other or the relationships with others (e.g., family, social network)?

- Have future relationship boundaries been clearly defined for all participants?
- How will participation affect their future relationship with a (potential) child?

An additional consideration in evaluating the known donor arrangement is when the infertility counselor must evaluate both the recipient and donor, and information forthcoming during the joint session causes a conflict. In most cases, the recipient couple are the contracting couple and, as such, take financial responsibility for the evaluation process. It is important to clearly define the role of the infertility counselor and address the possibility that the outcome of the evaluation is not something the counselor or recipient can predict. Recipients should be prepared for the possibility that the outcome may not be in their favor for a variety of reasons. In some situations, the identified donor may not be able to refuse the request for donation without disturbing the relationship. Consequently, the infertility counselor must take responsibility for the donor not proceeding in order to protect the well-being of the donor, and the donor/recipient relationship.

Addressing Disclosure Issues

The issue of whether a potential child should or should not be told about the method of his or her conception is often a subject of debate among professionals in this field (see Chapter 25)[24-26]. It should not be surprising to anyone therefore that it may be a subject of some debate among couples entering into this treatment. Historically, couples considering sperm donation were encouraged by their medical treatment team to keep the information about the donor conception private, not to tell anyone, including children born from the treatment. The donor was generally anonymous and the couples and resulting families rarely knew anything about him. This picture has changed considerably with OD, as evidenced by the consideration given in this chapter to the debate and discussion about whether couples are planning to use an anonymous or known donor. When OD first emerged as a viable treatment option, the use of anonymous donors was recommended by organizations such as the American Society for Reproductive Medicine, but the difficulty in obtaining donors led that body to recommend, 'for pragmatic reasons', the use of nonanonymous donors as well[27]. Clinicians working with couples entering OD programs are hearing a different story from those choosing nonanonymous donors: they made the choice because they wanted to know the donor!

What is yet to be determined is whether couples who choose known donors (or who recruit their own donors to have more information about them) plan to disclose this information to their potential children. Whether or not they plan to disclose, it is an issue that needs to be considered at the outset. Infertility counselors, while not purporting to have all the answers, can be very helpful to couples struggling with this question. What couples need to hear is that the issue of disclosure is one for consideration and discussion long before they undertake the process of using donated oocytes. Couples also need to hear that their thinking about where they stand on the issue is also a process, one that will eventually evolve as they discuss it between themselves. Helpful interventions from clinicians include education about what is known and is not known, educational materials, and papers and articles on both scientific and psychological studies of this family-building method. Couples can also make use of lay information, especially written materials from other parents who

have had this experience (see Chapters 18 and 25).

FUTURE IMPLICATIONS

'The future is now' is in many ways an apt phrase for this reproductive technology—meaning that much of the work that is taking place currently dictates the consequences for the future, certainly to the children born of this technology. Infertility counselors working with couples participating in OD need to consider not only their clients' wishes—the desire to have a family—but the needs and desires of their potential children. Such considerations should include thoughts about children born to couples well past normal childbearing age, children born to women who have been very ill and who possibly face a serious recurrence of their illness or early death, and children born with limited knowledge of their genetic heritage. What we know so far is that these children are faring well, and their parents are very grateful for this exciting technology[28].

We also need to consider the health of young women who are donating their eggs. Hopefully, future studies will determine that OD has not in any way jeopardized their future fertility and that donating eggs so that other women may give birth has not caused them any long-term psychological sequelae, health problems, or regrets.

The recent medical breakthrough of cryopreservation of oocytes may, in many ways, change the face of OD by making it available to a wider spectrum of women and altering the use of, or even need for, identified donors. Within a short time, the face of oocyte donation may resemble sperm donation more than ever before. By the same token, women wishing to postpone childbearing, may be able to cryopreserve or 'bank' their own oocytes (or ovaries) for use at a later date. Such developments may further expand and extend the childbearing possibilities for women in ways yet unforeseeable.

SUMMARY

- OD is increasing in frequency as a treatment for women without ovarian function.
- Studies thus far have shown oocyte recipients to be psychologically healthy.
- Recipients of donated oocytes confront a myriad of ethical dilemmas, such as choosing between anonymous and known donation, and disclosure versus nondisclosure.
- Psychological intervention and support are recommended for all participants in these programs.
- Infertility counselors can be particularly helpful in recipient evaluation, preparation, and education.

REFERENCES

1. Lutjen P, Tounson A, Leeton J, et al. The establishment and maintenance of pregnancy using in vitro fertilization and embryo donation in a patient with primary ovarian failure. *Nature* 1984;307:174

2. Rosenwaks Z Donor eggs: Their application in modern reproductive technologies. *Fertil Steril* 1987;47:895–909

3. Kennard EAD, Collins RL, Blankstein J, et al. A program for matched anonymous oocyte donation. *Fertil Steril* 1989;51:655–60

4. Sauer MV, Paulson RJ Human oocyte and preembryo donation: An evolving method for the treatment of infertility. *Am J Obstet Gynecol* 1990;163:1157–60

5. Society for Assisted Reproductive Technology, American Society for Reproductive Medicine in the United States and Canada: 1993 Results Generated from the American Society for Reproductive Medicine/Society for Assisted Reproductive Technology Registry. *Fertil Steril* 1995; 64:13–21

6. Meldrum DR. Oocyte donation. *Infertil Reprod Med Clin North Am* 1993;4:761–8

7. Sauer MV, Paulson RJ, Lobo RA. A preliminary report on oocyte donation extending reproductive potential to women over 40. *N Engl J Med* 1990;323:1157

8. Navot D, Beigh PA, Williams MA, et al. Poor oocyte quality rather than implantation failure as a cause of age–related decline in female fertility. *Lancet* 1991; 337:1375–7

9. Levran D, Ben–Shlomo I, Dor J, et al. Aging of endometrium and oocytes: Observation on conception and abortion rates in an egg donation model. *Fertil Steril* 1991;56:1091–3

10. Burton G, Abdalla HI, Kirkland A, et al. The role of oocyte donation in women who are unsuccessful with in vitro fertilization treatment. *Hum Reprod* 1992;7:1103–4

11. Mahlstedt PP, Greenfeld DA. Assisted reproductive technology for donor gametes: The need for patient preparation. *Fertil Steril* 1989;52:908–14

12. Schover LR, Tein J, Collins RL, et al. The psychological evaluation of oocyte donors. *J Psychosom Obstet Gynaecol* 1990;11:583–90

13. Braverman A. Survey results on the current practice of ovum donation. *Fertil Steril* 1993;59: 1216–20

14. Bartlett JA. Psychiatric issues in non-anonymous oocyte donation. *Psychsomatics* 1991;12:433–7

15. Greenfeld DA, Mazure CM, Greenfeld DG, Keefe DL. Social and psychological characteristics of donor oocyte recipients. *Fertil Steril* 1995;(suppl):251 abstract P346

16. Bertrand-Servais M, Letur-Konirsch H, Raoul-Duval A, Frydman R. Psychological considerations of anonymous oocyte donation. *Hum Reprod* 1993;874–9

17. Horney K. *Feminine Psychology.* New York: WW Norton, 1967

18. Sandelowski M. *With Child in Mind: Studies of the Personal Encounter with Infertility.* Philadelphia, PA: University of Pennsylvania Press, 1993

19. Mahlstedt PP. The psychological component of infertility. *Fertil Steril* 1985; 43:335–46

20. Winston R, Handyside AH. New challenges in human in vitro fertilization. *Science* 1993;260:932

21. Paulson RJ, Thornton MH, Francis MM, Salvador HS. Successful pregnancy in a 63-year-old woman *Fertil Steril* 1997;67:949–51

22. Schover LR. Psychological aspects of oocyte donation. *Infertil Reprod Med Clin North Am* 1993;4:483–502

23. Burns, LH. An overview of the psychology of infertility. *Infertil Reprod Med Clin North Am* 1993;4:433–54

24. Klock SC, Jacob MC, Maier D. A prospective study of donor insemination recipients, secrecy, privacy, and disclosure. *Fertil Steril* 1994;62:477–84

25. Daniels K. Artificial insemination using donor sperm and the issue of secrecy: The views of donors and recipient couples. *Soc Sci Med* 1988;27:377–83

26. Pruett KD. Strange bedfellows? Reproductive technology and child development. *Infant Ment Health J* 1992;13:312–18

27. American Fertility Society Guidelines for Gamete Donation: *Fertil Steril* 1993;59:s1

28. Applegarth L, Goldberg NC, Choist I, *et al.* Families created through other donation: A preliminary investigation of obstetrical outcome and psychosocial adjustment. *J Assist Reprod Genet* 1995;12:574–80

20

The Donor as Patient: Assessment and Support

Linda D. Applegarth, EdD, and Sheryl A. Kingsberg, PhD

All I know is, as a 'donor', I received an acknowledgment of 'the success of the experiment' ... the offspring of my loins ... I feel your absence only as I might feel amputated limbs.

James Kirkup

The gamete donor plays a unique role in infertility treatment as both a patient and a provider of genetic material. The Guidelines for Gamete Donation: 1993[1], published by the American Society for Reproductive Medicine (ASRM), point to differences between male and female gamete donors. At present, there are no published guidelines for embryo donation. Within the existing guidelines, there is a recommendation for psychological counseling for all parties involved in oocyte donation, but the same does not hold true for sperm donation. Nonetheless, these guidelines, and those offered by the Mental Health Professional Group of the ASRM (see Appendix 7), provide a foundation for the practice of donor counseling and assessment that can potentially have legal, psychosocial, and ethical implications.

This chapter provides a general overview of what is currently known about gamete donation from the donor's perspective, with the purpose of:

- understanding the theoretical issues involved in the screening and counseling of gamete donors

- defining the clinical issues, as well as the criteria for acceptance or rejection of donor candidates.

The role of mental health professionals appears to be of utmost importance because of the need to protect the emotional well-being of donors, and to help them understand as fully as possible the meaning and longer-term psychosocial implications of deciding to donate their genetic material to another individual or couple.

HISTORICAL OVERVIEW

The use of donor gametes and embryos has become increasingly more common in reproductive medicine. *Donation* refers to a wide range of transactions involving either anonymous or known sperm, oocytes, or embryos. While sperm donation dates back to antiquity, reference to the medical use of therapeutic donor insemination (TDI) for male-factor infertility dates to the early part of this century[2]. Oocyte donation is still a relatively new reproductive option, having developed in the last 15 years as an

357

extension of the use of in vitro fertilization (IVF) technology[3]. Embryo donation is newer still, with programs only recently able to consider offering this option reliably with the development of successful cryopreservation techniques.

Sperm Donation

With an estimated 30,000–40,000 babies born each year in the United States as a result of TDI[4], sperm donation appears to be an accepted and well established practice. The indications for TDI include male-factor infertility, severe semen abnormalities, genetic abnormalities, and untreatable ejaculation dysfunction. In addition, the use of TDI is increasing among single women and lesbian couples who want children[5]. With this growing demand for donor sperm, the business of recruiting donors and banking semen to sell to infertility programs and the general public is booming.

Over the last decade, sperm banks have been using more stringent guidelines for evaluating potential donors and have been screening for infectious diseases, particularly human immunodeficiency virus (HIV), and genetic defects. In fact, sperm banks use only cryopreserved semen to allow reassessment of infectious disease status months or years after the donation[6]. However, little attention continues to be paid to the motivation and later psychological adjustment of sperm donors. In striking contrast to oocyte donors, there is typically little, if any, psychological assessment or discussion regarding donors' feelings/motivations about donation.

Sperm donation is noninvasive and requires relatively little time and physical effort. There is virtually no risk of current or future physical harm from the process of donation. Only recently has research begun to look at the psychological effects of sperm donation on donors[6,7]. The success rate for TDI is 70–75%, with the majority of women conceiving within six cycles of treatment[5]. Although there are no significant differences in the use of fresh versus frozen sperm with regard to pregnancy outcome[5], there is a higher rate of conception per cycle using fresh sperm. Compensation for sperm donation varies by program and by country, with ranges from $0–$70.00[8]. Some countries prohibit any compensation for sperm donation and a few require the donor to be identified.

Oocyte Donation

Trounson and colleagues[9] reported the first use of oocyte donation as a treatment of infertility in 1983, and Lutjen and associates[10] published the first report of a successful pregnancy using donor ova in a woman with ovarian failure in 1984. Since this first successful pregnancy using oocyte donation, infertility programs offering IVF technologies have been rapidly including oocyte donation as an option for their patients. Just over a decade since it became a reproductive option, the prevalence of programs offering oocyte donation has equaled that for sperm[11] and has created a significant need for oocyte donors. For example, a world survey reported on 4486 cycles of oocyte donation from approximately eight countries[12]. Indications for the use of oocyte donation include:

- ovarian agenesis or gonadal dysgenesis (incidence, 1:10,000 in females)
- premature ovarian failure (incidence, 1–5%)
- postmenopausal women
- women with morphologically abnormal ova
- genetic abnormalities (including significant autosomal-dominant or sex-linked disorders or autosomal-recessive disorders in a couple reluctant to use donor sperm).

Further, the development of transvaginal ultrasound retrieval has helped increase the availability of oocyte donation[13]. When it was initially developed, it required laparoscopic retrieval, and the necessity for donors to undergo surgery kept the pool of potential donors limited. The main source of donors were women undergoing IVF who donated excess ova, women undergoing tubal ligation, or close relatives or friends willing to risk surgery. Another method of retrieval, also developed in the early 1980s, involved artificial insemination of the donor with the recipient male's sperm and washing the embryos from the uterus for transfer to the recipient female's uterus. This method is no longer used, as it had limited success and numerous problems, including donor infections and retained pregnancies[14]. As cryopreservation of embryos became available, the supply of ova from women going through IVF virtually dried up. Couples chose to fertilize all retrieved eggs in order to cryopreserve embryos for their own future use[15]. Fortunately, within a similar time frame, transvaginal ultrasound retrieval was developed, greatly reducing the risk to donors and their recovery time and thus opening up an entirely new potential pool of donors: young anonymous donors, analogous to the typical sperm donor. With this change, the majority of IVF centers in the United States began recruiting donors in some fashion, and businesses are developing as suppliers of egg donors, recruiting and evaluating potential donors to be selected by IVF programs or women/couples. Nevertheless, there is still considerable effort required from the donor, such as timed injections, blood work, ultrasound examinations, and timing of her cycle with the recipient's[16]. The major sources of oocyte donors to date are anonymous donors recruited by IVF programs or private recruiting organizations, known donors brought to the IVF program by recipients, personalized anonymous donation[17] (couples bringing their own donor to be used anonymously for a different recipient couple), and egg sharing (women also undergoing IVF). In England, some programs provide free tubal ligation in exchange for donated ova[5].

Currently, donors undergo standard IVF, a complicated, intrusive medical procedure that includes stimulation with a combination of folic hormones injected over a period of days prior to retrieval. With ultrasound guidance, ova are harvested through a needle inserted transvaginally into the ovarian follicles. Ova are then inseminated with the recipient partner's sperm, and fertilized embryos are transferred to the recipient's uterus. As of 1991, the clinical pregnancy rate was 31% per oocyte donation cycle[18].

Embryo Donation

Like oocyte donation, embryo donation also became a reproductive option with the development of IVF technology. Prior to the establishment of cryopreservation and storage, excess embryos obtained during an IVF cycle were sometimes offered for donation. As was the case in oocyte donation, with cryopreservation as an option, most couples now choose to freeze embryos for their own future use. However, there are still some couples who, for ethical reasons, do not wish to cryopreserve embryos and would prefer to donate. There are also unusual medical or other life crises that may prevent a completed transfer, and excess embryos may be a potential source for donation. The largest source of potential donor embryos is from couples who have cryopreserved additional embryos and decide, for any number of reasons, that they do not want to use them. For example, many couples may have completed their families, while others choose donation as a disposition of their excess embryos in case of death (of one or both partners) or divorce. There has been tremendous media attention on the surplus of cryopreserved embryos stored in IVF programs; for example, a report[19] from Britain in 1996 revealed the destruction of 5000 embryos. In addition to excess embryos, another source of embryo donation is recruitment of anonymous oocyte donors and anonymous sperm donors for the purpose of creating embryos for donation[5].

REVIEW OF LITERATURE

Gamete Donors

The literature is quite limited regarding the emotional and psychosocial status of the gamete donor. Novaes[20] stressed that in general almost no research is available on the long-term psychological impact of being a gamete donor. Haimes[21] considered the issue of sex in gamete donation and pointed out that gender is utilized as a resource for organizing the meanings attached to the processes. She suggested that historically semen donation has been associated with 'deviant' sexuality (masturbation, adultery, illegitimacy), though paradoxically the actual nature of sperm donation was subsequently used to justify the acceptance of oocyte donation. The assumptions about gender and reproduction lead to oocyte donation's being considered in a familial, clinical, and asexual context, whereas sperm donation is seen in an individualistic, unregulated context of dubious sexual connotations. These assumptions also would appear to have significant implications regarding donor recruitment, secrecy, and overall social acceptance of third-party reproduction.

Broderick and Walker[22] identified 10 major methodological limitations regarding the psychosocial literature on information access when donated gametes and embryos are used. As a result, these flaws prohibit any firm conclusions about whether or not donors and recipients should disclose information, should have access to information, want to have access to information about each other, or want to have information about themselves disclosed to the other party. The lack of well designed social research precludes any conclusions about deeper psychological motives for donating sperm, ova, or embryos.

Sperm Donors

Although family-building through the use of sperm donation is used extensively in this country and others, there is very little information about the psychosocial impact of this procedure on the donors themselves. Until the mid-1980s, the work of identifying and screening semen donors was a private and an individual one[23]. In other words, physicians would typically identify medical students, residents, or other graduate level males, test them for sexually transmitted diseases, and match them accordingly by phenotype. As HIV infection and hepatitis have become more prevalent, semen has been cryopreserved and quarantined for 6 months. The donor must then retest negative before the frozen semen can be released. With the improved techniques of sperm cryopreservation, there has been a large increase in the number of sperm banks with standardized basic quality assurances. Nonetheless, Schover[24] pointed out that in the ASRM's 1993 guidelines for gamete donation[1], there is a suggestion that 'psychological counseling be offered to all parties involved in oocyte donation', but no specific recommendation that semen donors undergo psychological screening other than to consider sexual history factors that might increase a man's risk for sexually transmitted diseases.

In a recent study of 54 sperm banks conducted by Gillis and Rausch[8], for example, it was found that few centers include mental health professionals as part of the personnel and only one center utilized psychological testing. Informal assessments were made by staff personnel by attending to attitude, personality, ambivalence, or 'inappropriate motivation' on the part of potential sperm donors. Psychological factors that would lead to rejection of a donor were depression, psychosis, anxiety, or 'too neurotic'. The authors therefore pointed out that 'the interpersonal impression of the potential donors was important in determining their rejection and acceptance after other medical criteria were met'[8]. They added that potential donors are given little information from sperm banks about the nature of donating and/or future psychological sequelae.

In a 1991 report[25] surveying sperm donors themselves, 60% stated that they would agree to some type of personal contact when the offspring reached the age of 18. They were also found to be willing to provide in-depth personal, medical, and psychosocial information to recipient families.

Daniels and coworkers[26] extensively studied semen donors in Europe and found that there is a need to take into account the views of donors in forming policies concerning assisted reproduction, as well as a need for the interests of the child to be paramount. In another study, Daniels and colleagues[27] considered whom sperm donors had told about their donation, who they thought should be told, and whether they thought recipient couples should tell the offspring about their conception. These authors thus challenged the dominant view that donor insemination is a practice of medical or legal importance by looking at the attitudes of donors toward both their own family and the family to which they have contributed their genetic material.

Swedish donors who were investigated were found to be less likely than donors in other countries to have told people about their involvement in donor insemination, including their partners and their children. Daniels and colleagues[28] also stressed the need for greater social acceptance and endorsement of donor insemination and of the man who would provide his sperm. They suggested that an appropriate goal would be to acknowledge semen donors as men who donate rather than sell their sperm, with the basic motivation of wanting to assist infertile couples. They added that the policies and methods used by clinics and staff play a critical role in the way in which sperm donors are thought of and recruited. In assessing the views and feelings of sperm donors, it was reported that donors perceive DI families as being normal and are very supportive of the autonomy and privacy of these families, but they also have concerns about the needs of the offspring[26].

Oocyte Donors

There is more information available about the psychosocial issues regarding oocyte donors. These donors, for example, are much more likely to undergo a clinical interview and psychological testing than are their male counterparts. Schover and associates[29] evaluated 26 oocyte donor candidates and found that they were significantly more likely than controls to have experienced at least one emotional trauma related to reproduction or at least one family event such as death of a parent, parental divorce, chemical dependency or psychiatric disorder in a relative, or sexual abuse. Oocyte donors themselves had also experienced a significantly greater number of reproductive traumas or family problems than controls. On follow-up[30], 23 women were surveyed with respect to donor satisfaction. Ninety-one percent were moderately to extremely satisfied with the experience; transient adverse psychological symptoms were reported by two donors but resolved with medical or psychological treatment. Although psychological risk factors predicted potential donors' decisions to participate and their compliance, they were not predictive of donor satisfaction on follow-up. Lessor and associates[31] also considered social and psychological characteristics in 95 women who volunteered to be oocyte donors and found, on the basis of clinical interviews and psychological test performance, that 73% were acceptable as donors. They noted that the incidence of dysfunction (abandonment, abuse) in family of origin or family of orientation was unremarkable.

One study[32] assessed the *motivations* of 10 oocyte donors and found that they were guided by an overall ethic of giving. However, there also appeared to be a need for those who had unresolved feelings about past abortions to compensate in some way for those past experiences. Schover and colleagues[6] also compared semen and oocyte donors and found that financial compensation was significantly more important to the men than to the women, while women's primary motivation was most often altruistic. They concluded that these differences may reflect the greater discomfort and medical risks associated with oocyte donation, as well as the comparatively smaller financial reward.

Brill and Levin[33] stressed the importance of *careful screening* and *counseling* of donors. In addition to a clinical interview, donors should be given the Minnesota Multiphasic Personality Inventory (MMPI). They pointed out that although this standardized measure was originally designed to determine psychopathology in a psychiatric population, there is now growing consensus among mental health professionals that the MMPI-2 or similar well researched measures provide a degree of standardization regarding psychopathology in potential donors. Schover[34] also indicated that the MMPI was useful in identifying oocyte donors with significant psychopathology and noted that profiles suggesting anger and rebelliousness may indicate risk for noncompliance during the medical procedure.

The use of *known versus anonymous* oocyte donors is also worthy of discussion. Brill and Levin[33] posited that known donors often wish to donate their ova because of the close relationship that they share with a sister or good friend. The mental health professional's role is to evaluate and counsel the donor so as to rule out recipient or family coercion, guilt, or the need to 'undo' past reproductive losses. Research[34,35] that has considered donors with past reproductive losses, however, suggests that carefully selected oocyte donors who are counseled about such losses may actually feel at follow-up that donating did console them. In essence, there is very little research addressing the particular psychosocial or emotional needs of the known oocyte donor or the special concerns of the 'identified' oocyte donor. Unlike the known oocyte donor, the identified donor has no familial or social relationship with the recipient couple. Instead, she has been recruited as a donor either by the couple themselves, by a broker or intermediary organization, or by the medical facility. The identified donor then meets with the recipient couple before the donation occurs and a mutual arrangement is made with respect to the donation. Again, there are no known data regarding this particular population other than anecdotal information with respect to outcomes or satisfaction following the donation. As with other types of oocyte donors, a thorough psychosocial evaluation, including psychological testing, would appear imperative.

Embryo Donors

There is no research regarding the psychological impact of embryo donation on either donor couples or recipient couples. As embryo cryopreservation has become an integral part of IVF programs, the availability of frozen embryos for donation to other infertile couples has become a viable family-building option. One research study[36] surveyed patients with cryopreserved embryos regarding hypothetical disposition decisions and found that 72% of men and 65% of women felt that couples should have the right to donate their embryos to a 'needy' couple. Laurelle and Englert[37] also queried 200 couples about to undergo IVF and embryo transfer and learned that donation was the most frequent choice made by couples. Donation was highest among couples who stress education more than genetic lineage in parental bonding. Cooper[38] pointed out, however, in her 'unofficial' research that what couples choose prior to IVF may change following the procedure. She contends that 'perhaps "successful" IVF couples look at their children and cannot imagine giving up a potential child like the one they see in front of them'.

In an essay on ethical and legal issues, Robinson[39] stated that a prime consideration in the willingness to donate supernumerary embryos will be the couple's 'fears and fantasies about the consequences of their act'. Whether or not couples are informed about the outcome of their embryo donation will also be a psychologically charged issue.

THEORETICAL FRAMEWORK

There is no clear theoretical framework underlying the psychological assessment and emotional support of gamete donors, nor has there been any apparent theory development in this area. Perhaps, the most obvious theoretical approaches are *altruism*, defined as 'behavior carried out to benefit another without anticipation of external reward'[40], and *exchange and reinforcement theory*, in which individuals are thought to give to others in order to obtain certain rewards for themselves. Altruism and exchange and reinforcement theories address the question of whether individuals are capable of making major sacrifices to help another person simply because of a wish to be helpful or a desire to remove distress for a person or to gain personal reward or payment[41].

In a very comprehensive investigation, Simmons and colleagues[41] addressed organ donation (particularly kidney donation) from the perspective of significant life decision-making for individuals and families under stress, with an assessment of the impact and consequences of the donation on the donor. Many individuals appear to find meaningful, altruistic acts deeply and intrinsically rewarding, primarily from the pleasure of viewing the benefit to the recipient and from the happiness at realizing one's capacity of making a sacrifice to help another. However, donors may experience less positive psychological effects if they are less able to perceive the consequences of the gift or less invested in the recipient. This certainly may be the case for anonymous gamete donors who have no emotional connection to recipients or are never given information about the outcome of their donation.

Donor decision-making was found to be based on moral decision-making (with an emphasis on the right thing to do), instantaneous choice (vs. deliberation of alternatives), and postponement (or decision avoidance)[41]. Although organ donation was seen as a positive act that emphasized the resilience of individuals and families, it was also determined that some persons were vulnerable to postdonation distress and the potential for family conflict. Research indicated that family donors who reacted more negatively postdonation were more likely to (1) be emotionally less tied to the recipient, (2) experience direct or indirect family pressure to donate, (3) not experience gratitude from the recipient or other family members, (4) feel less obligated to donate (or be helpful), (5) experience high levels of ambivalence about the donation, and (6) have lower self-esteem and overall happiness.[41] It would seem that each of these factors should be carefully considered in the use of known gamete donors. One might also understand how altruism might not be a primary motivation for donating in the case of anonymous donation.

There are also clear actual and conceptual differences between organ donation and gamete donation. The gamete contains the genetic code of the individual and does not give or prolong the life of the recipient; instead, the gamete is intended to create another human being. This idea may have a very different meaning, both favorable and unfavorable, to the donor. The theory of altruism may be most saliently seen, however, in the case of embryo donation. An infertile couple who donates excess cryopreserved embryos, with no financial reward, may feel a strong desire to help another couple who is unable to have a child. The donating couple may indeed sense great pleasure in believing that they can potentially contribute to the happiness of others.

CLINICAL ISSUES

The psychological considerations on which one views the gamete donor as patient are based in good part on sound clinical judgment, as well as on potential ethical and legal imperatives. It would appear that health and mental health professionals have an important role in creating the nature and meaning of gamete donation for both donors and recipients. This is accomplished through an understanding of the motivations for donating, as well as the reasons for psychological screening.

Motivations

The extent to which financial compensation is a motivating factor in providing gametes should be explored. The financial rewards that result from the donation may contribute to the donor's denial about the longer-term implications of the donation. Novaes[20] pointed out that if material reward was not available, the 'donor may feel compelled to reflect on the meaning that he (or she) attributes to this altruistic action'. She added therefore that financial remuneration could 'in the long run be an unethical means of obtaining the donor's consent'.

For the time being, however, it appears that the policy of financial compensation for gamete donation is here to stay, at least in the United States. As a result, it would seem that it is the responsibility of infertility counselors to help donors understand the meanings and implications of the donation and to protect the donors, as well as recipients, from making inappropriate decisions about gamete donation. Thus, current guidelines recommending psychological consultation and screening for oocyte and embryo donors should also be, in theory, the same for sperm donors (see Appendix 7). In essence, mental health professionals act as the donor's advocate.

Psychological Assessment: Rationale

The clinical bases underlying the need for psychological consultation and evaluation of gamete donors are essentially fivefold (Table 1). First, as Schover[24] pointed out, psychological screening provides some *protection for the recipient couple*. The clinical interview and standardized psychological testing help rule out major psychiatric

Table 1 Issues to include in a thorough, structured clinical interview of oocyte donors

Discussion of donor's motivation

Unrealistic expectations of the psychological benefits of donation

Financial pressures leading to donation out of desperation for money

Past history of reproductive loss and related expectations about donation

Risk for obsessing about unknown outcome for recipients

Risk for grieving the loss of perceived potential offspring

Guilt for past elective abortion or adoption

General coping with emotional losses

Realistic expectations about physical discomfort of shots and side effects, time requirements, discomfort/risk of oocyte retrieval, and hyperstimulation should it occur

History of somatization that might put her at risk for developing physical symptoms during donation cycle

History of involvement in a lawsuit related to her medical care

Significant pressure from family, spouse, partner, or friends regarding donation

Comfort with donation, evidenced by discussion of it with someone close to her

Assessment of sources of happiness and satisfaction

Assessment of stresses that could impact compliance

Demonstration of stability and goal-directedness

Past history of physical, sexual, or emotional abuse that may make her vulnerable to feeling victimized

Evidence of stable and happy relationships

Ability to comply with abstinence from sex during ovarian hyperstimulation and oocyte harvesting

Past history or current evidence of major psychopathology or chemical dependency, or first- degree relative with major psychopathology or chemical dependency

(Adapted from ref. 34, with permission)

disorders believed to have a genetic component such as schizophrenia or bipolar disorder. The evaluation by the mental health professional may reveal significant mental illness in the donor's own history or that of a first-degree relative. The social history and evaluation of the donor's lifestyle can also assist the medical team in determining whether or not a donor may be at risk for HIV infection or other sexually transmitted diseases.

Second, it is important, particularly in the case of oocyte donors, that they *understand and comply with the medical procedures* required during the donation.

Psychological testing and the clinical interview enable the infertility counselor to ascertain more fully the chances that the donor may not follow through with the donation. An unstable family history, sociopathy and/or legal difficulties, an erratic school or work history, or ambivalence about the donation may lead to noncompliance. This situation leads to frustration (and expense) for medical personnel and, more important, to great disappointment and upset on the part of the recipient couple.

A third, and very important, rationale behind thorough assessment and counseling of the gamete donor is the *protection of* the donor. As Schover[24] noted, 'Donors who are motivated to participate in order to gain restitution for a perceived loss or mistake in the past may be at risk for emotional disappointment or regrets about giving away a potential child'. Women and men who donate gametes, fantasizing that the donation gives them a sense of biological immortality or provides them the narcissistic pleasure of having provided the world with an offspring, may have problematic or inappropriate motivations to donate. There is no way that one can predict accurately how a donor will feel about the donation in the months or years to come.

Fourth, there are often questions on the part of recipients about the *matching of donors on the basis of intelligence and/or personality characteristics*. Although the extent to which these traits can be inherited is unclear[42], it is apparent that some heritability does exist. This is a complex issue and may ultimately put the infertility counselor in a difficult, if not impossible, position with respect to matching gamete donors and recipients. Often, recipients state a preference for donors to be matched to them on intelligence and personality traits rather than on physical characteristics.

Fifth, for recipients using anonymous gamete donors, there is often a desire to have as much *nonidentifying information* as possible about the donor. The infertility counselor can provide recipients additional information regarding a donor's family, education, and employment and social history, so as to make the donor more 'real' to them. Having this personal data may also be especially helpful in their efforts to disclose information to their offspring about the donor conception.

Ultimately, the donor's welfare must be a high priority for infertility counselor. Carefully exploring and understanding a donor's motivations for providing gametes may be the single most crucial element in counseling donors with respect to their emotions about the decision to donate. At the same time, the structured clinical interview serves as a vehicle for helping donors consider their feelings about any potential offspring that may be created, particularly when they are donating gametes to a close friend or relative.

THERAPEUTIC INTERVENTIONS

Several distinct clinical issues are relevant to gamete donation. These include the selection and psychological screening of potential donors (including criteria for acceptance or rejection), gender differences and attitudes toward donation, anonymous versus known donation, and the impact of donation.

Selection and Screening of Donors
Medical and Genetic Screening

The medical selection and screening process for sperm and oocyte donors is rigorous and very thorough. Thus, an unanticipated consequence of this for donors is the discovery of medical or genetic disorders that otherwise would not have been detected until sometime in the future, if ever. For some, this may be beneficial and protective, while for others such a discovery may cause significant psychological distress.

Sperm Donor

Selection. The ASRM guidelines[1] include the following: (1) donor age, 18-40 years, (2) good health status, (3) absence of genetic abnormalities, and (4) established fertility preferred but not required. A 1993 survey of Society of Assisted Reproductive Technology (SART) programs indicated an age range of 18–46. Most programs limit the number of pregnancies by one donor to 10 or fewer in order to avoid increasing the risk in consanguinity. There are no legal regulations in the United States limiting the number of donations or offspring per donor.

Screening. The ASRM guidelines recommend evaluating several semen samples 1–2 hours after ejaculation. Sperm are evaluated on volume, motility, concentration, morphology, and cryosurvival. In addition, most programs require genetic screening of potential donors, with some requiring a complete chromosomal analysis. The ASRM guidelines provide the requirements for a minimal genetic screening for gamete donors. A complete medical and genetic history should be taken and donors should be in good health with no hereditary or familial disease history. Donors are screened for the presence of diseases, especially hepatitis, sexually transmitted diseases, and HIV infection. Donors are tested initially for HIV antibodies, the semen is quarantined, and the donor is retested after 180 days. Thus, fresh sperm is no longer used for TDI.

Payment. Donors are compensated financially in differing amounts, but the ASRM guidelines recommend that the amounts not be such that 'monetary incentive is the primary factor in donating sperm'. In countries where donors are not financially compensated or legally required to be identified there has been a significant drop in available donors.

Oocyte Donor

Selection. The ASRM guidelines recommend that donor age be over 18 and, if over 34, that any recipient be informed of this. Most programs require that donors be between 18 and 35, although some known donors may be older than 35. The age range in one survey[11] of SART programs was found to be 18–41 years. Although younger donors are preferable for success rates, there is reasonable concern about using women under age 21 regarding their ability to give true informed consent. It is unlikely that younger women or men are at a sufficient point in their adult development, particularly as it pertains to reproduction, to be able to give true informed consent to donate their gametes. In addition, regardless of age, caution should be used with donors who have not yet at least begun their own family-building (or similarly have made a decision not to reproduce).

Donors should be in good physical health, and established fertility is preferred, but not typically required. Minimal genetic screening, as noted in the ASRM guidelines, is required. Limitation on the use of a single donor so as to avoid consanguineous marriages is the same as that of sperm donors. However, the risks from repeated ovarian hyperstimulation and oocyte retrieval should also be considered.

Screening. In accordance with ASRM guidelines, oocyte donors are screened for risk factors related to HIV infection such as intravenous drug use or sexual partners who are intravenous drug users. Serological testing is recommended for syphilis, hepatitis B and C, and HIV-I and -II. Donor ova cannot be quarantined for 180 days because ova have only limited success with being frozen. However, the ASRM guidelines suggest that recipients be offered the option of having resulting embryos frozen and quarantined and then having the donor retested for HIV 6 months later. A complete medical and genetic history should be taken to assess hereditary or familial disease history, but at present medical standards for oocyte donors are not as standardized as those for sperm donors.

Payment. ASRM guidelines recommend compensating donors for the direct and indirect expenses of their participation, the inconvenience and time, and the risk and discomfort. They also recommend that a contractual arrangement be established for the financial responsibilities in the event of unanticipated complications or medical expenses. Financial compensation is not to be so excessive as to be considered undue coercion, and it should not be based on the number of ova donated.

Embryo Donor

Selection, Screening, and Payment. Although embryo donation has been done, it remains a relatively new reproductive option, and therefore no guidelines have yet been established regarding donor selection and screening. However, it is likely that the guidelines would be similar to, if not the same as, those for each of the gamete donors involved. In the case of embryo donation, cryopreservation is possible, and thus it is likely that donor embryos will be recommended to be quarantined, with each donor being retested for HIV after 6 months. Further, couples who donate excess embryos would not receive financial compensation. In the case of anonymous gamete donation for the purpose of creating embryos for donation, compensation would be the same as that for sperm and oocyte donation.

Psychological Screening

Although psychological screening is a necessary component to all forms of gamete donation, there are clear gender differences. In contrast to the rigorous medical screening of potential sperm donors, men are rarely evaluated regarding their psychological status, nor are they screened regarding their motivation to donate or their feelings about donation. It is unusual for sperm donor partners to be interviewed or needed for informed consent, unless it is a known-donor situation. Most oocyte donation programs use a mental health professional for

screening purposes and are likely to attempt to assess psychological problems, substance abuse, and motivations for donation; some attempt to evaluate psychological risk of donation. In addition, some oocyte donation programs require an interview with spouses of donors, who must also provide informed consent. The ASRM guidelines are consistent with this gender difference with their recommendation that psychological counseling be offered to all parties involved in oocyte donation, but not sperm donation. Some explain this gender difference as reflecting the greater medical risk for oocyte donors and the greater likelihood of coercion (if known donor), given the limited supply of willing donors.

Although most programs acknowledge the need for psychological screening of all gamete donors, there is difficulty in determining the factors to be assessed, inclusion and exclusion criteria (Table 2), and variability in the use of standardized psychological testing tools. It has been reported that only 60% of oocyte donor programs have stated psychological criteria for donor rejection and only 59% interview the donor's partner[11].

Interview and Counseling

The psychological interview is a crucial component in the evaluation of gamete donors. First, it helps screen out individuals with major psychopathology. Second, it permits infertility counselors to address motivation and informed consent issues for the protection of the potential donor; that is, the infertility counselor must assess whether the donor's motivations and expectations are realistic and psychologically healthy. Other than altruism as a stated motivation to donate, it is difficult to establish a consensus on psychologically healthy motives. Therefore, it may be easier to rule out unhealthy or unrealistic motivations than to look for the 'right' list

Table 2 Psychological indications for acceptance or rejection of a gamete donor

Positive indicators	Negative indicators
Absence of significant psychopathology	Significant DSM-IV axis I or II disorder, including standardized psychological testing score that is two standard deviations above mean
Absence of unusual life stressors	Significant current stress
Use of adaptive coping skills	Chaotic lifestyle, impulsiveness, poor coping skills and judgment
Ability to provide informed consent and understand medical protocols when necessary	Inability to provide informed consent and understand medical protocols when necessary
Supportive and stable interpersonal and/or marital relationships	Marital instability, lack of social support system
Economic stability	Significant economic instability or financial need
Standardized psychological testing within normal limits	Positive history or family history of heritable psychiatric disorders or substance abuse/dependence
Educational/employment stability	Significant history of erratic educational background or employment
	Current use of psychotropic medications
	History of sexual or physical abuse with no professional treatment for donor
	History of legal difficulties/sociopathy

Objection to gamete donation on the part of the donor's partner should be grounds for at least deferment, and probably cancellation, of the donation. The donation should never interfere with or create problems in the relationship between partners or significant relationships.

of motivations. Potential gender differences should be considered when motivations to donate are addressed. Men appear to be motivated more by financial compensation, whereas for women the primary reason to donate appears to be altruism[6]. The interviewer must also address any sources of coercion, financial or emotional, and evaluate a potential donor's ability to give informed consent regarding realistic expectations about the medical procedures and to cope with the stress of donation, never knowing its outcome, and the emotional consequences in the near and distant future. Partners of potential donors should also be interviewed and provided with education and information to assist

them also in giving informed consent to gamete donation.

The psychological screening is often the only opportunity for the potential donor and infertility counselor to have contact. As a result of this and the emotionally charged issues that must be covered in the screening interview, infertility counselors may often feel pressure to pursue simultaneous roles of interviewer/educator and therapist. Although the process of educating a potential donor to be able to provide true informed consent may in and of itself be therapeutic, it is important for infertility counselors to limit their role to screening and education in this setting. If psychological problems in a potential donor are identified during the screening process a referral for care to another mental health professional is warranted.

Psychological Testing

An efficient and effective method of screening potential donors is to use standardized psychological testing and a structured interview by an experienced mental health professional who has extensive knowledge of reproductive issues. Schover[34] developed one of the most comprehensive and useful screening methods for oocyte donors and lists a number of issues that should be assessed by the mental health professional during the interview (see Table 1).

In addition, the Mental Health Professional Group of ASRM developed recommendations for screening potential oocyte donors and embryo donors (see Appendices 7 and 8). There are no equivalent published screening recommendations for sperm donors, but these may be adapted for men.

Psychological testing using well validated objective measures of psychopathology and psychological adjustment is strongly recommended for use in conjunction with the interview. Testing can both identify psychopathology that the interviewer missed and validate the results from the interview. It may also provide content areas for further discussion during the interview.

Gender Differences

There is no doubt that clear differences— more accurately, a double standard— currently exist in attitudes toward male versus female gamete donation in both the medical community and society at large. It is difficult to identify the source, but a number of possible variables may have an impact on this perceived difference:

- TDI has been available decades (if not centuries), longer than oocyte donation, and thus older, less stringent screening and counseling standards are in place for sperm donation.
- The simplicity of TDI and its long-standing availability have helped with the acceptance of sperm donation by some, whereas oocyte donation and its reliance on high-tech reproductive technologies may be disconcerting. In contrast, others are uncomfortable with sperm donation because it is too closely tied to intercourse and adultery, whereas oocyte donation and IVF are so high-tech that the idea of sexuality and adultery are far removed and thus more acceptable.
- Many people may conceptualize sperm, which come by the millions in a small sample, differently from ova, which come one each month (or at most several with fertility medications). That is, some may conceptualize ova as 'more' unique and thus easier to see as a potential child. Therefore, there would be greater discomfort or negative judgment toward women who would give up their ova, compared to men who would give up their sperm.
- Women may be expected to have stronger emotional ties to their gametes than men, and thus oocyte donors may appear less maternal.

Anonymous versus Known Gamete Donors

The use of anonymous versus known donors remains controversial and once again reinforces the idea that gender programs historically used predominantly anonymous donors, oocyte donation began with mostly known donors[11]. The difference exist in gamete donation. While sperm donation reasons given to justify anonymous sperm donation as preferable to known donation have historically focused on protection of the recipient male, that is, protection of the self-esteem of the recipient and the relationship of the recipient father to the child[7,43]. Little attention was paid to the impact on donors. When the protection of donors was considered, the main concerns were fear of legal liability for resulting offspring, offspring claiming inheritance rights, or donor liability if medical problems developed with offspring[5]. Other concerns included fear of invasion of future family life by offspring. The ASRM guidelines for gamete donation recommend the use of anonymous gametes. However, with oocyte donation, the limited number of potential donors initially made the use of known donors the only available option for many. Anonymous sperm donation remains the standard, and anonymous oocyte donation is rapidly increasing as more programs increase their attempts at recruiting potential donors. It is interesting to note that the majority of anonymous gamete donors report that if their identity could be revealed to offspring at the age of majority, they would still choose to donate[6].

With the use of known oocyte donors, there has developed an interest/concern in the impact of known donation on the donor, both male and female. It is extremely important to discuss the issues surrounding known donation in the counseling of potential donors. Therefore, in addition to psychological screening, infertility counselors must help potential donors consider the following:

- How will they feel about any resulting children, since they will most likely have close contact (e.g., many will be donating to siblings)? Are they at risk of perceiving the offspring as their own?
- How might this donation impact the relationship between donor and recipient? Will it improve the relation-

ship, or is it likely to put a strain on it?
- What is the plan for disclosure? If disclosure to family/friends is planned, how does the donor think people will react? If disclosure is not planned, can the donor live comfortably with this secret?
- Does the donor feel coerced or pressured to donate because of the close relationship to the recipient?

Each of these issues should be thoroughly processed in the context of predonation counseling to insure the donor's ability to give informed consent and to decrease the risk of later regret or relationship difficulties with recipients.

Impact of Donation

Although little research has been done to assess donor satisfaction after donation, it suggests that most donors are satisfied and experience few negative psychological consequences. To keep donor satisfaction high, careful assessment of the psychological status of donors, their motivations, and their expectations is important for excluding those at risk for negative consequences. In the rare situations in which a donor experiences significant psychological distress after donation, an infertility counselor can often be of help. Brief counseling at this time is appropriate and may help the donor understand the source of the distress and enable achievement of a healthy closure to the experience.

Another related impact of donation is the attempt to donate that results in exclusion from a program. If exclusion is due to psychological reasons, it may be necessary for the infertility counselor to have a follow-up interview. The infertility counselor may need both to explain the reason for exclusion in a way that is protective of the donor's self-esteem and recommend further counseling with a referral to another mental health professional if the interview or testing is suggestive of psychopathology, emotional or interpersonal distress, and/or significant unresolved conflict.

FUTURE IMPLICATIONS

As mental health professionals become increasingly involved in reproductive health, it is likely that they will be called upon to provide psychological screening and support to all gamete donors. The growth of third- (and fourth-) party reproduction as a parenting alternative has led to the need for increased research into the motivations of donors, as well as an understanding of the short- and long-term implications of donating genetic material for the creation of new life.

The use of gamete donation in family-building also brings with it certain ethical issues that affect not only the decision to donate but also the work of mental health professionals in assessing and counseling gamete donors. Not surprisingly, the very essence of gamete donation begs the question of parenthood: does parenthood come with the contribution of genetic material, with gestation, or with raising a child?

Similarly, in caring for the psychological well-being of the gamete donor, one must ask what the rights of the donor are. Should the donor be told the outcome of the donation? Is the medical risk taken by young women donors too great? Does a young college-aged donor truly comprehend the meaning of the donation if he or she has never had a child? Does the known donor have rights or privileges that are different from those of the anonymous donor? These and other compelling questions will continue to confront mental health professionals, as well as ethicists and health care professionals.

Lastly, as the assessment and counseling of gamete donors becomes more well-defined, it is likely that recipient couples will increasingly request more information about anonymous and identified donors. This need may be based not only on the wish to provide offspring as much information as possible but also on a powerful desire to have the donor matched to the recipient on the basis of personality traits and intelligence, as well as on phenotype. As noted previously, these factors may enable the recipient to feel more emotionally tied to the donor. It may also be an attempt to mitigate the losses inherent in the need for the use of gamete or embryo donation.

SUMMARY

- Historically, the use of gamete donation (sperm) dates back thousands of years. However, there is little information about the motivations underlying the decision to provide genetic material to another person(s). In addition, the data are limited regarding the short- and long-term implications for the donor of providing gametes.

- Embryo donation has also become a disposition alternative for couples who have excess cryopreserved embryos following IVF cycles. The decision to donate embryos to another infertile couple has a powerful emotional as well as ethical impact.

- Current research on gamete donors suggests that little is actually known about motivations, the impact of the use of known versus anonymous versus identified donors, and the effects of the donation on the donor's partner and family over the long term. The need for more, well researched information is evident.

- Although there is no specific theoretical framework underlying the need for psychological assessment and support of donors, some of the theory regarding organ donation may be

372

useful in our understanding of gamete donors. The concepts of *altruism* and *exchange and reinforcement* are helpful, but they do not fully take into account the donation of genetic material to create a child for another family.

- Clinical issues in the psychological evaluation and counseling of gamete donors include the need to protect both the recipient and the donor. Infertility counselors attempt to assess psychological problems, substance abuse, motivations for donation, and the potential psychological risk of donation. Donors are also counseled about issues regarding being informed of the outcome of the donation and the relationship with the recipient (known donation) and the potential offspring. Follow-up with donors is also recommended.

- It appears that mental health professionals will continue to play a significant role in the area of third- and fourth-party reproduction. The need for further data about gamete donors appears crucial in light of the ethical and psychosocial ramifications of these reproductive procedures.

REFERENCES

1. Practice Committee of the American Fertility Society. Guidelines for gamete donation: 1993. *Fertil Steril* 1993;59 (suppl):1s–9s

2. Rubin B. Psychological aspects of human artificial insemination. *Arch Gen Psychiatry* 1965;13:121–32

3. Rosenwaks Z. Donor eggs: Their application in modern reproductive technologies. *Fertil Steril* 1987;47:895–909

4. Office of Technology Assessment. *Artificial Insemination Practice in the U.S.* Washington, DC: US Government Printing Office, 1988

5. Schenker JG. Sperm, oocyte, and pre-embryo donation. *J Assist Reprod Genet* 1995;12:499–508

6. Schover LR, Rothmann SA, Collins RL. The personality and motivation of semen donors: A comparison with oocyte donors. *Hum Reprod* 1992;7:575–9

7. Klock SC, Maier D. Psychological factors related to donor insemination. *Fertil Steril* 1991;56:489–95

8. Gillis MW, Rausch DT. Survey results on the current practice of sperm banks. Unpublished manuscript, 1997

9. Trounson A, Leeton J, Besanko M, Wood C, Conti A. Pregnancy established in an infertile patient after transfer of an embryo fertilized in vitro. *Br Med J* 1983;286:835–7

10. Lutjen P, Trounson A, Leeton J, Findlay J, Wood C, Renou P. The establishment and maintenance of pregnancy using in vitro fertilization and embryo donation in a patient with ovarian failure. *Nature* 1984;207:174–6

11. Braverman AM. Survey results on the current practice of oocyte donation. *Fertil Steril* 1993;59:1216–20

12. Gianaroli L, Bertocci G, Ferraretti AP, Mencaglia L. World survey of oocyte donation: Abstracts from 10th world congress on IVF and assisted reproduction. *J Assist Reprod Genet* 1997;14(suppl):32s

13. Sauer MV, Paulson RJ, Lobo RA. Reversing the natural decline in human fertility. *JAMA* 1992;268:1275–9

14. Sauer MV, Paulson R J. Human oocyte and preembryo donation: An evolving method for the treatment of infertility. *Am J Obstet Gynecol* 1990;163:1421–4

15. Leeton J, Harman J. The donation of oocytes to known recipients. *Aust N Z J Obstet Gynaecol* 1987;27:248–50

16. Braverman AM. Oocyte donation: Psychological and counseling issues. *Clin Consult Obstet Gynecol* 1994;6:143–9

17. Raoul-Duval A, Letur-Konirsch H, Frydman R. Anonymous oocyte donation: A psychological study of recipients, donors and children. *Hum Reprod* 1992;7:51–4

18. Society for Assisted Reproductive Technology, the American Fertility Society. Assisted reproductive technology in the United States and Canada: 1991 results from the Society for Assisted Reproductive

Technology generated from the American Fertility Society registry. *Fertil Steril* 1993; 59:956–62

19. Ibrahim YM. Ethical furor erupts in Britain: Should Embryos be destroyed? *The New York Times* August 1, 1996

20. Novaes SB. Giving, receiving, repaying: Gamete donor and donor policies in reproductive medicine. *Int J Technol Assess Health Care* 1989;5:639–57

21. Haimes E. Issues of gender in gamete donation. *Soc Sci Med* 1993;36:85–93

22. Broderick P, Walker I. Information access and donated gamete: How much do we know about who wants to know? *Hum Reprod* 1995;10:3338–41

23. Seibel MM. Therapeutic donor insemination. In: Seibel MM, Crockin SL, eds. *Family Building Through Egg and Sperm Donation: Medical, Legal, and Ethical Issues.* Sudbury, MA: Jones and Bartlett, 1996;33–52

24. Schover LR. Psychological evaluation and counseling of gamete donors. In: Clinical Assessment and Counseling in Third-party Reproduction (XIII). Proceedings of Annual Postgraduate Course of the American Society for Reproductive Medicine; Montreal, Quebec, Canada; Birmingham, AL: ASRM. October, 1993

25. Mahlstedt PP, Probasco KA. Sperm donors: Their attitudes toward providing medical and psychosocial information for recipient couples and donor offspring. *Fertil Steril* 1991;56:747–53

26. Daniels KR, Curson R, Lewis GM. Families formed as a result of donor insemination: The views of semen donors. *Child Fam Soc Work* 1996;1:97–106

27. Daniels KR, Ericsson HL, Burn IP. Families and donor insemination: The views of semen donors. *Scand J Soc Welfare* 1996;5:229–37

28. Daniels KR, Curson R, Lewis GM. Semen donor recruitment: A study of donors in two clinics. *Hum Reprod* 1996;11:746–51

29. Schover LR, Reis J, Collins RL, Blankstein J, Kanoti G, Quigley MM. The psychological evaluation of ovum donors. *J Psychosom Obstet Gynaecol* 1990;11:299–399

30. Schover LR, Collins RI, Quigley MM, *et al.* Psychological follow-up of women evaluated as oocyte donors. *Hum Reprod* 1991;6:1487–91

31. Lessor R, Cervantes N, O'Connor N,

Balmaceda J, Asch RH. An analysis of social and psychological characteristics of women volunteering to become oocyte donors. *Fertil Steril* 1993;59:65–71

32. Berg BJ, Lewis V. Motivations of oocyte donors: A preliminary investigation. Poster presentation at the annual meeting of the American Society of Psychosomatic Obstetrics and Gynecology, Charleston, SC, March, 1993

33. Brill M, Levin S. Psychologic counseling and screening for egg donation. In: Seibel MM, Crockin SL, eds. *Family Building Through Egg and Sperm Donation: Medical, Legal, and Ethical Issues.* Sudbury, MA: Jones and Bartlett, 1996;76–93

34. Schover LR. Psychological aspects of oocyte donation. *Infertil Reprod Med Clin North Am* 1993;4:483–502

35. Bartlett JA. Psychiatric issues in non-anonymous oocyte donation. *Psychosomatics* 1991;32:433–7

36. Greenfeld DA, Nero FP, Greenfeld DG, *et al.* Distribution of frozen embryos: A patient survey. Poster presentation at the 7th world congress of IVF and assisted procreations, Paris, France, June, 1991

37. Laruelle C, Englert Y. Psychological study of in vitro fertilization-embryo transfer participants' attitudes toward the destiny of their supernumerary embryos. *Fertil Steril* 1995; 63:1047–50

38. Cooper S. The destiny of supernumerary embryos? *Fertil Steril* 1996;65:205. Letter to editor

39. Robinson JA. Ethical and legal issues in human embryo donation. *Fertil Steril* 1995; 64:885–94

40. Macaulay J, Berkowitz L, eds. *Altruism and Helping Behavior: Social Psychological Studies of Some Antecedents and Consequences.* New York: Academic Press, 1970

41. Simmons RG, Klein SD, Simmons RL. *Gift of Life: The Social and Psychological Impact of Organ Transplantation.* New York: Wiley, 1977

42. Plomin R. Environment and genes: Determinants of behavior. *Am Psychol* 1989;44:105–11

43. David A, Avidan D. Artificial insemination by donor: Clinical and psychological aspects. *Fertil Steril* 1976;27:528–32

44. Burns LH. An overview of the psychology of infertility. *Infertil Reprod Med Clin North Am* 1993;4:433–54

21

Surrogacy and Gestational Carrier Participants

Hilary Hanafin, PhD

The only gift is a portion of thyself.
Ralph Waldo Emerson

HISTORICAL OVERVIEW

Surrogate parenting has taken place informally throughout time. Although the practice of surrogacy dates back to the Old Testament, it was not practiced in contemporary American society formally until the 1970s. In 1977 the first contractual surrogacy was presented as an option to a wide range of infertile couples. *Surrogate parenting* was defined as an arrangement in which a woman was artificially inseminated with the semen of the husband in an infertile couple and the resulting baby was relinquished to the father and his infertile wife. By 1980, at least three private infertility clinics in the United States were offering services to infertile couples that included the advertisement for and introduction to women who would conceive a child for a contracting couple. By 1986, there were at least seven clinics available to couples and potential surrogates; approximately 500 children had been born as a result of these new and controversial arrangements.

This new alternative to childlessness continued despite the public controversy that erupted around it. Public concern about this new industry and the legal and ethical dilemmas it presented became the focus of much debate. The psychological repercussions of surrogacy for the surrogate and for the children involved was of primary concern to many. Some argued that intentionally creating children who were to be separated physically and legally from their birthmothers and half-siblings was contrary to public and social policy. Additionally, the curiosity about the enigmatic nature of women who became surrogates or gestational carriers was a concern. The media, legal community, and feminist community took an interest in these early volunteer birthmothers. In the psychological community, only a small number began to address the complex issues, and to this day there is a paucity of psychological research on surrogate mothers or gestational carriers, the infertile couples who contract with them, and children born as a result of this technology.

As the debates via courtroom and television continued, the practice of surrogacy grew and broadened in definition. The technical advances in in vitro fertilization (IVF) were applied to the practice of surrogacy so that in 1987 a surrogate mother delivered, via embryo transfer, a baby who was not genetically related to her. Women volunteered to be the host uterus—*gestational carriers*—for an infertile couples' genetic embryo. Excitement about this new medical success was accompanied by controversies about the legal and social definitions of mother and motherhood. To some, the lack of genetic connection between the baby and carrying mother made a significant difference; to others it was irrelevant. Physicians and hospital ethics committees began debating the ethics of participating in the implantation of patients' embryos into gestational carriers. While some IVF centers elected not to provide such a service to their patients, others did so on a case-by-case basis, while a few clinics actually offered the service of finding and matching their patients with carriers or surrogates.

The practice of surrogacy has continued despite the controversies and the paucity of research. By 1997, there were approximately 6000 births by surrogate mothers, according to statistics compiled by the Center for Surrogate Parenting and Egg Donation[1]. There is no central reporting of such contractual arrangements, so the actual number is unknown. Of the births, approximately 500 are the result of the more medically complicated method of conception, IVF gestational-carrier surrogacy.

Language and appropriate definitions in the field of third-party reproduction have been the source of debates among mental health professionals, ethicists, lawyers, physicians, and feminists in a struggle to agree on what words accurately describe the various roles of the patients involved. The word *surrogate* was seen as accurate to some because it reflected the intent of the women and how they reportedly perceived themselves. To others, *surrogate* was offensive in that the woman was indeed the mother. There has been a tendency by some to eliminate the word *mother* in third-party reproduction in order to reinforce the concept of the surrogate as

having no status or intention to be parent. However, others contend that the word *mother* is important so as not to minimize the value and integrity of the woman's role. The choice of terminology became more confusing with the application of IVF, embryo transfer, and gamete and embryo donation to the world of surrogate parenting. Centers across the country have chosen different terms to describe the woman who gestates another couple's embryo: *host surrogate, gestational carrier,* and *IVF surrogate.* Furthermore, the infertile couples are most often referred to as *prospective parents, intended parents,* or *contracting parents.* The traditional term *adoptive parents* has not been widely employed in surrogate practices, primarily to differentiate the practice of adoption from surrogacy wherein the resulting child was conceived for a specific couple and typically has a genetic relationship to at least one of the parents. More recently, *prenatal adoption* has been used to refer to gamete donation parenthood. In this book, *gestational carrier* has been used to refer to a woman who carries a pregnancy (embryo) conceived by IVF for a contracting couple who are also the intended parents. *Surrogate* has been used to refer to a woman who conceives via artificial insemination (AI) using the semen of the contracting husband. The term *intended parents* has been employed when referring to the contracting or prospective couple who are usually the infertile couple. In addition, *surrogacy* has also sometimes been used to refer to both surrogate and gestational carrier pregnancies.

This chapter will address:

- current practices in psychosocial evaluation and screening of third-party reproduction participants
- the roles of the mental health professional working with surrogates, gestational carriers, and intended parents

- common psychosocial problems encountered in third-party reproduction agreements and procedures
- legal and contractual considerations for the mental health professional working in this unique new field.

REVIEW OF THE LITERATURE

During the 1980s there was a dramatic increase in the literature on surrogate parenting, most of which addressed ethical and social policy issues. The literature and research as it pertains to the dynamics of surrogate mothers, gestational carriers, and the resulting new families was limited. To date, most research has focused on the psychological dynamics and motivations of surrogate mothers and gestational carriers. Franks[2] and Parker[3], in the first published research in the early 1980s, presented brief articles that explained and described the enigmatic population of surrogate mothers. Parker expanded his work with Reame in 1992 writing a description of 44 surrogacy pregnancies[4]. In addition, in 1992, the first descriptive study about the new IVF gestational-carrier surrogates was published by Mechanick-Braverman and Corson[5], while Hanafin[6] and Resnick[7] conducted doctoral dissertations in the 1980s that attempted a broader explanation of the psychological dynamics in third-party reproduction. All researchers were strikingly similar in their conclusions about the motivations and the demographics of surrogate mothers. Most importantly, none of the research found psychopathology in the participants. Resnick had one of the more interesting of the early studies, including a comparison of psychosocial histories between surrogates and nonsurrogates. There was no difference between the two groups' histories of attachment and abandonment.

Much needed long-term studies are slowly emerging as this field grows. In 1987, Hanafin[8] reported on 37 surrogates and 16 new families that had completed a surrogacy program. Ciccarelli[9] conducted a long-term follow-up study of 14 surrogate mothers and Reame[10] is collecting long-term data via interviews with surrogates who gave birth gave birth ten years ago. Preliminary findings in both studies are similar to Hanafin's[8]. In summary, surrogate mothers overall do not regret their involvement, and their satisfaction is positively correlated with a respectful and comfortable relationship with the parents. The respect shown by the parents and the contact with them appears to have significant consequences for the surrogates' long-term comfort.

THEORETICAL FRAMEWORK

The most applicable theoretical framework to this new field is probably traditional psychological assessment. In psychological assessment the clinician assesses human behavior in a given situation or arena of concern, often with the help of psychological testing. The main focus is usually problem-solving and decision-making. 'The clinician must have knowledge concerning problem areas and, on the basis of this knowledge, form a general idea regarding behaviors to observe and areas in which to collect relevant data.'[11]. The role of the mental health professional in third-party reproduction (as in other areas of infertility treatment) involves assessment and evaluation, patient preparation and education, and occasionally psychotherapeutic intervention. Assessment is often defined as screening, or more pejoratively as 'gate-keeping' in infertility and third-party reproduction but is nevertheless a fundamental to infertility counseling.

Mental health professionals providing evaluations and counseling services for surrogacy and gestational carrier arrangements tend to play several roles:

- The professional trying to determine what is best for all of the parties involved, including the existing children
- The professional asked to predict human behavior in a field where the well-being of children and family are at stake
- The professional able to foresee the range of problems that occur in third-party reproduction and pregnancy and to apply these to the unique circumstances of the person's life.

The involvement of mental health professionals in surrogacy has historically been inconsistent, with the majority of surrogacy programs not including mental health professionals as part of the treatment team. Typically the mental health professional evaluated the potential surrogate or gestational carrier prior to formally contracting with the infertile couple, although psychological evaluation was typically optional. In most programs, the mental health professional's role ended after the evaluation. However, a few of the early programs implemented mental health services as a standard component of their programs. The infertility counselor evaluated potential surrogate/carriers as well as intended parents, and provided individual and group counseling with both parties throughout the process.

This role of evaluator, gatekeeper, and counselor of surrogates, carriers, and infertile couples presents considerable dilemmas for the mental health professional. First, it was suggested that the mental health professional was colluding in an unhealthy, perhaps pathological process. Some believed that simply being involved endorsed the intentional conception of a child who would be placed for adoption, which was in and of itself an unethical role for mental health professionals. A frequent criticism was that it supported or encouraged the 'planned abandonment' of a child. Second, there was no research or

literature on which mental health professionals in the field could rely because the field was so new. Adoption literature was a primary source, although the psychological assumptions about adoption issues were in transition. Assumptions that secrecy was best for family members and that adoption issues were easily resolved had come under scrutiny. The writings of Sorosky[12], Brodskinsky[13], and Kaplan-Roszia[14] and others challenged these long-standing assumptions, thus impacting surrogacy work as well.

The impact of new adoption perspectives were most clearly seen when looking at the openness between surrogate/carriers and the intended or contracting parents. Adoption experts addressing issues of the adoption triad, the need to know, and the importance of psychological resolution all have had an important impact on third-party reproduction. As the adoption literature addressed the negative impact of anonymity, the field of third-party reproduction adopted a more open process in which the exchange of information and the relationships between families focused on long-term adjustment of all participants. The majority of third-party reproduction professionals choose an open format in which couples and surrogate/carriers meet each other and arrange a contract often including contact throughout the pregnancy. However, a few programs continued to prefer anonymous third-party arrangements. Finally, third-party reproduction clearly proved to be a successful social experiment, in which mental health professionals provided assessment and support using the open relationship model.

CLINICAL ISSUES

Screening of Surrogates and Gestational Carriers

Psychological screening of surrogate or gestational carrier candidates is an optional process from a legal standpoint. However, all parties including patients, physicians, and mental health professionals have more legal protection if an evaluation has been done. Ultimately, the role of the mental health professional is to help a candidate decide if being a surrogate or gestational carrier will serve a positive, satisfying purpose or a negative, dysfunctional purpose in her life. She needs to be able to give informed consent, be at peace with the relinquishment of the child, and leave the program whole and unharmed. In an effort to serve both parties, the mental health professional assesses the surrogate/carrier candidate's motivations, her ability to accurately perceive situations, her personality, and her intellectual competency.

Over 90% of programs only accept women who have given birth and parented at least one child. If a woman has not given birth and/or has not parented, she is less likely to be able to give informed consent. A woman with no childbirth experience may encounter unknown medical risks and will not be able to fully understand the physical demands that she is undertaking. A woman with no parenting experience may not be as able to predict her own behavior and emotions as they relate to the intended child. Another demographic criteria held by most programs is that of financial stability. If a candidate is participating strictly out of acute financial need, her decision-making process could be dangerously clouded.

As stated in the literature review, researchers report similar motivations across many sample groups. It appears important that a surrogate/carrier achieve something for herself beyond financial remuneration. Pregnancy itself is often cited as a motivation: many women report an attraction to the pregnancy experience. The opportunity to do something important, unique, and life-affirming is often stated. Most candidates express empathy for childless couples and speak about the joy given them by their own children. For some, empathy is increased by having had contact with infertile couples and having witnessed the pain and struggle first-hand. A relatively small percentage of candidates report that being a surrogate/carrier is an act of healing or 'redoing' some event or issue in their past. Sometimes this attempt to 'undo' or 'redo' a piece of their history is related to reproductive losses such as abortion, miscarriage, or adoption. It is important to help a candidate realistically assess whether her goals are attainable.

Related to motivations and goals are a woman's expectations and concerns about her relationship with the prospective couple (intended parents). It is crucial to explore the surrogate/carrier's hopes for contact and need for openness with the couple. A discussion of her wishes surrounding the relationship with the couple and with the future child will reveal many psychodynamics, as well as insure that she work with a couple with similar wishes. Unrealistic expectations, attempting to use surrogacy or being a carrier to fill a void, issues of mistrust, and a lack of clarity about boundaries need to be assessed. What she is looking for in the intended parents and how she sees herself in their lives are important issues to address early on in the process.

Personality assessment is the most important aspect of the assessment process. Being a surrogate or gestational carrier will present many ambiguous and potent situations. Predicting how a surrogate/carrier will respond to and resolve issues is key to protecting her and the families involved. A nonpathological personality that is resilient, adaptable, empathic, and intellectually competent and has good ego-strength is ideal. A psychosocial interview is fundamental to assessing her decision-making processes, her social and family relationships, her manner in resolving problems, and her ability to take care of herself and her children. Special consideration needs to be given to loss and trauma in her history.

Mental health professionals employ psychological testing to further understand candidates. There is no standard test that is used by every program. The challenge in testing surrogate/carriers is that their test norms are often similar to the general population. The Minnesota Multiphasic Personality Inventory 2 (MMPI-2) does help to eliminate psychopathology, but because the scores are usually within normal limits, other measures are often employed. Administering projective tests and tests based on nonpsychiatric populations is most helpful. Evaluators consistently report that the surrogate/carrier population typically tries to look their best in testing. This dynamic often results in a repressed or a 'fake good' analysis. Wolfe[15] analyzes test data for a large number of surrogates and reports that the Rorschach has provided rich information about candidates. She finds that it provides insight about life stresses, self-perception, the role emotions play in decision-making, and distortions in perceptions.

Additionally helpful in evaluation of the assessment is consideration of a candidate's support system, resources, and immediate family. It is standard to interview a candidate's partner, if any. It is anticipated that the partner will make many sacrifices during the process and will be thrust into vague and tenuous circumstances. The strength of the marriage and his motivation for supporting her should be assessed. Furthermore, her children are of utmost concern. Discovering how a candidate plans to explain the situation can reveal her own understanding of and empathy for her children. One may consider her participation more carefully if her children

have endured considerable loss and/or trauma. Mental health professionals have a responsibility to protect children psychologically. Robertson[16], who has counseled surrogates/ carriers since 1987, reports that she proceeds more cautiously and will do additional testing if the interview reveals painful histories for the candidate and/or her children.

One might consider doing references checks and/or criminal background investigations. If there is a history of prior psychological care, it is advisable to get a release of information and request a copy of the counseling records or have a conversation with the therapist. This information is especially important if the counseling has been recent. In addition, history of chemical dependency, eating disorders, depression, anxiety, and/or obsessive/compulsive disorder especially related to pregnancy or postpartum should be carefully assessed. Additional assessment information can be attained by the attendance at surrogate/carrier support group meetings. It is imperative that a candidate be educated about the protocols and problems that she may encounter. The educational and informed consent process is enhanced by speaking with surrogates actively participating in the process. Support group meetings prior to and throughout participation can be helpful for both the surrogates/carriers and counselors.

Lastly, the focus of the assessment interview may differ, depending on which program the woman is considering. Women who are IVF gestational carriers may need to be able to manage a burdensome amount of medical information and logistical inconveniences, as well as give herself injections for weeks or months. Furthermore, beliefs about fetal reduction and perspectives on multiple gestation are germane. On the other hand, interviews with AI surrogates typically focus on the feelings and fantasies about the genetic birth child. Though many surrogates tend to minimize the birth-family issues, it is important to explore their expectations, especially as they relate to their own children, the half-siblings. Additionally, traditional surrogates may have to endure more negative feedback and criticism than gestational carriers, who are genetically unrelated to the baby they carry.

Screening the Intended Parents

It should be briefly noted that there is a long-standing difference in the evaluation of intended parents, compared to the evaluation of surrogates and gestational carriers. The inequity with which these two populations are screened is due to several factors. First, women volunteering to be surrogate mothers are perceived to be more unusual and more difficult to understand than infertile couples, who are pursuing the common desire to parent. Second, surrogacy programs typically present themselves as providing a service to infertile couples and do not want to make these potential clients uncomfortable. In addition, most physicians and programs are philosophically opposed to the role of gatekeeper. Lastly, surrogates and gestational carriers are often perceived as having tremendous power and, consequently, as more threatening. Most programs do interviews of intended or contracting parents, although to date few programs include psychological testing of them.

Psychological screening of prospective parents, as with the surrogates, attempts to assess their general mental health and marital stability. For the third-party arrangement to be truly successful it is important that a couple be empathic, adaptive, and resilient. Participants who are overly intrusive or controlling, who are not comfortable with the concept of surrogacy, or who have personality disorders, put the surrogate and the program, as well as the child, at risk. The ability to trust, contain anxieties, and be generous in spirit serves couples well. The clinical interview should focus on their histories, decision-making processes, coping abilities and strategies, and marital adjustment. Observing how they treat the professional and other team members can be revealing and predictive of future behavior.

Often, the tool that is most revealing is a full discussion of the issues surrounding surrogacy. It is important to discuss how they came to this choice. Questions should reveal whether or not it is a joint decision, whether their choice is an informed one, and what they believe surrogacy can realistically provide for them. Education is an important part of the assessment. As with a surrogate or carrier, the motivation to choose surrogacy can be both healthy and unhealthy. Most couples choose surrogacy because of a desire to be connected genetically, to participate in the pregnancy, and to know the child's birth-mother. In addition, they often wish to avoid failed adoptions and/or the lack of opportunities to adopt in their country or state.

Perhaps, the most telling information comes from a couple's perception of the surrogate or carrier and their comfort level with contact with her. It is critical for them to have a reasonable degree of resolution about their infertility. The ambiguous process of choosing a surrogate or carrier, the intense and complicated means of conceiving, the long pregnancy, and the years of parenting all require a couple to be comfortable with the process and with their surrogate or carrier. The couple's capacity to trust and empathize with the surrogate or carrier can be predictive of the degree of tranquillity during the process and after birth. Conflicts are less likely to be exacerbated if the couple can contain themselves, seek assistance, and empathize with the carrier's or surrogate's situation. If the intended parents cannot envision themselves having some contact with the surrogate or carrier, then they should not proceed.

The evaluation and consultation with the intended parents usually include a discussion of the future and what they may tell the child, as well as what they anticipate telling family and friends. This discussion needs to be culturally sensitive. Often, educating the couple about child development and the myths and realities of adoption research is included. The consultation is typically spent sifting through the feelings about openness and imagining future discussions with the child. Encouraging couples to take the time to create a positive legacy for their child helps empower them to act with integrity and clarity.

Additionally, follow-up interviews can be conducted. If there is a concern, a second assessment by a colleague can be helpful, or interviewing spouses separately can be enlightening. To increase their comfort and their ability to give informed consent, it is advisable to have prospective parents speak with other parents and to do some reading. Most programs also require documentation regarding medical conditions and marital status.

The Joint Session

The meeting between the prospective parents and the surrogate/carrier and her husband, if any, provides a fruitful opportunity to identify any contra-indications to going forward. It is imperative that the surrogate/carrier candidate and her husband meet both intended parents. This meeting is important both legally and psychologically. If they do not have a history together, it is helpful to exchange what motivated them to pursue surrogacy. It is helpful for the surrogate/carrier to share her motivations,

reactions of her children and family, and her concerns about possible negative effects. The infertile couple should share their histories, their families' reactions, and what their day-to-day life is like, so as to build a connection and provide the surrogate/carrier with information for making her decision.

Medically, the joint session includes a review of the surrogate/carrier's pregnancy history and general health. It is helpful to provide the opportunity for the participants to discuss concerns about prenatal care (e.g., diet, lifestyle, caffeine, travel). Even among family members, there are different beliefs about what affects prenatal development. Other medical issues are those of physician, hospital care, and prenatal testing. It is not uncommon for intended parents with a history of painful losses to be vigilant, especially about medical care. The joint session should include a review of the surrogate/carrier's genetic history. Medical insurance issues can be complicated and should be reviewed very carefully. Lastly, a legal contract in which each party is represented by separate legal counsel is recommended. Issues addressed in the contract such as reimbursement arrangements, bedrest, premature labor or delivery, multiples, and miscarriage may be addressed in the joint sessions.

The discussion of fetal reduction and pregnancy termination dilemmas is critical, as the ethical, moral, and medical dilemmas are weighty. Though not all participants will be able to predict exactly how they will deal with these issues, it is important that the participants consider them and are clear on the decision-making process. They need to have similar approaches regarding how such difficult decisions will be made.

In surrogacy, almost every issue has a psychological component. A consulting mental health professional needs to raise the topic of finances, especially if the families are working outside of a program. If a couple and surrogate/carrier have found each other independently or if they are family or friends, the organizing of financial matters reduces the potential for anger and disappointment. Nevertheless, it is recommended that a intermediary trust office hold the funds and be in charge of distribution. The goal is to minimize discussion of and confusion about money. Power struggles can be avoided if an objective liaison is employed and if each party feels secure in the other's integrity and respect.

A joint session should also include a walk-through of the relationship that each participant envisions. As previously discussed, clients' assumptions about the role of openness in surrogacy are an ongoing issue. The desire for contact is part of the criteria on which they choose to work together. It is sad, stressful, and hurtful when two families have dramatically different agendas. Surrogate/carriers most often need to see the couple's responding like parents throughout the pregnancy. Their reward and comfort with relinquishing the baby are all increased if they know that the couple is eagerly preparing for the baby and is interested in her well-being. Achieving some clarity about contact during and after the delivery prevents psychological stress and harm. Even within family arrangements, there can be different assumptions about the wish for involvement before and after birth. Contact after the birth is often the most vague because of the incorrect application of adoption myths, the change in relationships, and the lack of structure. It is helpful to provide structure and definition in the relationship before and after birth which helps to reduce ambiguities, as well as misinterpretations of the others' behavior. It is advisable for the parties to have an additional consultation prior to delivery. The transition of the

child, the decision-making at the hospital, and the respect for closure are all important topics to be addressed.

Lastly, there needs to be a discussion about the surrogate/carrier's children. Is the couple willing to spend time with the surrogate/carrier's children? What will her children be told about this unique pregnancy? Does she anticipate any difficulties with members of either family? Additionally, if the intended parents already have a child, it is important to address the same questions.

Though sometimes these matters will remain vague, it is helpful to have some clarity about future issues with the intended child. Will the child be told about the unique birth? How will the role of the surrogate/carrier be explained? Will parents permit contact if so desired? How will the adults insure that there is an exchange of medical information as needed? What are each person's fears and concerns about the future? Are there issues of contact with extended family? A discussion of possible actions the families could take early on to minimize long-term issues is useful. These actions may include, for example, writing keepsake letters, assigning an intermediary for contact or emergency issues, and documentation of history. Of course, the critical variable for the child's long-term well-being is likely to be the degree of respect, warmth, and integrity between the two families.

THERAPEUTIC INTERVENTIONS

Common Problems

The problems than can evolve from a surrogate/carrier arrangement are endless. An important step in minimizing problems is to have a *proactive* planning stage. Many issues that need to be addressed in the planning stage have already been discussed. The inevitable common problems usually fall within three categories: (1)

struggles with mother nature, (2) struggles with the relationship, and (3) struggles with logistical surprises.

One of the most trying and disappointing problems for all families is the continual failure of mother nature to successfully and safely bring the child into the world. Miscarriages, high-risk pregnancies, birth defects, and illness all intrude, despite the best laid plans. One of the psychological issues stems from the disparate life experiences that the two couples have had with reproduction. They not only have different views of success with fertility but may have cultural differences as well. Speaking to these issues directly increases empathy and minimizes painful misunderstandings. The pains of infertility do not end with conception. Where surrogate/carriers tend to feel positive and invincible, the prospective parents may feel cautious and hypervigilant. Without understanding the other's perspective, there can be additional strain in the discussion of medical care, prenatal care, and the enthusiasm for exciting but tenuous news.

Beyond these disparate views of mother nature, there is the dynamic of 'my body, your baby' or 'my baby, your body'. The prospective parents come to surrogacy having surrendered a great deal already. Given that the issues of trust and control are central struggles in surrogacy (as well as infertility), it is inevitable that there will be conflict surrounding prenatal and medical care. The intended parents must decide both when to let a concern go and when to raise it. This discussion sounds simple at first but can be very taxing to everyone involved. A prospective couple is best served first by having accurate medical information and then choosing their confrontations carefully. As in any relationship, especially one in which trust is a primary component, one needs to make confrontations wisely. A surrogate/carrier

and a couple may cause each other great strain if they are not clear about the other party's limitations and what really matters to them. It is especially important to reaffirm with all parties that medical caregivers cannot be expected to mediate these differences. A mental health professional can be instrumental in deciphering when 'to let it go' and when to make an issue of something. Controversies usually evolve around travel, diet, money, illness, choice of doctor, and labor and delivery options.

Clients' assumptions about what type of contact and relationship they will have can be a common source of problems. It is exhausting and hurtful when the two parties have different agendas. Again, providing accurate information and increasing empathy for the other's perspective is usually constructive. It is important that the parties remain on the same team and adversarial positions be avoided. They need each other to make this work, and they need to create a positive legacy for the children. It is a common mistake for couples to mistrust the surrogate/carrier's integrity and consequently offend her. It is a common mistake for a surrogate/carrier to misread a couple's genuine enthusiasm and instead see anxiety or aloofness.

Perhaps, one of the clearest and most important roles that professionals can take is helping the families address issues of closure. Mental health professionals understand the importance of goodbyes and good endings. Given the understandable awkwardness, exhaustion, and anxieties inherent in surrogacy, it is helpful to clearly plan the birth, hospital stay, and postpartum contact. Giving attention to each family's needs and to simple rituals can be critical in assisting the families leaving whole and happy. Surrogates/carriers, as we all do, need to feel validated and trusted. A surrogate/ carrier and her family should not feel rushed and pushed aside. Couples need to have closure, so they feel safe and clear about the psychological dynamics of their child's birth-mother. A respectful, warm, and appreciative closure minimizes feelings of exploitation and emptiness for a surrogate/carrier. Attention to closure helps a couple feel secure in the relinquishment and provides a positive story to tell their child.

Legal and Contractual Considerations

Mental health professionals involved in surrogacy have several sets of legal paperwork with which they need to be concerned. One is a contract between the couples and the other are the legal documents between the professional and all of the clients.

It is important for mental health professionals as counselors and educators to refer clients to legal counsel prior to beginning attempts at conception. Being involved in third-party reproduction carries the responsibility of referring clients to other professionals so that they can better protect themselves. Legal consultation will protect clients from making poorly informed decisions, provide accurate information, and assist in creating a basis for an informed consent argument, if necessary. It is important for the clients to know the laws in their state and what legal issues can arise. Most surrogate/carrier arrangements involve a contract that outlines the responsibilities and intent of all parties. It also addresses issues of confidentiality, insurance, financial reimbursements, termination, misrepresentation, contact, etc. In addition to being legally significant, the task of reviewing important issues on paper is a revealing and clarifying psychological process.

Like clients, mental health professionals should seek legal counsel. The field of psychological assessment and third-party reproduction is legally complex. Professionals in this field are usually presented with two sets of clients, each with their own agendas, concerns, and need for confidentiality. The control of information—who is entitled to know what—can be tenuous and difficult when such evaluations are provided. It is recommended that professionals address these issues early in the consultations so that they are acting ethically and legally.

Three documents that mental health professionals may employ are a retainer, a psychological informed consent, and a conflict-of-interest waiver (See Appendices 9, 10, 12–14). A *retainer* may include such points as the professional's role, its limitations, the financial remuneration to be paid, and the nature of services to be provided, as well as the manner of action to be taken if there is a dispute. The *informed consent* outlines the understanding of the clients' roles and the guidelines of the professional's relationship with them. A confidentiality form also needs to be considered so that it is clear that the professional does, or does not, have permission to speak to other professionals and to the other client in the arrangement. The other document that is recommended is a *conflict-of-interest waiver*. Third-party reproduction and surrogacy/gestational carrier arrangements, in particular, most typically involve the controversial dilemma of one therapist's serving two parties. The waiver outlines this very dilemma. It informs the clients that there can be conflicts surrounding what will be withheld and what will be shared with the other party. Additionally, the waiver outlines the possibility that a counselor could give advice that is contrary to the other party's wishes. It is important to define who the client is. These documents do not waive professional liability, which can not be waived.

In this emotional and pioneering field, it is important for the mental health professional to consider serving clients only with whom they feel comfortable and qualified to assist. It is appropriate and ethical to refer cases to another professional if the decisions to be faced or the personalities involved do not appear to be ones that can be confidentially treated. A final means of protection for professionals is to receive consultation on a case and document that they have done so. It is in everyone's best interest to be informed about the legal issues and the profession's code of ethics.

FUTURE ISSUES

Third-party reproduction including surrogacy and gestational carrying is here to stay. The number of surrogate/carrier pregnancies increases each year. Mental health professionals are consulting with parents of young adolescents and school age children about the issues of their unique and once controversial beginnings. Research needs to be done on the families of surrogate/carrier arrangements, so that there will be more confident guidelines about the best ways to proceed.

Future issues will also include the new blended families. With the increase of options for family-building, there is an increase in the ways in which siblings come to their parents. One family can have children that are homemade, adopted, egg donor, and born to a gestational carrier. There are a growing number of families that have three children, each having had a different manner of conception and gestation. These new, blended families will be the source of helpful information, while simultaneously challenging the traditional definition of family.

Related to this issue is the increasing number of children born with four or five adults involved in bringing the child to fruition. Now that physicians can intervene at each step of conception, infertile couples and physicians can find donors to serve each separate step. New questions are being asked about the increasingly sought means of conception wherein an egg donor and/or a sperm donor are employed and the resulting embryo is implanted into a gestational carrier. The carrier relinquishes the baby to the contracting couple who are the intended parents. The birth of children involving the contribution of three women—an egg donor, a gestational carrier, and the contracting mother—has increased significantly since 1994. Furthermore, some centers report several families having been created by egg donor, sperm donor and gestational carrier, resulting in a child that has no genetic connection to the contracting couple who become the child's parents. Deliberations about these new multidonor conceptions are ongoing and are certain to be center stage in the future.

A correlate to the issue of egg donor embryos being implanted into gestational carriers is the increasing concern about multiple gestation in surrogacy. In traditional surrogacy there is no greater medically significantly risk of multiples than the world of homemade babies. However, with IVF and now IVF with young donor eggs, there is an increase in gestational carriers having twins, triplets, or more. The implication of young mothers conceiving high-risk pregnancies at the hands of IVF clinics on behalf of infertile couples (who may wish an 'instant family') certainly raises concerns of exploitation and poor judgment among participants. The new forms of conception and resulting multiple pregnancy are also likely to highlight the tensions surrounding prenatal care decision-making and medical insurance.

Lastly, there are certain to be new legal test cases and an ongoing debate about the definition of *mother* and *father*. As the number of surrogate/carrier arrangements grow with various combinations of gamete donation, it is certain that legislators, judges, and governments will become increasingly involved in defining *family* and family relationships.

SUMMARY POINTS

- It is important for all participants involved in third-party reproduction to have legal, medical, and psychological consultations.
- Empathy and integrity are key personality traits in the screening of surrogates, gestational carriers, and intended parents.
- The positive adjustment of all parties and the tranquillity of the case can be increased if the participants are well matched and invest in preconception discussions.
- Mental health professionals should encourage participants to clearly define the relationship through legal agreements and counseling sessions. When disagreements arise they should not expect medical personnel to mediate them, but instead address them with the mental health professional.
- The paucity of research highlights the need for all professionals to proceed cautiously in this new and ever-changing field.
- Mental health professionals providing evaluations and counseling services for surrogacy and gestational carrier arrangements tend to play several roles: (1) the professional trying to determine what is best for all of the parties involved, including the existing children; (2) the professional asked to predict human behavior in a field where the well-being of children and family are at stake; (3) the professional able to foresee the range of problems that occur in third-party reproduction and pregnancy and to apply these to the unique circumstances of the person's life.
- The inevitable common problems usually fall within three categories: (1) struggles with mother nature, (2) struggles with the relationship, and (3) struggles with logistical surprises.

REFERENCES

1. Synescu K. Personal conversation. Los Angeles, CA. 18 November 1997
2. Franks D. Psychiatric evaluation of women in a surrogate mother program. *Am J Psychiatry* 1981;138(10):1378–9
3. Parker JP. Motivation of surrogate mothers: Initial findings. *Am J Psychiatry* 1983;140:117
4. Reame N, Parker JP. Surrogate parenting: Clinical features of forty-four cases. *Am J Obstet Gynecol* 1990;162:1220–5
5. Mechanick-Braverman A, Corson SL. Characteristics of participants in a gestational carrier program. *J Assist Reprod Genet* 1992;9:353–7
6. Hanafin H. *The Surrogate Mother: An Exploratory Study. Dissertation*, Los Angeles, CA: California School of Professional Psychology, 1984
7. Resnick R. *Surrogate mothers: Relationship between early attachment and the relinquishment of the child*. Dissertation. Sanata Barara, CA: Fielding Institute, 1989
8. Hanafin H. Surrogate parenting: Reassessing human bonding. Paper presented at the American Psychological Association Conference, New York, NY, 1987
9. Ciccarelli J. *The surrogate mother: Post-birth follow-up*. Dissertation. Los Angeles, CA: California School of Professional Psychology, 1997

10. Reame N. Personal conversation. University of Michigan, Ann Arbor, MI. 18 August 1996

11. Groth-Marnat G. *The Handbook of Psychological Assessment*. New York: John Wiley & Sons, 1997:5

12. Sorosky A, Baron A, Pannor R. *The Adoption Triangle*. Garden City, NY: Anchor Press, 1978

13. Brodzinsky DM, Schechter MD, eds. *The Psychology of Adoption*. New York: Oxford University Press, 1990

14. Kaplan-Roszia S. *Cooperative Adoption*. Westminister, CA: Triadoption Publications, 1985

15. Wolfe C. Personal conversation. California, MD, 19 January 1997

16. Robertson D. Personal conversation, Sonoma, CA, 28 September 1996

VII. ALTERNATIVE FAMILY BUILDING

22

Adoption after Infertility

Linda P. Salzer, MSS

I did not plant you, true. But when the season is done—
Then I will hold you high, a shining sheaf above the boughs and seeds grown wild.
Not my planting, but by heaven my harvest—my own child.

Carol Lynn Pearson

HISTORICAL OVERVIEW

The world of adoption has changed significantly over the past 30 years. Prior to the 1970s, adoption was a more viable option for building a family than it is today. In years past, a greater number of healthy infants and children was available for adoption, for a variety of reasons—less use of birth control measures, fewer abortions, and greater social stigma attached to single motherhood[1]. The recent decrease in the number of children available for placement has led to significant changes in the adoption process and greater anxiety on the part of prospective adoptive parents. Today, adoption involves not only traditional adoption of infants and children but the non-traditional view of 'prenatal adoption' of gametes or embryos in conjunction with various forms of assisted reproductive technology and/or third-party reproduction.

Perhaps influenced by assisted reproductive technologies, attitudes toward adoption have become more open in recent years, and there is greater awareness of adoption issues, including knowledge about the emotional effects of adoption on birthparents, adoptive parents, and adoptees. Until recent years, most adoptions were arranged in secrecy, generally with anonymity and little exchange of information between birthparents and adoptive parents. Birthmothers were expected to 'forget' what had happened and move on with their lives. Adoptive parents were often unaware of the significance of birthparents in their children's lives or reluctant to acknowledge their impact. The issue of adoption was rarely discussed, and sometimes children were not even told of their adoption, perhaps unexpectedly learning of this secret later in life. Even when this knowledge was shared, feelings were typically not openly addressed. Adoptees were often given little information about their past and were limited in their ability to attain more information (e.g., search). Today, all members of the adoption triangle—birthparents, adoptive parents, and adoptees—are more vocal in addressing their feelings and needs. Birthparents are now asking for greater participation in the adoption plan and sometimes in ongoing contact. Adoptive parents are frequently given more background information about their children and opportunities to meet birthparents. They are being helped to become more comfortable with the differences that adoptive parenting brings. Adopted children often have mementos from a birth-mother—a letter, pictures, or special gift—and some answers to their questions of identity. Although there are many levels of openness in adoption today, the existence of better communication among all parties and increased awareness of the emotional impact of adoption has generally brought a healthier and more trusting atmosphere. This chapter will address:

- theoretical understandings of adoption and changing psychological perspectives over the past century
- common fears and psychological changes regarding adoption among infertile couples including the need to address unresolved infertility issues
- developmental tasks of adoptive families
- issues infertile couples must address in considering adoption as an option
- the different types of adoption options available today.

REVIEW OF LITERATURE

There are many fears about adoption that infertile individuals and couples must carefully address. A common concern is whether or not one can love an adopted child to the same degree as a biological child. Many fear that a blood relationship is necessary for an intense, close, and committed relationship. It is often helpful for prospective adoptive couples to discuss this issue with those who have already adopted and to observe their relationship. Parent-child bonding is not determined by a biological link. Despite these fears, one study[2] found that 95% of adoptive parents interviewed experienced a strong attachment to their child.

Another common fear is that an adopted child will ultimately reject his or her adoptive parents in favor of the birth-parents. Opportunities to search for biological parents are becoming more available through mutual disclosure registries, private investigations, and opening of birth records. Registries of sperm and oocyte donors in other countries may reflect this move toward increased openness in adoption. However, motivations and experiences vary widely when adoptees search. Some are disappointed because they have idealized this contact and/or potential relationship and it falls short of their expectations. Others who have positive experiences with their birth-parents find that it only enhances the relationships in their adoptive family. Many children seek contact primarily to obtain information about their heritage and their placement, in order to deal with identity issues. These are needs that cannot be met by the adoptive parents. A search does not imply inadequacy on the part of the adoptive family.

A third concern of prospective adoptive parents is whether an adopted child will be at risk for increased psychological difficulties. Studies on this subject have had conflicting results. A 1994 study[2] involving 715 adoptive families found that adolescents adopted in infancy were no more likely to suffer from mental health or identity problems than nonadopted teenagers. Several earlier studies showed similar results[2]. Others, however, have found that adopted children are overrepresented in the mental health system. Although less than 2% of children under age 18 in the United States have been adopted by unrelated parents, adoptees account for 5% of patients in psychotherapy and 10-15% in residential treatment[2]. There are several possible explanations for this overrepresentation. Adoptive parents, who have dealt extensively with medical and social service professionals during infertility and adoption, may be more likely to seek help should problems arise than those in the general public. Also, children who were adopted at an older age, often with a history of abuse or neglect, are certainly more likely to participate more extensively in the mental health system. Adopted children in general may experience periods of anger or depression in dealing with their loss and yet successfully resolve these issues.

Recent studies do indicate that adopted children are at increased risk for learning and attentional problems; 20-40% of adoptees are thought to have attention deficit disorder, compared to only 3-5% of nonadopted children[3]. Studies also indicate a higher risk for a variety of learning disabilities[4]. This may be due to hereditary factors, poor prenatal care including prenatal maternal drug or alcohol use, or complications during pregnancy or delivery.

THEORETICAL FRAMEWORK

Applicable theoretical frameworks include grief and loss, family systems—particularly family development, and attachment theory. The key issues affecting adoptive families are:

- grief and loss
- attachment and entitlement
- identify formation
- unmatched expectations
- shifts in the family system[5].

Grief and Loss

The experience of infertility brings many losses: loss of genetic continuity, the physical experience of pregnancy and birth, the breast-feeding experience, a life goal and expectation, a love child that a couple has conceived together in the traditional fashion, self-esteem, sexual identity, and control. Infertile couples approaching adoption need to mourn these losses to succeed as adoptive parents. Grieving is the ability to let go of unfulfilled dreams and

replace them with a comfortable reality. Not all grieving will occur before an adoption is completed, but couples should have resolved many of these feelings.

Adoption is an avenue to parenthood but not a cure for infertility. For most couples, adoption is a second (or even third) choice toward parenthood, and the losses from infertility must be emotionally resolved. When this fails to happen, problems will often develop in the adoptive family.

Adoptive couples must understand and work through the many losses that infertility entails. They must also acknowledge why they chose to adopt and come to terms with those feelings. It is important for them to identify their personal and often selfish needs in adoption, rather than focusing on any savior fantasies of rescuing a child from unfortunate circumstances or creating the perfect child through specially selected gametes. Infertility creates a tremendous loss of control, and many who fail to come to terms with this will try to reestablish control by overinvolvement with or overprotection of their child. Continuing fears of loss can also lead to overcontrol of the child or one's self as a parent. In general, 'there is ample evidence to suggest an identifiable association between resolution of infertile feelings and family functioning . . . Failure to come to grips with such feelings may result in an atmosphere of tension for the adopted child and the family as a whole'[6].

Attachment and Entitlement

Attachment theory (based on Bowlby's[7] work) is based on the premise that the infant's attachment to the mother or a primary person provides the security necessary for the child to explore his or her environment, and failure to form an attachment in the early years can be related to an inability to develop close personal relationships in adulthood. Attachment theory provides an understanding of affectional bonds and their meaning as well as who and what is lost by infertile couples: a biological child, fantasy child, parental roles, ties to spouse and extended family, or personal identity. Factors in attachment that are particularly important concepts in adoptive parenting include: bonding (the process of attachment), claiming, and entitlement. Claiming refers to the mutual process by which an adoptive family and an adoptee come to feel that they *belong* to each other. Entitlement refers to the adopted parents' sense that they have both a legal and emotional right to be parents to their child. In many respects bonding, claiming and entitlement are inextricably intertwined processes in the adoptive family.

Building a sense of entitlement means acknowledging that adoption is different from traditional biological parenthood. Biological and adoptive parenthood share more similarities than differences. When a child has been adopted, the parents have the same responsibilities as any parent in caring for and guiding that child. The parent-child feelings are equally loving and intense, and the child becomes an unconditional member of the family. A basic question to be considered by all adoptive parents and their children, however, is 'Who are the *real* parents of this child'? Adoptive parents must develop a sense of security in their role as the *real* parents both for their own sake and for the comfort/security of the child. Developing this sense of *entitlement* means that they believe that a child is really theirs and that they are really the parents.

Identity Formation

Identify formation is an individual's core sense of self, self-worth and identifiable boundaries[8]. It begins in childhood, develops within the context of the family, and is consciously shaped in adolescence. Adopted children (and parents) may have more difficulty with identity formation because they have incomplete or inaccurate information about their genes or birth family history, they do not feel they have full membership in the adoptive family, or because as they establish their personal boundaries they must cope with the ultimate attack on self-worth—'abandonment' by their birth families. Adoptive parents must recognize the particular issues of identity formation for their children, as well as their own issues of identity formation as the parents of adopted children, which may involve children of different races, cultures, assisted reproductive technologies, or other unique qualities that set them apart. Within this context adoptive parents cannot rely on traditional means of identifying with their children or with other parents.

Unmatched Expectations

Unmatched expectations may be a form of grief and loss, in that adoptive parents and/or children have expectations of the relationship, themselves, or each other that are unrealistic or out of synch with one another[8]. New parents may expect the rewards of parenthood in general or adoptive parenthood specifically to be greater than they actually are. They may express expectations of themselves as parents or of their child that are unrealistic or irrational, based on expectations that developed during infertility or beliefs about what is owed to them having weathered the storms of infertility or the adoption process. For many infertile couples this includes a relinquishment of the 'ideal' child that they had hoped to have or feel they deserve.

Family Systems and Developmental Tasks of Adoptive Families

Family system theory provides the ability to recognize how events in the family—nodal happenings—can affect the family's development. Family transitions and other nodal events such as marriage and parenthood require families to reorganize and adapt. Infertility typically occurs at a junction between developmental stages, that of a newly married couple and of a family with young children; and becomes an obstacle that challenges the completion of life goals and developmental tasks resulting in stress and requiring adaptation and reorganization on a number of levels.

Every adoption is made within the framework of the family system of those involved. It involves the creation of a new kinship network that forever links two families together through the child, who is shared by both. As in marriage, the new family created through adoption does not signal the absolute end of one family and the beginning of another, nor does it sever the psychological ties of the earlier family. Instead, it expands the family boundaries of all those involved[8].

Use of the genogram to identify extended family history will often reveal issues that affect feelings about adoption and aid in assessment of the couple's family system. How do family members view adoption? What significance does genetic continuity have in the extended family? How do the relationships with one's parents and the parenting that one received as a child affect the desire for a biological child? These are just a few of the many questions raised by exploration of family history and family system dynamics.

The developmental tasks of the adoptive families are: (1) resolving feelings about infertility, (2) recognizing and accepting the differences that adoption brings, and (3) learning to deal with society's negative views of adoption (including being able to handle the many questions and comments that accompany adoption). Canadian sociologist and adoptive parent H. David Kirk[9] was the first to present a theoretical framework of adoption that did not involve a psycho-analytic approach. Kirk contended that an adoptive family is exposed to different tasks and challenges that must be resolved in order for satisfactory adjustment to be achieved. Adaptive adjustment in adoptive families involve two different forms of acknowledging the difference of adoptive families: *acceptance of difference* and *rejection of difference*[9]. Kirk contended that adoptive parents who are able to strike a balance in their behavior are generally the most healthy. They accept the difference by not trying to pretend that adoption is 'just the same' as biological parenthood. However, at the same time, they do not dwell on the differences; they recognize that adoption and biological parenthood are more alike than different. In addition, Kirk was one of the first in the field to promote greater openness in the adoptive parent-child relationship, especially in the telling process, and greater openness and honesty in the placement process.

Another category of behavior in adoptive families, identified by David Brodzinsky, is *insistence of difference*[8]. Typical of this category are people who continuously raise the topic of adoption with others, constantly dwell on it, and always identify themselves and/or their child in terms of adoption. Such behavior generally indicates a sense of insecurity and difficulty with a sense of entitlement.

Learning to deal with adoption within the context of society is a third important step in reaching a sense of entitlement and family adaptation. Those who are secretive and continue to feel uncomfortable or embarrassed about being an adoptive family are exhibiting problems in this area.

They may see adoption as 'second best' or are fearful of being viewed differently or negatively as an adoptive parent. Negative societal views do exist, and the public is naturally curious about adoption or assisted reproductive technologies as different forms of family-building. Adoptive parents have a responsibility to act as educators and to dispel inaccurate or prejudicial information.

CLINICAL ISSUES

For most infertile people, the decision to adopt or use third-party reproduction (e.g., donated gametes or embryos) does not occur quickly or easily. During early medical treatment, when couples are hopeful of success, any mention of adoption can produce panic, that is, fear that they might not succeed in their quest for a biological child. Anger can also occur, as others insensitively and simplistically remark, 'Well, you can always adopt'. The general public fails to understand the complex emotional issues, the time required to make this decision, the financial expense of adoption, and the lack of availability of healthy infants or embryos.

Although fantasies of an ideal biological child are common during infertility, couples must put these dreams to rest and accept that there is no 'perfect child', either biological or adopted. When a person has not dealt realistically with this issue, the tendency is to continually compare the adopted child with the fantasy. Accepting a child for who he or she is, with his or her unique characteristics, is in large part what makes adoption (and parenthood) successful.

In resolving infertility, a couple must recognize that they can find tremendous happiness and fulfillment as parents, despite their inability to produce a biological or genetically-related child. They need to understand that bearing a child does not make one a parent. Rather, it is the day-to-day guidance, love, and care given that are the determining factors in parenthood.

In preparation for adoption, individuals need to acknowledge any signs of unresolved infertility. Again, it should be noted that resolution is a process and some of these feelings may not fully disappear until well after traditional or prenatal adoptive parenthood has occurred. Indications of unresolved infertility might include:

- sadness or anger around pregnant women that continues to be intense
- refusal to acknowledge grief or disappointment at being infertile
- inability to spend time around others' children
- strong fear that an adopted or donor gamete/embryo child will fall short of family standards
- ongoing fantasies about the perfect biological or genetic child
- continuing resentment of infertility and sense of feeling cheated
- discomfort in discussing adoption or donor issues
- inability to share adoption or donor plans with others out of shame or embarrassment.

Some of these feelings will continue throughout the adoption process but need to be acknowledged and eventually worked through to a comfortable conclusion.

When individuals are unable to resolve the painful feelings surrounding infertility and fail to develop a sense of entitlement, it can affect their parenting. For example, they may be uncomfortable providing appropriate discipline for their child. This may stem from a belief that they are not *real* parents who should have this role or authority. They may also feel insecure in the relationship and thus be fearful of their child's not loving them. Feelings of inadequacy, stemming from infertility, may also lessen their sense of competence. Sometimes, feelings about birthparents interfere with developing a sense of entitlement. Adoptive parents may have feelings of competition or believe that the birthparent would be a more adequate parent. Some empathize so much with the birthparent's loss, feeling their devastation, that they are unable to experience their own happiness and fulfillment as fully-fledged parents. In addition, some adoptive couples will have excessively high expectations of themselves, feeling that they must become perfect parents to compensate for their previous reproductive failures. A parent who is overprotective or overanxious, never allowing a child any independence, may also be exhibiting some difficulty with establishing a sense of entitlement.

When a couple resumes medical treatment for infertility after adoption, this may or may not indicate their failure to resolve infertility issues and accept adoption as a family-building option. Major developments in medical science continue to occur, and new advances can suddenly become a viable option for achieving genetic parenthood or couples may be offered various forms of prenatal adoptive parenthood. Those who adopt and then quickly reenter the medical arena, within weeks or months of becoming a parent, are clearly demonstrating unresolved infertility and adoption issues. These couples have taken little time to enjoy their child, adjust to parenthood, and/or to bond with their child and are giving a strong message that adoption has not fulfilled their needs. These families have unique adjustment, kinship, and attachment issues that need to be explored and resolved to ensure healthy family and individual adjustment.

Unfortunately, adoptive couples may need to contend with negative or uneducated views of adoption voiced by the general public. Infertile couples need to become knowledgeable about adoption and comfortable with their role as adoptive parents, so they can educate others about any misconceptions. It is not uncommon for others to make remarks such as 'Now that you've adopted, maybe you'll have one of your own', 'Who are his real parents?' or 'You're lucky you didn't have to go through pregnancy and delivery'. All of these comments reflect ignorance and/or a negative view of adoption or third-party reproduction. Those adoptive parents who view adoption as second best or who have not resolved their anger and grief surrounding infertility will continue to have difficulty handling the inappropriate comments of others.

As prospective adoptive parents, a couple must accept the reality of the child's birthparents or donor and their significance in the child's life. For some couples, the idea of a birthmother placing her child or voluntarily donating genetic material is incomprehensible. They may be unable to differentiate between the circumstances that they themselves are in (ready and willing to have a baby but unable to do so) and those of the birth-parents (physically able to have a child but unprepared in all other ways). It is not unusual for a woman enduring infertility to feel anger at others who get pregnant easily, unexpectedly, or unintentionally. Some prospective adoptive parents may continue to feel anger and resentment toward a birthmother who was able to conceive yet never wished to have a child. Being happy that a birthmother has decided to place her baby is not the same as being able to empathize with her predicament and her difficult decision. Often, when adoptive parents meet a birth-mother, they can better understand her situation by recognizing her as a 'real' person with 'real' problems and feelings. Negative attitudes about birthparents can interfere with the ability of adoptive parents to establish an agreement with the birthparents, develop a sense of entitlement, and to later comfortably discuss adoption with their child. Feelings of competition with the birthparents and/or fears of them reemerging in a child's life can also be problematic. These are normal worries for prospective adoptive parents and need to be addressed.

Couples also need to determine what kind of relationship, if any, they wish to have with the birthparents. Whereas adoption and donor gamete conception were historically shrouded in secrecy and anonymity, today's world brings a variety of 'open' adoption options. Frequently, birthmothers now want a more active role in the placement of their child and sometimes in future contact. This might include talking to or meeting with prospective adoptive parents, exchanging extensive information, sending letters and/or pictures on an ongoing basis, or remaining in physical contact with visits and telephone calls. Couples must assess their level of comfort with an anonymous, semi-open, or fully open placement. A fully open relationship typically involves ongoing communication and contact among all parties, including birthparent(s), adoptive parents, and child. The terms of the placement, including the degree of openness and extent of future contact, needs to be clarified before the adoption occurs. Those approaching adoption for the first time are often wary of contact with the birthmother and may feel threatened by her presence. Despite such fears, it is important that prospective adoptive parents obtain as much information as possible about the birthparents at the time of placement. Many couples find that as they feel more secure in their parental role, their fears begin to dissipate. They often later regret that they did not take the opportunity to meet the birthmother or obtain additional information. Meeting face-to-face with birthparents, gathering information, taking pictures, and asking a birthmother for a letter to her child at the time of birth can be invaluable in future years, when a child is interested in learning more about his or her origins.

THERAPEUTIC INTERVENTIONS

Considering Adoption as an Option

Most people who consider adoption will travel through numerous emotional stages before making this decision, including: (1) initial consideration of adoption as an option, (2) forming a decision as a couple, (3) soul searching (questioning personal beliefs, needs, and fears), (4) grieving over the unborn biological child, and (5) gathering information. These stages do not occur in a structured, straightforward manner and are not mutually exclusive. Rather, they are pieces of the complicated emotional path toward reaching parenthood.

Couples generally move from infertility treatment to adoption in one of two ways. Some feel the need to complete every medical option available before they can begin to consider adoption. They want to determine that biological parenthood is definitely beyond their grasp. Unfortunately, this approach is difficult because the field of infertility treatment is constantly changing and expanding, with new treatment options available at an increasingly rapid pace. Rarely will a couple be told that their situation is hopeless and that no further medical treatment can be offered. This makes it very difficult to end treatment and pursue adoption strictly from a medical point of view. A confounding factor is that patients are often offered medical treatments that are actually forms of adoption (e.g., donor insemination, oocyte donation, or embryo donation) and may fail to consider the psychosocial issues of adoption in their decision-making. Other couples begin to consider adoption while in the midst of infertility treatment. They may be frustrated with their failures in treatment and experiencing diminished hope, but they have not yet reached the end of medical options. They know, however, that they want to become parents and are considering future choices. These couples may be realistic or panicked about their slim chances for biological parenthood and concerned about the passage of time.

Should couples pursue adoption before ending their medical treatment? It is advantageous for couples to discuss the possibility of adoption while still in treatment and to begin exploring this vast field. The prospect of adoption can be overwhelming because of its complexity and the diverse avenues available (e.g., international vs. domestic, independent vs. agency). It often takes considerable time to evaluate all the alternatives and forms of adoption. Not only will it accelerate the process if a couple later pursues adoption wholeheartedly, but many find that it relieves the stress of medical treatment by assuring them that parenthood is ultimately possible. In the meantime, if medical treatment is successful, a couple has simply educated themselves about adoption.

Since many domestic agencies have lengthy waiting lists, it can be beneficial for couples to begin the adoption process while still in medical treatment. However, if a couple is planning to pursue independent adoption, they should be nearing the end of treatment. Independent placement can occur quickly, and couples must be emotionally and physically prepared for this possibility. This also applies when an agency with a shorter waiting list or with a portfolio service is used. *Actively pursuing both adoption and infertility treatment is not recommended.* Couples must allow time to educate themselves about adoption, for example, birthparent issues, talking to children about adoption, handling social

situations, resolving lingering feelings about infertility, and understanding the psychological impact of being an adoptive parent or an adopted child. Couples must also prepare physically and emotionally for the arrival of a child. Understandably, they may be apprehensive about making purchases for a baby or preparing a nursery, but these early joys should not be missed. Those who continue with treatment may not be able to invest their time and emotions in anticipation of a child's arrival. An unwillingness to stop treatment may also indicate failure to resolve infertility issues, an inability to accept adoption as a joyful and fulfilling path to parenthood, or a reliance on others (e.g., physician) for life's decisions.

Forming a Decision as a Couple

Partners often begin to consider adoption at different points in their infertility treatment and they may initially disagree about the decision to adopt. It is normal for partners to view this option differently. Couples often panic when they express dissimilar points of view, and this fear can impede further communication. Partners need to share their fears and skepticism with one another in an honest and open fashion. Adoption does require a leap of faith and can be both an exciting and frightening proposition. Often, the differences that partners express are not as disparate as they initially seem. For example, couples may agree on the next step in their decision-making process (e.g., going to an informational meeting about adoption) but be at odds on the timing of the decision (e.g., doing it immediately or waiting until after the next course of medical treatment). In addition, individuals often do not accurately express what they feel. For example, a partner might state, 'I could never adopt', when actually what he or she means is, 'I'm not ready to stop treatment'. It is important for partners to listen carefully to one another and to attempt to understand the feelings behind a differing point of view.

Often, conflict between partners develops because each has an internal conflict or ambivalence that is not being honestly expressed. The infertility counselor can serve as an objective and supportive third party, helping the couple to unravel these issues. During early discussions, couples often try to balance each other's point of view, consciously or unconsciously. One may take a strong proadoption stance with no expression of anxiety or ambivalence, while the other counteracts with a firm negative standpoint. Counseling can help couples identify points of agreement—similar fears, desires, objectives, or needs—that are often present. They can be given the task of making individual lists of pros and cons regarding adoption and then comparing these lists with one other. This is often helpful in clarifying differences and similarities. Infertility counselors should emphasize that talking about adoption does not mean that the individuals must pursue it.

When couples hit an impasse, it may be necessary to retreat from the conflict and to agree on a future date for further discussion. This may be several weeks or even months later. Placing the issue on hold, with the purpose of exploring individual feelings and gaining greater knowledge, often brings a change in perspective and more openness in future talks. Couples should be told that opinions about adoption often change over time as individuals deal with their feelings, reassess their situation, or learn more about adoption. It is not unusual for a person to adamantly oppose adoption at one point and later successfully adopt.

Soul-Searching (Exploring Personal Needs, Beliefs, and Fears)

When partners are in disagreement over adoption, they must allow time to privately consider the issues and gather information. Each person should determine how the losses of infertility have affected them personally. Which losses are most significant to each of them, and which of these losses could be addressed by making a decision to adopt? Each must assess his or her needs and be able to separate the experience of pregnancy from that of becoming a parent. Although most infertile people desire both the pregnancy and parenting experience, many have a primary focus. Most couples who ultimately choose adoption find that their desire for parenthood is more important. If the need for genetic continuity and/or a longing to experience pregnancy are the most significant factors, adoption will not fulfill these needs—although some couples may wish to consider using donor gametes as a means of meeting the latter.

Those considering adoption must carefully assess their views on the role of genetic factors versus environment in affecting the development of a child. Recent studies indicate the growing significance of genetic inheritance not only in determining physical characteristics but also personality traits, intelligence, and interests. Environment clearly plays a role in a person's development, but all children will display specific inherited characteristics. These traits may be significantly different from those produced in one's biological child, but not necessarily worse.

Helping Couples Grieve

Often, infertile couples become 'stuck' in their inability to grieve and cannot move comfortably toward adoption. Infertility counselors can help individuals and couples identify their reasons for their failure to grieve:

- *extreme anger*: inability to accept that infertility is a situation over which they have no control
- *unresolved guilt*: a view that they are 'bad' people deserving of their infertility
- *shame and embarrassment*: a belief that infertility is too personal, shameful, or embarrassing to admit to others
- *fear*: a need to remain in control, due to fear that grief will be devastating
- *denial*: inability to admit that severe infertility exists, an unwillingness to accept a negative prognosis from multiple specialists, or unrelenting and unrealistic pursuit of assisted reproduction.

In addition, some people are unable to grieve because the losses of infertility are too intangible. In such cases, couples may develop a ceremony for mourning, in which they mark the end of their treatment efforts and embark in a new direction.

For individuals who have been unable to grieve, infertility counselors may need to 'push' them into feeling. Therapists can ask them to picture their fantasy biological child. Who would he or she look like? What color hair and eyes would the child have? What would they name him or her? The infertility counselor may have them imagine different experiences with parenting and ask them to consider how their life would be different if infertility had not been an issue. If individuals are experiencing difficulty with verbalizing these thoughts, they may find it easier to express themselves in writing or in an artistic endeavor. The therapist might ask clients to write a letter to their unborn child. Sometimes, these feelings will also emerge in dreams. Interpretation of these dreams

can be helpful in addressing previously unspoken feelings.

Many couples become 'stuck' on the idea of a biological child because they have idealized what that child would be like. They imagine their own best qualities and believe that their offspring will be a composite of all their positive characteristics. It is important for couples to address the unlikelihood of this perfect fantasy. One way is to have couples list the worst characteristics of themselves and their family and then imagine their biological child as a composite of these traits. Couples will hopefully realize that this scenario is just as unlikely as the perfect child.

One of the most important aspects of grieving and ultimately resolving infertility is 'coming out of the closet', that is, being able to communicate openly about infertility with one's partner, close friends, and family. Infertility counselors should encourage clients to join an infertility support organization or a preadoption group. For those who have been secretive about infertility, a group 'normalizes' their experience, giving them the opportunity to share feelings with others who intimately understand the infertility crisis and to learn how others have handled this experience (see Chapter 7). When infertile people become isolated, they often feel 'damaged' or 'unworthy'. Participating in a group can help the infertile person view this crisis in a more constructive manner with less self-blame, anger, and isolation. For those who find a group logistically or emotionally impossible, the Internet is another means of connecting with others as well as gaining information.

Gathering Information

When people first consider adoption, many are overwhelmed by the scope of the field—the wide variety of avenues to pursue and the extensive psychological issues that need to be considered and addressed. Most have just emerged from the frustration and devastation of infertility, having educated themselves in the complexities of the medical world only to find that adoption brings an equally great challenge, another maze. Early on, the quest of adoption seems to raise more questions than answers.

One of the most important stages in the adoption process is information gathering. Couples need to understand the many options available and the psychological issues of adoption before they can proceed further. Infertility counselors should recommend that couples read extensively on all aspects of adoption, for example, how-to-adopt-guides, books from the perspective of the birthparents, books about life as an adoptive parent, and literature geared to children. Because adoption is often more difficult to accomplish now than in years past, prospective adoptive parents will need to avail themselves of all educational opportunities. They should attend adoption conferences, join an adoption support organization, network with friends, relatives, and professionals, and openly share their goals. An adoption support group is a valuable resource for meeting others who have adopted, becoming familiar with issues in adoption and obtaining information on the how-to options (e.g., referrals to agencies, attorneys, or knowledgeable professionals). Most support organizations offer monthly informational meetings, newsletters, videotapes, annual conferences, referral services, informal peer or professionally led support groups, Internet Websites, and library services.

Although many adoptions proceed quickly and smoothly, the adoption process is most often frustrating and time-consuming. Babies and children *are* available for adoption, but couples need to be creative and patient in their efforts. Most who persevere will successfully adopt, but there may be disappointments and dead ends along the way. Infertility counselors can be helpful in offering much needed encouragement and support during the course of adoption. For those couples who experience disappointment and may be on the verge of abandoning their plans, it is important to emphasize that persistence will ultimately succeed. Many begin to feel persecuted—first by their reproductive failures and failed infertility treatment, and then by their lack of success in adoption. Helping couples understand that such disappointments are common in the adoption process can help normalize their experience.

Finally, the more active a couple is in their quest to adopt, the faster it is likely to occur. Some will be most comfortable on an agency waiting list, but they should also continue to share their goals with others and explore additional options. Networking is exceedingly important because adoption leads can come unexpectedly from any source. Very often couples attempt to 'equalize' the infertility experience through adoption: the partner undergoing the least medical treatment is the one who takes responsibility for or does the lion's share of effort toward adoption. This strategy can be helpful when spirits or energies lag, especially for couples investigating adoption while completing medical treatment.

Kinds of Adoption

The numerous options available in adoption today can be confusing and overwhelming. However, this range of choice does allow prospective adoptive parents to determine what best suits their needs and their family values. Each has advantages and disadvantages that need to be carefully considered.

Domestic Adoption: Agency

There is a variety of agencies throughout the United States. In a traditional agency adoption, the birthmother (or birthparents) places the child with an agency, which then selects adoptive parents from its waiting list. The prospective couple may express their particular desires or needs, but the agency determines the match. In many cases, the birthparents and adoptive parents remain anonymous to each other, although nonidentifying information is generally exchanged. In recent years, some traditional agencies have begun to offer limited contact between the parties.

Agencies generally establish rules for their placements, and these can be interpreted in a positive or negative light, depending on one's needs. For example, many traditional agencies will place a baby in foster care prior to making an adoption placement. This is to ensure that the birthparents have relinquished their parental rights before the placement occurs. Adoptive parents then do not have to worry about bringing a child home and subsequently having the birthmother change her mind. It is a drawback, however, in not being able to care for the child immediately from birth. Many agencies also have restrictions regarding age, religion, marital status, length of marriage, criminal background, and medical or mental health history. On occasion, an agency might also stipulate that one parent plan to stay home on a full-time basis. Counseling is often provided to the birthmother when working with an agency. Although counseling can also be arranged in an independent placement, it occurs more routinely in an agency adoption.

In recent years, many nontraditional private agencies have emerged with innovative approaches to placement. Some, for example, encourage open placements, with meetings between adoptive parents and birthparents, extensive exchange of history and identifying information, and plans for future communication or visitation. Some agencies also operate with a portfolio system, in which prospective adoptive parents complete a portfolio that is then shown to birthparents who select the people with whom they wish to place their baby.

Agency Adoption: Special-Needs Children

One unique area of agency placements is the adoption of special-needs children. These include children who have significant emotional and/or physical problems or are mentally challenged, as well as sibling groups and older children, who often have a history of abuse or neglect. Children with special needs require exceptional parents. They must be flexible people who are willing to commit a tremendous amount of time, money, and effort to their child. Extra resources, including counseling, academic assistance, and medical help, are often necessary—although some states offer these families additional resources. Although the rewards are potentially great, it can be stressful and emotionally draining to care for these children. They often arrive with physical and emotional scars as a result of abuse and neglect and may have difficulty establishing close relationships. A stable, loving home, by itself, may not 'cure' these kinds of problems. Couples who pursue this option should have a realistic understanding of what to expect and an enormous degree of patience and resources.

Independent Adoption

Independent adoption (also referred to as private adoption) occurs when an individual or couple locates a birthmother and makes an independent arrangement for placement of the baby. This is generally in exchange for pregnancy and delivery-related expenses. No state allows actual payment for the baby. Sometimes, the contact is made through an intermediary (often a physician or attorney). In other situations, the prospective adoptive parents have advertised in a magazine or newspaper or used networking to locate a birthmother. Networking might include: (1) talking to friends, relatives, colleagues, and professionals; (2) sending out resumes, letters, or brochures; (3) obtaining contacts through the Internet; or (4) posting calling cards or announcements on bulletin boards, in newspapers, and in other community areas.

Independent placements are legal in most states; but at present they are not legal in Connecticut, Delaware, Massachusetts, and Michigan. There is a wide range in cost, depending on the extent of medical, legal, and other pregnancy-related expenses. If a birthmother has insurance or Medicaid coverage for her medical care and the legal costs are contained, an independent adoption can be relatively inexpensive. However, when birthparents request payment for living costs during the pregnancy, as well as extensive medical and legal fees, the cost can be significant.

There is a wide variation in waiting time as well. Independent placements can occur quickly, but some couples will advertise or network for long periods of time without locating a birthmother. Luck clearly plays a role. Because of this unpredictability, no one should embark on independent placement without being emotionally, physically, and financially prepared for a sudden response or the disappointment of 'false starts'.

One of the advantages of independent adoption is that many feel a greater sense of control than they might in an agency placement. They are actively working to locate a child and are fully involved in making the decisions surround placement. Although there are still many aspects of the process that are beyond one's control, some find it preferable to sitting on a waiting list.

Individuals and couples can also adopt without the restrictions found at many agencies. Another advantage is that there is the opportunity to adopt a baby immediately after birth, since most infants will go directly from the hospital to the adoptive home without the need for an interim foster care placement.

Although some independent placements can be completed anonymously, many birthparents and prospective adoptive parents pursue this option because of their desire for greater involvement between parties and increased sharing of information. Adoptive parents can determine, along with the birthmother, how much (if any) contact and what kind of communication they wish to maintain in the future.

Unfortunately, there are also significant disadvantages with independent adoption. Emotional and financial risks are both higher in an independent placement than in a placement with a reputable agency. The greatest risk is that until parental rights are terminated, birthparents can reclaim the child. States have different laws regarding the amount of time until relinquishment of parental rights, so it is important to know the specific laws in the state where the adoption will take place. Although most adoptions will proceed smoothly once a baby has gone home with the adoptive parents, there is significant risk of a birthparent changing his or her mind at the time of birth or shortly thereafter. It is not uncommon for an adoption plan to fall through at any point during the time of pregnancy or delivery. A related risk is that any expenses already paid to a birthmother may not be refunded should she change her mind regarding the placement. This makes it extremely important to carefully watch expenditures prior to placement and to get advice from a reputable attorney. Although most birthmothers are legitimate, well-meaning individuals, there have been scams, unfortunately, in which dishonest people have taken advantage of desperate infertile couples. The unpredictability of cost is an additional disadvantage. The costs of advertising varies widely, depending on the length of time necessary to locate a birthmother and the avenues used. The final costs for medical and legal services may also be unclear until the delivery and placement are completed.

Identified Adoption

Identified adoption is a combination of independent and agency adoption and can be especially useful in states that do not allow independent placements. It occurs when an individual or couple locates a birthmother through independent means and then contacts an adoption agency to oversee or facilitate the placement. All or part of the agency services are provided to the parties in involved.

Transracial Adoption

During the past 25 years, there has been considerable controversy over the adoption of African-American children by Caucasian individuals or couples. In 1972, the National Association of Black Social Workers presented strong opposition to transracial adoptions, and, as a result, the majority of states and agencies instituted policies that favored placements within the same race. However, although these policies still exist, there have been an inadequate number of African- American or minority families for same race placements. Therefore, some agencies now place African-American or other minority children with white or other non-white parents, in lieu of having them remain in foster care. Recent studies indicate that 'adopted children placed transracially do just as well, in all respects, as children placed in same-race homes'[10].

International Adoption

As with domestic adoption, international placements can be completed through an American agency, an agency or orphanage in a foreign country, or an adoption attorney/intermediary (i.e., independently). Fees for international adoption are comparable to a domestic placement, generally in the rage of $15,000–$30,000. Waiting times vary, ranging from 6 months to 2 years, but are often shorter than for a domestic agency adoption. Options exist in many countries in Latin American, eastern Europe, and the Far East. Travel requirements vary from country to country. Some countries and agencies have restrictions on age, marital status and length of marriage, number of biological children presently in the family, criminal history, health factors (including obesity), and/or work status (e.g., requiring one parent to be at home full-time). It is important to get up-to-date information on countries currently allowing placements in the United States. Changes often occur due to political events, government policy, and issues related to the adoption process. It is not unusual for countries to suddenly terminate placements, providing little information about when their doors will reopen.

In an international adoption, parents are not simply adopting a child but also a culture, heritage, and ethnicity from which that child originates. Infertility counselors must help clients assess their ability to deal with these 'differences'. Couples need to determine how they feel about parenting a child who will probably not resemble them and who may differ in other ways. They also need to consider how a child will look not only as an infant but when fully grown. Those who adopt internationally must be willing to help their child identify with both American culture and the child's country of origin. As couples assess their own feelings, they will also need to consider how their extended family, friends, and community will respond to their child being 'different'. Societal challenges may be a prominent factor in an international adoption, with the possibility of rude or intrusive questioning, staring, occasional discrimination, and greater attention from the public whether positive or negative. Those who successfully adopt from another country generally view the racial or ethnic diversity of their family as an enriching experience.

The children most often available for international adoption are 6 months of age and older. There is frequently little background information available, and the pediatric history of the child's early months may be limited. It is not unusual for children to arrive with health problems that were heretofore unnoted. Therefore, it is important to deal with a reputable agency, intermediary, or orphanage and to obtain as much information as possible beforehand. Adoptive parents must also be certain that appropriate health care can be obtained in their community.

Many who turn to international adoption are attracted by the availability of children for placement and the relative lack of risk related to birthparents. It is unlikely that birthparents will be involved in an international placement, and in fact they are often not known or identified. For those who worry about a birthmother changing her mind or later appearing in the child's life, international adoption may have some appeal.

There is no question that international placements require considerable paperwork and may involve extensive red tape. However, with guidance from an agency, attorney, and/or adoption support organization, prospective adoptive parents can follow the steps to placement without much difficulty.

Home Studies

Anyone in the United States who wishes to adopt must complete a home study or assessment. The process of the home study varies considerably, depending on the agency and/or social worker completing it. The traditional idea of home study was of an intimidating 'white glove' approach to evaluating a couple and their home for potential parenthood. In recent years, many professionals have restructured the home study into a process of parental preparation, in which the couple and social worker work together to help the couple become knowledgeable and effective adoptive parents. Many agencies now provide, in addition to interviews and home visits, the use of parent groups, meetings with birthparents (to obtain some perspective on their feelings and points of view), and a variety of other support or educational opportunities.

Regardless of the home study format and the degree of compassion shown by the social worker, most prospective adoptive parents find it to be a threatening experience. This, again, represents a loss of control for the couple. They are not able to move toward parenthood without the approval or intervention of others. Many prospective adoptive parents feel resentful, since the rest of the world does not need to be evaluated for parenthood. Frustration and a sense of powerlessness can reemerge, as well as resentment of the invasion of privacy: Issues often reminiscent of infertility. It is important that adoption workers understand these reactions and not set up an adversarial relationship with those wishing to adopt. It can also be helpful for infertility counselors to explain the nature of the relationship or act as an advocate for adopting couples. Traditionally, adoption workers have been advocates for the child, and certainly this is a significant role. However, it is equally important for these professionals to be a support system to the adoptive parents. When couples feel a supportive, positive relationship with the social worker (and/or infertility counselor), they are often more willing to communicate openly, discuss their anxieties, better educate themselves regarding the unique aspects of adoptive parenthood, and ask for help when needed.

Although some view the home study as unfair, it can be very beneficial. Adoptive parenthood resembles biological parenthood in many ways, but the differences are significant and as such, need to be understood and prepared for.

Waiting to Adopt

Infertility counselors working with adoptive couples need to understand that once a child has been identified, the waiting period can be extremely stressful. Not only are there normal anxieties about parenthood, but there is also fear that the adoption plan will not succeed. Will the birthmother change her mind? Will the child be healthy? In international adoptions, will the political situation of the country remain stable and the rules remain unchanged? If travel to the country is required, adoptive parents often have a number of logistical worries in addition to the adoption itself. How long will they have to stay in the country? Where will they stay? The sense of failure and pessimism that developed during infertility often leads to feelings of insecurity and pessimism about the adoption. Couples need tremendous support and encouragement during the waiting period. Infertility counselors should recommend that couples remain busy with constructive goals (e.g., working on home improvements, learning more about adoption or parenthood, meeting with other adoptive parents, going to baby care classes). It is also important for partners to spend positive time together. Infertility can easily erode a relationship, and this waiting time may be an excellent opportunity to renew previous interests and to recharge their intimate relationship.

Prior to placement, it is important for couples to begin educating friends and family about adoption issues. Significant others may be interested in reading some of the literature that the prospective adoptive parents have found to be helpful. It is important that adoptive parents, significant others, and professionals learn to use correct adoption terminology. For example, the terms *real* or *natural* parent should be replaced by the words *birth* or *biological* parent. In reference to the termination of parental rights, the phrases 'give up' or 'give away' should not be used. More correctly, a birthmother can be described as 'making an adoption plan' for her child. The term *illegitimate* should be replaced by *born to single parents*.

FUTURE IMPLICATIONS

Research that identifies the effects of adoption on birthparents, adoptive parents, and especially adoptees will continue in future years, offering clinicians an increased understanding of the needs and feelings of each group. Although *open adoption* remains controversial, the trend toward openness continues. It is expected that much research will focus on the long-term effects of *open adoption*, especially in situations in which there is frequent and ongoing contact among all members of the triad.

It is hoped that adoptive families and support organizations will continue to confront negative stereotypes of adoption found in the media and general public. The goal is for adoptive families to be viewed as equally loving, cohesive, and 'real' as those families with biological children. Adoption, like infertility, is becoming more visible in the community, through the increasing openness of those in the adoption triangle. This visibility should help to break down misconceptions and better educate the general public about adoption.

As the medical options in infertility treatment continue to expand, those struggling with infertility may find it increasingly difficult to end treatment and move toward adoption. At the same time, adoption avenues remain complex, expensive, and often time-consuming. Although large numbers of children with special needs and of nonwhite background are in need of permanent homes, the quest for the white, healthy infant remains difficult. The recent adoption tax credit in the United States has brought some financial assistance to prospective adoptive parents, but for many adoption remains a financially prohibitive venture.

Finally, there is an increasing awareness of the parallels between traditional adoption and the nontraditional view of prenatal adoption of gametes and/or embryos. While the process is different in prenatal adoption (i.e., conception and birth occur with the use of donated gametes or embryos), many of the psychological dynamics are the same as in traditional adoption (i.e., raising a child that is not genetically connected to one or both parents). Hence, as the face of adoption continues to change and evolve, it will no doubt grow to increasingly include the use of third-party adoption as a family-building alternative with similar psychosocial issues. Furthermore, it is assumed that each form of adoption will continue to influence the other (for better or worse) drawing parallels and contrasting lessons about family adaptation and growth.

SUMMARY

- The world of adoption has substantially changed in recent years. Although it is a positive and fulfilling path to parenthood for many, the decreased number of healthy babies available for adoption has made it more difficult to accomplish.

- Most couples eventually succeed with adoptive placement, but they often must persevere longer in their efforts to adopt and utilize more creative avenues. Disappointments with failed placements are common, with high emotional and financial risks.

- The traditional secrecy in adoption is giving way to greater openness at the time of placement and in post-placement years. In both agency and independent placements, birthparents and adoptive parents are increasingly making contact—meeting one another, sharing extensive information, and often maintaining ongoing communication.

- Those who move from infertility to adoption need to grieve for their many losses and resolve the issues of infertility in order to successfully move on. They must also accept that there are differences between adoptive and biological parenthood.

- Society continues to hold negative stereotypes of adoption, and, as a result, adoptive parents have the responsibility of educating others as well as effectively advocating for themselves and their children. Those who effectively address these issues will be the most successful in their adoptive family functioning.

- Couples are increasingly considering less traditional forms of adoption such as the use of donated sperm, oocytes, or embryos as a means of becoming parents. The psychological issues of adoption are similar to those couples becoming parents through these less traditional forms of adoption.

REFERENCES

1. Editorial. Social costs of teenage sexuality (social science and the citizen). *Society* 1993;30 (Sept/Oct):3–4

2. Bower B. Adapting to adoption: Adopted kids generate scientific optimism and clinical caution. *Science News* 1994;146 (Aug):104–5

3. Melina L. Prenatal drug exposure affects school-age child's behavior. *Adopted Child* 1996;15(Jan):1–4

4. Melina L. Children with learning disabilities need help understanding adoption. *Adopted Child* 1994;13(Sept):1

5. Reitz M, Watson KW. *Adoption and the Family System: Strategies for Treatment*. New York: Guilford Press,1992

6. Smith J, Miroff F. *You're Our Child: The Adoption Experience*. Lanham, MD: Madison Books, 1987

7. Bowlby J. *Attachment: Attachment and Loss*. New York: Basic Books, 1982

8. Brokzinsky DM, Schechter MD, eds. *The Psychology of Adoption*. New York: Oxford University Press, 1990

9. Kirk HD. *Shared Fate: A Theory and Method of Adoptive Relationships*, 2nd edn. Port Angeles, WA: Ben-Simon Publications, 1984

10. Alexander-Roberts C. *The Essential Adoption Handbook*. Dallas, TX: Taylor Publishing, 1993

23

Involuntary Childlessness: Deciding to Remain Child-Free

Gretchen Sewall, RN, MSW

Farewell dear child, thou ne'er shall come to me

Anne Bradstreet

The inability to become a parent is an experience of profound loss and suffering for both men and women. Gender influences the way this loss is felt, expressed, and resolved. Female reproduction mandates a significant investment of time, energy and, in some instances, health. While biology may in fact play a role in a woman's love for children and in her propensity for nurturing, society has reinforced and supported a woman's primary roles as mother and wife. Most women today want children and cherish the idea of motherhood. For these women, childlessness strikes at the heart, challenging the essence of their identity and their place in society.

Although most men desire fatherhood, historically their primary role has been that of provider for the family. It is rare for a male to seek therapy for reproductive issues. The vast majority of those seeking infertility counseling are women. This chapter's exploration of involuntary childlessness focuses on women, while client interventions are intended for both women and men. This chapter will address:

- Incidence and pathways to childlessness in the USA
- Historical and current societal perspectives of childlessness

- Psychological theories of women that influence adjustment to childlessness
- Clinical issues of childlessness including grief and loss, decision-making, gender differences, pronatalist societal pressures, impact on relationships, and cross-cultural issues.

HISTORICAL OVERVIEW

For early European settlers in the United States, fertility was not an optional matter of personal choice and pleasure: children were a religious and political obligation, as well as an economic necessity. The colonists believed that bearing children was a woman's natural calling. 'Prayers, laws that regulated sexual behavior, early marriage, basic medical principles, and folk wisdom all encouraged procreation'[1]. The average colonial woman gave birth to eight children[1]. Generally, she continued to give birth and raise children until she or her husband died or were too old.

It is estimated that about 1 in 12 colonial women was barren[1]. Male sterility was typically not acknowledged, and when reproduction failed, the woman was suspect. Myths and stereotypes plagued women who were not blessed with children. It was often infertile women or those who suffered miscarriage or stillbirth who were

411

accused of witchcraft. In colonial times, one of the few Americans who wrote of her feelings as a barren woman was the poet, Anne Bradstreet. She assumed that her sinful ways had caused her affliction, and she prayed for forgiveness for her lapses in piety[1]. Barrenness was also considered a test of faith. Religious leaders advised barren women to strengthen their faith and find other ways to lead a more godly life. 'Rather she should be more fruitful in all the good works of Piety and Charity'[1].

This culture of procreation changed dramatically in the early years of the new American nation. In the 18th century, towns and cities expanded, while the industrial revolution made large families unnecessary because economic endeavors moved out of the house and into separate places of work. The family home became a private retreat from the challenges of the world[1]. Procreation shifted from a matter of survival to a source of expansion, national identity, and personal happiness[1]. 'Men were the builders of the nation, women the vessels of propagation, and children the hope of the future'[1].

In 1903, Theodore Roosevelt put reproduction on the national reform agenda when he stated that Americans were committing 'race suicide'. He saw that immigrants were pouring into the country and reproducing faster than middle and upper class white Americans. 'Directing his remarks to female citizens, he compared women's reproductive obligation to the noble male sacrifice of military service and condemned the viciousness, coldness and shallow-heartedness of any woman who avoided her duty[1].'

Roosevelt's pronouncements marked the birth of the eugenics movement, which resulted in political, institutional, medical, and legislative measures designed to encourage some Americans to reproduce, while controlling the reproductive rights of others: immigrant and black Americans.

Some couples were childless by choice and worked to defend themselves publicly against the pronatal norms of the time. For the infertile, medical treatment offered little hope as treatment was still extremely limited and generally unsuccessful. Adoptions were rare, often illegally arranged, and/or involved taking in orphaned immigrant children who were valued more for their economic potential as workers than for the emotional rewards of the parent–child relationship.

Due to poverty and poor health, African-Americans in the 1940s suffered double the rate of childlessness of more affluent white women. Childless rates for African-Americans rose from 16% in 1910 to 26% in 1940[1]. Over time, the economy improved; resulting in better health care delivery and a decline in the rate of childlessness for all ethnic groups. This decline was further fueled by powerful patriotic overtones. With World War II behind them, the daughters of the first career women of the 1920s and 1930s were being drawn back to the home. Now, childlessness took on psychological significance. The childless woman was viewed as a maladjusted woman who did not conform to appropriate gender roles. Fatherhood became not just a matter of pride but also an important responsibility and evidence of maturity, patriotism, and citizenship. Motherhood was thought to be the only worthy occupation for women after the war. It was idealized and glorified. Having and raising children embodied the hope for the future and the ultimate achievement of happiness and personal fulfillment (see Chapter 13).

This postwar baby boom ostracized childless adults in a way that had never before been experienced. Intentional childlessness during these years was so stigmatized that demographers assumed it was practically nonexistent[2]. Childless couples had two choices: infertility treatment or adoption. Only about half of the infertility cases could be accurately diagnosed and about one-third of them treated. Adoption agencies found children for childless couples in an effort to restore their 'self respect'[2].

As a result of the pronatal forces of the 1940s, family size again increased during the 1950s. Women who were not mothers were considered selfish and in some way deficient—or worse; defiant or deviant. A prevailing theory on the cause of infertility came from the psychoanalytic community. Without a physical diagnosis, not having children was thought to be the result of a woman's unconscious desire to avoid parenthood and her unresolved conflict with her own mother[2]. It was also believed that education and a career could hinder a woman's reproductive potential[2]. Clearly, voluntary childlessness was not an acceptable possibility for most women at this time.

REVIEW OF THE LITERATURE

Incidence of Childlessness in America

The rate of childlessness has varied significantly throughout American history. The lowest rate reported by the National Center for Health Statistics occurred in 1975, when 9% of women between the ages of 20 and 44 were childless. In 1993 this percentage had risen to 16%. It has been projected that this figure may climb to as high as 20% by the year 2000. The only other time such a high rate of childlessness occurred was during the Depression years (1929 to 1934): 22% of women remained child-free[3].

Historically, most childlessness was believed to be caused by poor health or not being married[3]. Present-day childlessness is increasing in incidence for other reasons. It is difficult to accurately assess the number of women who are childless by choice and/or circumstance, compared with those suffering from biological infertility. Current estimates are that one in six couples in their childbearing years are infertile. Of these couples, 40-60% will become parents through medical assistance, adoption, and, in some cases, over time[1,2]. Those women who do not become mothers through treatment or adoption remain childless along with women who lack a suitable partner, do not choose to parent alone, or encounter economic, social, or other barriers to parenthood. There are many possible causes of involuntary childlessness and the number of women affected is sizable and appears to continue to be growing.

Paths to Childlessness

Ireland[4] found that of the 105 women she interviewed, those who had not 'given up' and had spent years in infertility treatment were more traditional in their values than those who sought little or no medical treatment. These 'traditional women' identified with a feminine sex role (evaluated by the Bem Sex Role Inventory) and planned to devote a major part of their adult life to motherhood[4]. Career was more often secondary to the primary role of motherhood. For these women, the central issue became one of mourning. 'The mourning process is necessary if the traditional woman is to be able to view herself and others like her in positive, rather than damaged terms'[4]. Infertility treatment can create an extended period of denial as each month renews the hope of motherhood, when it is perhaps more appropriate to face the reality of infertility.

THEORETICAL FRAMEWORK

Women who are involuntarily childless must alter their life goals along with their personal identities. Matthews and Matthews[5], sociologists and experts on involuntary childlessness, assert that 'Nonparenthood is likely to have as significant an impact on family and personal identity as parenthood itself'. Mathews and Mathews conclude that the transition to *nonparenthood* is as important and demanding a transition for families and individuals as the more traditional transition to parenthood. Ireland[4] wrote extensively on the topic of female identity and motherhood in her book *Reconceiving Women: Separating Motherhood from Female Identity*, explaining that traditional gender identity is based on an incomplete view of the nature of women. A fulfilled life without motherhood exposes mistaken assumptions about female identity. Ireland optimistically asserted that a personal identity based on an expanded view of femaleness allows a woman to develop to her full potential.

Psychoanalytic theory has for the most part offered a pathological view of women without children. It has influenced the way others represent childless women in society, and has limited the way these women think of themselves. Ireland suggested a variation of object-relations and Lacanian[6] theory to begin to understand the woman who is not a mother. Object-relations theory, based on the work of British theorists Melanie Klein, W. R. D. Fairbank, and D. W. Winnicott, emphasizes that women have had the primary caretaker role for both female and male offspring. This has impacted identity formations, as girls have the challenge of formation and maintenance of an identity separate from their mothers. 'Unlike the male, who must reject his early identification with mother and shift his identification to father, the daughter's identity evolves through a path of continual relatedness; she will never have to completely relinquish her earliest maternal identification'[7]. Consequently, the desire or need for recreating the mother-child bond is intimately tied to a woman's identity formation and maturation. Unfortunately, because the childless woman identifies with her mother, it is difficult for her to see herself in roles of competency and independence beyond the role of motherhood.

Simply put: all mothers are women, but not all women are mothers. It is important to recognize a mother's multifaceted personality, not just her 'good' or 'bad' mothering. This gives her daughter more opportunity to identify with and be influenced by her mother's personality without viewing motherhood as the defining component of a woman's identity. Lacan[8], a controversial analyst, emphasized human subjectivity in terms of the way in which language structures identity, and the reformation of the roles of the father. Lacan perceived the father as facilitating the shift from the fused unit of the mother-infant bond to two separate beings. According to Lacan, acquisition of language is key to assuming a separate identity, opening a reflective space between one's self and one's immediate experience. The problem is that experience is symbolically represented through language based on a patriarchal society. The female experience is not fully represented linguistically. An example of this is seen in many countries, including the United States, with family lineage in which only the male is symbolically represented through his surname. Therefore, it is the father who must assist his daughter by supporting a new voice and language in our society.

Both object-relations and Lacanian theories regard a place of absence (the empty uterus) as a locus of desire and creativity. It is by encountering one's lacking or transitional space that one becomes more fully present and creative. Erickson's[9] generative task of midlife can also expand beyond childbearing to include the birth of a multitude of creative endeavors and expressions of feminine influence in the world.

CLINICAL ISSUES

Changes in American society have greatly altered the nature of the family. Rising female participation in the labor force and ideals of sexual equality have challenged traditional gender roles. Sexual activity before marriage, cohabitation, and delayed marriage have increased options and altered expectations for many women. These changes first took root in the 1960s and early 1970s with the rebirth of the women's movement. Economic forces, legalization of abortion, and advances in technology and medicine (i.e., reliable contraception and assisted reproductive technologies) have released some women from reproductive obligation. Unfortunately, with delayed childbearing, the opportunity to parent may be lost. Advanced maternal age has now become a common cause of infertility, and an increasing number of patients are seen at infertility clinics for this reason. However, donor ovum conception may cross this biological frontier, allowing women well into menopause to have children.

The danger of childlessness due to voluntary delay or ongoing but unsuccessful medical treatment lies in the possibility of never making the decision to live without children. Endless treatment options can keep the wound open and delay healing. Year after year the grief persists and festers. Fulfillment and happiness become as elusive as parenthood. The focus of the woman's identity becomes a sense of not having, not belonging, and not sharing. The cost of unresolved grief can be the additional losses of relationships, marriage, jobs, career, and other lifeplans. There is also a substantial risk of depression, anxiety, and other mental and physical health problems[10].

Defining and understanding a client's pathway to childlessness is the first step to a therapeutic working relationship. In infertility practices, the most common cause of childlessness is biophysical infertility, which accounts for approximately 4.5 million couples in the United States[10]. The cause of infertility, ages of partners at the time of diagnosis, treatment options, and resources available all influence the couple's attitudes about childlessness and their willingness to consider the possibility of never having children.

For a growing number of women entering their fourth and fifth decades of life, social and economic factors have resulted in more childlessness. 'At some point, all are awakened by an internal voice or external event that calls their attention to the timeline of their lives; they realize that motherhood is not going to happen'[1]. For some, this results in panic, fear and a sense of loss of control, which may last for as little as a day or for years.

These 'transitional' women, according to Ireland[4], want a career and family. Flemming[11] sheds light on this cause of childlessness in her book *Motherhood Deferred*. Like many women today, Flemming delayed childbearing until it was biologically too late. For some, the delay is caused by marrying later in life or marrying a partner who does not want children, is not ready for children, or already has children. Single women may suffer from involuntary childlessness, as well as the absence of marriage or a committed life partner. Many of these women are admittedly ambivalent about motherhood. Without actively seeking motherhood, a woman can drift into her middle and later years without children. As she passively waits, she misses her opportunity to fully realize her creative and nurturing self. By not making a conscious choice and acknowledging her role in her circumstances, a woman may struggle to maintain a positive and coherent sense of self.

Another obstacle to childbearing is homosexuality. Many lesbian women and gay men have a deep desire to become parents, raise children, and enjoy family life. Prevailing social norms and values, discrimination, and reproductive biology all impact chances of becoming parents for sexual minorities. There are no laws that sanction gay or lesbian marriage. Adoption is difficult, if not impossible, in most states for same-sex couples, and medical intervention may be no easier. Lesbians may not have access to medical facilities for donor insemination. Surrogate arrangements can be complex and beyond financial means. In addition, medical intervention does not guarantee pregnancy and parenthood. These couples must also consider the potential effect of prejudice on a child growing up in a homophobic society. Involuntary childlessness for sexual minorities is not generally acknowledged by our society. A prevailing belief is that the individual chooses his or her sexual orientation, and, therefore the pain and suffering of childlessness are self-imposed. Some people believe that same-sex couples do not deserve the right to become parents. Gay and lesbian couples may need significant help coping with childlessness, as well as living as sexual minorities in a homophobic society[12] (see Chapter 14).

Stepparenthood is a state of being both with and without children. In most families the biological mother cannot be replaced in children's hearts and minds. Frequently, a stepmother's efforts at trying to fulfill the role of the mother breeds resentment[2]. Stepmothers and stepchildren can become rivals for the husband and father's attention, money, and love. Some stepfamilies do make a smooth transition into blended families, generally when the stepmother finds significant roles to play with the children, other than mother[2]. For this reason, being a stepmother may not satisfy a woman's desire to become a mother (see Chapter 16).

Less common causes of childlessness include significant genetic disorders, health problems (e.g., positive HIV status of one partner), and physical and mental health disabilities. Again, understanding each client's personal journey to childlessness is the key to comprehending the meaning of their loss and beginning the healing process (see Chapters 10 and 11).

THERAPEUTIC INTERVENTIONS
Facilitating Grief and Loss

Letting go of the possibility of having children involves an unfocused grieving. There are many losses. It is mourning the loss of an experience rather than an actual death. One must face the loss of the dreamed-of child, the loss of whatever part of one's identity is wrapped up in those dreams, and the loss of a destiny that one always assumed would be achieved. It also includes the abstract loss of hope and a sense of control in life[1]. This grieving is lonely and isolating because childlessness brings to the surface losses that are largely unrecognized by others. Generally, the longer a woman has pursued pregnancy, the longer she mourns her failure to conceive[13]. The pain can hurt and paralyze its victims until it is dealt with[1]. If the loss is denied or minimized, there is a risk of becoming psychologically impaired.

In her book on loss across the lifespan, Judith Viorst[14] states that loss is part of adult life: we must all develop the skill to accept loss to allow for growth and to regain control over our lives.

> *Throughout our life we grow by giving up our deepest attachments . . . [and] certain cherished parts of ourselves. We must confront, in the dreams we dream, as well in our intimate relationships, all that we never will have and never will be.*

Shapiro[15] wrote: 'Couples can't rein in control over their emotions and private lives until they cease their quest for a baby'. With the many treatment options available today, deciding to stop treatment can be more difficult than staying on the treatment treadmill. Medical intervention locks a person into a cycle of hope, followed by the crushing despair of failure. Patients often feel they cannot give up and think that if they keep trying, eventually something will work. Only the honest acceptance of their circumstances allows their hope and energy to return.

When there is little choice associated with a couple's situation or there has been ambivalence about parenthood, the transition to a child-free existence can occur without an emotional crisis. This was often the case in previous generations, when treatment options were limited and generally unsuccessful. Now with the use of a younger woman's eggs and intracyto-plastic sperm injection, treatment options can extend into the fifth and sixth decades of both men and women. For couples seeking treatment today, ending the medical quest for pregnancy can be emotionally traumatic.

To be effective clinicians, we must understand our clients' personal experience of loss within the societal and cultural context of the times. With this knowledge and understanding, clinicians can help clients acknowledge their losses, guide their decision-making and assist the transformation of identity in pursuit of new life meaning. The goal of each client is consciously to accept and find fulfillment in their child-free life.

Facilitating Decision-making

Carter and Carter[13] wrote: 'Choosing to be child-free after infertility is not giving up hope, it is finding hope of a good life again, only this time without children'. *Child-free* is a hopeful word used to describe the positive potential in life[13]. A conscious, deliberate decision to live child-free does not mean resigning oneself to a life without children. Rather than drifting into lifelong childlessness, one can believe that for every loss there is a potential gain. This decision allows for new growth and new goals, and the ability to invest renewed energies into work, family, and hobbies. To live child-free is a choice that requires honest thoughts, feelings, and communication before becoming acceptable to both partners. Living child-free is a way to fulfill the goals of parenthood in other positive, constructive ways. People with the desire to nurture and love can find ways to do this without having children. The move to a child-free life is a creative adaptation from sorrow, pain, and loss[1].

Difficulties in making decisions about options for family-building, or conflicts over these options, are common presenting problems for clients seen in clinical practice. Either of these problems can lead to the decision to remain child-free. Couple counseling is recommended if the couple has not been able to come to an agreement on being child-free. Each person needs an opportunity to verbalize and have his or her feelings acknowledged. Compromise is always the goal but may not be possible if one partner is determined to be a parent and the other partner is equally invested in *not* being a parent. By helping the couple appreciate each other's views and by renewing their commitment to each other, possible solutions emerge. Generally, the client(s) and the therapist will agree to a time-limited contract with clearly defined goals. Typically, goals will be met within two to ten sessions.

After years of dashed hopes and recurrent disappointments, denial of or the inability to feel and identify feelings is common. This emotional whitewash has the potential of leading to clinical depression. Using solution-focused therapy or a cognitive-behavioral framework, therapists can help clients reconnect with their feelings in a safe and supportive environment. Sessions end with homework

Table 1 Client exercises

Exercises to access feeling and acknowledge losses
What is it about parenting that drives you?
Describe your infertility crisis beyond your diagnosis and treatment.
What are some of the stereotypes of childless people?
Compare yourself to these stereotypes. Do they fit?
What makes it difficult for you to consider living child-free?
What do you grieve the most?
What is the difference between not having children and not being a parent?

Exercises to end treatment and say goodbye to the dream child
What do you need to do to finish treatment?
How have your feelings about treatment changed over time?
Could your desire to parent be met in other ways?
Develop a ritual or ceremony to say goodbye to your dream child.
Develop a plan and vocabulary for explaining to others why you do not have children.
Look at how your life is set up. What changes have you already made and what changes do you
    need to make to accommodate a child-free life (i.e. house, career, pleasure activities)?
What opportunities lie ahead of you?

---

assignments from either therapeutic modality. Table 1 provides a list of exercises that can be used during or between sessions. For clients suffering from long-standing depression or dysthymia, a thorough assessment may lead to a referral and further evaluation for pharmacological intervention in conjunction with longer-term insight-focused therapy. As the depressive symptomatology recedes, the work in therapy returns to active decision-making within an outcome-focused framework.

As stated earlier, confronting loss is the first step in deciding to remain child-free. Telling one's 'story' offers an opportunity to identify losses. Verbalizing personal motivations to parent is also valuable. Work outside the session can be as simple as listing losses or as elaborate as creating a ritual or ceremony to say 'good-bye' to the dream child. For some, creative expression such as drawing, painting, poetry, or collage can be helpful as well.

Basic strategies for decision-making involve taking control of one's life, developing a positive identity, and reasserting goals and priorities[13]. Rubin[16] offers a very useful model for helping clients with decision-making. Assessment starts with looking for and identifying possible 'decision blocks'. Some blocks identified by Rubin include: (1) resignation or holding on to pain, (2) believing there is only one correct decision, (3) holding onto all possible options rather than choosing any one path, (4) procrastination, and (5) guilt over previous decisions. The work in therapy is to identify a client's particular obstacles and, through the use of therapeutic interventions, overcome these blocks to allow the process of decision-making to unfold.

The next task in Rubin's[16] model is to establish a foundation for decision-making based on personal values. When consumed by the blindfold of infertility, perception and definition of self become myopic. It is suggested that either during or between sessions the clients take the time to create a list of priorities. Possible items on the list might be health, quality of life, religion, education, and security. As clients develop a list, they see themselves as full human beings with the ability to alter their behavior to match their values and create or follow other lifeplans not involving parenthood[13].

The final task entails committing to the decision. This means operationalizing, which in this case is the decision to stop treatment and move from being childless, or the state of having less, to the position of choosing a child-free life. For most couples, this is a gradual process that happens over time. They may find it takes months or even years before being child-free starts to feel right. Then, everything begins to fall into place, and concrete evidence of moving on appears. Perhaps, a house is purchased without a large family room and four bedrooms, or an application to graduate school is completed or a career move is made. For others, it might be new hobbies, meaningful volunteer work, new friends, or a renewed focus and commitment to their marriage.

Addressing Pressures of Pronatalism

Once a women confronts and deals with her own feelings about not having children, she must deal with everyone else's feelings about her decision. In 1955, only 1% of women expected to remain childless[2]. By 1988, 10% claimed they did not expect to have children and another 15% were not sure[2]. Gradually, it has become somewhat easier and more acceptable not to have children. Still, the pressure from parents, friends, casual acquaintances, and society cannot be denied. Stereotypes persist, the most common being that the childless couple or woman is self-centered. Those who choose to remain childless are often called upon to justify their decision, while prospective parents are rarely asked why they want a baby. Some women without children think their lives symbolize a threat to people whose daily lives are largely mandated by their role as parents. The reality of why children are conceived

nowadays is worth examining: to please parents, cement a marriage, fulfill traditional roles, prove youthfulness by reproducing, have someone to love and be loved by, and have someone to care for them in their old age. Although having children may satisfy many of these desires, children require years of endless responsibility, hard work, and money and can be a threat to a couple's relationship. Marital satisfaction tends to follow a U-shaped curve, starting out high, dropping when children are young, and climbing again after children leave home[17]. One must consider whether today's motives for having children are perhaps narcissistic and self-serving. It is ironic that these are often the adjectives used to describe childless individuals.

One of the fears often verbalized about childlessness is the fear of loneliness and regret in old age. Also of concern is the loss of connection with the next generation. Studies have shown, however, that older childless women have found other goals and interests to give their lives meaning. Having children has been found to contribute neither to happiness nor to overall satisfaction in later life[2]. Gerontologists describe the effects of being childless in later life as 'benign'[2].

One of the most difficult aspects of childlessness is coping with the disappointment of would-be grandparents. Children try to gain parental approval even as adults. Several women in Lang's[2] study described tension in their relationships with their mothers, who interpreted their daughters' rejection of motherhood as 'a spitting in their face'. As women move into their 40s, peer pressure eases. People stop asking about children. Lang found that the older women that she interviewed expressed very little concern about stigmas and stereotypes and did not feel devalued for not having children.

Carter and Carter[13] described being child-free as a 'closet choice'. Couples are reluctant to discuss their choice because infertile couples find it threatening, parents are disappointed, and friends generally do not understand. Typically, couples find little support and must find solace from their own resolution[2]. It is likely that over time others will accept their choice as they see the peace and renewed energy in a couple's life. Women at a local infertility support group (RESOLVE) spoke of the peace and relief they experienced as the transition to a child-free life was made. They said they were once again masters of their own destiny and had moved beyond tragedy to acceptance and opportunity.

For some, the use of birth control or sterilization helps to avoid dissonance. This ensures that the door to parenthood is, indeed, closed and hopes for the future are directed elsewhere. Birth control also prevents an unexpected pregnancy from happening after a couple has made new lifeplans without children. As friends' children grow up and leave home, childlessness becomes less of an issue. Choosing to be child-free does not mean permanent liberation from feelings of loss. It means becoming big enough to embrace both loss and gain and exercising the human ability to adapt to life's circumstances[10].

Addressing Impact on Relationships

A necessary and distinctive characteristic of the child-free life is the possible presence of new and meaningful relationships. As a couple works through the decision to stop treatment and accept a child-free life, they are forced to reexamine the choices, goals, and dreams that they made together. The partners' new hopes and aspirations may be different from one another. One person may even decide to continue with the quest to have children in his or her life, while the other is pleased to have new opportunities and experiences without children. Clinical

experience suggests that couples staying together tend to recommit to each other and direct their energy toward the marriage and each other rather than toward treatment and children.

For the single woman, friendships often become the most important kinship link. As she drifts away from friends with children, she develops new connections. Holiday traditions and special events are created and shared with a family of friends. Relationships with children may play an significant and new role in her life. Many women become active and involved aunts, or mentors to children or young adults. Women in the helping professions have an opportunity to enjoy children through their work. Many women find themselves as role models to younger women or seek older child-free women for guidance and support. Older or more mature women become 'permission givers' that legitimize a chosen path.

Addressing Cross-Cultural Issues

Infertility and childlessness have very different significance in other cultures. For example, within some cultures, it is socially acceptable for a husband to divorce his wife or take another wife if his wife does not bear him children, regardless of the cause of infertility. Some couples choose to hide their childlessness from family and friends by continuing medical treatments (albeit minimal) in order to continue their marriage and cultural status. Cultures or religions that emphasize children make the choice of child-free particularly difficult. Further, the status of marriage, women, and/or the couple without children can be one of discrimination, stigma, or significant isolation (see Chapter 13).

Mental health professionals and medical staff working in the field of reproductive medicine are increasingly being called on to address cross-cultural issues whether patients come from minority American cultures or patients from other countries come to American clinics requesting medical treatments for infertility. As such, professionals must consider language, religious values, cultural norms, and individual beliefs when considering both medical and mental health care of infertile men and women. Fundamentally, the cultural and religious acceptability and feasibility of childlessness as an alternative for these couples will shape and direct both medical treatment plans and counseling goals—a fact about which the infertility counselor must be keenly aware.

FUTURE IMPLICATIONS

Infertile men and women have a right to pursue treatment options in an effort to become parents. They should also have a right to accept the limits of their bodies and medical science and find other outlets for their nurturing. The goal must be their welfare rather than a medical cure. As the incidence of voluntary childlessness and delayed childbearing increases, men and women will have more opportunities for fulfilling and satisfying lives without children. Infertility counselors will be called upon to help them to accept their childlessness with courage, and aid them in finding meaning and fulfilling lives without children. They will also be needed to help patients take responsibility for their decisions for or against children, rather deciding through avoidance or a decisional drift of repeated treatment trails and failures.

Individuals and institutions of America today must continue to question prevailing pronatalist norms and values and recognize the possibilities for ourselves and society as a whole. Will women be valued by themselves and others as complete, mature, and feminine women without the rite of passage of childbirth? Can we support men

and women who uncover meaningful ways to contribute and nurture without becoming parents? Can society tolerate families without children? Will we value a woman's opportunity to devote herself to a career which feeds her spirit and soul, as well as our nation? Can we create a new definition and expression of 'family values' that truly nurtures and improves the family of humankind? Therapists working in the field of reproductive health must address these questions. This is our work and our opportunity.

SUMMARY

- The client's pathway to childlessness sets the stage for grief process, decision-making, and the transition to a child-free life. Culture, religion, and ethnicity serve as road maps for the therapist.
- The greatest danger of childlessness lies in the possibility of never making a decision to live without raising children. Drifting and waiting leads to a poor self image, feelings of unfulfillment and not belonging, and compromised relationships.
- Losses must be recognized, acknowledged, and ultimately accepted before negatives can be changed to positives.
- Gender and role definition and identity are closely tied to the desire to have children. A child-free life requires redefining one's identity and life goals.
- Decision-making may occur over several days or several years. The steps include: identifying and overcoming decision blockers, clarifying priorities, committing and investing in the decision.
- Historical and present-day societal pressure to procreate is based on pronatalism, a force required for the continuation of the species.
- A child-free life includes reevaluating

and committing to significant relationships. Communication and nurturing are core elements in a meaningful and satisfying life.

- The increasing number and greater visibility of women who do not give

birth and raise children will help to encourage a broader definition and expression of meaningful, creative, and successful lives for women.

REFERENCES

1. Tyler EM. *Barren in the Promised Land*. New York: Basic Books, 1995
2. Lang SS. *Women Without Children: The Reasons, the Rewards, the Regrets*. New York: Pharos Books, 1991
3. Hastings DW, Gregory RJ. Incidences of childlessness for United States women, cohorts born 1891–1945. *Soc Biology* 1914;21:178–84
4. Ireland M. *Reconceiving Women: Separating Motherhood from Female Identity*. New York: Guilford Press, 1993
5. Matthews R, Matthews AM. Infertility and involuntary childlessness: The transition to nonparenthood. *J Mar Fam* 1986;48:641–9
6. Lacan J. *Four Fundamental Concepts of Psychoanalysis*. New York: Norton, 1978
7. Klein M. Early stages of the oedipus complex. *Int J Psychoanalysis* 1928; 9:167–80
8. Lacan J. *Feminine Sexuality*. New York: Norton, 1985
9. Erickson E. *Identity and the Life Cycle*. New York: Norton, 1980
10. Anton HL. Never to be a Mother: A Guide for All Women Who Didn't—or Couldn't—Have Children. San Francisco, CA: Harper, 1992
11. Flemming B. *Motherhood Deferred: A Woman's Journey*. New York: Putnam's Sons, 1994
12. Waldal L, Sewall G. Donor egg conception for lesbian and heterosexual women. *J Naturopathic Med* (forthcoming)
13. Carter JW, Carter M. *Sweet Grapes. How to Stop Being Infertile and Start Living Again*. Indianapolis, IN: Perspectives Press, 1989
14. Viorst J. *Necessary Losses*. New York: Ballantine, 1986
15. Shapiro C. *Infertility and Pregnancy Loss: A Guide for the Helping Professionals*. San Francisco, CA: Jossey-Bass Publishers, 1988
16. Rubin TI. *Overcoming Indecisiveness: The Eight Stages of Effective Decisionmaking*. New York: Harper and Row, 1985
17. Renne KS. Childlessness, health and marital satisfaction. *Soc Bio* 1976; 23:183–97

VIII. POSTINFERTILITY COUNSELING ISSUES

24

Pregnancy after Infertility

Sharon N. Covington, MSW, and Linda Hammer Burns, PhD

If I could only feel the child! I imagine the moment of its quickening as a
sudden awakening of my own being which has never before had life.
I want to live with the child, and I am as heavy as a stone.

Evelyn Scott

The pregnancy following infertility treatment is a 'premium' pregnancy: precious, priceless, and precarious. It is also a 'high stakes' pregnancy, usually representing a considerable investment of time, emotion, energy, money, and medical treatment. Furthermore, the pregnancy after infertility may be the result of medical treatments facilitating conception, such as in vitro fertilization (IVF), donated gametes, or pregnancy in a gestational carrier or surrogate. The postinfertility pregnancy may be impacted by the side effects of assisted reproductive technologies, such as complicated multiple gestation, multifetal reduction, high-risk pregnancies/deliveries, and the ultimate risk—loss of the whole pregnancy. Pregnancy after infertility is more than a planned pregnancy: it is a deliberate pregnancy. Once achieved, it can be a distressing realization that it involves a myriad of new challenges and perils demanding considerable psychological and physical adjustments.

This chapter will address the unique aspects of pregnancy after infertility and:

- define how the pregnancy after infertility is different from other pregnancies
- outline the psychological tasks of the postinfertility pregnancy

- address issues of psychopathology and its psychiatric treatment in the post infertility pregnancy
- delineate the unique characteristics of the postinfertility pregnancy, including multiples, third-party reproduction, and pregnancy in the older mother
- specify therapeutic interventions for helping the previously infertile couple manage the typically precious and highly valued postinfertility pregnancy.

HISTORICAL OVERVIEW

Simkin[1] reviewed how childbearing has evolved during the 20th century and how social changes have influenced the experience of pregnancy for American women. At the turn of the century, women rebelled against the Victorian custom of confinement during pregnancy and entered society, bringing about the introduction of maternity clothes and bottle feeding. By the 1920s, in a further attempt to gain control of their reproductive lives, women were limiting pregnancies through the widespread use of birth control. In the 1930s, 50% of deliveries were taking place in a hospital rather than at home. During the 1950s, natural childbirth and childbirth education became popular following reactions to an article in the *Ladies Home Journal* decrying cruelty in the maternity ward. By the 1970s, fathers had entered the delivery room, abortion was legalized, and maternal–infant bonding was advocated. This was also a time of burgeoning medical technology, including the development of ultrasound, amniocentesis, genetic counseling, neonatology as a new medical specialty, and the first baby conceived by IVF. The 1980s continued the trend of delayed and controlled childbearing, with increasing emphasis on 'the perfect baby'.

The decade of the 1980s also saw a number of firsts in reproductive technology: the first child conceived by a donated oocyte, the first pregnancy carried in a gestational carrier, the first surrogate pregnancy, and the first conception using intracytoplasmic sperm injection. By the end of the 20th century, parenthood and pregnancy could involve deceased parents (pregnancy maintained in a brain-dead mother or pregnancy achieved by sperm harvested from a deceased father), cloning of embryos, the birth of twins several months apart, and genetic testing of embryos before implantation. At the beginning of this century, women were attempting to reject reproductive destiny by gaining greater control of their reproductive lives. Now, at the end of the century, women are attempting to gain even greater control of reproduction by extending their childbearing lives through the use of donated gametes and volunteer carriers.

As the 21st century approaches, the meanings of pregnancy, conception, motherhood, and parenthood have been forever changed and altered. Traditionally, there has not been a distinction between biological or genetic parenthood and psychological or social parenthood. However, conception and pregnancy now entail various forms of prenatal adoption, donated gametes or embryos, surrogacy, gestational carrier, 'intentional' versus 'biological' parenthood, and conception after death. Traditional means of determining parenthood, such as genetics, blood-lines, or physical pregnancy, have given way to 'parenthood by intention'[2,3], altering the experience of pregnancy and ultimately parenthood. Thus, while pregnancy after infertility has much in common with 'normal' pregnancies, there is also much about it that sets it apart.

REVIEW OF LITERATURE

While the psychology of infertility has received considerable research attention, investigation of psychological factors in pregnancy after infertility has been limited. Research has traditionally focused on obstetrical outcomes, especially following particular fertility treatments such as donor insemination conceptions and assisted reproductive technologies. One early pre-IVF study[4] investigated obstetrical complications in 122 pregnancies in previously infertile women and reported an increased incidence of pregnancy complications: 64% of the infertility group experienced complications compared to 46% of the control group. Pregnancies following assisted reproductive technologies have been found to have a greater risk of pregnancy complications and problem deliveries, including increased incidence of preterm labor and delivery, multiple gestations, and cesarean deliveries[5,6]. Pregnancy and delivery problems may be the result of the initial infertility diagnosis, multiple gestations, advanced maternal age, prenatal testing, or multifetal reduction.

Increased anxiety and cautious attachment to the postinfertility pregnancy have been a frequent research finding. Garner[7] noted that reactions to pregnancy after infertility fell between two extremes: denial/avoidance (women who denied pregnancy and failed to seek appropriate prenatal care for several months) and hypervigilance (women who called the clinic constantly with exaggerated fears over each minor event in the pregnancy). Anxiety has been described as a 'waiting to lose' period, when previously infertile pregnant women are constantly alert to signs of impending miscarriage and have little confidence that a baby actually will be born[8]. In addition, a prior reproductive loss has been identified as significantly increasing anxiety for both partners, resulting in difficulty in coping as they anticipated a negative outcome and withdrew from investment in the pregnancy[9-11]. One study[12] reported that previously infertile pregnant women avoided preparing for their baby and attempted to control every aspect of the pregnancy in an effort to distance normal feelings of trepidation, ambivalence, and fear of the unknown. They were also found to have elevated depression scores compared to never-infertile women.

A large longitudinal study[13] of IVF parents and their children in Australia examined psychological adjustment during pregnancy and found no significant differences in mood, marital satisfaction, neuroticism, or self-esteem between the control group and women who became pregnant following infertility. However, the previously infertile women showed greater external locus of control and were more likely to keep feelings of anxiety, depression, and anger to themselves as opposed to expressing them. At 30 weeks of pregnancy, the previously infertile women were found to be significantly more anxious about the survival of the pregnancy and the well-being of their baby. And while they expressed stronger feelings of identification with pregnancy as a positive and fulfilling experience, they tended to deny the significance of psychological and

physical difficulties of the pregnancy, were less interested in seeking information about childbirth and parenting, and were less likely to engage in active preparation for parenthood through classes and/or reading. Furthermore, they expected their babies to be more difficult, reported fewer conversations with their baby in utero, and delayed preparation of the nursery. This research may support Garner's[7] findings that previously infertile pregnant women cope with the complex feelings of pregnancy through avoidance or hypervigilance, with avoidant coping resulting in less preparation for parenthood and more complicated transition to motherhood.

Research also indicates that previously infertile women have difficulty letting go of the rituals of infertility, separating from the infertility team, developing a new support network, and investing in a pregnancy that they might yet lose[14]. Relinquishing infertility 'involved efforts to let go of the negative identity, feelings, and thought patterns developed over the course of the struggle to conceive'[14]. Previously infertile women also reported a higher incidence of guilt and shame that they associated with their formerly infertile status[15]. These women continued to harbor feelings of failure and malformation about their reproductive ability or, if the baby was conceived by donor gametes, embarrassment about the circumstances of the child's conception. Guilt was associated with their relationships with their friends who remained infertile. Glaser and Strauss[16] found that previously infertile women struggled with three issues during pregnancy: (1) *selflessness*, defined as the belief that all their energy and effort should be devoted and directed toward the baby; (2) *lack of entitlement*, defined as having no right to complain or expect more because they had what they wanted—a baby; and (3) *vulnerability*, defined as their feeling that they were more at risk than they had ever been and perceived their baby to be at greater risk as well.

Olshansky[17] contends that difficulty in letting go of the infertility experience contributes to the 'paradoxes of pregnancy after infertility:' simultaneous feelings of contradictory emotions. The paradoxes involve the 'embrace of contraries', such as happiness about pregnancy and fear of loss or perception of self as defective due to infertility. The 'normalization of pregnancy' for the previously infertile woman consists of a complex identity shift from an infertile and childless state to one of pregnancy, and ultimately motherhood. It involves the ability to experience pregnancy as a normal developmental process that is gratifying and involves its own set of tasks, responsibilities, and goals.

Little is known about men's responses to pregnancy after infertility. In one study[18] of previously infertile husbands' responses to pregnancy in their wives, the men experienced couvade symptoms (sympathetic pregnancy-type symptoms) consistent with the incidence in the general population. Nevertheless, a husband's responses to pregnancy may be influenced by the circumstances of conception, the demands of pregnancy such as bedrest or hospitalization, the emotional stability of the expectant mother, and his own psychological well-being.

Although sexual functioning during infertility has been the topic of considerable investigation, no research to date has specifically addressed sexual functioning during the postinfertility pregnancy, and little is available on sexuality in pregnancy in general. However, an anecdotal report[19] about the impact of infertility on sexual functioning during pregnancy indicated both positive effects (no longer having to plan sex to achieve pregnancy) and negative effects (fear of pregnancy loss or impact of sexual intercourse on the fetus).

THEORETICAL FRAMEWORK

While early literature focused on the psychoanalytic interpretation of the symbolic meaning and experience of pregnancy[20,21], pregnancy is now considered a normal developmental process signaling arrival into adulthood and acceptance of adult roles. Pregnancy and parenthood represent a bridge between generations central to the human experience and to a woman's sense of self, gender identity, and self-esteem[22]. Physical, intrapsychic, and interpersonal adaptations are needed to successfully adjust to pregnancy, delivery, and ultimately parenthood.

Pregnancy is a time when profound physical and emotional changes occur within a short period. During pregnancy, a woman faces monumental issues: the sharing of her body with another, changes in her body image, changes in her relationship with others, attachment to the baby she is carrying while at the same time preparing to separate from it, and feelings about motherhood in general, herself as a mother, and the mothering she received as a child[23]. The physical demands and emotional stresses of pregnancy can impact a woman's coping ability and style, her relationship with significant others, especially her spouse/partner, and her psychological adjustment, including her individuation, ego development, and consolidation of self .

Even when a pregnancy is wanted, some ambivalence is normal and probably universal. During pregnancy, women often feel a sense of accomplishment, heightened self-esteem, increased feelings of femininity, and comradeship with other women. At the same time, there may be feelings of resentment and even hostility about the changes taking place that are beyond a woman's control. When things go well, pregnancy can be a narcissistically rewarding period—a gratification of the body's performance—or if there is a problem, a narcissistically wounding period—anxiety and distress about the body's competence during pregnancy and delivery. Feelings of ambivalence, anxiety, or fear may increase self-doubt and lower self-confidence, thereby complicating adjustment to pregnancy and parenthood. Furthermore, adjustment to pregnancy is affected by a number of factors in a woman's life, including previous life experiences, prior psychological adjustment, the meaning of this pregnancy in her life, her dependency needs, and her relationship with her partner and others[23]. Physical and emotional dependence on her partner may clash with a woman's own desire for independence and self-sufficiency during pregnancy. These issues may arise when the pregnancy is complicated by bedrest or other medical restrictions.

The meaning of the pregnancy after infertility varies and is highly individual. It may represent hopes, dreams, miracles, expense, overinvestment, success, fulfillment, or even a burden or hindrance. Following years of infertility, the developmental transition to parenthood can be difficult and stressful for a couple. The postinfertility pregnancy may involve its own unique challenges: fears of pregnancy loss, the strains of a medically complicated pregnancy, and attachment to a non-genetically related baby or a baby being carried by someone else. Fundamentally, the tasks of pregnancy are influenced by the experience of infertility in general and the previously infertile pregnant woman's experience of this pregnancy. Ultimately, not only do previously infertile couples arrive at pregnancy differently, but their experience of pregnancy is significantly different.

Psychological Tasks of Pregnancy after Infertility

The abrupt transition from long-standing infertility to potential parenthood is a psychological challenge requiring a rapid revision of identity and internal reconfiguration[24]. Olshansky[25] described the identity shift in the formerly infertile woman as a confusing psychological state in which the expectant mother with a history of infertility simultaneously straddles the two worlds of infertility and pregnancy. She has difficulty seeing herself as a normal pregnant woman and feels that her experiences with infertility, medical treatment, and childlessness set her apart from other pregnant women. She may feel that she has no right to complain about the physical demands of pregnancy because either her support network is tired of hearing about her not being pregnant or she herself feels that she should feel only gratitude for this pregnancy. Some women pregnant after infertility are unable to relate to the 'whining' about the discomforts of pregnancy from women who have had no problems with conception.

Unique to the pregnancy after infertility are donated gametes, surrogate mothers, or gestational carriers, resulting in confused physical and psychological boundaries. Here one is 'circumventing rather than "overcoming" infertility', for although pregnancy may be achieved, the original infertility diagnosis or problem is not 'cured'[15].

The developmental tasks of normal pregnancy include[26]:

- *validation of pregnancy*: This is difficult after infertility because confirmation and affirmation of the pregnancy are less an event than a process, often involving repeated pregnancy tests, ultrasounds, and examinations. Acceptance and assimilation of the reality of the pregnancy may be more tentative and difficult, especially if the process involves a significant period of time.

- *fetal embodiment*: The expectant mother's incorporating the fetus into her body image may be especially difficult if she perceives her body to be defective or unreliable after the experience of infertility or prior problem pregnancies. Recognizing the baby as part of her body may be threatening, which is reinforced if there are complications during the pregnancy.

- *fetal distinction*: Recognition of the fetus as a separate entity is actually the beginning of parental bonding, attachment, and acknowledgment of the baby's individuality and separateness. Sometimes, fetal distinction is delayed or suspended until the final status of the pregnancy has been determined, as in cases of threatened miscarriage, possible fetal reduction, or waiting for results of prenatal testing.

- *role transition*: This involves redefinition of the self as a parent and integration of the baby as a separate person within the family. This may be a formidable task when a couple has been defined as childless in a child-filled world. The wounds from infertility may make it difficult to bond with the 'miracle' baby or deal with the infant's many needs.

Lederman's[27] model of psychosocial adaptation to pregnancy concluded that it is a psychological process that keeps pace with and complements the physical development of the fetus. There are seven dimensions of maternal development during pregnancy: (1) acceptance of pregnancy, (2) identification with motherhood role, (3) relationship to one's own mother, (4) relationship with spouse or partner, (5) preparation for labor, (6) prenatal fear of loss of control in labor, and (7) prenatal fear of loss of self-esteem in labor.

According to Colman and Colman[28], the psychological tasks of the childbearing years are defined in terms of pregnancy as a developmental stage that inaugurates a much longer one: parenthood. The six tasks of pregnancy are (1) accepting the pregnancy, (2) accepting the reality of the fetus, (3) reevaluating the older generation of parents, (4) reevaluating the relationship between the two partners, (5) accepting the baby as a separate person, and (6) integrating the parental identity. Each of these tasks can have special meaning and challenge to the previously infertile couple who may have difficulty acknowledging the reality of the pregnancy or baby, have experienced long-term marital adjustment problems, or have unrealistic expectations of self as a parent or of their child.

The pregnancy after infertility has its own unique challenges and tasks. Glazer[29] defined the tasks of pregnancy after infertility in terms of how it differs from 'normal' pregnancy: (1) fear of loss of the pregnancy, (2) fear of having a baby with defects, (3) difficulty in becoming an obstetrical patient (as opposed to an infertility patient), (4) feeling neither fertile nor infertile ('in a no-person's land'), and (5) fear of having a high-risk pregnancy. She further defined the issues of the postinfertility pregnancy as[30]:

- *ambiguity*, referring to the process versus the event of pregnancy confirmation in normal pregnancies, although it can apply to other forms of ambiguity in the postinfertility pregnancy, such as the ambiguity of genetic ties to the pregnancy (e.g., donor gametes)

- *isolation*, referring to feelings of alienation and not belonging to either the fertile or infertile worlds

- *fear* or *anxiety* about the pregnancy, including fears about pregnancy outcome and parenthood but possibly also anxiety about one's ability to manage the pregnancy or delivery or fear of the response of others, should they discover the circumstances of conception

- *loss*, fundamental to infertility, involves the multiple losses of pregnancy after infertility, including the potential for pregnancy loss, the necessity of fetal reduction, the loss of a 'normal' pregnancy experience, and/or the loss of a support network, such as friends left behind in the world of infertility after pregnancy is achieved
- *technological bewilderment*, defined as the myriad medical technologies that contribute to creation and/or maintenance of the postinfertility pregnancy.

CLINICAL ISSUES

Psychopathology During Pregnancy After Infertility

Early investigations[31] into the incidence of psychiatric hospitalizations during pregnancy found a decrease, supporting the belief that normal pregnancy is a time of relative calm, providing protection from psychiatric illness. However, more recent research has shown either a small decrease or an unchanged incidence of major psychiatric illness during pregnancy[23]. The most significant factor predictive of psychiatric illness during pregnancy is prior history of mental illness[23]. The significance of psychiatric illness during pregnancy primarily involves its potential effect on obstetrical outcome (prematurity, low birth weight, and subsequent child morbidity), disturbances of mother–infant relationship, and inability to comply with medical care or appropriately care for oneself or the pregnancy[32,33].

Mood, Anxiety, and Personality Disorders

Although a first episode of major depression is unlikely to erupt during pregnancy, *reoccurrence* of major depression during pregnancy is a possibility which both patients and caregivers must be aware of. Apart from a history of a prior major depressive episode, additional risk factors include presence or absence of prior children, instrumental support during pregnancy, prior pregnancy loss, disturbed marital relationship, stressful life circumstances, and medically high-risk pregnancy[23]. Because a history of major depression is such a significant predictor of depression during pregnancy and postpartum, it has been suggested that women with a history of depression should be carefully screened before conception, as well as during pregnancy and postpartum. In addition, preparing women by educating them about risk factors, symptoms, and treatment options can provide understanding and preventive care. Depression during pregnancy can be particularly painful for a previously infertile pregnant woman who may have (mistakenly) believed that the long-awaited pregnancy would be a time of happiness and health. Furthermore, depression can be surprising and distressing to the women's spouse, family, and caregivers. However, patients and caregivers can be reassured by the availability of a variety of treatment options that have been found to be successful, including interpersonal therapy, cognitive-behavioral therapy, and medications[32]. In addition, recent research has shown that some psychotropic medications (e.g., Prozac) has no detrimental impact on the fetus and can be relatively a safe, effective treatment approach[35].

Although pregnancy does not appear to increase the risk of depression during pregnancy, several studies found that depression during pregnancy is a significant predictor of postpartum depression[36,37]. Other predictive factors for postpartum depression include lack of social support, stress in terms of increased 'daily hassles', unstable relationship with the baby's father, family history of depression and/or alcoholism, and more difficult pregnancy, labor, or delivery[38–40]. The experience of infertility combined with stressors such as high-risk pregnancy, loss of social support postinfertility, relationship problems, and the effects of ovulation-inducing medications may increase vulnerability for depression in previously infertile pregnant women. In addition, research[41] has indicated higher rates of depression in women following miscarriage (11% vs. 4% of community women), indicating another potential risk factor.

Just as with depression, women with prior anxiety disorders are not 'protected' from panic disorders during pregnancy[42] and may be at increased risk for triggering or worsening of anxiety disorder and obsessive-compulsive disorder postpartum[43–45]. Although some anxiety during pregnancy is typical, especially if the focus is on the fetus rather than the woman herself, overwhelming anxiety that impairs functioning is not. For postinfertility pregnant women, certain levels of anxiety are common and predictable, although a comprehensive psychiatric history or objective measures with attention to prior episodes of panic and anxiety attacks may be the best diagnostic tool.

The impact of personality disorders during pregnancy has not been investigated, but the developmental tasks of pregnancy may be profoundly influenced by characterological disturbances; these include assumption of adult roles, revival of unresolved developmental or childhood conflicts, ambivalence toward the fetus, changes in internal boundaries and body image, reactivation of separation–individuation struggles, and resurgence of mother–daughter conflicts[46]. Personality disorders involve a pervasive, persistent, and maladaptive pattern of perceiving one's environment and behaving. As such,

these disturbances can significantly affect patient behavior and care, especially during a stressful postinfertility pregnancy[47]. Overdependence, violence, grandiosity, hypervigilance, emotionality, self-aggrandizement, wariness, and sociopathy are common presenting features in women with personality disorders. The risks of these problems involve a patient's vulnerability to overwhelming feelings of despair, hopelessness, and anxiety; reduced functioning; and/or increased pathological behavior that may endanger the pregnancy or her ability to receive appropriate care as a result of her disturbing behavior[47].

Eating Disorders and Hyperemesis Gravidum

Eating disorders, contrary to popular belief, do not diminish in intensity during pregnancy. They may in fact trigger more intense risky eating behaviors, endangering the infant's life, maternal health, and intrauterine growth, reducing infant birth weight, and increasing congenital anomalies[23,48,49]. When symptoms of disordered eating diminish as the pregnancy progresses, they frequently resurface postpartum[50]. One study[51] found that compared with women whose eating disorders were in remission, women with an active eating disorder during pregnancy gained less weight and encountered more pregnancy complications.

Although not a psychiatric disorder, hyperemesis gravidarum is a rare condition of intractable vomiting resulting in dehydration, ketonuria, weight loss, and/or electrolyte imbalance and may require hospitalization. It is common for women to be so debilitated that they are unable to function normally, even when vomiting does not require hospitalization. Furthermore, the severe emotional and physical distress of hyperemesis gravidarum can be demoralizing to the point of a major depressive episode. Psychological management usually includes supportive counseling, psychoeducation, progressive relaxation, visualization, hypnosis, accupressure, relief of guilt, identifying and lessening exacerbating factors, and assisting patients with self-assertion to limit contact with experiences and individuals who worsen symptoms[52]. Occasionally, psychotropic medication is also appropriate.

Interestingly, one study[53] of patients with hyperemesis gravidarum found a history of an eating disorder in 50% of women who had presented to an infertility clinic for ovulation-induction treatment and had failed to disclose to their caregivers that they suffered from an eating disorder. Given the high prevalence of disordered eating in the infertility population, it has been suggested that all infertility caregivers address the issue of eating disorders and dieting behavior before proceeding with treatment[53, 54].

Pseudocyeses and Pregnancy Denial

Pseudocyesis (false pregnancy) is a syndrome in which an otherwise nonpsychotic woman firmly believes that she is pregnant and develops physical signs of pregnancy when she is not pregnant. Although there are no firm psychological or physical explanations for pseudocyesis, it has been postulated that cultural pressures to have children, an inordinately strong desire to be pregnant, and the strain of infertility may be causative factors[23,55].

Denial of pregnancy is characterized by refusal to accept the pregnant state, failure to affiliate with the fetus, and no evidence of preparatory behavior (e.g., wearing maternity clothes, acquiring things for baby)[56]. Denial may range from subtle failure to adjust one's lifestyle to frank psychotic denial of pregnancy in the face of physical evidence. For previously infertile pregnant women, some denial of pregnancy or delayed acceptance of the pregnancy is normative, often the result of an ambiguous pregnancy confirmation process that contributes to disbelief or unreality. Attainment of certain landmarks of pregnancy such as a certain number of weeks of gestation, confirmation of fetal heartbeat, or fetal movement may help validate the reality of the pregnancy for a previously infertile couple. Often, women are consciously aware of denying or avoiding the pregnancy as a means of self-protection against pregnancy loss, even though they remain involved in caring for the pregnancy. In more serious situations, women may avoid or refuse medical care or directly jeopardize the pregnancy through risky behaviors while professing a desire for a child, indicating significant internal conflicts and psychological disturbance[57]. This phenomenon is more common in patients who thought to try IVF one last time but did not expect it would work.

Complicated Pregnancy After Infertility

Although most pregnancies after infertility are uneventful, many are not. A woman who becomes pregnant after infertility is at a one-third greater risk than the general population of experiencing pregnancy complications and loss[58]. Complications may be due to preexisting conditions or to factors unique to this pregnancy. The original infertility diagnosis (e.g., uterine fibroids, luteal phase disorder, or cervical problems) may contribute to pregnancy complications, or complications may be related to conception (e.g., multiple gestation or ectopic pregnancy). Other problems of pregnancy include complications of advanced maternal age, gestational diabetes, toxemia, hyperemesis gravidarum, hypertension, or preexisting medical problems, such as multiple sclerosis, arthritis, or obesity. All of these complications increase the risk of pregnancy loss and vulnerability of both mothers and infants, and highlight how the pregnancy following infertility is not 'normal'.

When pregnancy complications arise, psychological distress in both mother and father is common. The mother-to-be may have to relinquish her work, restrict her activity, abdicate the care of her other children, and submit to varying degrees of medical intervention, while experiencing anxiety about the baby and her own health. Wohlreich[59] described how obstetrical complications shatter previous plans and hopes for the pregnancy while exposing the mother to a confusing array of medical information, tests, and treatments. Women who become pregnant after infertility often feel cheated of a normal pregnancy and delivery, an experience that many feel is owed to them after the trials and tribulations of infertility. They often experience pregnancy complications as another blow to self-esteem and confidence in their ability to perform basic life tasks or their body's ability to function in a normal fashion. Ruminating about the cause of the pregnancy problems, many women blame themselves for real or imagined wrongdoing, such as failure to comply with minor medical instructions, sexual intercourse, or temporary ambivalence about the pregnancy.

Nausea and Vomiting

Nausea and vomiting occur in the majority (50–90%) of pregnancies and are at best nuisances that dispel some of the magic of the precious pregnancy[23]. Occasionally, nausea and vomiting continue episodically or continuously throughout the pregnancy, although not severe enough to be considered hyperemesis gravidarum. Nevertheless, feeling unsettled and sick is distressing for a previously infertile expectant mother, often increasing her anxiety about her baby, dampening her enjoyment of the pregnancy, and potent-

ially contributing to pregnancy complications by retarding maternal weight gain and fetal growth. Furthermore, although nausea and vomiting are common and normal in early pregnancy, these symptoms may trigger a recurrence of anorexia or bulimia in women with a history of an eating disorder. And while food aversions and cravings are typical and normal in pregnancy, they too may trigger the reemergence of disordered eating[52]. Women experiencing difficulty in eating during pregnancy due to nausea, vomiting, or food aversions/cravings may find it helpful to consult a nutritionist for guidance.

Pregnancy Bedrest

Bedrest, a common prescription for the problem pregnancy, can be physically and psychologically demanding. Restriction of activity and limited social interaction can contribute to emotional distress, including regression, anxiety, resentment, vulnerability, and feelings of sadness and helplessness. Loss of control, one of the issues of particular significance during infertility, often reemerges during a pregnancy that requires bedrest and/or hospitalization. Boredom, although usually unidentified and underestimated, can be a true nemesis of the bedrest pregnancy, affecting compliance with medical care and the emotional well-being of the mother-to-be. Financial problems, dependence on the care of others (often parents and in-laws), relinquishment of roles (e.g., employee, parent), and loss of social network at the workplace are additional stressors. Furthermore, husbands may become restless, resentful, or overwhelmed, further stressing the marital relationship, especially when the demands of caring for other children or assuming the wife's relinquished duties may impair their well-being. Creative ways of coping with the demands of the bedrest pregnancy include telephone networking with other bedrest mothers, reading materials, college courses on television, visits from home health care providers, and computers for work or networking with others[60].

Whether pregnancy complications require surgery, bedrest, extended hospitalization, or simply activity restrictions, an expectant mother may experience a myriad of negative emotions, further 'spoiling' her pregnancy and robbing her of the normal pregnancy experience she expected or felt she deserved. Extended hospitalization may increase the mother's ambivalence about the pregnancy or the baby, especially if she feels like a 'living intensive care incubator' in which the baby's well-being is a higher priority than her own. Failure to bond or delayed bonding to the baby may result from the mother's fears about her own well-being, ability to carry the pregnancy, or loosing the pregnancy. By contrast, hospitalization with the constant availability of medical care may give some women a false sense of security and confidence about the outcome of the pregnancy. They may find the hospital environment so reassuring that they react with profound disbelief and despair if the pregnancy outcome is negative.

Some women are better able to handle the psychological stressors of the complicated pregnancy, whereas others find it beyond their ability to cope, precipitating extreme psychological or marital crisis. Some women willingly tolerate the discomforts and restrictions of a bedrest pregnancy, while others consider the rigors of the complicated pregnancy punishment or simply intolerable. Some expectant mothers experience the sacrifices of a bedrest pregnancy as a means of being a good mother, psychologically facilitating the transition to motherhood. For other women, high levels of anxiety, guilt, ambivalence, or conflicts about dependency needs result in noncompliance with care,

increased conflict with caregivers or loved ones, or decreased confidence in herself as a mother.

A history of infertility may place a pregnant woman at risk for psychological problems that may be further exacerbated by a complicated pregnancy. Obstetrical risk factors for depression during and after pregnancy include toxemia, hyperemesis, malpresentation, hydramnios, placental defects, and multiple gestations[61]. Whether the complications of pregnancy after infertility are physical or psychological, they take a toll on the woman, her partner, her relationship with her baby, and her caregivers. Pregnancy complications stress marital relationships, compromise and even endanger the expectant mother's health, threaten the well-being of the pregnancy, and impede the developmental tasks of pregnancy, including attachment to the infant and transition to motherhood. Furthermore, pregnancy complications after infertility highlight the qualities of isolation, ambiguity, loss, fear, and technological bewilderment unique to the pregnancy after infertility.

Multiple Pregnancy

Pregnancies following infertility are frequently the result of ovulation-enhancing medications and/or assisted reproductive technologies, in which multiple gestation is a common consequence. Multiples are, in effect, 'too much of a good thing', contributing to preterm labor and delivery; fetal growth restriction and low birth weight; obstetrical complications such as toxemia, gestational diabetes, and cervical incompetence, resulting in extended bedrest or long-term hospitalization; and neonatal disabilities or mortality. Multiple gestations following assisted reproduction have increased as much as 40% over the past 20 years, placing a heavy burden on obstetrical care and neonatology units[62]. One study[63] comparing international outcomes in assisted reproduction found the incidence of twins to be 20–25%, triplets 2–5%, and quadruplets 2.8% or more, and reported that multiple gestation was the major factor contributing to high perinatal mortality rates.

The risk of the multiple or 'super-twin' pregnancies is unfortunately often beyond comprehension for infertile couples, even when they have been informed of the possibility. Frequently, infertile couples respond to the news of a multiple pregnancy with delight and without apprehension, even though the reality is that these pregnancies are risky for both mother and babies. In fact, in a study[64] of attitudes regarding multiple births, previously infertile women were significantly more positive about having multiple gestations than the noninfertile control group. However, the previously infertile woman expecting multiples expressed greater worry about losing the pregnancy and more concern about potential consequences to their health, attractiveness, and marital relationship.

Couples facing a multiple pregnancy need assistance in understanding the risks, consideration of pregnancy options, preparation for the birth, and ultimately education about the issues and demands of raising multiples. One of the remedies for multiple gestation is multifetal pregnancy reduction (MPR)[65]. It involves the termination of one or more fetuses in the first trimester, usually with reduction to triplets or twins, thereby, increasing the possibility for a successful pregnancy. However, MPR is not a procedure without risk, as the entire pregnancy may be lost and there is an increased risk of preterm delivery and fetal growth restriction[66].

For many previously infertile couples, the concept of terminating a much longed-for pregnancy is particularly offensive and disturbing. Marital conflict and frustration are understandable, as are individual responses of distress and sadness. Feelings of panic and dismay are also common as couples consider challenging decisions regarding the pregnancy and termination. Some couples choose to reduce a twin pregnancy to a singleton because they had not anticipated the possibility of multiples or because of economic or social reasons—often to the shock and dismay of caregivers. Other couples reluctantly accept a procedure that is in opposition to their personal wishes and/or moral beliefs. Some women experience MPR as the loss of another child, not unlike miscarriage, stillbirth, or a chemical pregnancy following IVF. Furthermore, it is a loss that usually occurs in isolation, without the support or knowledge of family and friends, within a social context of stigma and censure regarding pregnancy termination. Still others refuse MPR, choosing to take their chances—hoping to beat the odds of the pregnancy they have.

Despite the obvious emotional side effects of MPR, recent research[67,68] has shown that women who have undergone the procedure handle it fairly well. Ideally, all couples pursuing assisted reproduction should be educated early on, preferably before conception, about the possibility of a multiple pregnancy and the option of MPR, so that they can consider and prepare for possible decision-making (see Chapter 12).

Although women may not be at greater risk of psychiatric illness following MPR, its impact should not be minimized or maximized, but should be avoided whenever possible with proper prepregnancy educational counseling and appropriate medical treatment. It cannot be overlooked that the 'super-twin' pregnancy is an iatrogenic condition, often resulting from overzealous caregivers or infertility patients who decide to transfer multiple embryos or proceed with conception attempts when multiple follicles developed despite caregiver recommendations to the contrary.

Pregnancy and Third-Party Reproduction

An issue of pregnancy after infertility that is unique to the previously infertile is third-party reproduction, which includes pregnancies conceived using donated sperm, oocyte, or embryos and pregnancies in a surrogate or gestational carrier. Although studies of obstetrical outcome following donor insemination conception have revealed no increased obstetrical risk of problematic outcomes, this has not been the case for other forms of third-party reproductive technologies. While the advent of oocyte donation has provided a means for women without ovarian function to experience pregnancy and delivery, there is some evidence that pregnancies conceived via oocyte donation, especially in women with ovarian failure, should be considered obstetrically high-risk because of the higher incidence of pregnancy complications and multiples[69].

Third-party reproduction involves physical and psychological complexities that can complicate a pregnancy and the transition to parenthood and strain the well-being of the partners and the marriage[70]. If the pregnancy is the result of donated gametes or embryos, the psychological tasks include attachment to an infant to whom one or both parents are not genetically related, genealogical bewilderment, resolution of issues regarding secrecy versus disclosure, and psychological adjustment to feelings of ambivalence, anxiety, resentment, confusion, and apprehension[71–73]. If the third-party pregnancy is carried by a gestational carrier or surrogate, the psychological tasks for the intended parents include attachment to the fetus, establishment of appropriate boundaries with the gestational carrier or surrogate, management of fear and anxiety regarding the pregnancy and its outcome, and management of social attitudes[74].

Pregnancy in the surrogate or gestational carrier involves a whole different set of psychological tasks. Preliminary research on the psychological adjustment to surrogate pregnancy has shown a strong prenatal attachment between the surrogate/carrier and the fetus[75]. In addition, some surrogate mothers may experience grief responses at the time of relinquishment, resulting in feelings loss or abandonment after the birth or resentment at no longer being the 'center of attention'[74] (see Chapter 21).

For the intended parents, surrogate/carrier pregnancies may enhance feelings of powerlessness, lack of social support, and uncertainty about parenthood. Running parallel with the desire and need to attach to the expected child are the parents' fears that the surrogate/carrier may change her mind, not surrender the child, or not take proper care of herself, thereby endangering the pregnancy or baby. Research[76] has indicated that intended (vs. carrier) mothers have a high need for affection and may need to feel that the surrogate carrier cares about them and their husband. Furthermore, the intended mother may attempt to shape and nurture her child by forming a positive relationship with the surrogate carrier.

Infertility counselors can provide assistance to intended parents and the surrogate/carrier by defining and facilitating the tasks of pregnancy and by supporting the individuals as they move through them. These tasks include preserving the autonomy of the carrier/surrogate; protecting the rights and responsibilities of all parties; preventing any adverse maternal outcomes for the carrier/surrogate; avoiding psychosocial traumatization of all parties, particularly the disadvantaged carrier/surrogate; facilitating attachment between the intended parents and the baby; and providing ongoing counseling for all parties, especially the carrier/surrogate for at least 6 weeks postpartum[77]. It is a delicate balance for infertility counselors between preventing exploitation and protecting autonomy for the carrier/surrogate, while protecting the rights and responsibilities of the genetic or intended parents[78] (see Chapter 21).

The pregnancy achieved through donated gametes involves unique tasks of pregnancy. Before conception, the infertile couple must assimilate complex medical information, cope with one parent's loss of genetic contribution, as well as the loss for both partners of the genetically-shared pregnancy, and undergo varying levels of medical treatment. During pregnancy, the expectant mother must come to terms with carrying a fetus that is not genetically related either to her or to her husband, often harboring secret fears about the baby's appearance or normalcy. Just after the birth, new parents may experience heightened anxiety attributable to fears that the baby's physical characteristics will be distinctively different from the parents, somehow publicizing the circumstances of the conception[75].

Secrecy about the means of conception is a unique feature of the donor gamete pregnancy, because this pregnancy is not visibly different from any other pregnancy. This factor can be both a positive, in that it enables the 'normalization' of pregnancy and parenthood, and a negative, in that it makes it easier to avoid the differentness of this pregnancy. Hence, decisions about disclosure that began before conception will continue to be revisited during the pregnancy and long afterward.

The issues of the postinfertility pregnancy—ambiguity, isolation, fear, loss, and technological bewilderment—are most apparent in third-party reproduction. The ambiguity of these pregnancies involve ambiguous bloodlines, loyalties, and relationships, as well as new definitions of parenthood, kinship, and family roles. Intended parents may not share the circumstances of the conception or pregnancy with family and/or friends, leading to increased isolation and/or feelings of stigma. The fears of this pregnancy are more complex: will the carrier or surrogate relinquish the child? Will the donor be of the same race? Could there be a laboratory mix-up of gametes or embryos? Will the use of donor gametes become an issue for a spouse, the child, or the family in the future? The losses of the third-party pregnancy are also unique, including loss of control of the prenatal environment, loss of predictability, and even loss of the pregnancy experience.

Finally, technological bewilderment is fundamental to third-party pregnancies—donated gametes, donated embryos, gestational carrier, surrogacy—resulting in a myriad of complexities for both parents and children, boundary violations, and confusion between the fetus, surrogate/carrier, and intended parents[79]. Although reproductive technologies provide family-building opportunities previously unimaginable, they are not without dilemmas, ethical challenges, and confusion about parental roles, definitions, and kinship ties. Not surprisingly, parents-to-be in third-party reproduction often feel ill-prepared for the challenges of these pregnancies or the stresses of parenting under such unique circumstances. Although there has been an increasing demand from both infertility patients and mental health professionals to improve patient education and preparation, provide appropriate psychological support and evaluation, and better equip patients for these unique pregnancies, the majority of women and their partners remain ill-prepared for their third-party pregnancies[80].

Pregnancy in the Older Mother

There is a growing trend toward pregnancy in older mothers, especially in the infertile population. Medically termed *elderly gravida*, it encompasses pregnant women over the age of 35. However, with the advent of donated oocytes, women have given birth after age 60, a practice not generally recommended or condoned for social, ethical, and medical reasons. The risks of pregnancy in older mothers include gestational diabetes, macrosomia, hypertension, toxemia, preeclampsia, and pregnancy loss[81]. In one study[82], first-time mothers over 35 had no greater risk of preterm delivery, infants small for gestational age, perinatal death, or infants with an Apgar score of less than 7 at 1 or 5 minutes. However, they were found to have an increased risk of gestational diabetes, pregnancy-induced hypertension, gestational bleeding, abruptio placentae, and placenta previa. Although infants born to older mothers may be at no greater risk, older first-time mothers *are* at significantly greater risk.

If the pregnancy in an older mother involves her own gametes, the fetus is at increased risk of a variety of problems related to increased maternal age, such as chromosomal abnormalities, molar gestations, and monozygotic twining (see Chapter 11). Consequently, prenatal testing is seriously recommended for older mothers, often affecting her feelings about the pregnancy and/or attachment to the fetus. Some prenatal testing, such as serum alpha-fetoprotein testing, involves a simple blood test and is less invasive. Other genetic tests such as amniocentesis, chorionic villus sampling, fetoscopy, and percutaneous umbilical blood sampling are more invasive and involve some risk of loosing the pregnancy.

The whole issue of the 'less than perfect' baby is another consideration of these pregnancies and can be a significant psychological hurdle. Terminating a much longed-for pregnancy is never easy but can be even more challenging if it represents the end of one's childbearing possibilities or ending a pregnancy achieved after considerable investment of time, treatment, finances, and emotional energy. Equally difficult or challenging can be the care of a disabled or handicapped child after years of infertility when one or both parents are well into middle-age. In one study[83] of previously infertile couples undergoing amniocentesis, prenatal testing contributed to feelings of adversity, uncertainty, and hope that reprised elements of the infertility experience and affected the pregnancy experience in a negative way. Interestingly, the majority of the infertile women under age 35 in this study refused amniocentesis, reflecting, in the authors' opinion, a greater sense of the value of the pregnancy and baby.

Older first mothers typically represent a last chance at parenthood, frequently following a quest for a 'baby at any price'. They often willingly risk their own health and well-being for the longed-for pregnancy and baby, reasoning that, if the baby is healthy, complications or risks to their own health are acceptable[84]. Apart from the medical considerations, the complex social situation of older primigravidae—remarriage, stepchildren, adult children from previous marriages, older or younger spouse, aged parents—frequently complicates their adjustment to parenthood and parental satisfaction[85-87].

Pregnancy Following Secondary Infertility

Pregnancy in the secondarily infertile woman has not been investigated but has its own set of experiences and issues. Secondary infertility may follow a period of prior infertility, complicated pregnancy, or pregnancy loss, so that additional infertility treatment was foreseen. By contrast, previous conceptions and pregnancies may have been uneventful, while this pregnancy was achieved after considerable medical intervention. If a woman's other children are younger and still require considerable care, this precious pregnancy may be more difficult to safeguard and manage—especially if bedrest is required. On the other hand, the comfort of a child may ameliorate feelings of anxiety, distress, and worry about this pregnancy[88].

Of special consideration in the post-secondary-infertility pregnancy is the conception achieved via donated gametes or carried by a surrogate/gestational carrier, while previous conceptions were genetically-shared pregnancies. The post-infertility third-party pregnancy highlights 'the new blended family' composed of children, each with a unique reproductive beginning. But it can be a mixed blessing: although it provides a longed-for child, it presents parenting and relationship challenges. The third-party postsecondary-infertility pregnancy involves ambiguous genetic ties, more complicated pregnancy management, and a redefinition of family and kinship meanings. Furthermore, the postsecondary-infertility mother-to-be may be unable to interact with her social support system in the same manner in which she did during prior pregnancies, and obstetrical care may be based on inaccurate assumptions from her prior pregnancy history, enhancing feelings of ambiguity, isolation, and technological bewilderment.

THERAPEUTIC INTERVENTIONS

Pregnancy after infertility is an exciting, terrifying, delightful, frightful time for couples. Infertility counselors can play a special role in assisting patients in moving from infertility through the transition to becoming expectant parents to eventually new mothers and fathers. There are six areas in which counselors can facilitate and support the adaptation to pregnancy and the preparation for parenthood: (1) facilitating the adjustment to pregnancy, (2) assisting in decision-making about prenatal care and testing, (3) developing and strengthening coping skills, (4) assessing for potential psychopathology and intervening, (5) identifying and providing support resources, and (6) advocating with caregivers.

Facilitating the Adjustment to Pregnancy

Moving from the identity of an infertile person, to that of an expectant parent, and finally to the long-awaited identity as mother or father occurs in rapid succession once pregnancy is established. Couples often need help from infertility counselors in making the transition. The psychological tasks of pregnancy—validation, fetal embodiment, fetal distinction, and role transition—occur in a maturational process that counselors can help to facilitate through education, support, and discussion. Understanding the unique aspects of pregnancy after infertility will also help in the adjustment. Mothers have to be able to take in their developing baby as part of themselves before they can separate from the infant during the birth process and see it as an individual.

Recognizing that there are unique challenges in pregnancy after infertility, couples also need encouragement to find as many opportunities as possible to 'normalize' the pregnancy experience for both partners. One area that will need to be addressed is a couple's sexual relationship, which often is negatively affected by years of infertility. Renewing sexual intimacy encourages closeness, pleasure, and communication on which new parents can draw. However, couples may have many fears about sex during pregnancy and will need reassurance and concrete information that an orgasm does not precipitate labor or premature rupture of membranes in nonproblematic pregnancies. In addition, minimal spotting after intercourse is not harmful or troublesome[89]. This is an example of one of the many ways in which, through education and support, infertility counselors can dispel myths and fears that can and often do interrupt healthy adjustment to pregnancy.

Facilitating Decision-making

Once pregnancy is established, the formerly infertile couple often faces a new set of medical experiences and decisions. They must make decisions about use of a mid-wife, obstetrician, or high-risk perinatologist, about hospital or birthing facility, and about the extent of medical intervention and diagnostic and prenatal genetic testing that they will want done. Making the shift from the infertility practice, where the couple may have been involved for years, to an unknown obstetrical practice is often difficult for patients. It becomes yet another loss, as they leave behind caregivers who have shared in the most intimate aspects of their lives and may have become part of their primary emotional support system. There may be concerns that the new caregivers will not appreciate the preciousness of this pregnancy or be as 'invested' in their care. A 'pregnancy support group' sponsored by the reproductive medical practice is an ideal method for assisting infertility patients in these transitions by providing an understanding environment of the special issues involved in the pregnancy, as well as continuing connection to the clinic.

The pregnant couple may also be faced with decisions about prenatal testing and MPR, requiring support and understanding about their feelings and values, which are often conflicted and ambivalent. In addition, couples will have to explore and examine the risks of the procedures compared with the benefits that they will obtain. For example, if a couple knows that they would not terminate the pregnancy of a genetically defective fetus, it may not be worth the risk of having testing that has the potential of jeopardizing the pregnancy. With any of these decisions, it is always better that couples be educated, informed, and prepared for the possibilities well before having to make the choices. Even so, infertility counselors can provide additional support as a familiar anchor, aware of their personal situation and knowledgeable of who they are apart from this crisis.

Strengthening Coping Skills

Pregnancy after infertility could well be called the definition of 'the anxious pregnancy'. Couples often need assistance in identifying and strengthening coping mechanisms during this anxious and challenging period. Nine months often feels like nine years to the previously infertile pregnant couple. Thus, one of the first tasks may be to help them adopt the Alcoholics Anonymous motto 'one day at a time', as looking too far down the road and considering all the 'what ifs' can be overwhelming. Breaking the pregnancy into a more manageable time frame, such as trimesters, may help to compartmentalize worries and fears, adjusting to the current demands versus the potential ones.

Increased anxiety and vigilance are common in the pregnancy after infertility, perhaps representing a long-standing dependency on medical technology or a need to maintain contact with caregivers who have become a primary source of support and reassurance. Hypervigilant coping is often represented by repeated requests or demands for reassurance or repetition of tests or by difficulty in relinquishing the infertility treatment team for more appropriate obstetrical care. The result of hypervigilant coping may be an overreaction to the normal symptoms and physiological changes of pregnancy such as nausea, heartburn, or backache and misinterpreting them as signs of problems with the pregnancy or the baby. Hypervigilance often includes requests for weekly physician visits, repeated ultrasound examinations, special medications, self-imposed bedrest, or sexual abstinence. Cognitive-behavioral interventions, including stress relaxation techniques and keeping a journal, may be useful in managing this acute anxiety and worry.

It may be that couples with a history of infertility are more aware of what can go wrong with a pregnancy[90]. Hence, they seek out ways of ensuring the safety of the pregnancy, even when there is no evidence that it is endangered. Other couples use avoidant coping to handle their numerous fears. Coping through avoidance may include not telling friends and family about the pregnancy, delaying or refusing to use maternity clothing, resisting transfer to obstetrical care from the infertility clinic, not following medical advice, and consciously resisting bonding with the baby. Furthermore, avoidant coping impedes problem solving and mastery of the tasks of pregnancy, further diminishing self-esteem and self-confidence as an effective parent.

Assessing Emotional Distress

Infertility counselors may be called on to assess and intervene with emotional problems, which may be preexisting or precipitated by this pregnancy. Women with a history of depression or other mood disorders, anxiety or panic disorder, eating disorders, or other psychological problems may need to be followed more closely during pregnancy and postpartum. In addition, these women (and their families) need to be educated early in the pregnancy about risk factors, treatment options, warning signs, and action plans in order to minimize the effects of the illness. Further,

marital problems may surface after the years of infertility and will need to be addressed as couples prepare for the transition to parenthood, the next great marital stressor.

Sometimes, women who become pregnant after infertility react with feelings of bitterness toward the pregnancy or the baby. They may feel that they have 'paid their dues' during infertility treatment and are 'owed' an effortless pregnancy or delivery. Resentment about the additional physical demands and psychological stresses of pregnancy or even resentment of the baby itself may surface, much to the alarm of the woman, her partner, and caregivers. In extreme situations, newly pregnant infertility patients may be so overwhelmed and disturbed by the experience that they demand an abortion or act out their distress in equally alarming ways. Careful and immediate assessment and intervention are needed to understand the basis for this extreme reaction and provide appropriate diagnosis, treatment, and support.

Since depression and anxiety are common concerns in the pregnancy after infertility, several tools have been developed for assessing depression during pregnancy as a means of predicting postpartum depression; these include the Antepartum Questionnaire[91] (see Appendix 4) and the Antenatal Questionnaire[92]. High scores indicate not only increased anxiety and depression during pregnancy but are also predictive of postpartum depression. However, standardized measurements for depression may be just as effective in assessing depression, especially administered repeatedly during the pregnancy.

Providing Resources

Many postinfertility pregnancy patients need assistance in accessing and utilizing pregnancy resources, which often feels like unfamiliar and foreign territory. It is important that couples be encouraged to 'normalize' the pregnancy as much as possible and become involved with the same support resources as the noninfertile pregnant group—childbirth classes, pregnancy exercise programs, support groups, preparation for parenthood classes, and parents of multiples organizations. Couples also need access to information and reading materials on pregnancy, prenatal testing, normal obstetrical care, or special problems of this unique pregnancy. Support groups now exist in many places, and the Internet has become a helpful resource for many issues related to infertility, as well as pregnancy. 'Surfing the net' may help lessen feelings of loneliness and isolation that follow infertility and help prepare for parenthood. However, caution must be used, as information received on the Internet may not be accurate.

Advocating with Caregivers

The history of a woman pregnant after infertility may include physical and emotional losses following failed medical treatments, marital disruption, sexual dysfunction, or even serious psychiatric illnesses such as depression, anxiety, or obsessive-compulsive disorder. She may have idealized pregnancy as a state of bliss and fulfillment or fantasized that her baby would be perfect in every way or that she would be the perfect all-knowing, all-caring mother. Furthermore, a woman's own stage of life may influence her adjustment to pregnancy. For example, the first-time mother in her late 20s will experience pregnancy differently from the woman who is pregnant in her 40s after a period of secondary infertility. As a consequence, women may need assistance from infertility counselors in navigating and negotiating the pregnancy path. This may mean advocating for patients, when they are unable, with physicians, other caregivers, employers, or family members. For example, an infertility counselor may want to be in contact with the obstetrician to coordinate care and help the physician better understand the patient and her past infertility experience. Often, infertility counselors are bridges between the worlds of infertility and obstetrical caregivers and, as such, are able to explain or discriminate normal and abnormal responses to pregnancy in a previously infertile patient[93].

FUTURE ISSUES

Though pregnancy is as old as mankind, the way conception is achieved has changed drastically in the last few years. However, the future may hold more changes in the ways in which babies are carried to term. Third-party reproduction with gestational carriers and surrogates has already been an example of some of these changes. The next century may see babies gestated in vitro rather than in vivo, in a manner not unlike that envisioned in Aldous Huxley's *Brave New World*. Continued research is needed to understand the psychological adaptation to pregnancy after high-stakes infertility treatment. Olshansky[15] outlined three possible future directions for research on pregnancy after infertility:

- delineation of the differences in experiences of infertility and correlation of those different experiences with subsequent experiences of pregnancy
- more diverse sampling in research on those pregnant after infertility, including the various reproductive technologies, cultural perspectives and pregnancy experiences
- gender differences in responses to pregnancy after infertility.

Other resources need to be developed to assist this special population (targeting the special needs of the previously infertile pregnancy). Educational materials are needed on normal pregnancy, pregnancy complications, delivery, and parenting. Support resources, especially pregnancy support groups, childbirth education classes, and preparation for parenthood classes for the previously infertile pregnant couple are sorely needed. There must also be education and training of obstetrical staff about the special nature, needs, and unique characteristics of women who become pregnant after infertility.

SUMMARY

- The pregnancy after infertility is a premium pregnancy with additional potential medical and psychological hurdles to overcome before a successful outcome is achieved.

- The psychological tasks of pregnancy—validation, fetal embodiment, fetal distinction, and role transition—are challenged and complicated by the infertility experience.

- The psychological tasks of pregnancy after infertility involve addressing the issues of ambiguity, isolation, fear, loss, and technological bewilderment[30].

- The pregnancy after infertility is at higher risk for complications, including multiple gestation, advanced-maternal-age-related problems, premature delivery, low birth weight, and perinatal loss.

- The postinfertility pregnancy is often marked by high anxiety, hypervigilance, or denial as typical coping mechanisms. In addition, there may be an increased risk of depression, anxiety, obsessive-compulsive disorder, and other psychiatric illness in the post-infertility pregnancy.

- There are six areas in which infertility counselors may assist pregnant couples: (1) facilitating in adjustment to the pregnancy, (2) assisting in obstetrical decision-making, (3) strengthening coping mechanisms, (4) assessing and treating maladaptive responses, (5) providing additional resources, and (6) advocating for patients.

REFERENCES

1. Simkin P. Childbearing in a social context. *Women Health* 1989;15:5–21

2. Gordon ER. Blended families: Adopted, ART, and natural children. In: Postgraduate Course XII: ART Parents and Children. American Society for Reproductive Medicine; Seattle, WA, October 7–8, 1995;78–83

3. Macklin R. Artificial means of reproduction and our understanding of the family. *Hastings Cent Rep* 1991;21:5–11

4. Poulson AM, Bryner WA. The obstetric complications of the infertility patients. *Obstet Gynecol* 1977;49:174–9

5. Applegarth L, Goldberg NC, Choist I, *et al.* Families created through ovum donation: A preliminary investigation of obstetrical outcome and psychosocial adjustment. *J Assist Reprod Genet* 1995;12:574–80

6. Spensley JC, Mushin D, Barreda-Hanson M. The children of IVF pregnancies: A cohort study. *Aust Paediatr J* 1986;22:285–9

7. Garner CH. Pregnancy after infertility. *J Obstet Gynecol Neonatal Nurs* 1985; 14(suppl):58–62

8. Harris BG, Sandelowski M, Holditch-Davis D. Infertility and new interpretations of pregnancy loss. *J Matern Child Nurs* 1991; 16:217–20

9. Phipps S. The subsequent pregnancy after stillbirth: Anticipatory parenthood in the face of uncertainty. *Int J Psychiatry Med* 1985;15:243–64

10. Cuisinier M, Janssen H, de Graauw C, *et al.* Pregnancy following miscarriage: Course of grief and some determining factors. *J Psychosom Obstet Gynaecol* 1996;17:168–74

11. Bernstein J, Lewis J, Seibel M. Effect of

previous infertility on maternal-infant attachment, coping styles, and self-concept during pregnancy. *J Women's Health* 1994; 3:125–33

12. Bernstein J, Mattox JH, Kellner R. Psychological status of previously infertile couples after a successful pregnancy. *J Obstet Gynecol Neonatal Nurs* 1988;164(suppl):404–8

13. McMahon C, Ungerer J, Tennant C, *et al.* Psychosocial adjustment and the mother–baby relationship for IVF mothers. Symposia of the Mental Health Professional Group, presented at the American Society for Reproductive Medicine, Boston, MA; November, 1996

14. Sandelowski M, Pollock C. Women's experiences of infertility. *Image J Nurs Sch* 1986;18:140–4

15. Olshansky EF. Identity of self as infertile: An example of theory-generating research. *Adv Nurs Sci* 1987;9:54–63

16. Glaser BG, Strauss AL. *The Discovery of Grounded Theory*. Chicago: Aldine Press, 1967

17. Olshansky EF. Pregnancy after infertility: An overview of the research. Course XII: ART Parents and Children. American Society for Reproductive Medicine; Seattle, WA, October 7–8, 1995;5–13

18. Holditch-Davis D, Black BP, Harris BG, *et al.* Beyond couvade: Pregnancy symptoms in couples with a history of infertility. *Health Care Women Int* 1994;15:537–48

19. Bing E, Colman L. *Making Love During Pregnancy*. New York: Farrar, Straus, and Giroux, 1977

20. Benedek T. Parenthood as a developmental phase. *J Am Psychoanal Assoc* 1959;7:379–417

21. Deutsch H. *The Psychology of Women*, vol 1. New York: Grune & Stratton, 1944

22. Notman MR, Lester EP. Pregnancy: Theoretical considerations. *Psychoanal Inq* 1988;8:139–59

23. Miller LJ. Psychiatric disorders during pregnancy. In: Stewart DE, Stotland NL, eds. *Psychological Aspects of Women's Health Care*. Washington DC: American Psychiatric Press, 1993;55–70

24. Raphael-Leff J. *Pregnancy: The Inside Story*. London: Jason Aronson, 1993, 1995

25. Olshansky EF. Psychosocial implications of pregnancy after infertility. *NAACOG Clin Issues Perinat Womens Health Nurs* 1990; 1:342–7

26. Clark AL, Affonso D, eds. *Childbearing: A Nursing Perspective*. Philadelphia: FA Davis, 1976

27. Lederman RP. *Psychosocial Adaptation in Pregnancy*, 2nd ed. New York: Springer Publishing, 1996

28. Colman LL, Colman AD. *Pregnancy: The Psychological Experience*. New York: Noonday Press, 1991

29. Glazer E. *The Long-Awaited Stork*. New York: Lexington Books, 1990

30. Glazer E. Parenting after infertility. In: Seibel MM, Kiessling AA, Bernstein J, *et al*, eds. *Infertility and Technology: Clinical Psychological, Legal, and Ethical Aspects*. New York: Springer-Verlag, 1993;365–72

31. Pugh TF, Jerath BK, Schmidt WM, *et al.* Rates of mental disease related to childbearing. *N Engl J Med* 1963;268:1224–8

32. Gise LH. Psychiatric implications of pregnancy. In: Cherry SH, Barques R, Kale N, eds. *Rovinksy and Gutmacher's Medical, Surgical, and Gynecologic Complications of Pregnancy*, 3rd ed. Baltimore, MD: Williams & Wilkins, 1985;614–54

33. Callahan EJ, Desiderato L. Disorders of pregnancy. In: Blechman EA, Brownell KD, eds. *Handbook of Behavioral Medicine for Women*. New York: Pergamon Press, 1988;103–15

34. O'Hara MW, Rehm LP, Campbell SB. Predicting depressive symptomology: Cognitive-behavioral models and postpartum depression. *J Abnorm Psychol* 1982;91:457–61

35. Chambers CD, Johnson KA, Dick LM, *et al.* Birth outcomes in pregnant women taking fluoxetine. *N Engl J Med* 1996;335:1010–15

36. O'Hara M, Zekoski E, Phillips L, *et al.* Controlled prospective study of postpartum mood disorders: Comparisons of childbearing and nonchildrearing women. *J Abnorm Psychol* 1990;99:3–12

37. O'Hara MW. Social support, life events, and depression during pregnancy and the puerperium. *Arch Gen Psychiatry* 1986; 43:569–73

38. Powell S, Drotar D. Postpartum depressed mood: The impact of daily hassles. *J Psychosom Obstet Gynaecol* 1992;13:255–63

39. O'Hara M, Rehm L, Campbell S.

Postpartum depression: A role for social network and life stress variables. *J Nerv Ment Dis* 1983;171:336–41

40. O'Hara MW, Zekoski EM. Postpartum depression: A comprehensive review. In: Kumar R, Brockington IF, eds. *Motherhood and Mental Illness*. London: Butterworth, 1988

41. Neugebauer R, Kline J, Shrout P, *et al.* Major depressive disorder in the 6 months after miscarriage. *JAMA* 1997;277:383–8

42. Villeponteaux VA, Lydiard RB, Laraia MT, *et al.* The effects of pregnancy on pre-existing panic disorder. *J Clin Psychiatry* 1992;53:201–3

43. Neziroglu F, Anemone R, Yaryura-Tobias JA. Onset of obsessive-compulsive disorder in pregnancy. *Am J Psychiatry* 1992;149: 947–50

44. Brandt KR, Mackenzie TB. Obsessive-compulsive disorder exacerbated during pregnancy: A case report. *Int J Psychiatry Med* 1987;17:361–6

45. Cowley DS, Roy-Byrne RP. Panic disorder during pregnancy. *J Psychosom Obstet Gynaecol* 1989;10:193–210

46. Notman MT. Reproduction and pregnancy: A psychodynamic developmental perspective. In: Stotland NL, ed. *Psychiatric Aspects of Reproductive Technology*. Washington DC: American Psychiatric Press, 1990; 13–24

47. Stotland NL. Personality disorders. *Prim Care Update Ob/Gynecol* 1997;4:57–60

48. Abrams BF, Laros RK. Pregnancy weight, weight gain and birth weight. *Am J Obstet Gynecol* 1986;154:503–9

49. Hollifield J, Hobdy J. The course of pregnancy complicated by bulimia. *Psychotherapy* 1990;27:249–55

50. Lacey JH, Smith G. Bulimia nervosa: The impact of pregnancy on mother and baby. *Br J Psychiatry* 1987;150:777–81

51. Stewart DE, McDonald OL. Hyperemesis gravidarum and eating disorders in pregnancy. In: Abraham S, Llewellyn-Jones D, eds. *Eating Disorders and Disordered Eating*. Sydney, Australia: Ashwood House, 1987;52–5

52. Downey J, Whitaker A. Nausea and vomiting of pregnancy: Behavioral aspects of diagnosis and management. *Clin Consult Obstet Gynecol* 1994;6:258–64

53. Stewart DE, Robinson GE, Goldbloom DS, *et al.* Infertility and eating disorders. *Am J Obstet Gynecol* 1990;163:1196–9

54. Abraham S, Mira M, Llewellyn-Jones D. Should ovulation be induced in women recovering from an eating disorder or who are compulsive exercisers? *Fertil Steril* 1990;52:566–8

55. Ladipo OA. Pseudocyesis in infertile patients. *Int J Gynaecol Obstet* 1979;16:427–9

56. Brezinka C, Huter O, Biebl W, Kinzl J. Denial of pregnancy: Obstetrical aspects. *J Psychosom Obstet Gynaecol* 1996;15:1–8

57. Miller LJ. Psychotic denial of pregnancy: Phenomenology and clinical management. *Hosp Community Psychiatry* 1990;41:1233–7

58. Bernstein J. Pregnancy after infertility. *Serono Reprod Med Infertil Nurses* 1986;Sept 27–28:68–81

59. Wohlreich MM. Psychiatric aspects of high-risk pregnancy. *Psychiatr Clin North Am* 1986;10:53–68

60. Johnson SH, Kraut DA. *Pregnancy Bedrest: A Guide for the Pregnant Woman and Her Family*. New York: Henry Holt, 1990

61. Nadelson CC. 'Normal' and 'special' aspects of pregnancy: A psychological approach. In: Nadelson CC, Notman MT, eds. *The Woman Patient, Medical and Psychological Interfaces*, vol. 1: *Sexual and Reproductive Aspects of Women's Health Care*. New York: Plenum, 1978;279

62. Levene MI, Wild J, Steer P. Higher multiple births and the modern management of infertility in Britain. *J Obstet Gynaecol* 1992;99:607–13

63. Lancaster PA. International comparisons of assisted reproduction. *Assist Reprod Rev* 1992;2:212–21

64. Leiblum SR, Kemmann E, Taska L. Attitudes toward multiple births and pregnancy concerns in infertile and non-infertile women. *J Psychosom Obstet Gynaecol* 1990;11:197–210

65. Greenfeld DA, Walther VN. Psychological consideration in multifetal reduction. *Infertil Reprod Med Clin North Am* 1993; 4:533–43

66. Silver RK, Ragin A, Helfand BT, *et al.* Multifetal reduction increases the risk of preterm delivery and fetal growth restriction in twins: A case-control study. *Fertil Steril* 1997;67:30–3

67. McKinney M, Downey J, Timor-Tritsch I. The psychological effects of multifetal pregnancy reduction. *Fertil Steril* 1995; 64:51–61

68. Schreiner-Engel P, Walther VN, Mindes J, *et al*. First trimester multifetal pregnancy reduction: Acute and persistent psychological reactions. *Am J Obstet Gynecol* 1995;172:541–7

69. Bilieu A, Abdatia H, Wren M, *et al*: The outcome of ovum donation pregnancies. *J Assist Reprod Genet* 1995;12:74–80

70. Bertrand-Servais M, Letur-Konirsch H, Raoul-Duval A, *et al*. Psychological considerations of anonymous oocyte donation. *Hum Reprod* 1993;8:874–9

71. Pados G, Camus M, Van Steirteghem A, *et al*. The evolution and outcome of pregnancies from oocyte donation. *Hum Reprod* 1994;9:538–42

72. Braverman AM. Oocyte donation: Psychological and counseling issues. *Clin Consult Obstet Gynecol* 1994;6:143–9

73. Schover LR. Psychological aspects of oocyte donation. *Infertil Reprod Med Clin North Am* 1993;4:483–502

74. Parker PJ. Motivation of surrogate mothers: Initial findings. *Am J Psychiatry* 1983;140:117–18

75. Braverman AM, Corson SL. Characteristics of participants in a gestational carrier program. *J Assist Reprod Genet* 1992;9:353–7

76. Braverman AM. Surrogacy and gestational carrier: Psychological issues. *Infertil Reprod Med Clin North Am* 1993;4:517–33

77. Reame NE. The surrogate mother as a high-risk obstetrical patient. *Jacobs Inst Women's Health* 1991;1:151–4

78. Reame NE, Parker PJ. Surrogate pregnancy: Clinical features in 44 cases. *Am J Obstet Gynecol* 1990;162:1220–5

79. Lester EP. Surrogate carries a fertilised ovum: Multiple crossings in ego boundaries. *Int J Psychoanal* 1995;76:325–34

80. Mahlstedt PP, Greenfeld DA. Assisted reproductive technology with donor gametes: The need for patient preparation. *Fertil Steril* 1989;52:908–14

81. Hansen JP. Older maternal age and pregnancy outcome: A review of the literature. *Obstet Gynecol Surv* 1986;41:726–42

82. Berkowitz GS, Skovron ML, Lapinski RH, *et al*. Delayed childbearing and the outcome of pregnancy. *N Engl J Med* 1990; 322:659–64

83. Sandelowski M, Harris BG, Holditch-Davis D. Amniocentesis in the context of infertility. *Health Care Women Int* 1991; 12:167–78

84. James C. Impact the psyche of the cycle: Pregnancy after forty. In: Postgraduate Course XI: American Society for Reproductive Medicine; Seattle, WA, October 7–8, 1995;135

85. Windridge KC, Berryman JC. Maternal adjustment and maternal attitudes during pregnancy and early motherhood in women of 35 and over. *J Reprod Infant Psychol* 1996;14:45–55

86. Berryman JC, Windridge KC. Pregnancy after 35 and attachment to the fetus. *J Reprod Infant Psychol* 1996;14:133–43

87. Frankel SA, Wise MJ. A view of delayed parenting: Some implications for a new trend. *Psychiatry* 1982;45:220–5

88. Rosenblatt PA, Burns LH. Long-term effects of perinatal loss. *J Fam Issues* 1986;7:237–53

89. Shapiro CH. Is pregnancy after infertility a dubious joy? *Soc Casework J Contemp Soc Work* 1986;67:306–13

90. Reamy KJ. Sexuality in pregnancy: An update. *Clin Consult Obstet Gynecol* 1994;6:265–73

91. Posner NA, Unterman RR, Williams KN, *et al*. *Antepartum Questionnaire: APQ*. Albany, NY: Department of Obstetrics & Gynecology, Albany Medical Center, 1996

92. Cooper PJ, Murray L, Hooper R, *et al*. The development and validation of a predictive index for postpartum depression. *Psychol Med* 1996;26:627–34

93. Burns LH. Pregnancy after infertility. *Infertil Reprod Med Clin North Am* 1996; 7:503–20

25

Parenting after Infertility

Linda Hammer Burns, PhD

Your children are not your children. They are the sons and daughters of life's longing for itself ... you may strive to be like them, but seek not to make them like you.

Kahil Gibran

The legacy of infertility extends beyond the children and families created through medical treatment and reproductive technologies; the impact may be experienced in the long-term adjustment and psychosocial development of the family system and its individuals. The legacy of infertility often includes multiple losses, prolonged yearning for a child, intrusive reproductive technologies, possibly third-party reproduction, a tenuous, highly anxious pregnancy, and/or an exorbitant investment of time, energy, and money to have children. Exceptionally determined and purposeful, previously infertile parents may be aware of their reasons for wanting to be parents but less cognizant of the potential challenges and actual joys of parenthood. Once parenthood is achieved, these parents are often equally determined about parenthood as they were about infertility. Their goal is often to be the world's best parents and they are not satisfied with being simply good enough parents. Furthermore, most previously infertile parents believe that parenthood is worth it: they value their children, take the responsibilities of parenthood seriously, savor the pleasures of their children, and do their best to act in the best interests of their children. Nevertheless, many previously infertile couples refer to their history

of infertility as 'the shadow', a legacy that resurfaces long after parenthood is achieved and emerges in various ways long after the maelstrom of infertility has passed. While adoptive and single parenting are addressed in other chapters (see Chapters 14 and 22), this chapter will address:

- the unique psychosocial issues of and the transition to parenthood after infertility
- special parenting situations including the older parent
- parenting after secondary infertility
- parenting multiples
- parenting children conceived through donor gametes
- the issues surrounding disclosure of third-party reproduction.

HISTORICAL OVERVIEW

Motivations for parenthood or reasons for wanting children are enigmatic and timeless, representing biological drive, cultural norm, religious mandate, status symbol, attainment of adulthood, affectional ties, economic utility, role fulfillment, ego gratification, or power. Motivations for wanting children in infertile couples have also been identified as a couple's desire for happiness and well-being[1], motherhood and identity-development for women, and marital completion for men[2,3]. While infertile couples are often impressively determined in their struggling to have children, research indicates that infertility triggers in them a process of thinking and rethinking their reasons for wanting and having children[3].

Historically, it was thought that previously infertile parents would be more appreciative and conscientious parents— reinterpreted as more overprotective and overinvested parents. In 1943, a study of overprotective mothers concluded, 'Mothers who suffer the trials of prolonged anticipation of the first born, long periods of relative sterility, or spontaneous miscarriages or stillbirths, are rendered obviously more apprehensive and protective in their attitude toward the offspring than if childbirth occurred without these circumstances'[4]. By contrast, it was speculated that a history of infertility resulted in parents who were more hostile, abusive, or neglectful of their children—perhaps acting on lingering feelings of shame, self-reproach, frustration or long-standing marital conflict about infertility. One case report[5] went so far as to conclude that child abuse and abortion were manifestations of parental hostility toward children resulting from prior infertility and reproductive failure. Finally, it was theorized that a history of parental infertility could produce disturbances in children and the family system. In a 1971 investigation of child-centered family systems, Bradt and Moynihan[6] concluded that prematurity and adoption (as evidence of reproductive failure) increased the risk of a child's becoming disturbed and the 'emotional focus' of a family, as evidenced by a child's 'acting out' to escape the pressure and responsibility of the family's happiness. However, none of these theories or speculations ever produced conclusive evidence that families with a history of infertility were at greater risk for psycho-logical disturbance in the children, family system, or parents.

REVIEW OF LITERATURE

Although interest in postinfertility families has grown among reproductive health professionals, it has yet to capture the curiosity of the broader community of mental health professionals and researchers. As a result, the field has been plagued by lack of funding, uncooperative participants, poor research design, and lack of standardized measures. Research has been characterized by small numbers, lack of control or comparison groups, and investigation of very young children— primarily to assess incidence of developmental delays. To date, no research has addressed the child's perception of parenting or family dynamics; older children, adolescent or adult offspring; family dynamics and adjustment; parental attitudes; comparisons of expectations before and after parenthood; or the long-term impact on families created through third-party reproduction.

Part of the problem is the tendency of postinfertility parents to blend with the larger population of parents, so that other professionals are unaware of the legacy of infertility and the difficult issues faced by these parents. In addition, infertility has been treated as a medical, not a psychosocial, problem and, as such, has been the focus of attention within the medical community but less so within the mental health community. For these reasons, it has been difficult to formulate a research agenda or define research questions that address the long-term adjustment of family members, especially since the goal of medical treatment has been achieved and consequently both professionals and patients anticipate no further problems.

Investigations historically have focused on medical treatments facilitating parent-hood, less on actual parenting, and rarely on the child. Obstetrical outcome and infant development, especially following assisted reproductive technologies and/or donated gametes, have been a common research interest, but more often as a means of program evaluation than as a means of assessing family adjustment. An inordinate amount of research has focused on parenthood achieved by donated gametes, looking at consumer satisfaction, parental adjustment, marital well-being, and disclosure decisions. More recently, a few studies have addressed the psychological adjustment of previously infertile parents and investigated the ease of adaptation to new parenthood following infertility.

Obstetrical Outcome

Early studies on donor insemination investigated obstetrical outcomes, incidence of problems in infants (developmental delay, congenital anomalies, genetic disorders), and parental satisfaction with donor insemination as a family-building alternative[7-9]. Pregnancies following donor insemination were found to be at no increased risk of obstetrical complications or emotional problems in parents[10,11] and children were found to be normal and at no greater risk of developmental difficulties or psychosocial problems[12,13]. Marriages were found to be impressively stable, and divorce rates were remarkably lower than the general population[14]. High levels of parental satisfaction were found, as well as no increased risk of emotional problems in the parents, despite early assertions by some psychiatrists[15] that participation in donor insemination in itself was indicative of an emotional disturbance dooming the family to disturbed adjustment. More than half of the respondents in one study[11] thought that pregnancy after donor insemination had improved their marriage, whereas only 3% thought it had had a detrimental effect. A recent review[16] of empirical literature on donor insemination families and their children found that research failed to reveal major psychological problems: parents were well adjusted and had stable marital relationships, and the children did not show significantly more emotional disturbances than controls. Furthermore, the quality of the parent-child relationship was better in the donor insemination families than in controls of naturally conceiving parents.

Studies[17-21] of obstetrical outcome following in vitro fertilization (IVF) consistently report increased incidence of obstetrical complications attributable to the effects of multiple gestation, resulting in increases in cesarean deliveries, prematurity, and low birthweight infants. However, these infants were found to be at no increased risk of developmental problems, except in multiple gestations[22-28]. Similar findings have also been reported with oocyte recipients: an exceptionally high rate of cesarean deliveries but with no developmental delays in offspring[29]. While no major developmental disorders were found in children born following IVF, one study[30] reported increased sleep disturbance in children and increased depressive symptoms in mothers at 9 months, although symptoms had dissipated by 36 months.

Adjustment to Parenthood

Parenthood achieved through IVF has been found to affect parental perceptions of their child(ren), usually for the better. Greenfeld and colleagues[31] found, in a survey study of parents who had conceived following IVF, that half (52%) of the mothers reported that the IVF process had created special feelings of attachment to their child, causing some difficulty in initial parent-child separation. Mushin and colleagues[24], in a study of 52 post-IVF children, found no cases of child neglect, abuse, or severe disturbance in the child, although three couples felt that IVF had altered their perceptions of their child. Another study[32] compared a group of 20 parents via IVF to 20 procreation parents and found no differences between the two groups in emotional health or marital adjustment. However, the IVF parents gave higher positive ratings for feelings about their babies and their 'personal freedom', while more also reported feeling 'over-protective' toward them.

Research indicates that previously infertile parents are satisfied with their parental roles but have more difficulty adjusting to parenthood. In a comparison study of 174 infertile couples, Abbey and colleagues[33] found that previously infertile mothers experienced greater global well-being, while previously infertile fathers (but not mothers), experienced greater home-life stress. The complexity and challenges of parenthood broaden with multiple births, indicating increased psychological distress. In a matched comparison study of 158 parents of preschool twins conceived spontaneously, with infertility treatment, or via IVF, Monro and colleagues[34] found that the IVF parents, especially the mothers, reported more difficulty in social relation-ships following parenthood. In a study evaluating psychological well-being in mothers of multiples following IVF, Garel and Blondel[21] reported that, at 1 year, the majority of mothers experienced consider-able fatigue, stress, social isolation, and strained marital relationship. In addition, they felt their relationship with the children was often disturbed and that it was difficult to give adequate attention to each child.

Maternal identity after infertility has also been the focus of investigation. Dunington and Glazer[35] found no sig-nificant difference in prenatal maternal identity between previously infertile mothers and noninfertile mothers. How-ever, previously infertile mothers lacked self-confidence in their ability to perform mothering tasks, sought more reassurance about the normalcy of their baby, and showed more identity confusion between career and maternal identities. In a preliminary evaluation from a study of children born by anonymously donated oocytes, Olshansky[36] found that previously infertile mothers were more likely to report feelings of guilt and shame, which they associated with their formerly infertile status. These women continued to harbor feelings of failure and malformation about their reproductive ability and felt embarrassed by the circumstances of the child's conception.

In the first longitudinal study of mothers and their infants conceived by IVF, McMahon and colleagues[37] investigated psychosocial adjustment, child behavior, and the quality of the mother-child attachment during pregnancy and postpartum. They found no significant differences between the IVF mothers and noninfertile mothers on satisfaction with motherhood or marriage. However, during pregnancy, the IVF mothers expected their babies to be more difficult, talked less to their babies in-utero, and delayed preparation for the baby. At 4 months postpartum, IVF mothers reported lower self-esteem and diminished self-confidence in their ability to care for their infants. In the second part of this study, Gibson and colleagues[38] evaluated mother-infant inter-actions. They found that IVF babies at 4 months engaged in higher levels of fussing and escape behaviors, which were con-sistent with the mothers' rating of their infants' temperament. When mothers and infants were assessed at 12 months, IVF mothers of first-born singleton babies and control group mothers reported compar-able levels of parenting stress, anxiety, and depression, as well as similar attachment to their child. However, even though IVF mothers reported more difficult behavior and reactivity in their children, no observable behavioral differences were found between IVF infants and control group infants.

For previously infertile parents, the transition and adjustment to parenthood are often more challenging and complex than for noninfertile parents. In two studies of young children (age range: 15 months to 8 years), researchers compared parents via assisted reproductive technologies to procreation parents. Golombok and colleagues[39] compared 41 children conceived via IVF and 45 children conceived via donated sperm to two control groups: 43 children conceived via pro-creation and 55 children adopted at birth. Researchers found that on the issues of warmth, emotional involvement with the child, and parent-child interaction, the quality of parenting was superior in the IVF and donor-insemination parents. In a study evaluating perceptions of parenthood in previously infertile parents who had become parents via conception or adoption but not assisted reproductive tech-nologies[40], no significant differences were found between adoptive or procreation parents. However, in comparison to a control group, the previously infertile parents were more likely to be satisfied with their marital relationship than with their parenting ability.

Third-Party Conception/Gestation Disclosure

A major issue of postinfertility parenthood achieved through third-party reproduction (e.g., donated gametes, gestational carrier, surrogacy) is disclosure versus secrecy: to tell or not to tell the child about the circumstances of his/her conception and/or birth. While the use of donated sperm has been in practice for nearly a century in the USA, the use of donated oocytes has only been available for 10 years. Nevertheless, a plethora of studies have investigated infertile couples' beliefs and practices regarding the disclosure to their child of his/her donor-gamete conception. Now, this issue has broadened to include disclosure issues about other forms of third-party reproduction (e.g., donated embryos, gestational carrier, and surrogacy) and, although there have been some noticeable changes, the issue of disclosure remains controversial, especially for families created through these reproductive technologies.

Research continues to show that the vast majority of donor-recipient parents do not plan to tell their child the circumstances of his/her conception and/or birth. Over the past decade, rates of disclosure for sperm recipients around the world have remained similar despite differing policies and practice: in the United States 14–29%[10,41,42], Canada 30%[43], and New Zealand 22%[44]. A British study[45] reported higher disclosure rates among oocyte recipients (32%) than sperm recipients (12%), while a French study[46] of oocyte recipients found a 52% disclosure rate among identified oocyte and a 26% rate among anonymous oocyte recipients. These findings were supported by a recent review[16] of empirical literature on donor insemination that reported that the vast majority (47–92%) of donor insemination parents intended to keep their child's donor origin secret.

Nevertheless, there appears to be a gradual shifting of public opinion and practice regarding disclosure, although only two countries worldwide (New Zealand and Sweden) have legislated an 'openness' approach to donor gametes[47]. A 1988 New Zealand study[48] showed that only 5% of couples believed a child had *a right to know* the identity of the donor and 41% believed children *did not* have a right to know the circumstances of his/her conception. However, a recent American study[49] found that 87% of couples believed a child had the need or right to know but only 58%

planned to tell their own child. However, what couples *plan* to do and what they *actually* do is often very different. In an ongoing longitudinal study[50] of donor-insemination families, the majority of parents did not plan to tell their child the circumstances of his/her donor origin, even though many of the parents had told family and friends before or during the pregnancy. Furthermore, over time, these parents were *more* disinclined to disclosure, despite their earlier stated plans to do so.

Couple disagreement about disclosure may occur, often with one partner preferring openness and the other preferring privacy. Klock[50] found that 16% of couples disagreed on whether or not to tell others about their use of donor insemination. Nachtigall and colleagues[42] reported a 22% disagreement rate, with the vast majority (14 of 17) of disagreements involving indecision in one partner and only 3 of 17 involving opposing opinions on disclosure. Schover and colleagues[41] found a higher percentage of women than men supported disclosure (26% v. 20%), reporting that wives worried about their husband's attachment to the child, although husbands reported very little perturbation about loving their donor-conceived child. In a New Zealand study[44] of partner agreement regarding disclosure decisions, similar disagreement rates (29%) were reported. The authors also described a pattern of women's giving way to men's feelings, needs, or beliefs regarding disclosure; they attributed this to: (1) a protective/facilitative/compromising approach on the part of wives in an attempt to assist husbands' denial of infertility, (2) wives' belief that husbands need psychological protection regarding infertility, and (3) men's feelings of marginalization regarding the reproductive/insemination process. In short, it appears that although a minority of couples disagree about disclosure decisions, disagreements may represent more funda-mental issues with infertility, donor conception, or marital interaction patterns.

Finally, factors influencing couples disclosure decisions have become of increasing interest. One recent study[12] found that a couple's disclosure decisions were not linked to parental bonding with the child or to the quality of the interparental relationship, concluding that nondisclosure is not harmful to family relationships or a symptom of family problems. Factors that increased a couple's likelihood of disclosure included younger age, azoospermia, lower stigma scores, and having more than one child by donated sperm. These researchers also found that whether couples decided for or against disclosure, they perceived their motives to be the same: in the best interest of their child.

THEORETICAL FRAMEWORKS
The Tasks of Parenthood

Parenthood is recognized as a major developmental milestone in the lives of men and women, often marking a symbolic entry into adulthood. Parenthood implies a certain stability, maturity, and willingness to assume adult roles and responsibilities. Physical, interpersonal, and relational adaptations are required to successfully adjust to pregnancy, delivery, and parenthood. While some well-adjusted previously infertile couples anticipate and adapt to the demands of parenthood quite well, others arrive at parenthood with unrealistic expectations, utopian fantasies, or idealized perceptions of their child or themselves as parents. In short, adjustment to parenthood after infertility involves all of the 'regular' tasks of parenthood in addition to the unique tasks of postinfertility parenthood.

Fundamentally, parenthood involves the physical and psychological care of a child ensuring his/her well-being, growth, and development from infancy to adulthood. It involves setting behavioral standards for the child and providing for the child a culture of the values of family and society. The six stages of parenthood according to Galinsky[51] are:

- image-making stage
- nurturing stage
- authority stage
- interpretive stage
- interdependent stage
- departure stage.

The *image-making stage,* beginning in pregnancy or preadoption, involves fantasizing about the child who is to arrive and envisioning oneself as a parent. The *nurturing stage,* lasting from birth until the child learns to say 'no', involves cementing attachment to the child and reconciling the real infant with the imagined infant. During the *authority stage,* the child enlarges his/her environment, and the primary parental responsibilities are to keep the child out of danger, while still allowing enough freedom and independence to explore the world. An important issue for parents is how to enforce limits and manage conflict with the child, avoid battles of wills, and adapt to changes in the child. During the *interpretive stage* (latency age), parental tasks involve explaining the culture and physical world to the child so that he or she absorbs parental views of society and the world. An additional parental task is keeping up with the child's physical, emotional, and intellectual growth. The *interdependent stage* begins just before puberty and, for parents, involves reconciling two images: their self-image as parents of a maturing child and their image of their child versus the child's self-image. During this stage, punishment and communication must adapt to the child's increased autonomy and maturity. The *departure stage* is marked by the child's leaving home and taking personal responsibility for his/her life, during which parental tasks are letting go and accepting the child's separation and individuation. During this stage, parents often have the mistaken belief that 'this is it; we're done', not realizing that departure is often a coming and going process that can evolve over several years.

Some issues of parenthood are often more challenging for previously infertile parents, especially those regarding a child's autonomy, separation, and individuation; parental acceptance of the child's identity, independence, and maturity; and parental authority, discipline, and enforcement of age appropriate limits. Each stage of the child's development represents specific challenges for previously infertile parents, highlighting how infertility presents difficulties to parents long after the crisis has passed.

Tasks of Parenthood for Previously Infertile Parents

The process of the transition to parenthood for previously infertile parents involves, according to Sandelowski and colleagues[52], four different tasks:

- *facing infertility*: the process of revealing, concealing, and accommodating the consequences and meaning of infertility
- *mazing*: the recursive, iterative, and capital-intensive process of the pursuit of parenthood
- *relinquishing infertility*: involves a couple's efforts to divest themselves of the infertility identity, thoughts, feelings and behavior patterns
- *reconstructing infertility*: the process in which a couple seeks to understand and gain interpretive control of their infertility experience.

All of these tasks are fundamental to adaptation not only to the infertility experience but also to parenthood as the couple incorporates infertility into their history and relinquishes it in preparation for parenthood.

Glazer[53] presents another theoretical model on the tasks and transition to parenthood for previously infertile parents. She defined the tasks as:

- giving up of the fantasized child
- developing a realistic approach to bonding
- accepting ambivalence
- redefining and realigning the family.

Accordingly, previously infertile parents must surrender the child they had anticipated or felt that they deserved in preparation for acceptance of the child they will actually parent. A form of *relinquishing infertility*, giving up the fantasy child involves grieving the child whom the infertile couple dreamed of having, often an idealized child who is perfect in every way. *Developing a realistic approach to bonding* involves recognizing that bonding is not 'love at first sight' but an attachment process that takes on average 18 months.

While all new parents experience some ambivalence, previously infertile parents are often frightened or distressed by their doubts about parenthood, themselves as parents, or their child. During infertility, many women and men make a private bargain to be perfect parents if just given the opportunity, only to discover, once they actually become parents, that they have made an impossible bargain. Glazer[53] suggested that this bargain is an example of 'magical thinking' that parents must relinquish to experience the real feelings of parenthood—ambivalence, disappointment, discouragement, and confusion—along with its joys.

Finally, *redefining and realigning* the family, similar to Sandelowski and colleagues' reconstructing infertility, involves postinfertility parents' recognizing how their family and children may be different than traditional definitions of family. The postinfertility family may be the result of assisted reproductive technologies, third-party reproduction involving donated gametes, surrogacy, or gestational carrier; or adoption. These family-building technologies challenge traditional definitions of kinship and relatedness—defined by Gordon[54] as the 'new blended family'. In the new blended family, each child may enter the family via a unique reproductive beginning or adoptive process that differs from other siblings' origins and even the parents' reproductive beginning. Still, despite the fact that these families have complex biogenetic origins, their social and experiential relationships are more like those of traditional nuclear families than of stepfamilies.

CLINICAL ISSUES AND THERAPEUTIC INTERVENTIONS

The transition to parenthood, loosely defined as the period from pregnancy through the first year of the life of a first-born, is always a period of change and stress as the parents, marriage, and new infant adjust to one another. This transition for previously infertile parents may involve a number of risk factors and challenges during both pregnancy and parenthood. Previously infertile parents may arrive at parenthood having exhausted their coping abilities, diminished their marital satisfaction, and experienced depression or psychological distress[55]. The elongated anticipation of parenthood may have contributed to overidealization of the child or parenthood, resulting in unrealistic expectations of one's self or spouse as a parent, or misperceptions of 'normal' infant behavior[29,55–57]. By contrast, previously infertile parents may be buffeted from normal decreases in marital satisfaction following parenthood because they are typically older, better educated, married longer, and less likely to define their marriage solely in romantic terms[24,55,57].

Furthermore, the experience of infertility may have required more egalitarian relationship patterns and problem-solving, and both partners may have become more comfortable with the expression of sensitive feeling[55,59]. Previously infertile new mothers, although lacking self-confidence, may be more comfortable turning to their husbands for support and encouragement and establishing a team approach to parenthood that fosters skills attainment in both partners[29,30,32,33].

Facilitating Adaptation to Parenthood after Infertility

Adapting Galinsky's[51] stages of parenthood, infertility counselors can assist previously infertile couples in their transition to parenthood. During the *image-making stage* of parenthood, previously infertile parents must relinquish both the fantasy child and their infertile identity, thoughts, feelings, and behavior patterns. Lack of social support during pregnancy and/or parenthood, stigma (especially if parenthood is achieved through donated gametes), and altered self-concept involving feelings of incompetence or inadequacy are frequent and familiar feelings for previously infertile parents. In addition, relinquishing infertility may include letting go of important relationships—medical staff at the infertility clinic, friends from support organizations, or enjoyable activities such as get-togethers with childless friends. Bernstein[56] suggested that disturbances of parenting after infertility may be related not only to psychosocial distress during infertility treatment (see Table 1) but to the lack of appropriate role models for parenting after infertility; to delayed attachment to the baby, especially during pregnancy; and to cognitive dissonance, a disparity between what was imagined about parenthood/the baby and the actual experience.

Table 1 Potential impact of infertility

Transition to parenthood
Increased anxiety levels during pregnancy and/or adoption period
Lack of role models
Possibility of delayed bonding
Cognitive dissonance: gap between ideal and real self and between fantasy and real child
Ethical and emotional issues related to means of achieving parenthood

Factors affecting parenting
Decreased self-esteem and self-efficacy
Altered body image and self-concept
Impaired marital communication, loss of sexual intimacy and pleasure
Isolation from family and friends
Grieving over losses associated with infertility: anxiety, depression, and anger management issues

(Reproduced from ref. 56, with permission)

During the *nurturing stage*, previously infertile parents must establish a comfortable means of bonding to their child, such as through baby massage, bedtime rituals, and special lullabies. In addition, parents need to come to terms with and understand the normalcy of their ambivalence about parenthood (e.g., fatigue, no time to oneself) and their baby (e.g., colicky, unlikeable characteristics). Previously infertile parents may become overprotective—enmeshed, excessively involved, infantilizing the child, preventing independent behavior, and stunting the child's emotional growth[4]. Often, the child does not view the parents' overprotection as an indication of their insecurity and self-protection but as a justifiable lack of confidence in the child's ability to manage in his/her life or to venture into the world.

For previously infertile parents, the *authority stage* can be particularly challenging as parents recognize the need to set limits, determine discipline, and define their roles as authority figures for their children. Some of the potential problems for previously infertile parents include overprotective parenting, difficulty with appropriate discipline, and unrealistic expectations of parenting or the child[10,53,57]. They may become hypervigilant or over-indulgent, while attempts at discipline are half-hearted and inconsistent. They may manage their feelings of loss and grief about infertility by holding the child too close or by limiting the child's attempts at increased self-sufficiency and self-reliance.

Discipline problems in postinfertility families often represent two extremes: rigid, strict control of the child or the inability to set appropriate behavioral limits. Previously infertile parents may be hesitant to become angry with their child out of a mistaken belief that it is inappropriate, may feel guilty about their angry feelings at their longed-for child, may fear that it will damage the child or the parent-child relationship, or may misperceive anger as an unacceptable emotion. Some parents may recognize that their anger is disproportionate to the situation but have little insight into the factors influencing this response, such as unrealistic expectations of the child, inappropriate behavior in the child, disappointment that the child is not more emotionally rewarding, or frustration that parenting is not easier. These parents often need assistance in learning how to set appropriate limits and boundaries with their children and in recognizing how doing so is positive and helpful for the child.

During the *interpretive stage*, parents of children born as a result of donated gametes, gestational carrier, or surrogacy face issues of disclosure and interpreting the culture of reproductive technology for their child. Questions of whether the child has a moral right to know and privacy as a primary family value must be considered, agreed upon by both parents, and interpreted for the child. For previously infertile parents and their children, the interpretation of reproductive technology (even IVF) or family-building options (e.g., donated gametes, adoption) may mean realignment of the family. These families must adapt to new definitions of kinship and relatedness, normalize parent-child relationships, and acknowledge the child's unique origins and circumstances in the family. Just as important, families with a history of infertility must recognize the ways not only in which they are unique and different but in which they are much the same as other, more traditional families.

Adolescence, or the *interdependent stage* of parenthood, is often a challenging time for both parents and their children. It involves the reconciling of two images: the parents' self-image and their image of the child as he or she is. During this stage, punishment and communication must adapt to the child's increased autonomy and maturity. Reemergence of common psychological responses to infertility may occur including grief, anxiety, depression, feelings of isolation, and diminished self-esteem as the child challenges the parents' values, belief systems, and limits. Previously infertile parents may have difficulty allowing or acknowledging their child's increased independence and may actively or unconsciously infantilize (prevent appropriate movement toward adulthood) the young person's separation by impeding individuation, autonomy, and assumption of responsibility for his/her own life and destiny.

Frequently, parental impediments to a child's maturation involve the issues of the child's sexual development, sexual behavior, and/or reproductive ability. For previously infertile parents, their child's sexual development can be a bitter reminder of infertility and reproductive losses. They may respond to the child's developing sexuality by avoiding issues—failing to prepare the child for menstruation or failing to provide them with sex education or birth control information—thereby covertly fulfilling their own reproductive hopes and dreams. Finally, after infertility, family meanings about sex and reproduction may over-emphasize procreation and ignore the other meanings of sex, such as commit-ment, caring, sharing, or play.

Finally, the *departure stage* is marked by the young adult's leaving home either temporarily (e.g., going to college) or permanently (e.g., marriage). For many previously infertile parents who devoted extensive time and money to having child(ren), departure may entail a reexam-ination of these prior decisions: Was it worth it? What will their own financial stability be in retirement or old age? What are their obligations or responsibilities to the child after a certain age? Departure represents an acknowledgment of the discrepancy between what they hoped their family/child would be and who their child actually has become for better or worse.

Unrealistic expectations place an undue burden on parents and pressure children to be perfect, grateful, successful, and emotionally rewarding—an impossible feat. Danger signs of disturbed parenting after infertility are: overemphasis on excellence or exceptionality in the child or self as a parent, inability to see the child in realistic or objective terms, belief that the child is perfect and flawless, inappropriate expec-tations of the parent–child relationship to meet the parents' emotional needs, imposition of the parents' hopes and dreams onto the child, splitting of parents, parent-child enmeshment, parental inabil-ity to allow age-appropriate or peer-appropriate behavior, infantilizing the child, refusal to allow or train the child in age-appropriate problem-solving, extreme conflicts with the child regarding separation and individuation, inadequate or inappropriate discipline, parental

rejection, neglect or abuse, and repeated boundary violations.

Special Parenting Issues after Infertility

Parenting after infertility presents some special clinical issues for older parents, the only child after secondary infertility, multiple birth, and third-party repro-duction. Further, questions regarding disclosure to a child born through donor gametes, surrogacy, or gestational carrier are a major concern to parents.

Older Parenthood

Although only 0.06% of live births occur in women over the age of 45 in the United States according to data from 1994[60], older parenthood has received increasing attention, often facilitated by the use of donated sperm or oocytes. Older parent-hood has medically and traditionally been defined as first-time motherhood after age 35, although increasingly it involves motherhood after age 55 or fatherhood after age 75. Recently, the case of a 63-year-old woman, who gave birth through ooycte donation, caught world-wide attent-ion; both the mother and 60-year-old father were first-time parents[61]. Motivations for older parenthood may be lack of oppor-tunity earlier in life, repeat parenthood in a subsequent marriage, replacement of a child lost to death, assuagement of a new partner, or an attempt to maintain youth and postpone aging. Older parenthood is often experienced within the context of numerous responsibilities and life demands concurrent with other midlife events such as aging parents, high work demands, peers' adjusting to 'empty nests', and friends facing major life crises[62].

A major issue for older parents and their children is the parents' health and life expectancy. An elderly parent may not survive to see or participate in the important milestones of a child's life, while the younger spouse must assume primary parenting responsibilities if the older spouse becomes ill or aged, or dies. A younger surviving spouse may face the emotional, financial, and physical challenges of single parenthood that are enhanced by the financial drain of earlier medical treatments for infertility, children from previous marriages or relationships, or the care of the older or infirm spouse. Retirement may not be possible, work must be continued, and/or the standard of living may need to be adjusted to meet the demands of older parenting.

The impact of older/elderly parenthood on children has rarely been investigated, especially when related to infertility. Furthermore, issues of age and impact on children are often met with resistance and even hostility by potential older parents. One study[63] found that older parents exhibited increased anxiety about all decisions relating to their children and had a tendency to overemphasize all aspects of the parent-child relationship. In an interview study[64] of adult 'last-chance-children' raised by older parents, adult children spoke about the pros (parents with greater patience and more life experiences) and cons (parents unable to participate in physical activities) of having older parents. In summary, older parenthood after infertility entails a number of significant issues and challenges that are often minimized or ignored by the potential parents (see Chapter 15).

Parenting the Only Child after Secondary Infertility

Secondary infertility may come as a surprise to parents or may be expected after prior infertility treatment. However, couples experiencing secondary infertility are not expecting to be parents of only children and often have difficulty relinquishing the family of their dreams. While a child at home may ameliorate some of the pain of infertility, he or she may also exacerbate it by reminding parents of the joys and possibilities of parenthood. The challenges of parenting an only child involve distinguishing the parents' wish for another child from the child's wish for a sibling, addressing the child's feelings (pro and con) about being an only child, coping with the grief of not having another child or the ideal family size, managing societal pressure for a larger family, educating oneself about the advantages of an only-child family, guarding against over-indulgence or overinvestment in the only child, closing the family boundaries and moving on, and managing the feelings of vulnerability regarding an only child[62].

One of the challenges of secondary infertility for parents is protecting their child from internalized parental longing and grief for the wished-for baby. Parental conversations about another child, medical treatments, doctor visits, medications, and infertility treatments may be misinterpreted by the child. If younger than 2 years, he or she may not be aware of or affected by infertility treatments. However, older children may be acutely aware of what is happening in the family and feel distressed by it[65]. Young children may interpret their mother's constant medical care as evidence that she is very ill and respond with fears of her death[65]. Children may experience parental distraction and emotional distance as dissatisfaction with them. Further, they may believe that something is wrong with them or feel responsible for the parents' inattentiveness. Children, feeling 'Aren't I enough?' or 'What's wrong with me?', may respond with overcompliance, hypervigilance of the parent, or rebellious uncooperativeness and acting-out in a bid for attention and affirmation (see Chapter 17).

Historically, having an only child has been considered a negative family constellation producing self-centered and socially impaired children. However, current research does not support this belief. Only children have been found to have more social skills than children with siblings, especially later-born children, and to be psychologically very stable[66]. Research on only children as adults has consistently found few significant differences in behavioral outcomes between them and children raised with siblings. In addition, only children are more likely to be more educated than non-only children[66].

Parenting Multiples

Twins, triplets, and other multiples have become increasingly common after infertility treatment and are usually considered a blessing, albeit mixed, by many previously infertile parents. After a lengthy period of childlessness, many formerly infertile parents find caring for an instant family an enjoyable immersion experience in which both parents are actively and energetically involved[67]. They often enjoy the special attention that their family and children receive, as well as the additional involvement of their own parents, family members, and friends. The parenting challenges of raising multiples after infertility include possible prematurity, special needs and disabilities in the children, financial burdens including the loss of the mother's income, the mother's loss of her social network at the workplace, public attention and invasions of the family's privacy, breastfeeding and childcare decisions, unanticipated family configuration, separate individuals versus 'packaging' multiples as a group, absence of a one-to-one relationship with each child, adequate family help, and household arrangements to accommodate multiples[62].

Previously infertile parents of multiples face a number of significant challenges, including management of limited resources (time, money, energy, attention) and the well-being of all family members, especially other siblings who are not included in the aura of 'specialness'. Unique issues for twins and more include establishing their individuality, managing issues of separation and independence not only from their parents but from each other, twin talk, and the special twin (or multiple) bond[68]. Despite these distinctive factors, research indicates that multiples are at no increased risk of more difficulty with issues of individuality, separation, and independence than singletons[68,69].

Parenthood and Third-Party Reproduction

Parenthood after third-party reproduction—donated gametes, embryos, gestational carrier, or surrogate—is unique, as it separates biological (genetic) from psychosocial (rearing) parenthood. A baby may be genetically related to both psychosocial parents yet carried by another woman (gestational carrier) or genetically related to the psychosocial father and carrying mother but not the psychosocial mother (traditional surrogate). Or a child may not be genetically related to either psychosocial parent yet be carried by the psychosocial mother (donated embryo). A child may be genetically related to the father but not to either the psychosocial or the carrying mother (donated oocyte) or genetically related to the carrying mother but not to the psychosocial father (donor sperm). The inequity of the biological or genetic contribution of each psychosocial parent can contribute to marital conflict, differing feelings of 'ownership' or investment in the child, and divergent opinions on disclosure, impacting family dynamics and kinship definitions. All of these variations of biological and psychosocial parenthood make third-party reproduction more psychologically complex and create confusing dilemmas for families.

Infertile couples often choose donated gametes (sperm or oocyte) as a family-building option because, in comparison to adoption, it is expeditious, typically more economical, less socially obvious, allows control of the prenatal environment, and offers genetic or biological connection to one partner. Parenthood achieved by donated embryos has been referred to as 'prenatal adoption' and is psychologically similar to traditional adoption (see Chapter 22). Infertile couples often choose parenthood via third-party reproduction to avoid some of the pitfalls of adoption, such as involvement or relationship with the relinquishing mother. However, research shows that most parents who use a surrogate or carrier meet and spend time with her both before and after the birth of the child[70,71]. Consequently, an important task for these parents involves defining appropriate boundaries and relationship parameters for ongoing interactions between them and the surrogate/carrier[62,72].

One of the most significant challenges of parenthood via surrogacy or gestational carrier is how it impacts the legal definition of motherhood. While it is banned in several countries, in many states, genetic mothers are legally required to 'adopt' the child born to a gestational carrier or a surrogate[71]. Gestational carriers and surrogates may be a previously unknown woman hired to carry a pregnancy or may be a compassionate friend or family member volunteering to be a surrogate or gestator. Dual relationship in third-party reproduction, including family members who donate gametes, may increase the psychological perplexities within the family and contribute to potential problems for parents, child, and the family later in life. Clearly, a pregnancy carried by someone else can delay maternal bonding, contribute to lingering feelings of loss, and enhance feelings of insecurity, anxiety, and loss of control. Highlighting boundary

issues prevalent in third-party reproduction are the continuing relationships surrogates and carriers may have with the new family after the birth[70,71].

Simply, the more complex the method of achieving pregnancy and the more participants involved in the conception/birth, the more complex the psychological implications and emotional reverberations for all participants: child, rearing parents, and contributing parents[72,73]. Families must decide how they will integrate these relationships into their life, often within a social context of stigma, secrecy, and ambiguity. Thus, third-party parents must come to terms with feelings of isolation and differentness and with the lack of societal support or a peer group[74]. They must also address the potential and actual psychological impact on their child of his/her unique biological beginning, a beginning that Sants[75] referred to as resulting in 'genealogical bewilderment'. Infertility counselors may be an important ongoing resource to these families as they grow and deal with the issues of third-party reproduction.

Disclosure and Third-Party Reproduction

Disclosure is a major parenting issue for couples who have become parents via third-party reproduction. Recent research has shown that parents' reasons for disclosure versus privacy involve beliefs about the child's inherent right and need to know his or her biological origins versus a belief in the virtues of privacy[42]. Whatever the parents decided, they approached the decision-making process from the same perspective—the best interests of the child. Interestingly, there were no differences found on quality of parenting or attachment to the child.

The decision to disclose will be influenced by the situation, family structure and history, and social milieu: nuclear two-parent family, single mother, lesbian couple, or stepparent family[76]. For example, the presence of older children who are aware of their parents' reproductive history may make nondisclosure impossible or very difficult. Further, an obvious pregnancy in a gestator or carrier usually makes it logistically impossible for infertile parents to maintain secrecy about the child's birth. Or a single mother or lesbian couple may have little motivation to keep a child's conception secret (see Chapter 14). For these couples, the issue is less about whether or not to disclose but rather about how and when to tell the child about his or her special beginning. In a rationale for nondisclosure, some mental health professionals believe that donor anonymity allows couples to impose their own identity patterns on the child and to introduce him or her in an unbiased way into their own lives and social network, thereby minimizing social stigma for all family members[77]. Many parents are opposed to telling because they wish to eliminate any feelings about the donor's involvement in their child's conception or birth. They fear that acknowledgment of another person's role will diminish their relationship and entitlement to the child. Furthermore, they feel that the information may be traumatizing to the child and damaging to the parent-child relationship. Some parents believe that what a child does not know will not hurt him or her, or that normal procreation is confusing enough to children and technical reproduction even more so. Many parents contend that without record keeping or significant information about the genetic parent, there is no reason to tell the child. Finally, parents believe that psychological, sociological, and legal factors favor secrecy or a measure of privacy[78].

By contrast, an increasing number of mental health professionals suggests that every donor child has both a *need* and a *right* to know the truth about his or her origins, as well as information about the donor, carrier, or surrogate[47,79–84]. They contend that concealment of the truth may potentially lead to further lies and deception tantamount to a 'family delusion'. The corrosiveness of secrets in families and psychological energy needed to maintain them is considered enough justification for increased openness[80]. Some families are simply not able to maintain a secret, so that the child may learn about the conception in an unplanned, destructive, and less controlled manner. Finally, it has been suggested that children often intuitively figure out that something is going on in the family and their suspicions (mother had an affair) or fantasies (result of a virgin birth) are more detrimental than the truth[84].

Since there has been no definitive research on the long-term effects of disclosure versus privacy on children or family well-being, it is unwise for infertility counselors unilaterally to recommend a specific approach. As a result, most infertility counselors recommend a neutral, parental self-determination approach in which parents are encouraged to weigh the pros and cons of both disclosure and privacy as applied to their particular situation and their child[42,85–87]. An infertility counselor can facilitate consideration of the various psychosocial issues impacting each family member, the family's values, and the social context in which the child will be raised (see Tables 2 and 3).

A couple's current decision not to disclose to a child does not have to be a final decision. Disclosure is usually an issue that parents revisit and reevaluate many times, taking into consideration the child's age, personality, and psychological stability, as well as their own opinions or circumstances which may have changed over time. *Disclosure is a not an event; it is a process that involves a series of discussions as the*

Table 2 Issues to address regarding disclosure and privacy

What role do you believe genetics plays in a person's personality, sense of humor, values, goals, etc.?

Are secrets necessarily lethal or detrimental?

Is there information that parents have a right to keep private?

Do you feel that a child has an inalienable right to know about his/her genetic origins?

Are there any dangers in telling your child about his/her donor conception?

Would you want to know if your parents used a gamete donor?

Can you live with a secret?

When are the parents' right to privacy superseded by a child's right to know?

Are feelings about disclosure or privacy entangled with the husband's or wife recipient's feelings of shame or discomfort about their fertility?

How will the child's family and community react to the use of donor?

How would you feel if your child 'discovered' the donor circumstances of his/her conception at some time in the future?

How important is it to you to manage or control the means of disclosure?

Given your situation, how feasible is it to maintain secrecy and for how long?

How will you/would you feel if family or community knew about the child's donor conception?

Can you imagine any circumstances in which donor conception as a secret could be used in a negative manner by your partner?

If the laws regarding donor gametes change, how comfortable would you be with your child having access to information about the donor?

How would you feel about a central donor registry?

(Adapted from ref. 72, with permission)

child gains greater understanding and sophistication (Table 4). It is best considered as an opportunity to educate the child, which can be facilitated by books for parents, storybooks for children, and support organizations for families created by third-party reproduction. As Leiber Wilkens[81] pointed out, learning is a process of integration, so that parents must be prepared to tell and retell the child's life story for him or her.

Baran and Pannor[80] suggested that the initial telling should be simple, straightforward, and include: (1) identification of the nongenetic parent's fertility restriction, (2) identification of the donor as a person, and (3) reassurance of the child's being loved by both psychosocial parents. Parents should begin with the simplest facts and gradually add information appropriate to the child's growing cognitive abilities, age, and emotional make-up[88]. During the initial telling, parents should provide basic information, elicit questions, and listen. They should not elaborate unnecessarily or barrage the child with more information than he or she can assimilate. They should be encouraged to reassure the child that the donor exists and is important as someone who genetically contributed to who the child is, but be assured that the donor has no role in nurturing, parenting, or taking

Table 3 Pros and cons of disclosure to children regarding third-party reproduction

---

For disclosure

Child has a fundamental right and need to know about biological genetic origins

Medical information is critical, and nondisclosure may limit the information received and/or may lead to wrong information being given about the recipient's genetic history

Secrets are lethal and may permanently hurt the family and/or the child

Children born using assisted reproduction will sense that there is something different, and this difference will affect their sense of self and their relationship with their families

Parents are able to control and manage the disclosure and prevent unintended disclosure

Manner in which child is told or discovers will impact child's relationship with parent more than disclosure itself

Parents agree that openness is a family value

Genetic and biological information are fundamental to an individual's sense of self and personal identity

Believe it is best for child

For privacy

Telling will undermine parental role and parental connection to child

Disclosure has potential of making parents' infertility public

May jeopardize parents' connection with the child

Beliefs and ideas regarding disclosure may change over time

Believe it is best for child

Individuals do not have a fundamental right to know about their genetic origins

Medical information can be incorporated into the child's and family's medical history to ensure accurate information

All families have secrets, and we do not know that this is a 'lethal' secret

Children born through donor gametes will not sense anything different when raised in a home where the parents are loving and unconflicted about the use of a donor gamete

Sperm donation has been commercially available for decades, and less formally for centuries, under the restrictions of privacy and these families appear to have managed well. In short, privacy seems to have worked for these families

---

(Adapted from ref. 78, with permission)

care of the child. Information about the donor, if it is available, should be shared with the child at an appropriate age, probably late adolescence. It has been suggested that donor disclosure can be normalized by making it a family story, not unlike the repeated story of the child's birth, the parent's wedding, or other family history[81]. Finally, each child's need for information and discussion is idiosyncratic and individual: Some will want more information; some will not.

Table 4 Discussing third-party reproduction with children

Early years
  Assure child of parent's unconditional love, how much he/she was wanted,
  happiness of parents when he/she was born
  Assess child's readiness for information about sexuality, reproduction, own story
  Explain simple facts of reproduction, various ways families are made
  Tell child the story of his/her own arrival in family
  Emphasize the nongenetic parents' role as parent
Middle years
  Reassure child of unconditional love of both parents
  Explain that child's place in family was something both parents wanted, that
  child would not be here if both parents had not made the decision together
  Build on basic facts of reproduction to explain difference in child's conception
  Reassure child that he/she was carried in mother's uterus, born like everyone else
  Reassure child about donor: good person wanting to help other people have
  children
Later years
  Reassure child of unconditional love of both parents and parent's shared wish for
  him/her
  Explain why parents choose this option to have children (because of infertility)
  Share information about how conception occurred (e.g., clinic, physicians,
  process, presence of father at insemination, reaction to pregnancy as part of
  child's own family story)
  Explain various reasons why donors decide to assist individuals to become
  parents
  Share available genetic history and information about the donor
  Normalize experience for child: there are many others who have been conceived
  in this fashion
  Recognize that the feelings of confusion, sadness, and pain are appropriate—
  may even reassure by explaining that parents had same feelings as child now has
  Explain that sharing this information with others is his/her choice; it may be
  difficult and not everyone will understand. Help child process who he/she would
  like to tell and why. Support child if he/she wishes to keep it private
  Offer child help in talking to others (e.g., therapist, pediatrician) if he/she wishes

(Adapted from ref. 82, with permission)

It is generally agreed that when children are told about their biological origins, it should be at an appropriate time, although there is disagreement about what the best time is. Very young children (ages 2–4) have difficulty understanding the abstract concepts of reproduction, let alone medical technology. Parents may mistake the typical curious questions about sex and reproduction as evidence that the disclosure discussions should begin. Most of the storybooks available are written for young children aged between 4 to 10 years.

Some mental health professionals have suggested disclosure to children during adolescence because the abstract concepts of third-party reproduction will be better understood. Others suggest full disclosure by early adolescence (ages 10–14), before the child's struggles for identity and independence are in full force[88]. Still others suggest disclosure in late adolescence (ages 15-18), as the information (like family history of alcoholism or adoption) is an important part of the child's history to which he or she is entitled[52,88]. However, adolescence is often tumultuous, emotionally traumatic time of identity establishment, confusion, separation, and individuation from parents, which results in increased parent-child conflicts. For this reason, some mental health professionals have suggested telling children at the age of 9–10[52,78], while others suggest beginning discussions before puberty (age 11–12) when the child is cognitively capable of abstract thinking yet is still fairly free of the difficulties and struggles of adolescence[88]. Finally, it should be apparent that these brave new babies are coming into a world in a manner that creates unique challenges and dilemmas for parents. Historically, professionals have recommended parents not tell a child, contending that secrecy is in the child's best interest and that if the child should accidentally learn about the truth, psychological difficulties would ensue[89]. However, there is no evidence of this. Nevertheless, more and more mental health professionals now view this approach with skepticism, recognizing the potential destructiveness of secrets, the demands of keeping them, and the problems of accidental discovery[90]. By contrast, privacy is not secrecy, and disclosure need not be a public announcement. Parents must be encouraged to assess their personal situation and values, the child's circumstances and personality, and the social and family context in reaching a decision on the complex issue of disclosure.

FUTURE IMPLICATIONS

Today, parenthood after infertility involves a variety of meanings, challenges, and responsibilities. In the 21st century, how post-infertility families and children adjust to the unique legacy of infertility and assisted reproductive technologies remains to be seen. Although there appear to be indications of risk factors and vulnerabilities in post-infertility families, there is also plenty of evidence to show that these families have adapted and adjusted in a healthy and positive fashion. Infertility counselors are in an excellent position to prepare postinfertility families for the challenges of adjustment, as well as conducting research on these parents and children.

Previously infertile parents may present soon after conception or birth, requesting assistance with adjustment to parenthood or at a later point in the child's or family's development—most often at points in the life cycle that involve separation, individuation, and autonomy. When problems occur, these parents are most likely to present for help to school psychologists, social workers at child mental health centers, family physicians, pediatricians, pastors, or mental health workers within the legal system. Unfortunately, these professionals are often unaware of the family's history of infertility, reproductive losses, and use of assisted reproductive technologies and therefore are often less likely to understand the child's unique legacy. Consequently, it is important to review with infertility patients, when appropriate, the unique issues of transition to parenthood and family adaptation. The role of infertility counselors may increasingly entail assisting parents, children, and families with the consequences of reproductive choices that provided miracle babies and life-long ramifications.

SUMMARY

- Parenthood after infertility is full of joys, challenges, and, at times, complications due to the circumstances of the conception/birth.
- Research indicates that, despite the protracted nature of infertility treatment, infertile families are no more vulnerable to psychological disturbance than noninfertile families. Further,

these couples evidence stronger marital satisfaction, have more egalitarian relationships, and are more emotionally expressive than their procreative counterparts.

- The developmental stages of parenthood, applicable to all couples, are: image-making, nurturing, authority, interpretative, interdependent, and departure[51].
- Previously infertile parents face unique psychological tasks in their transition to parenthood: giving up the fantasy child; realistic bonding; accepting ambivalence; and redefining the family[51,52].
- Special issues are faced by parents who are older, parenting multiples, or experiencing secondary infertility; are single, gay or lesbian, or adoptive; or who have children created through third-party reproduction using donor gametes, donated embryos, a surrogate, or a gestational carrier. These parents

may be isolated and lack a support system, may be exhausted physically, emotionally, and financially, and experience greater social stigma and shame regarding the means through which they achieved parenthood.

- Disclosure is one of the most perplexing areas of parenting for those who have used third-party reproduction. While cases can be made for openness and privacy in sharing a child's genetic origins or unique reproductive beginnings, infertility counselors need to present balanced information to allow client self-determination in the decision.
- Disclosure is a not an event, it is a process that involves a series of discussions as the child gains greater understanding and sophistication. It needs to be discussed in 'pediatric doses', in simple terms, and must be adapted to the child's age, maturity, and curiosity.

REFERENCES

1. van Balen F, Trimbos-Kemper TCM. Involuntary childless couples: Their desire to have children and their motives. *J Psychosom Obstet Gynaecol* 1995;16:137–44
2. Halman LJ, Andrews FM, Abbey A. Gender differences and perceptions about childbearing among infertile couples. *J Obstet Gynecol Neonatal Nurs* 1994;23:593–600
3. Newton CR, Hearn MT, Yuzpe AA, *et al.* Motives for parenthood and response to failed in vitro fertilization: Implications for counseling. *J Assist Reprod Genet* 1992;9:24–31
4. Levy DM. The concept of maternal overprotection. In: Anthony EJ, Benedek T, eds. *Parenthood: Its Psychology and Psychopathology*. New York: Little, Brown, 1970: 387–409
5. Calef V. Hostility of parents to children: Some notes on infertility, child abuse, and

abortion. *Int J Psychoanal Psychother* 1972; 10:76–96
6. Bradt JO, Moynihan CJ. Opening the safe: A study of child-focused families. In: Bradt JO, Moynihan CJ, eds. *Systems Therapy: Selected Papers: Theory, Technique, Research.* Washington, DC: Groome Center, 1971
7. Farris EJ, Garrison M. Emotional impact of successful donor insemination. *Obstet Gynecol* 1954;3:19–20
8. Jackson MH. Artificial insemination (donor). *Eugen Rev* 1957;48:203–11
9. Milsom I, Bergman P. A study of parental attitudes after donor insemination (AID). *Acta Obstet Gynecol Scand* 1982;61:125–8
10. Clayton CE, Kovacs CT. AID offspring: Initial follow-up of 50 couples. *Med J Aust* 1982;1:338–9
11. Amuzu B, Laxova R, Shapiro SS. Pregnancy outcome, health of children,

and family adjustment after donor insemination. *Obstet Gynecol* 1990;75:899–905

12. Kovacs GT, Mushin D, Kane H, *et al.* A controlled study of the psychosocial development of children conceived following insemination with donor semen. *Hum Reprod* 1993;8:788–90

13. Leeton J, Backwell J. A preliminary psychosocial follow-up of parents and their children conceived by artificial insemination by donor (AID). *Clin Reprod Fertil* 1982;1:307–10

14. Bendvold E, Skjaeraasen J, Moe N, *et al.* Marital break-up among couples raising families by artificial insemination by donor. *Fertil Steril* 1989;51:980–3

15. Gerstel G. A psychoanalytic view of artificial donor insemination. *Am J Psychother* 1963; 17:64–77

16. Brewaeys A. Donor insemination, the impact on family and child development. *J Psychosom Obstet Gynaecol* 1996;17:1–13

17. Fabis C, Licata D, Garzena E, *et al.* In vitro fertilization and intra-uterine growth retardation. *Paediatr Perinat Epidemiol* 1990;4:243–5

18. Tan SL, Doyle P, Campbell S, *et al.* Obstetric outcome of in vitro fertilization pregnancies compared with normally conceived pregnancies. *Am J Obstet Gynecol* 1992;167:778–84

19. Friedler S, Morgel N, Lipitz S, *et al.* Perinatal outcome of pregnancies following assisted reproduction. *J Assist Reprod Genet* 1994;11:459–62

20. Howe RS, Sayegh RA, Durinzi KL, *et al.* Perinatal outcome of singleton pregnancies conceived by in vitro fertilization: A controlled study. *J Perinatol* 1990;10:261–6

21. Garel M, Blondel B. Assessment at 1 year of the psychological consequences of having triplets. *Hum Reprod* 1992;7:729–32

22. Saunders K, Spensley JC, Munro J, *et al.* Growth and physical outcome of children conceived by in vitro fertilization. *Pediatrics* 1996;5:688–92

23. Bandes JM, Scher A, Itzkovits J, *et al.* Growth and development of children conceived by in vitro fertilization. *Pediatrics* 1992;9:424–9

24. Mushin DN, Barreda-Hanson MC, Spensley JC. In vitro fertilization children: Early psychosocial development. *J In Vitro*

Fertil Embryo Transf 1986;3:247–52

25. Spensley JC, Mushin D, Barreda-Hanson M. The children of IVF pregnancies: A cohort study. *Aust Paediatr J* 1986;22:285–9

26. Yovich JL, Parry TS, French NP, *et al.* Developmental assessment of twenty in vitro fertilization (IVF) infants at their first birthday. *J In Vitro Fertil Embryo Transf* 1986;3:253–7

27. Pruett KD. Strange bedfellows? Reproductive technology and child development. *Infant Ment Health J* 1992;13:312–18

28. Morin NC, Wirth FH, Johnson DH, *et al.* Congenital malformation and psychosocial development in children conceived by in vitro fertilization. *J Pediatr* 1989;115:222–7

29. Applegarth L, Goldberg NC, Cholst I, *et al.* Families created through ovum donation: A preliminary investigation of obstetrical outcome and psychosocial adjustment. *J Assist Reprod Genet* 1995;12:574–80

30. Raoul-Duval A, Bertrand-Servais M, Frydman R. Comparative prospective study of the psychological development of children born by in vitro fertilization and their mothers. *J Psychosom Obstet Gynaecol* 1993;14:117–26

31. Greenfeld DA, Ort SI, Greenfeld DG, *et al.* Attitudes of IVF parents about the IVF experience and their children. *J Assist Reprod Genet* 1996;13:266–74

32. Weaver SM, Clifford E, Gordon AG, *et al.* A follow-up study of 'successful' IVF/GIFT couples: Social-emotional well-being and adjustment to parenthood. *J Psychosom Obstet Gynaecol* 1990;14:5–16

33. Abbey A, Andrews FM, Halman LJ. Infertility and parenthood: Does becoming a parent increase well-being? *J Consult Clin Psychol* 1994;62:398–403

34. Monro JM, Ironside W, Smith GC. Successful parents of in vitro fertilization (IVF): The social repercussions. *J Assist Reprod Genet* 1992;9:170–76

35. Dunington R, Glazer G. Maternal identity and early mother behavior in previously infertile and never infertile women. *J Obstet Gynecol Neonatal Nurs* 1991;20:309–17

36. Olshansky EF. Parenting after infertility. In: ART Parents and Children. American Society of Reproductive Medicine, Seattle, WA, October 7–8, 1995;59–65

37. McMahon C, Ungerer J, Tennant C, *et al.*

Psychosocial adjustment and the mother-baby relationship for IVF mothers from pregnancy to 4 months postpartum. Presented at the American Society for Reproductive Medicine, Boston, MA, November 1996

38. Gibson FL, Ungerer JA, Leslie GI, *et al.* Psychosocial adjustment, child behavior and quality of attachment relationship at one year postpartum for mothers conceiving through IVF. Presented at the American Society for Reproductive Medicine, Boston, MA, November, 1996

39. Golombok S, Cook R, Bish A, *et al.* Families created by the new reproductive technologies: Quality of parenting and social and emotional health of the children. *Child Develop* 1995;66:285–98

40. Burns LH. An exploratory study of perceptions of parenting after infertility. *Fam Syst Med* 1990;8:177–89

41. Schover LR, Collins RL, Richards S. Psychological aspects of donor insemination: Evaluation and follow-up of recipient couples. *Fertil Steril* 1992;58:583–9

42. Nachtigall RD, Quiroga SS, Tschann JM, *et al.* Stigma, disclosure, and family functioning among parents of children conceived through donor insemination. *Fertil Steril* 1997;68:1–7

43. Berger DM, Eisen A, Suber J, *et al.* Psychological patterns in donor insemination couples. *Can J Psychiatry* 1986;31:818–23

44. Daniels KR. Artificial insemination using donor semen and the issue of secrecy: The views of donors and recipient couples. *Soc Sci Med* 1988;27:377–83

45. Bolton V, Golombok S, Cook R, *et al.* A comparative study of attitudes towards donor insemination and egg donation in recipient, potential donors and the public. *J Psychosom Obstet Gynaecol* 1991;12:217–28

46. Weil E, Cornet D, Sibony C, *et al.* Psychological aspects in anonymous and non-anonymous oocyte donation. *Hum Reprod* 1994;9:1344–7

47. Daniels K, Lewis GM. Openness of information in the use of donor gametes: Developments in New Zealand. *J Reprod Infant Psychol* 1996;14:57–68

48. Daniels KR, Lewis GM, Gillett W. Telling donor insemination offspring about their conception: The nature of couples'

decision-making. *Soc Sci Med* 1995;40:1213–20

49. Sewall G, Mason L. Parental acceptance, disclosure, and decision making amongst recipients in an anonymous donor oocyte program. Presented at the American Society for Reproductive Medicine, Seattle, WA, October 7–8 1995:s252–3

50. Klock SC. Psychological aspects of donor insemination. *Infertil Reprod Med Clin North Am* 1993;4:455–69

51. Galinsky E. *Between Generations: The Six Stages of Parenthood.* New York: Times Books, 1981

52. Sandelowski M, Harris BG, Black BP. Pregnant moments: The process of conception in infertile couples. *Qualitat Health Res* 1992;2:273–82

53. Glazer E. Parenting after infertility. In: Seibel M, Kiessling AA, Bernstein J, Levin SR, eds. *Technology and Infertility: Clinical, Psychosocial, Legal, and Ethical Aspects.* New York: Springer-Verlag, 1993:399–402

54. Gordon ER. Blended families: Adopted, ART, and natural children. In: ART Parents and Children. American Society of Reproductive Medicine, Seattle, WA, October 7–8, 1995:78–83

55. Klock SC. The transition to parenthood among fertile couples: A review of the psychological literature. In: ART Parents and Children. American Society of Reproductive Medicine, Seattle, WA, October 7–8, 1995:17–35

56. Bernstein J. Parenting after infertility. *J Perinat Neonatal Nurs* 1990;4:11–23

57. Bernstein J, Mattox JH, Kellner R. Psychological status of previously infertile couples after a successful pregnancy. *J Obstet Gynecol Neonatal Nurs* 1988;17:404–8

58. Salzer LP. *Surviving Infertility.* New York: HarperCollins, 1991

59. Benezon N, Wright J, Sabourin S. Stress, sexual satisfaction and marital adjustment in infertile couples. *J Sex Marital Ther* 1992;18:273–84

60. Abma JC, Chandra A, Mosher WD, *et al.* Fertility, family planning, and women's health: Estimate from the 1995 National Survey of Family Growth. *Vital Health Stat* 1997:23(19)

61. Paulson RJ, Thornton MH, Francs MM, *et al.* Successful pregnancy in a 63-year-old

woman. *Fertil Steril* 1997;67:949–51

62. Glazer ES. *The Long-Awaited Stork: A Guide to Parenting After Infertility.* New York: Lexington Books, 1990:3

63. Frankel SA, Wise MJ. A view of delayed parenting: Some implications for a new trend. *Psychiatry* 1982;45:220–5

64. Morris M. *Last Chance Children: Growing Up with Older Parents.* New York: Columbia University Press, 1988

65. Clapp D. Secondary infertility. In: Seibel M, Kiessling AA, Bernstein J, Levin SR, eds. *Technology and Infertility: Clinical, Psychosocial, Legal, and Ethical Aspects.* New York: Springer-Verlag, 1993:313–17

66. Falbo T. Only children: A review. In: Falbo T, ed. *The Single-Child Family.* New York: Guilford Press, 1984:1–24

67. Leiblum SR, Kemmann E, Taska L. Attitudes toward multiple births and pregnancy concerns in infertile and non-infertile women. *J Psychosom Obstet Gynaecol* 1990;11:197–210

68. Bryan EM. *Twins, Triplets and More.* New York: St. Martin's Press, 1992

69. Noble E. *Having Twins.* Boston: Houghton Mifflin, 1991

70. Cooper SL, Glazer ES. *Beyond Infertility: The New Paths to Parenthood.* New York: Lexington Books, 1994

71. Braverman AM. Surrogacy and gestational carrier: Psychological issues. *Infertil Reprod Med Clin North Am* 1993;4:517–33

72. Braverman AM. Oocyte donation: Psychological and counseling issues. *Clin Consult Obstet Gynecol* 1994;6:143–9

73. Sorosky AD. Lessons from the adoption experience: Anticipating times of developmental conflict for the ART child. In: ART Parents and Children. American Society of Reproductive Medicine, Seattle, WA, October 7–8, 1995:137–61

74. Clamar A. Psychological implications of the anonymous pregnancy. In: Offerman-Zuckerberg J, ed. *Gender in Transition: A New Frontier.* New York: Plenum, 1989:111–21

75. Sants HJ. Genealogical bewilderment in children with substitute parents. *Br J Med Psychol* 1964;37:133–41

76. Klock SC, Jacob MC, Maier D. A prospective study of donor insemination recipients: Secrecy, privacy, and disclosure.

Fertil Steril 1994;62:477–84

77. Bertrand-Servais M, Letur-Konirsch H, Raoul-Duval A, *et al.* Psychological processes in pregnancy and the earlier mother-child relationship. *Psychoanal Study Child* 1961;16:9–24

78. Braverman AM. Issues in privacy and disclosure in donor gametes. Presented at the Eighth National Conference for IVF Nurse Coordinators and Support Personnel, Serono Symposia, Boston, MA, May 28–20, 1995:63–8

79. Sokoloff BZ. Alternative methods of reproduction. *Clin Pediatr* 1987;26:11–17

80. Baran A, Pannor R. *Lethal Secrets.* New York: Warner Books, 1989

81. Leiber Wilkens C. Talking to children about their conception: A parent's perspective. In: ART Parents and Children. American Society of Reproductive Medicine, Seattle, WA, October 7–8, 1995:163–73

82. Probasco KA. Discussion with children about their donor conception. Insights into Infertility. Serono Symposia, Longwell, MA: Summer 1992:5,10

83. Snowden R. The family and artificial reproduction. In: Bromham DR, Dalton ME, Jackson JC, eds. *Philosophical Ethics in Reproductive Medicine.* Manchester: Manchester University Press, 1990:70–8

84. Snowden R, Mitchell GD. *The Artificial Family: A Consideration of Artificial Insemination by Donor.* London: Unwin Books, 1981

85. McWhinnie AM. Outcome for families created by assisted conception programmes. *J Assist Reprod Genet* 1996; 13; 363–5

86. Klock SC, Maier D. Psychological factors related to donor insemination. *Fertil Steril* 1991;56:489–95

87. Mahlstedt PP, Greenfeld DA. Assisted reproductive technology with donor gametes: The need for patient preparation. *Fertil Steril* 1989;52:908–14

88. Sherry SN, Sherry M. Explaining gamete donation to children. In: Seibel MM, Crockin SL, eds. *Family Building Through Egg and Sperm Donation: Medical, Legal, and Ethical Issues.* Boston: Jones and Barlett, 1996:274–7

89. Shapiro SA. Psychological consequences of infertility in critical psychophysical

passages in the life of a woman. In: Offerman-Zuckerberg J, ed. *Infertility: A Psychodynamic Perspective*. New York: Plenum, 1988:269–89

90. Waltzer H. Psychological and legal aspects of artificial insemination (AID): An overview. *Am J Psychother* 1982;36:91–102

IX. INFERTILITY COUNSELING IN PRACTICE

26

Integrating Infertility Counseling into Clinical Practice

Sharon N. Covington, MSW

Where no counsel is, the people fall: but in the multitude of counsellors there is safety.

Proverbs 11:14

Infertility counseling is a specialty that combines the fields of reproductive health psychology and reproductive medicine. Mental health professionals working in the field of infertility counseling include social workers, psychologists, psychiatrists, marriage and family therapists, and psychiatric nurses. The field of infertility counseling promotes the work of a multidisciplinary group of mental health professionals sharing a common interest and purpose: to 'counsel' (i.e., to advise) and to 'console' (i.e., to give comfort to) people encountering reproductive health problems. There is a wide range of health professionals providing medical treatment, as well as counseling and consoling, to infertility patients: physicians, nurses, laboratory technicians, administrative staff, and others. While the primary focus of these health professional's patient care is the medical diagnosis and treatment of infertility, it must entail 'treating the patient, not the disease'. By comparison, the focus of patient care for infertility counselors is the psychological care and treatment of the individual and/or couple within the context of the medical condition and infertility disorder.

Mental health professionals have become increasingly important in reproductive health care. This has been the result of technological advances in reproductive medicine and the recognition of the complex psychosocial issues and demands facing infertile patients. The role of infertility counselors in reproductive medicine extends beyond advising and comforting: It requires specialized skill, knowledge, and training in the inter-relation of the medical and psychological aspects of infertility. Infertility counseling includes psychological assessment, psychotherapeutic intervention, and psycho-educational support of individuals and couples experiencing fertility problems. This chapter:

- explores the role of mental health professionals in reproductive medicine
- provides a historical perspective on infertility counseling
- presents different views on the provision of counseling services
- discusses different practice frameworks for integrating infertility counseling into clinical settings.

HISTORICAL OVERVIEW

Although the psychological sequelae of infertility have been addressed in the literature as early as 50 years ago[1,2], it has only been within the last 20 years that infertility counseling has emerged as a recognized profession and a specialization within the mental health professions. Historically, the role of the mental health professional was to cure the neurosis that was thought to be the cause of a patient's (usually a woman's) infertility. However, as this approach fell into disfavor, counselors working in infertility clinics began increasingly to provide psychological support, crisis intervention, and education to ameliorate the stress of infertility and enhance quality of life[3]. Today, the role of infertility counselor has expanded to meet the psychological challenges of assisted reproductive technologies and now includes assessment, support, treatment, education, research, and consultation[4].

The importance of including infertility counseling as part of reproductive medical treatment was first addressed by several countries in the early 1980s as a consequence of an enormous technological leap: the first successful birth following in vitro fertilization (IVF) in 1978. In Australia, the Waller Report[5] was followed by legislation for IVF that included compulsory counseling. Infertility clinics providing reproductive technology treatments were required to provide counseling by accredited counselors under the Australian Infertility (Medical Procedures) Act of 1984. In 1991, in a nationwide summary of consumer perspectives, the National Bioethics Consultative Committee Report further defined the role of infertility counseling by recommending that counseling provide (1) education, (2) facilitation of decision-making, (3) personal and emotional counseling, and (4) therapeutic counseling. In 1992, the role of infertility counseling was further defined and supported by the Fertility Society of Australia Reproductive Technology Accreditation Committee, Code of Practice[6]. This report recommended that by 1995 all clinics have available for patient care professionally trained counselors in infertility, and it included specific standards for counseling staff.

During the same time period in Great Britain, the Warnock Report[7] of 1984 considered all aspects of assisted reproduction and recommended that counseling be made available to all infertility patients, at any stage of treatment, in both private and public health clinics. It further suggested that counseling should be nondirective and neutral and should be provided by a skilled, fully trained counselor. The Human Fertilisation and Embryology Act of 1990, which evolved from the recommendations of the Warnock Report, mandated licensure of all infertility clinics. As a provisions of licensure, all infertility clinics were required to make counseling available to patients for the opportunity to contemplate the implications of assisted conception. Furthermore, infertility counselors were to be considered an integral part of the 'treatment team'. Subsequently, a multidisciplinary committee was established to further define infertility counseling services and identify the qualifications of the infertility counselor. The King's Fund Centre Counselling Report[8] of 1991 provided guidelines and recommendations specifying the parameters of counseling and training of counselors. Three distinct types of counseling that should be made available to infertility patients were defined as (1) *implications counseling*, in which the implications of the proposed treatment for the individual, family, and potential child are discussed; (2) *support counseling*, which provides emotional support regarding the stresses of infertility; and (3) *therapeutic* counseling, in which the goal is to help people cope with the consequences of infertility and reach resolution, no matter what the outcome.

As preparation for similar legislation in Canada, in 1989 the Commission on New Reproductive Technologies[9] investigated current and potential developments in assisted reproduction and considered the social, ethical, health, research, legal, and economic implications, as well as the public interest. *Proceed with Care*, the two-volume final report of the Canadian commission, published in 1993, recommended that infertility counseling be an integral part of assisted-conception services and either be offered on-site or be referred out to appropriate professionals. It further recommended that standard written materials be used in counseling, including information about alternatives to medical treatment, exploration of questions related to the patient's values and goals, and the physical and psychological effects of treatment. However, legislation establishing a government authority or regulations regarding infertility treatment, which was supposed to come out of this report, has not be enacted.

The United States has lagged far behind other countries in legislation regarding infertility treatment and assisted reproductive technologies, as well as the integration of counseling into infertility services. Currently, there is no legislation in the United States mandating infertility counseling as part of reproductive medical treatment. However, there have been recent recommendations from two influential groups suggesting that infertility counseling services be made available to patients. The American Society for Reproductive Medicine[10] (ASRM) (formerly the American Fertility Society) in 1996 recommended in its *Guidelines for the Provision of Infertility Services* that infertility counseling services be available in tertiary

care programs, meaning programs offering assisted reproductive technologies. In addition, the National Advisory Board on Ethics in Reproduction[11] (NABER) recommended that potential oocyte donors and donated oocyte recipients receive counseling and that those providing counseling services be 'trained and skilled counselors who are independent of the physician involved in oocyte donation procedure'.

Combined with public awareness and consumer demand, this legislation, committee work, and guidelines from professional organizations have moved infertility counseling from the background to the forefront of patient care in reproductive medicine. Infertility counseling is no longer considered an elective adjunct service available to a minority of needy infertility patients. Nor do the services or skills of mental health professionals providing infertility counseling need to be further justified or defended. Infertility counseling is now recognized as a separate body of knowledge and professional services integral to reproductive medicine and patient care.

Professional Organizations for Infertility Counselors

In the United States, the need for a professional organization to address the psychological aspects of infertility started at the annual ASRM meeting in 1984, when a small group of mental health professionals working in the field met and began informal discussions. By 1985, a special interest group, now called the Mental Health Professional Group (MHPG), was established within ASRM, made up of mental health professionals, physicians, nurses, and allied professionals working in the field of infertility. In addition, mental health professionals from other countries (i.e., Canada and Mexico), where there are few infertility counselors and networking opportunities are more limited, have joined this organization. The MHPG has been consistent in promoting a knowledge base, research, and understanding of the psychological aspects of infertility and is today considered an essential part of the ASRM.

The MHPG provides continuing education in the form of annual postgraduate courses on the psychological aspects of infertility and related counseling issues, sets professional standards in the field, and recognizes outstanding research in the psychology of infertility. It has been instrumental in developing guidelines for psychological screening and counseling of recipients and potential donors in gamete and embryo donation, as well as surrogacy and gestational carrier programs[12,13]. Committee work within the organization has included development of the Comprehensive Psychosocial History for Infertility (see Appendix 2), under the direction of Burns and Greenfeld, for assisting professionals in the assessment and evaluation of infertility patients. Other committees have conducted survey research on the practice of oocyte donation and sperm donation[12,14]; developed counseling qualification guidelines (see Appendix 1), educational materials on infertility counseling for patients and professionals, and a professional bibliography available through the ASRM; addressed the continuing education needs of mental health professionals; and addressed and supported research within the field. As a collaborative and multidisciplinary group within a medical organization, it has set the standard of professional organizations with its shared vision and purpose, which has consistently focused on quality and empathic patient care.

Similar organizations of mental health professionals involved in reproductive medicine have developed in other countries, most prominently the Australia/ New Zealand Infertility Counselling Association (also known as ANZICA) and the British Infertility Counselling Association (BICA). In Great Britain, infertility counseling developed out of an ad hoc meeting of interested individuals in London in 1988 (interestingly convened by an infertility counselor from Australia) that led to the establishment of the National Association for Infertility Counselling, later becoming BICA. This organization was instrumental in contributing information and perspective to the Human Fertilisation and Embryology Act of 1990, the subsequent authority and code of practice of the King's Fund Centre Report. BICA established an outline for a training program in infertility counseling, produced a bibliography, and in 1991 published *Infertility Counselling Guidelines*[8]. Members participated in the King's Fund Centre Counselling Committee report and identified four elements integral to the provision of infertility counseling[8]:

- the welfare of the resultant child and other children who may be affected
- the needs of the infertile people
- the needs of the prospective donor
- the desire for assurance at a societal level that the infertility services are 'conducted responsibly'.

However, despite the groundbreaking work of BICA, which has been instrumental in establishing clear government and professional mandates for infertility counseling and defining the goals and roles of infertility counselors, the problems faced by infertility counselors in Great Britain are the same as those worldwide. The challenges that remain include providing even clearer definitions of professional standards, overcoming the resistance of other professionals, and establishing professional training programs in the field of infertility counseling[15].

Qualification Guidelines for Infertility Counselors

The expanded involvement of mental health professionals in infertility settings, or those interested in providing infertility counseling, led to a concern within the MHPG that guidelines needed to be developed that would identify a minimum standard of training for individuals wanting to work in the field[4]. In 1991, a multidisciplinary committee was formed to accomplish this task, resulting in the Qualification Guidelines for Mental Health Professionals in Reproductive Medicine, published in 1995 (see Appendix 1). The guidelines recommend that infertility counselors be licensed mental health professionals with additional training and knowledge of the medical and psychological aspects of infertility. States vary regarding requirements for licensure, but generally mental health professionals have at least a master's level graduate degree in a mental health field: psychology, social work, marriage and family counseling, or psychiatric nursing. Psychiatrists always have medical degrees, while psychologists usually have a doctoral degree (PhD or EdD). According to the guidelines, a qualified infertility counselor should be able to provide the following services: psychological assessment and screening, psychometric testing (psychologists only), decision-making/implications counseling, grief counseling, supportive counseling, education/ information counseling, support group counseling, referral/resource counseling, sexual counseling, crisis intervention, couple and family therapy, diagnosis and treatment of mental disorders, psychotherapy, and staff consultation. The guidelines suggest a framework for training to practice, set a standard for determining an individual's qualifications as an infertility counselor, and help ensure quality patient care.

Continuing education recommendations are also made.

While there has been some attempt to define infertility as a specialty with a given mental health profession, this has not met with overwhelming success. Within the field of social work, the National Association of Perinatal Social Workers has developed its *Standards for Social Work Services in Infertility Treatment Centers Offering Assisted Reproductive Technologies and the Use of Donor Gametes*[16]. Ten standards of social work practice are defined, based on the general principles of social work and infertility counseling. However, these standards are actually more recommendations for care because they do not involve specific training, the definition or attainment of a special body of knowledge, or qualifying examinations or internships. Within the American Psychological Association, specialization in the field of reproductive health and/or infertility counseling has come under increased consideration. However, efforts have been hampered by the very nature of infertility counseling: It does not represent any one, applicable theoretical framework, operate solely or primarily within a mental health field, or involve a specific body of knowledge (e.g., cognitive therapy) or clearly defined issue (e.g., sex therapy). As the field of infertility counseling and reproductive health psychology becomes more clearly defined, theoretical frameworks are developed, and research identifies clinical issues with effective interventions, it will be possible to establish a multidisciplinary training program for infertility counselors or specialization within specific mental health fields.

REVIEW OF LITERATURE

Early work in the area of the psychology of infertility and the role of mental health professionals centered on the psychosomatic basis of infertility and sterility[1,2,17-19]. Historically, gender bias regarding the woman as the cause of infertility was evident: Treatment was provided by psychiatrists (primarily male) who employed a psychoanalytic orientation, and the focus of treatment was on patients (almost exclusively women) who were seen as having unresolved, hostile feelings about motherhood or their relationships with their mothers. Thus, if infertility could not be identified in medical terms, it was viewed as a psychosomatic reaction requiring extended psychoanalytic treatment of the woman to 'cure' her neurotic response to her childlessness.

Gradually, a change occurred in the literature as the emotional distress of infertility was seen as a *consequence* rather than a *cause* of infertility. With this change came a growing recognition of the need for supportive counseling services for couples undergoing infertility treatment. One of the earliest articles, by Berger[20], discussed the role of psychiatrists consulting in an infertility clinic as both helping couples deal with the outcome of infertility treatment and identifying psychological factors as possible causative agents of infertility, particularly related to sexual function. Other articles[21-23] described counseling services provided at reproductive medical clinics by other mental health professionals, involving assessment of emotional symptomatology associated with infertility and enhancement of quality of life for patients. Thus, there was an increasing recognition of the psychological sequelae of infertility as a consequence of the emotionally intrusive and protracted nature of the medical treatment process[24,25]. As this recognition increased, so did the awareness of the need for skilled mental health professionals to provide these services.

The development of IVF and other assisted reproductive technologies facilitated the involvement of mental health professionals as part of the medical treatment team[26,27]. A number of authors[12,28,29] recommended the inclusion of psychological services for the evaluation and treatment of participants in the more involved fertility therapies. Recommendations have been suggested for provision of counseling services for patients undergoing assisted reproductive technologies including IVF; sperm, oocyte, or embryo donation; and surrogacy or gestational carrier participants. Other recommendations for counseling have been based on concern about marital or psychological functioning, the best interest of the child, inability to provide informed consent, or partner coercion.

THEORETICAL FRAMEWORK

Conceptualization of integrating infertility counseling into clinical practice may be viewed along a continuum of medical treatment. Covington[30] and Feldman[31] developed a theoretical framework for examination of counseling issues and provision of services within a six-phase model of infertility treatment. This model underscores the importance of integrating medical and psychological services throughout the process, thereby normalizing the counseling experience (Table 1). In *phase I*, the mental health professional, on a limited basis, provides support, reassurance about the normalcy of feelings, and preparation for what to expect with medical evaluation as patients begin to acknowledge their fertility problem. During *phase II*, the infertility counselor's role broadens to include increased understanding of a couple's psychosocial functioning in relation to their infertility diagnosis and treatment. Services may involve assessment, education, or psychotherapeutic interventions to promote effective coping and/or more adaptive behavior. In addition, infertility counseling

Table 1 Six phases of infertility treatment and counseling tasks

Phase[31]	Task
I. Acknowledging a fertility problem: seeking help	support education, information, and resources
II. Undergoing medical evaluation	psychosocial assessment and support education preparation for treatment
III. Treating infertility problems	support and education identifying coping mechanisms stress management emotional and therapeutic counseling preparing for outcome
IV. Further treatments: investigating and treating additional diagnosis	stress management and coping strategy emotional and therapeutic counseling exploring alternatives
V. Attempting noncoital conception: donor gametes and assisted reproductive technologies	emotional and therapeutic counseling implications counseling psychosocial assessment and support facilitating decision-making exploring alternatives preparing for outcome
VI. Deciding to end treatment and redefine family: adoption and childlessness	grief and therapeutic counseling pursuing alternative family-building preparing for outcome
Any stage: adjustment to pregnancy and parenthood	support and education redefining self/couple as parents emotional and therapeutic counseling

attempts to prevent problems in later phases by providing services and interventions early in the treatment process. In *phase III*, patients characteristically have a renewed sense of hope about the success of treatment plans, as well as increased stress as treatment begins or becomes more intense. Continued support and education are provided by the infertility counselor and involve managing treatment demands, enhancing coping strategies, and preparing for realistic expectations of treatment success. *Phase IV* may continue over several years, often dominated by feelings of frustration and failure or obsessive determination. During this phase, the infertility counselor helps patients deal with the consequences and chronicity of infertility, express or manage the myriad of negative feelings, and begin preparing for consideration of other family-building alternatives. Patients often enter *phase V* psychologically depleted, only to face complex decisions about assisted reproductive technology or third-party reproduction. Counseling is vital to assess psychological readiness, explore implications of decisions, and prepare for the outcome of treatment. Finally, in *phase VI*, the infertility counselor helps patients reach a decision about ending treatment, grieving the losses, and redefining family so that resolution and closure can occur. By giving meaning to the infertility and integrating it into the sense of self and the marital history, patients are able to 'let go' of infertility and move on without impairment or damage. During any phase of treatment, if pregnancy or the decision to adopt occurs, the counselor's role is to assist in the adjustment to pregnancy and parenthood, which is influenced by the infertility experience.

Another way of looking at the integration of infertility counseling in medical treatment of infertility has historically focused on patient symptomatology. Under this approach, the provision of counseling services is based on a more traditional medical model that focuses on evidence of patient symptomatology. Counseling is provided on an as-needed basis when the patient expresses or the caregiver identifies distress, or crisis intervention is provided when symptomatology has impaired patient functioning, particularly with compliance in medical treatment. A popular approach to integration of infertility counseling is to require or recommend counseling for specific treatments or certain populations (e.g., IVF, donor insemination, egg donation, single women)[28,29,32]. In this method, infertility counseling is defined to the situation and reflects a concern for patient preparation and education, understanding of the implications, and assessment of psychological readiness for treatment.

Still another approach to the integration of infertility counseling into clinical medical practice is to examine the framework for furnishing services. Mental health professionals providing infertility counseling services have three arenas for practice:

- independent clinical (private) practice
- independent consultant, or
- employee of the medical practice.

These practice frameworks are on a continuum from complete independence from the medical practice to complete integration into it as an employee. In each area, there are advantages and disadvantages for infertility counselors, patients, and the medical practice.

Independent Clinical Practice

Mental health professionals involved in their own independent private or group practice may serve as an outside referral source to a reproductive medical practice or physician. Patients are seen in the office of the counselor, which is separate and apart from the medical clinic where they receive care. Infertility counseling may be a small percentage of a general counseling and psychotherapy practice or the entire focus of the mental health professional's practice. In the independent clinical practice approach, the counselor operates completely independently of the referring physician or medical clinic, and communication between the counselor and medical team is limited and structured by traditional parameters of exchange of information. Fee-for-service arrangements are handled by the therapist and patient, and patients must sign appropriate authorization for release of information. Thus, the therapist's primary responsibility is to the patient, not the referral source. Boundaries of the relationship are clearly defined and separate, an understanding that is underscored by the separate facilities.

Because the therapist operates completely independently of the medical practice, there is little potential for therapist coercion or conflict of interest—a distinct advantage of this arrangement. Patients often find this arrangement more comfortable: They feel freer to express negative feelings about care, objectively assess medical treatment alternatives, and discuss issues that they worry will impact the availability of care or the alter the caregiver's positive feelings toward them. Disadvantages of this arrangement range from minor logistical problems to major impediments to care when patients refuse to sign an authorization for release of information or allow the therapist to share information with the medical staff that clearly impacts medical care or compliance.

Independent Practice Consultant

In this arrangement, the mental health professional is a consultant who works as an independent contractor to the medical practice. This arrangement represents a middle ground between the completely independent, off-site infertility counselor and the infertility counselor who is an on-site, practice employee. The infertility counselor usually sees patients at the medical practice, either renting office space from the medical practice or making some other arrangements for the use of office space. The counselor usually bills the patient on a fee-for-service basis, independently and separately from the medical practice. However, the infertility counselor may bill the medical practice for specific services that the clinic provides to patients, such as the initial counseling session, preparation for IVF, evaluation of oocyte donors or gestational carriers, or clinic support groups. The infertility counselor operates as an independent consultant and receives no benefits that an employee of the practice would normally receive.

The advantages of this arrangement include convenience for the patient and facilitation of crisis intervention and continuity of care because of therapist proximity. Since services are integrated as an accepted part of treatment, the counseling experience is 'normalized'. Being on the premises can also help the infertility counselor better understand the particular clinic's procedures and policies, which can facilitate patient education and preparation. In addition, the members of the treatment team may feel more comfortable consulting or discussing treatment problems with a counselor who is readily accessible. Infertility counselors often find the 'informal', curbside consultation one of the keystone's of educating medical staff about the psychology of infertility.

A further advantage is that there is minimal expense to the practice for providing infertility counseling services. Since fee for service is handled independently of the medical clinic, the issues of coercion and job security are less relevant, although the counselor is still dependent on the medical practice for referrals. This arrangement allows greater integration of care, as the therapist operates and interacts more as a staff member, while maintaining professional and financial independence. However, the therapist as a member of the treatment team may be advantageous in some situations (e.g., when a united front is required) or detrimental in other situations (e.g., when the counselor disagrees with medical treatment decisions).

The drawbacks of this arrangement often involve role misunderstandings, unclear boundaries, and boundary violations, particularly regarding confidentiality. Patients viewing the therapist as affiliated or associated with the practice may have more difficulty disclosing or establishing a therapeutic alliance, especially if they have disagreements with the medical practice. Boundaries of the relationships between the infertility counselor, staff, and the patient must be more clearly defined, discussed, and addressed early in counseling, so that issues of confidentiality and the therapist's role are clearly understood by all parties. This can be emphasized by the signing of appropriate release forms or written information that explicitly defines the counselor's relationship with the medical clinic. Nevertheless, the potential for confusion and misunderstanding is always there when counseling services are provided on the same premises as the medical clinic. When the therapist is on the premises, communication between the treatment team and infertility counselor is often less formal and may unwittingly involve unauthorized discussions or sharing of information.

Practice Employee

The third practice approach involves the mental health professional as a salaried employee of the medical practice and, as such, a formal member of the treatment team. This approach enables the integration of medical and psychological care with close collaboration between the members of the treatment team and the patient. Fees for counseling are billed by and paid to the medical practice, and the infertility counselor receives a predetermined salary. Because the counselor is a salaried staff member and consequently dependent on the practice for employment, there is some ethical concern that the counselor's judgment is vulnerable to coercion or undue influence from the employing medical clinic and may be susceptible to bias or lack of objectivity. The infertility counselor may feel that her/his job may be jeopardized by recommendations that are unfavorable to the practice or disagree with physicians. However, these concerns may not be as significant as they may seem at first in that the professional has ethical standards and legal requirements of licensure that supersede employment responsibilities. Although the infertility counselor is part of the treatment, professional standards of confidentiality and relationship boundaries

remain and should be clearly understood by all parties, including patients.

An advantage of this approach, as clearly defined by the British counseling system, is that the infertility counselor is perceived and operates as an integral and equal member of the treatment team, attending patient care conferences and participating, when appropriate, in treatment decisions. Patient care may be more comprehensive, as the counselor is in the clinic, readily available, and patients are encouraged to access this service. It is also thought that this approach legitimizes the importance of the psychological aspects of infertility making it 'OK' for patients to accept or take advantage of referrals for counseling. However, the disadvantages of this approach are similar to those described earlier, including boundary violations, conflicts of interest, and role confusion.

CLINICAL ISSUES

Infertility counselors serve as a resource to patients and staff by providing psychological services that support and enhance quality care. These counselors can provide a variety of services including[4]:

- assessment of patients' functioning in relation to their infertility
- evaluation of psychological appropriateness of participants for medical procedures, including recipients, gamete donors, surrogates, or carriers
- support, intervention, and treatment for the consequences of infertility or for underlying mental disturbances that could affect medical treatment
- education about psychological sequelae of infertility affecting individuals and families, and ways to deal with them
- research on reproductive psychology and on families created through advanced technology
- consultation with and support of the medical staff.

The role of the mental health professional may be divided between that of a counselor and that of an evaluator. Counseling in its purest form entails advising and guiding patients about their options and treatments. Ideas and feelings are expressed in an atmosphere of mutual respect, trust, and safety. In addition, counseling involves knowledge of human behavior, interpersonal relationships, and family dynamics. With the knowledge of people and of reproductive medical treatment, counselors can educate and assist patients with their choices and the possible consequences of their decisions[33]. Silman[34] delineated three areas of fertility counseling:

- helping the clients determine what it is they desire or seek
- exploring the implications of the desire, both physical and emotional, that might be overlooked in the 'excitement of the chase' for a baby
- supporting the decision with realistic information.

In the role of evaluator, infertility counselors may offer psychological screening of participants in various assisted reproductive technologies and third-party reproduction. Although there may be recommendations from national organizations in the United States on the screening of participants in assisted reproductive technologies, the decision concerning which patients should be screened and for which procedures is left to each individual fertility practice. Thus, available guidelines for assessment and evaluation are usually tailored to the specific requirements or preference of a particular medical practice. Whether a clinic adopts formal or recommended guidelines or chooses to develop its own, the clinic's policy regarding infertility counseling, screening, exclusion criteria, and so on should be clearly defined for the protection of the medical team, the infertility counselor, and patients[28].

Evaluation may involve certain groups of patients (e.g., those particularly vulnerable to stress) or certain treatments (e.g., participants in third-party reproduction). Currently, psychological screening is usually recommended for oocyte donors (both known and anonymous), as the procedures for donation are physically demanding and medically intrusive; for gestational carriers and surrogates; and for recipients of donated gametes (sperm, oocyte, or embryo), especially if the donor is known or related[11,12,28]. Other situations where individual practices may require screening involve patients undergoing IVF, single recipients of gamete donation, older infertility patients, lesbian couples, and patients considered psychologically or physically vulnerable[28,29].

When the mental health professional is in the role of evaluator, she or he becomes a gatekeeper recommending inclusion or exclusion of patient participation in treatment. Clearly, infertility counselors must be explicit with patients at the outset as to which role they will play—the counselor or evaluator. If a decision is made to withhold participation or treatment, the infertility counselor has a responsibility to inform the patient as to the reason for rejection and refer the individual or couple for follow-up counseling apart from the medical clinic[35]. Furthermore, the therapist who has had an ongoing counseling relationship with a patient must not attempt to change roles from counselor to evaluator, as the action raises serious ethical issues (e.g., dual relationships) and threatens the therapeutic alliance. In this situation, it is best for an independent counselor to the perform the assessment.

If a recommendation to withhold or postpone treatment is made by the infertility counselor, a team consensus for exclusion is preferable. In this sense, the counselor is not the gatekeeper; rather, the multidisciplinary team is, sharing responsibility for inclusion and exclusion. However, there may be situations in which the infertility counselor makes a recommendation for exclusion with which the team disagrees, or the team decides to overrule the counselor's judgment. In these situations, the mental health professionals should clearly document the reason for exclusion, including supporting information and evidence of notification to the treatment team for the recommendation of exclusion. It may be useful to look on these recommendations as *protection* of the parties involved rather than *rejection*, since it is the first responsibility of medicine and helping professionals 'to do no harm'.

The role of evaluator and/or exclusion decisions are often difficult, and some infertility counselors find them objectionable and against their ethical beliefs. Some counselors refuse to make clear recommendations and instead provide a patient profile leaving the decision for inclusion or exclusion to the medical team or attending physician. However, this can be particularly problematic when the medical team, unable or unwilling to assess complex psychosocial issues, expects or depends on the expertise of the mental health professional. Ultimately, if the infertility counselor is uncomfortable or opposed to screening or evaluation, she or he should not accept these referrals and should notify medical practitioners accordingly.

It bears repeating that patients need to be made aware, at the beginning of any interview required or recommended by the medical clinic, of the counselor's role as part of the treatment team and, specifically, how it pertains to this interview. Issues of confidentiality and sharing of information with the medical team should be discussed, and signed consent to share information (when appropriate) should be obtained. Fees and billing arrangements should be discussed, especially in cases of third-party reproduction, in which the contracting parents may be financially responsible for evaluations. Counseling records and notes should be kept separate from medical records and under the therapist's (not clinic's) control. If a report is to be written, shared with the medical team, and /or made a part of the medical record, the patient must be made aware of this. Finally, the results of psychological testing should be reviewed with the patient in a manner that is understandable to her or him. If there are clinic policies regarding testing, such as requirements that patients score within a certain range, the patient should be made aware of this policy.

In the United States, the decision of when infertility counseling is essential and when it is optional is left to the discretion of each medical practice. The medical treatment team may look to the infertility counselor for assistance in defining when counseling should be required or recommended. Or the medical practice may have its own ideas about the necessity or applicability of counseling—which may conflict with the counselor's opinions or the recommendations of institutions. Often, mental health professionals working in reproductive medicine spend a great deal of time educating the medical team about what they do and how best to use their services. Role negotiation and clarification seem to remain an important and fundamental task of infertility counselors[36].

FUTURE IMPLICATIONS

Reproductive medicine will continue to change as advancing technology presents increasingly complex options and choices for patients. As clinical practice has become more specialized, so has the need for more specialization of the staff members who make up the infertility treatment team. Infertility counselors provide psychological assessment, insight, and judgment that can assist the medical team in making increasingly difficult ethical and clinical decisions, as well as improving patient care.

To accomplish this task, infertility counselors must be highly skilled therapists who are knowledgeable about the medical and emotional aspects of reproductive medicine. There is an increasing need for training programs, practicums, and continuing education workshops on infertility counseling, especially its application within the specific mental health professions. In addition, there is a need for international collaboration with other mental health professionals working in the field of reproductive health psychology.

It is becoming increasingly important for infertility counselors to be involved in scientific research about the psychological aspects of infertility, the impact of reproductive technology, and the efficacy of various psychological interventions. Possibly the most important area of research is the long-range impact on offspring and families created by advancing reproductive technologies. Families are being created today through technologies that just a few years ago were thought to be fiction, not unlike Aldous Huxley's *Brave New World*. As much as infertility counselors may advise patients about the implications of these technologies, no one can predict how someone will feel tomorrow about his/her decisions, let alone 10 years from now. Age, experience, unexpected life events, and societal changes are only a few factors influencing feelings as time goes on. Thus, it is crucial for infertility counselors to be involved in and aware of research and clinical practice in ways that provide a greater understanding of families with affected by a legacy of infertility and/or created through assisted reproductive technologies.

SUMMARY

- Mental health professionals working in the field of infertility counseling include social workers, psychologists, psychiatrists, psychiatric nurses, and marriage and family therapists.

- Although all members of the reproductive medical team counsel and console patients, infertility counselors are mental health professionals who provide specialized services of psychological assessment, psychotherapeutic intervention, psychoeducational support, psychological research, and staff consultation.

- The growing recognition of the complex relationship between the psychological and medical aspects of infertility has made it important for mental health professionals to be part of the treatment team. In some countries, infertility counselors are required by law to be part of reproductive medical services.

- Mental health professionals need special training and experience to provide infertility counseling services as part of the treatment team.

- Infertility counseling is ideally viewed along a continuum of the medical process, where the medical and psychological aspects of infertility treatment are integrated.

- Infertility counseling services may be integrated into clinical practice in three ways: (1) referral to an independent, private practitioner who is outside the medical practice, (2) use of an independent contract consultant, who is affiliated with the practice, or (3) hiring of an employee, who is an infertility counselor and a staff member.

- Infertility counselors must explicitly define their role and responsibilities to patients and staff.
- Infertility counselors must be clear with patients during an evaluation. If they make a recommendation to withhold treatment, a decision preferably should come from a consensus on the multidisciplinary team.

- Infertility counselors must be involved in research on the psychological aspects of infertility, the impact of reproductive technologies, and the efficacy of psychological interventions.

REFERENCES

1. Marsch EM, Vollmer AM. Possible psychogenic aspects of infertility. *Fertil Steril* 1951;2:70–9
2. Rubenstein BB. Emotional factors in infertility: A psychosomatic approach. *Fertil Steril* 1951;2:80–6
3. Bresnick E, Taymor ML. The role of counseling in infertility. *Fertil Steril* 1979;32:154–6
4. Covington SN. The role of the mental health professional in reproductive medicine. *Fertil Steril* 1995;64:895–7
5. Waller Report—Committee to Consider Social, Ethical, and Legal Issues Arising from In Vitro Fertilisation. *Report on the Disposition of Embryo Produced by In Vitro Fertilisation.* Melbourne, Australia: Parliament of the State of Victoria, 1984
6. Fertility Society of Australia reproductive technology accreditation committee, code of practice, section B. *Standards for Counselling Staff.* 1992;11
7. *Warnock Report—Department of Health and Social Security Report on the Committee of Inquiry into Human Fertilisation and Embryology.* London: HMSO,1984
8. *Report of the King's Fund Centre Counselling Committee: Counselling for Regulated Infertility Treatments.* London: King's Fund Centre, 1991
9. *Proceed with Care: Final Report of the Royal Commission on New Reproductive Technologies,* vol. 1. Toronto, Canada: Ministers of Government Services, 1993
10. American Society for Reproductive Medicine. *Guidelines for the Provision of Infertility Services.* Birmingham, AL: American Society for Reproductive Medicine, 1996
11. National Advisory Board on Ethics in Reproduction. Oocyte donation: Recommendations of the National Advisory Board on Ethics in Reproduction. Washington, DC. *NABER Report* 1995;1:2–5
12. Braverman AM, Ovum Donor Task Force of the Psychological Special Interest Group of the American Fertility Society. Survey results of the current practice of ovum donation. *Fertil Steril* 1993;59:1216–20
13. Mental Health Professional Group. *Psychological Guidelines for Embryo Donation.* Birmingham, AL: American Society for Reproductive Medicine, 1996
14. Gillis MW, Rausch D. Survey results on sperm bank practices. Unpublished manuscript, 1997
15. Jennings SE, ed. *Infertility Counselling.* Oxford: Blackwell Scientific Publications, 1995
16. Standards committee. Washington, DC: National Association of Perinatal Social Workers, 1992
17. Benedek T. Infertility as a psychosomatic defense. *Fertil Steril* 1952;3:527–41
18. Fischer IC. Psychogenic aspects of sterility. *Fertil Steril* 1953;4:466–71
19. Ford ESC, Forman I, Willson JB, *et al.* A psychodynmic approach to the study of infertility. *Fertil Steril* 1953;4:456–65
20. Berger DM. The role of the psychiatrist in a reproductive biology clinic. *Fertil Steril* 1977;28:141–5
21. Rosenfeld DL, Mitchell E. Treating the emotional aspects of infertility: Counseling services in an infertility clinic. *Am J Obstet Gynecol* 1979;135:177–80

22. Sarrel PM, DeCherney AH. Psycho-therapeutic intervention for treatment of couples with secondary infertility. *Fertil Steril* 1985;43:897–900

23. Covington SN. Psychosocial evaluation of the infertile couple: Implications for social work practice. In: Valentine D, ed. *Infertility and Adoption: A Guide for Social Work Practice*. New York: Haworth Press, 1988;21–36

24. Menning BE. The emotional needs of infertile couples. *Fertil Steril* 1980;34:313–19

25. Mahlstedt P. The psychological component of infertility. *Fertil Steril* 1985;43:335–46

26. Greenfeld D, Mazure C, Haseltine F, DeCherney A. The role of the social worker in the in-vitro fertilization program. *Soc Work Health Care* 1984;10:71–9

27. Freeman EW, Boxer AS, Rickels K, *et al.* Psychological evaluation and support in a program of in vitro fertilization and embryo transfer. *Fertil Steril* 1985;43:48–53

28. Klock SC, Maier D. Guidelines for the provision of psychological evaluations for infertile patients at the University of Connecticut Health Center. *Fertil Steril* 1991;56:680–5

29. Covington SN. Preparing the patient for in vitro fertilization: Psychological consider-ations. *Clin Consider Obstet Gynecol* 1994; 6:131–7

30. Covington SN. The psychosocial evaluation of the infertile couple within the medical context. In: Counseling the Infertile Couple (IX). Proceedings of Twenty-third Annual Postgraduate Course; 1990 Oct 13–14; Washington, DC. Birmingham, AL: American Society for Reproductive Medicine (formerly the American Fertility Society), 1990;26–48

31. Feldman PR. Infertility: A view its medical and emotional aspects. In: Counseling the Infertile Couple (IX). Proceedings of Twenty-third Annual Postgraduate Course; 1990 Oct 13–14; Washington, DC. Birmingham, AL: American Society for Reproductive Medicine (formerly the American Fertility Society), 1990;2–23

32. Daniels KR. Management of psychosocial aspects of infertility. *Aust N Z J Obstet Gynaecol* 1992;32:57–63

33. Covington SN. Reproductive medicine and mental health professionals: The need for collaboration in a brave new world. *Orgyn* 1997;3:19–21

34. Silman R. What is fertility counseling? In: Jennings SE, ed. *Infertility Counselling*. Oxford: Blackwell Science, 1995;205–13

35. Covington SN. Ethical issues in infertility counseling. In: National Advisory Board on Ethics in Reproduction. Washington, DC. *NABER Report* 1996;2:4–6

36. Applegarth LD. The role of the mental health professional: What are the boundaries of our responsibilities? In: ART Parents and Children: An Integration of Clinical Experience and Psychosocial Research to Counsel the Next Generation (XII). Proceedings of Twenty-eighth Annual Postgraduate Course of the American Society for Reproductive Medicine; 1995 Oct 7–8; Seattle, WA. Birmingham, AL: American Society for Reproductive Medicine, 1995;175–82

27

Legal and Ethical Aspects of Infertility Counseling

Elaine R. Gordon, PhD, and Randi G. Barrow, JD, Esq.

Knowledge not based on ethics cannot ... bring real honor or profit to its master.

Marie de Jars

The boundaries of responsibility for mental health professionals working in reproductive medicine are increasingly challenged by the burgeoning needs of infertile patients and technologies. Of particular concern to infertility counselors are those options that separate the genetic, gestational, and rearing roles of parents through the collaborative use of donated gametes, surrogates, and gestational carriers. Technological innovations such as cryopreservation, posthumous collection, preimplantation diagnosis, cloning, and fetal reduction further complicate what is recognized as an ethical minefield, giving voice to an abundance of complex dilemmas and problematic situations in the evolving field of reproductive medicine.

No longer is it the infertility counselor's task merely to provide emotional support, education, or counseling to those struggling with the malady known as infertility. As the possibilities for treatment multiply, the infertility counselor is obligated to reach beyond the conventions of his or her respective license and to delve into uncharted territory where there are no precedents. Ethical, legal, and moral issues abound and have become part and parcel of an infertility counselor's professional domain as he or she is called on to screen,

evaluate, counsel, and educate individuals involved in these complicated family-building arrangements.

It is recognized that the psychology of reproductive medicine is an emerging field of study and application. The infertility counselor is besieged by problems, controversies, and moral dilemmas unique to this specialized area of medicine. Despite evidence of legal and ethical unrest concerning policy, the infertility counselor is not exempt from practicing due diligence in addressing the pertinent issues and protecting patients from harm, while remaining faithful to designated standards of care (Standard 1.14)[1].

It is not enough to be well versed in the governing guidelines prepared by the infertility counselor's respective licensing board. The area of reproductive medicine is so specialized that new knowledge and expertise are necessary to meet the growing demand. Infertility counselors must heed their professional guidelines[2-5], when interpreting and applying these dictates to the increasingly complex world of contemporary baby-making.*

As a profession they must design and develop new standards that meet the needs of this more visible patient population, while conforming to certain societal values.

This chapter is an effort to sort through and comprehend the pivotal role that an infertility counselor plays in this evolving field. It will:

- clarify legal and ethical obligations for all participants—patients, donors, surrogates, and carriers
- outline the fundamentals of ethical principles and their application to infertility counseling
- address the most important and relevant ethical issues for the infertility counselor.

HISTORICAL OVERVIEW

Women and men desirous of having children once engaged in fertility rites that included herbs, trees, sacred rocks, and holy wells[6]. Today, they no longer look to nature as the source or talisman of their fertility but to the technology of reproductive medicine. A long-standing criticism of reproductive medicine is the speed at which it develops and implements each new technology, offering up ways to intercede in the family-building arena. No sooner is an intervention put into place than queries emerge as to whether or not it is prudent. The impetus to move forward, whether it be consumer-driven or physician-driven, occurs long before there has been time to digest, assess, or reflect on the ramifications of a given medical breakthrough.

The last 40 years have seen profound and contradictory changes in the area of reproduction. In 1960, the United States Food and Drug Administration approved use of 'the pill', allowing women to successfully separate sex from reproduction[7]. The Roman Catholic Church fought back in 1968, reiterating its steadfast opposition to any form of birth control other than abstinence[8]. By 1972, the United States Supreme Court recognized American women's right to abortion[9]. Just 6 years later, the first 'test tube' baby, Louise Brown, was born in England. At the same time that technology was expanding and refining methods of conception in the West, China was implementing its 'one-child policy' to curb its burgeoning population growth[10]. The year 1984 brought the first successful oocyte donation[11]. The 'Baby M' case was decided in 1988, giving custody of a child to its biological father rather than to the surrogate and genetic mother who carried her[12]. A California court added to the surrogacy controversy by denying a gestational carrier any rights to the child she bore (but to whom she had no genetic connection)[13]. A final futuristic scenario was created when a court granted a woman ownership of the sperm willed to her by her dead lover, attempting what is referred to as 'posthumous conception'[14].

Taking conception out of the bedroom and putting it into the laboratory was pivotal in shifting what was once a private matter over to the public domain. This was a frightening and dubious prospect for many. The birth of the first 'test tube' baby was the wake-up call, met with admiration on the one hand and outrage on the other. Voices from many sectors were heard, quarreling about the future and how life would be viewed and created. We have yet to see what impact the latest reproductive feat will have on humankind: the birth of Dolly, a sheep cloned from a single cell of

---

* Ethical considerations have been formulated by the American Society for Reproductive Medicine but primarily address medical concerns as opposed to psychological concerns. The National Advisory Board on Ethics in Reproduction (NABER) (now defunct) published reports relevant to decision-making in reproductive medicine, addressing psychosocial concerns as well as medical issues.

its genetic mother and born to a gestational carrier[15].

Traditional family-building was believed by many to be undermined by these technological developments. John Robertson[16] stated, very succinctly, that one is damned either way; either for technologizing the intimate or for losing the very real benefits that this technology provides.

As the field evolved and family-building arrangements became increasingly complicated, the entire issue became a Pandora's box. Experts started to disagree as to the correct protocols for assisting people who wanted children. Questions emerged regarding patients' psychological health and well-being, as well as what responsibility the medical community held concerning the best interests of the children whom they were helping to create[11-17].

It became immediately clear that there were no answers to these difficult and complex questions. Medical practitioners increasingly began calling on mental health professionals to help address the complex concerns voiced by a distraught population of infertility patients. Furthermore, as third-party arrangements became more popular, legal experts were also asked for input on how best to proceed. Due to the lack of established standards in this growing field, the challenge was to formulate guidelines specific to the area and set precedents that could protect all parties involved, while at the same time remaining loyal to what is 'right'.

This necessitates working quickly in an attempt to catch up in a field that has taken us by storm in a very short period of time, with new innovations continually arriving: in vitro fertilization (IVF), gamete intra-fallopian transfer, zygote intrafallopian transfer, embryo transfer, assisted hatching, cloning. No sooner does the scrutinizing of one issue begin than a new issue emerges, further complicating any previous headway.

THEORETICAL FRAMEWORK

The applicable theoretical framework concerns the ethical principles in mental health and medicine that are usually defined as:

- personal autonomy
- veracity
- nonmalfeasance
- beneficence
- confidentiality
- justice[18].

Mental health professionals have the duty and obligation to serve clients and, at the same time, a responsibility to protect themselves from professional misconduct. As with most professional disciplines, mental health practitioners are obligated to adhere to the codes of conduct prescribed by their specific professional governing board. These codes dictate the professional's guiding principles and are comparable in intent. They speak to the philosophical principles of autonomy, beneficence, and justice[19,20]. Contributing to the welfare of others and doing no harm are code ideals fundamental to the field of mental health. In the attempt to respect a client's autonomy, a counselor is duty-bound to minimize the client's burden and increase their benefit in a fair and just manner. In addition, mental health professionals practicing in the field of reproductive medicine must be responsive to the standards of practice prescribed by this medical community in meeting patients' needs. The interpretation and application of these principles are often what wreaks havoc for infertility counselors working in this complex field.

Each mental health discipline (psychiatry, psychology, social work, marriage and family therapy, and psychiatric nursing) has stipulated standards for practice for which failure to comply could result in formalized sanctions. However, all too often, the conventional principles are difficult to apply so that all participants are equally and justly protected. More often than not, a counselor's responsibility involves balancing the interests of *more than one* client in any given situation. This can be especially true in third-party reproduction arrangements.

How to apply the mental health professional's code of conduct while serving the needs of patients and third-party participants is the quintessential question. Issues of dual roles, conflicts, confidentiality, record keeping, and access must be addressed. How do the principles of beneficence and autonomy get defined? Whose rights are being protected: the infertile, the embryo, the donor, or the potential child? Who is the client? The demands inherent to some family-building options dictate that there is more than one client at any one time, and the aim is to serve the multiple interests at stake. Egg donation procedures yield the obvious two-client scenario (recipient and donor)—but what about the embryo(s) or the child(ren) that will hopefully result? The needs presented by reproductive medical practitioners and their patients clearly challenge many of the traditional standards-of-care practices for counselors working in this field.

CLINICAL ISSUES

The diverse goals of birth control, abortion, IVF, egg and embryo donations, and surrogacy are all brought together under the vague ethical and legal heading of reproductive rights. Although law and precedent regarding the use of birth control and abortion are largely settled, laws governing egg donation, surrogacy, and gestational carriers are almost nonexistent[9,21-23]. A handful of states have outlawed surrogacy, and fewer still have addressed egg donation.*

Legislation on a controversial subject is often drafted piecemeal, usually in response to an especially egregious problem, leaving the primary legal rights and responsibilities unaddressed or ignored altogether. An example of this occurred when California Governor Pete Wilson vetoed passage of the Alternative Reproduction Act of 1992, which would have given concrete legal status to ovum donation and surrogacy, only to be haunted a few years later by the alleged unauthorized distribution of embryos to infertile couples by doctors at the University of California at Irvine. California State Senator Tom Hayden then introduced legislation to make that specific act illegal, but neither politician has introduced a law that would fully govern egg donation and surrogacy[24], reproductive medicine in general, or specific third-party reproductive matters.

This situation creates an endless source of potential liability for practitioners in the field, whether counselors, physicians, or lawyers. Infertility counselors are in a particularly difficult and vulnerable position due to the various roles played in assisting donors, recipients, and all parties in a surrogate or carrier arrangement. Self-protection is not a priority for most infertility counselors or for most practitioners in the helping professions. But understanding where the potential liability lies and avoiding it are essential to maintaining one's license and ability to practice. To do that, certain key concepts and their legal implications must be understood. The most critical are:

---

* For example, the laws of Arizona, Indiana, Michigan, New York, Utah, and under certain circumstances Louisiana, Nebraska, and Washington have outlawed surrogacy, and Florida, Oklahoma, and Texas have addressed issues of egg donation.

- competence
- confidentiality and the infertility counselor's role
- conflict of interest
- informed consent.

Although each topic will be addressed separately, these four issues often overlap.

Competence

The threshold question that a mental health professional has to answer is whether they have the proper training to justifiably be called an infertility counsellor or specialist in the field. The American Psychological Association's (APA) 'Ethical Principles of Psychologists and Code of Conduct'[2] mandated that psychologists perform only in areas in which they have formal training*.

However, to acquire the appropriate formal training in an emerging field such as third-party reproduction, counselors may have to use creativity. Consulting with or being supervised by a recognized expert would be ideal, but attending educational seminars, researching the literature, subscribing to journals, and joining professional associations are necessary[25]. It is also mandatory under the APA code (sec. 1.05) to maintain one's expertise[1]. Infertility counselors would be prudent to continue the educational efforts noted above, or risk formal sanctions for violation of a mandatory standard, which could include the loss of one's license[1].

Most lawsuits against counselors are based on claims involving their competence. These are generally malpractice suits based on a counselor's alleged negligence. The legal rule of thumb is that negligence may be based on the theory that the practitioner deviated from or fell below the standard practice of care in the

profession[26]. When mental health professionals hold themselves out to the public as specialists, the law too will hold them to that standard of expertise, when assessing liability[24]. The APA standard that one does not practice beyond one's boundaries of competence fits snugly into the legal framework of liability due to negligence, especially if counselors lack the expertise they advertise themselves as possessing.

Confidentiality and the Infertility Counselor's Role

Confidentiality and privileged communications are the hallmark of the therapeutic relationship (secs. 5.01, 5.02)[1,27]. The problem in third-party reproduction is that the infertility counselor's role is not one of the traditional therapist, but rather some combination of assessor, counselor, facilitator, and gatekeeper. To whom then do infertility counselors owe their duty? Third-party reproduction arrangements are analogous to group or family therapy in the respect that all participants are the clients and the infertility counselor is duty-bound to maintain all of their confidences (sec. 4.03)[1,27]. This must be made clear in writing and signed by all participants at the first meeting with the counselor, to avoid confusion about the counselor's role and claims of breach of confidentiality (sec. 5.05)[1].

The client 'holds the privilege', meaning his or her permission is needed to share information given to a counselor. An infertility counselor should have all parties sign a waiver of confidentiality, indicating exactly what information given by them will be shared and with whom (sec. 5.05)[1]. Verbal waivers are insufficient. *All exceptions and exclusions to confidentiality must be in writing* (see Appendix 11). Much of the

---

* The APA general principles are aspirational goals. The 102 rules of conduct that follow the principles are mandatory, and serious sanctions may be imposed for noncompliance.

information given to the counselor will be shared with physicians, clinics, and medical staff, and some information may automatically be entered into databases for statistical or research purposes. Special care must be taken by infertility counselors to exclude identifying information, unless a waiver has been signed (sec. 5.07)[1].

Three separate sections of the APA codes refer to the importance of keeping proper records, all of which further emphasize the importance of confidentiality (secs. 1.23, 1.24, 5.04)[1]. Counselors must 'maintain appropriate confidentiality in creating, storing, accessing, transferring, and disposing of records under their control', whether written, recorded, or in any other medium (sec. 5.04)[1]. One rule instructs that an even higher quality of records must be kept if counselors believe that the documents might one day be used in legal proceedings involving the participants (sec. 1.23)[1]. By following these rules carefully, counselors protect not only their clients but themselves. A precise written record of all meetings, tests, and interactions, made at a time when no conflict existed between the parties, carries great weight in a court of law. Finally, counselors will be paid for the services they provide to all parties by one of the parties. The *retainer agreement* should contain a disclaimer clarifying for the payer that the receipt of money does not obligate the counselor to refrain from screening him or her out of the program if that is appropriate (see Appendix 13). This simple precaution will protect practitioners from claims based on false assumptions about their role and loyalties.

Conflict of Interest

Even after a practitioner has clearly defined their role, employment, and duties in signed documents with the appropriate waivers, problems may still arise when one of the parties is denied services based on the counselor's recommendations. This places the counselor in direct conflict with the desire of one or all of their clients. Anger and blame should be anticipated. A disappointed client may argue that the rejection or delay of services reduced his or her chances of successful reproduction, even though statistics make it clear that a significant percentage of third-party reproductive efforts will fail even under the best conditions.

Although there is arguably a constitutionally protected right to procreate coitally without state interference, it is not clear that there is a comparable right to procreate noncoitally in a private medical setting[21-23,28]. This is especially true when there are sound medical or psychological reasons not to proceed. Third-party reproduction is first a medical phenomenon. If, for example, pregnancy over the age of 40 carries significant medical risks for mother and child, exclusion from the program may be the responsible decision. If the physician and infertility counselor are mandated 'to do no harm', legitimate reasons exist to screen out potential candidates, while avoiding claims based on discriminatory treatment (sec. 1.4)[1].

Some problems may be sidestepped by working only with clinics whose policies regarding age, health, marital status, and sexual orientation of potential third-party reproduction patients are on record and in place. The medical team will already be serving as gatekeeper, deflecting blame and possible liability away from the infertility counselor. However, an infertility counselor may be best served by maintaining their professional and financial independence from the physician or clinic providing medical services (see Chapter 26). This avoids claims that she is proceeding with an inappropriate match because of personal financial gain. Her duty to the client is uncompromised when this separation exists, and less pressure can be exerted by the clinic in cases of disagreement over decisions made by him or her. A clinic may also proceed with a reproductive arrangement against an infertility counselor's recommendation. In that case, infertility counselors who test appropriately, keep thorough records, and hold themselves separate from the medical team has reduced their liability substantially from any complaints brought after the delivery of services.

The use of standardized psychological tests, with result analysis that is the least susceptible to subjective interpretation, further protects the practitioner. Assessments should be made based on clearly defined medical and psychological standards (secs. 1.06, 2.02)[1]. Although 'gut feelings' and 'intuitions' are important, the infertility counselor is at greater risk if these are the major or only criteria used. Referencing guidelines such as those developed by the American Society for Reproductive Medicine[29] for egg and sperm donation add authority and credibility to the infertility counselor's assessment if challenged.

Assisted reproductive technologies have implications for the offspring born of successful third-party reproductive arrangements. The intense desire of recipients to have a biologically related child may also be felt by a child seeking their genetic parent in the future. As the children of anonymous sperm donors reach middle age, many are becoming more vocal in their outrage that no one considered their needs as human beings, when arranging some of the original third-party reproduction contracts[30]. While statutory law ignores the interests of these children, a careful practitioner should discuss the desires of recipients and donors regarding release of information to any child born from these procedures. The parties may

have conflicting interests that must be resolved and documented before the parties can move forward.

Informed Consent

A psychological informed consent should be signed by each member of the reproductive arrangement[31]. These documents are necessary to ensure that clients may intelligently exercise their judgment by balancing the probable risks against the probable benefits of their involvement[32]. These are similar to medical informed consent forms that clients sign with physicians, clinics, or hospitals, but the psychological informed consent is solely the counselor's responsibility. Not surprisingly, the concept breaks down into two parts: what it means to be informed and what it means to give consent.

What It Means To be Informed

To be properly informed, counselors must give clients 'all material information' regarding the known and potential psychological consequences of their involvement in the reproductive arrangement[33]. *Material information* means what would be regarded as significant by a reasonable person in the client's position when deciding to accept or reject involvement[29]. A clear presentation of the material could be broken down into three sections: the psychological evaluation, the psychological impact of reproductive technology, and future considerations.

Psychological Evaluation

This would include a description of the components of the evaluation, a listing of the possible effects and side effects, and the psychological risk.

Psychological Impact of the Reproductive Technology

This would include a statement of the psychological, social, and physical risks of involvement, including future reactions or triggering of past traumas. Included are risks that may be present if the procedure is successful or it is unsuccessful, with statements regarding possible effects on spouses, families, and children. The statement should also include the fact that the long-term physical effects of the procedure and medications are unknown but could be serious and/or affect future good health, with the accompanying psychological responses.

Future Considerations

It is important that it be clear that delayed reactions are possible, particularly when pregnancy occurs or if a client (or spouse) were to become infertile at some future point. It should be emphasized that social and personal attitudes may change about the procedure, along with the law, and that this may have a psychological impact on well-being (see Appendices 9 and 10).

What It Means To Give Consent

One must have the capacity to give consent; it must be voluntary and be given at the appropriate time[32]. By the exclusion of donors who are under 21 years of age and who have not had children, the argument for capacity is strengthened. To be voluntary, consent must be given freely, without duress[34]. This can be most tricky in third-party reproduction when the donor or surrogate is a relation or good friend of the recipient. Extra care should be taken to meet with the donor separately and probe these relationships and the unspoken demands of family and friends. All informed consent should be taken only after the screening process but before the person is enrolled in the program[35].

Informed consent should also include a statement that clients understand that the psychologist is not responsible for predicting or ensuring their current or future

response and that is not certain that they will receive any benefit from their involvement. It should be emphasized that there is no guarantee about the outcome of the evaluation nor that the experience will be a positive one. To avoid future complications, the donor or surrogate's spouse should also sign the informed consent form to reduce the possibility of claims that their interests were neglected, impinged on, or overridden. In short, patients must be fully informed, understand the risks, and freely assume them.

The uncertainty of the law in most areas of third-party reproduction means that all the contracts so carefully crafted and entered into may be declared null and void as against public policy and held to be unenforceable in the event of future conflict between the parties. The contract may be seen as evidence of the intentions of the participants, but without legislation steering a clear course, any outcome is possible. If all a judge has to look at is intention, the clarity of the documents and the records kept by a counselor will be the judge's guiding light, and perhaps the practitioner's saving grace.

THERAPEUTIC INTERVENTIONS

There are specific ethical considerations pertinent to the field of reproductive medicine for which no paradigm exists. They emerge as a consequence of the multiplying family-building options more readily available to patients. With the proliferation of third-party reproduction arrangements and the advances made in technological procreation, baby-making is no longer the exclusive domain of two people engaging in sexual intercourse who happen to conceive. Procreation takes on new meaning. Not only can conception take place outside the body, but the collaboration and contributions of other individuals make available Orwellian possibilities previously thought impossible. That a child can have five parents—the genetic mother, gestational carrier, sperm donor, rearing father, and rearing mother—is nothing compared to the complications brought on by posthumous procreation or transsexual conception, whereby the genetic mother is the rearing father. These very real situations boggle even the most forward-thinking mind.

The challenges infertility counselors face are monumental. Because of the unprecedented nature of these family-building scenarios, a counselor may find themself working in a quandary. They must address issues as they emerge, with little time to assess, evaluate, and confer thoroughly about each unique set of circumstances. Needless to say, the topical issues of today will tomorrow seem mundane, yet if infertility counselors are to practice wisely, there are critical ethical issues that must be addressed. The most important and relevant of these are:

- the infertility counselor's role
- personal bias
- collaborative arrangements
- terminating treatment
- best interest considerations.

The Infertility Counselor's Role: Wearing Multiple Hats

Infertility counselors are called upon to participate in helping infertility patients forge their way through the complicated maze of reproductive choices. The medical community is more willing to recognize the contribution infertility counselors can make not only for the struggling patient but for the medical practice as well.

It is important to distinguish the various roles an infertility counselor can have and ensure that all parties understand the differences. A clinician may be asked to engage in assessment, education, counseling, research, therapy, or organizational consulting (sec. 1.05)[1]. Not only can an infertility counselor serve in a number of capacities, but he or she may be providing services to several persons at any one time who are engaged in a semiformalized relationship, such as those demonstrated in collaborative arrangements: counselor to the surrogate, donor, or recipient.

The professional responsibilities involved in these activities are different with respect to what the purpose of the intervention is and who has access to what information. It is necessary at the outset that infertility counselors inform the relevant parties as to what the intent of the intervention is, what information will be shared, and what information will remain confidential.

One question that repeatedly resurfaces is the issue of 'gatekeeping'. Is it the infertility counselor's job to determine who should become a parent and who should not? Why should individuals seeking medical assistance be scrutinized in this way when those who can conceive in the traditional manner are not put to the same test? Most medical practices have very different standards for recipient patients who are attempting to have their own biological child than for patients who have to engage a third-party reproduction to help them in their quest. Even in these situations third-party providers, whether it be donors, surrogates, or gestational carriers, are evaluated and examined more thoroughly than third-party recipients.

Standards for acceptance or rejection vary from clinic to clinic. It is the responsibility of infertility counselors working with medical practices to establish guidelines relevant to their involvement. An infertility counselor who agrees to provide services for a medical clinic must clarify at the outset the nature of the relationship with the various interested parties (sec. 1.21)[1]. The medical team must have a complete understanding as to what role an infertility counselor will serve. Professional providers must be alert to the potential for conflict and do everything feasible to avoid such situations.

Together, the medical team and infertility counselor needs to determine how they will interface so that there are no unmet expectations concerning the counselor's professional responsibilities. It is wise to discuss whether the infertility counselor is to serve as a screener, therapist, counselor, or educator. If the infertility counselor is to screen prospective clients, the criteria utilized to make recommendations to the medical team should be established. The medical team will also need to understand that there might be some limits to confidentiality that must be respected (sec. 5.05)[1].

Recommendations made should be detailed and documented, so that there is little room for misunderstanding between infertility counselors and the medical team members. Further, the professional obligations of all service providers, mental health professionals, and medical staff must be clearly understood and delineated to avoid abdicating responsibilities. The goal is to minimize opportunities for miscommunication, conflict of interest, and professional impropriety to protect patients from harm[2].

In all professional relationships, it is the counselor's responsibility to inform clients as to what role the counselor will serve and clarify what services will be provided. Clients are entitled to know the purpose of the counseling endeavor and the means by which they are going to work toward that goal (secs. 1.07, 4.01)[1]. If the purpose is to counsel, then the infertility counselor is there to assist clients in making an appropriate decision regarding the reproductive treatment options available. This can be accomplished by examining the psychosocial implications of any given protocol with respectful regard for individual needs, feelings, and concerns.

The moral, ethical, and religious attitudes of clients can, and should, be integrated into the counseling process, so that they can best understand why they are choosing a particular path and why one route might be more appealing to them than another. It is never the counselor's job to tell a client what to do.

If, on the other hand, the infertility counselor's role is to screen with the intent of serving as gatekeeper, then this too must be established prior to the start of the evaluation process. Individuals who are required to submit to pyschological testing as part of a screening protocol have the right to know what the purpose of the testing is and what information is expected to be gleaned through the assessment process. The task here is to determine who will be included and who will be rejected. Usual grounds for rejection include psychological instability or pathology, and evidence of coercion. The ability to comprehend the implications of any decision made should also be considered by infertility counselors.

Clients must be informed as to how these decisions will be made and what tools will be used to make such determinations. Additionally, tests must be administered and interpreted only by persons qualified to do so (sec. 2.02)[1]. Test takers have the right to receive test results, and these results should be given out *only* by qualified individuals (usually psychologists) and never by adjunct program staff. Steps should be taken to insure that appropriate explanations for test results be given to designated persons in language that is understandable (sec. 2.09)[1].

It is professionally prudent to offer test results only to those taking the tests, except in certain situations wherein the appropriate releases were obtained prior to the actual screening process. Interested parties, such as recipients working with donors, should be informed whether or not test results are acceptable in an effort to ascertain the wisdom of working with any particular donor or surrogate candidate.

Persons who are screened out of programs should be given a reasonable explanation why they were rejected. If the rejection is based on psychological competency, this difficult information should be communicated by the infertility counselor. Patients have the right to know on what grounds they are being excluded and whether there is any avenue available to rectify the rejection. For example, if a couple is rejected because coercion has been ascertained, in that one partner is forcing the other to submit unwillingly to invasive procedures, subsequent therapy can be suggested to help the couple resolve their differences This ongoing counseling must be with an independent therapist to avoid any conflict of interest (sec. 1.17)[1].

Personal Bias: A Disaster Waiting to Happen

When counselors broach issues having to do with life-giving or life-denying events, moral issues inevitably seem to surface. Issues of morality are naturally interwoven with religious beliefs and church sanctions. Religion having entered the picture paves the way for governmental intervention, with discussions about public policy and legislative controls and regulation. Needless to say, once legislation is proposed, the judicial system must rule, with attorneys close at hand interpreting and arguing the law and its application. One can just imagine the sight of a bewildered infertile couple standing amid physicians, clergy, attorneys, bioethicists, mental health professionals, and special interest groups and crying out that they simply want a baby.

Infertility counselors hold the responsibility of putting this very chaotic house in order so that 'good decisions' are made for those involved. Because this is such a new field of inquiry, the opportunity for varying and conflict opinions and attitudes does exist. The infertility counselor is there to help participants sort through the multiple issues and controversies and move forward from an 'informed' place (sec. 1.09)[1].

Infertility counselors need to be thoroughly aware of their own prejudices relative to the current practices operative in reproductive medicine. It is crucial to preclude personal biases from influencing or contaminating professional responsibilities (sec. 1.08)[1]. Yet it is virtually impossible to avoid the sway that one's own life experiences present. Each infertility counselor must determine whether their particular bias will interfere with the decision-making process in each case. If one acknowledges having potentially damaging opinions with regard to one's work, it is necessary to address those concerns through supervision or perhaps to remove oneself from those seemingly troubling cases. For example, if a prejudice exist about nontraditional families (e.g., single parent, lesbian or gay couples), there is a professional obligation to refer such cases out.

More and more nontraditional families are being created as a result of the options made available through reproductive practices. Single men and women, as well as lesbian and gay couples, are choosing to parent. There are unique considerations that these families will face as their children grow. Psychological providers can help these nontraditional families grow healthy children in the context of mainstream society (see Chapters 14 and 25).

Collaborative Arrangements: Friends or Foes

Collaborative reproductive arrangements are those by which third parties assist those unable to have children in the traditional way, utilizing nontraditional means: egg donation, sperm donation, surrogacy, or gestational carrier. Infertility resolutions might involve utilizing state-of-the-art medical interventions or perhaps include the biogenetic contributions of third parties, be they cousins, children, friends, siblings, or strangers.

Third-party helpers, by virtue of adding another person to this traditionally two-person process, complicate the existing family-building equation. The needs of third-party participants must be respected as separate yet commensurate with the infertility patients seeking treatment. These helpers are viewed as patients by medical clinics, albeit on a very temporary basis.

Collaborative efforts raise ethical questions for which there are no easy answers or fast solutions. Two areas that incite the most controversy are the issues of intrafamilial donation and age appropriateness for recipients, donors, and surrogates. Infertility counselors are being asked to comment on what are reasonable parameters for inclusion or exclusion. Clearly, no groundwork exists, and opinions on these subjects are diverse.

Intrafamilial Donation/Gestation

Intrafamilial arrangements are chosen for seemingly sound reasons, including preserving some genetic continuity for the desired child or perhaps just feeling more comfortable working with someone who is known and familiar. Yet before such agreements are embarked on or endorsed, there are specific psychological issues that need to be systematically addressed. First and foremost, it is necessary to assess the relationship between the participants to establish whether the particular reproductive plan is in the best interests of those involved, including the child that they hope to create. If it is obvious that there are no underlying feelings or pathology that could

potentially contaminate the situation at some later time, are the relationships otherwise seemingly healthy and stable?

Gamete donation and surrogacy have made it possible for participants to cross generational lines. Mothers can carry pregnancies for their children. Fathers can donate sperm for their sons. It is possible for daughters and sons to donate gametes to their parents. Is it different for a son to donate sperm to his father than for a daughter to donate eggs to her mother? Does the invasive quality of an egg aspiration make the difference, or, as some believe, are they considered equitable?

In these situations, infertility counselors must look for coercion, whether subtle or more blatant, where one party feels obligated to the other. It is sometimes very difficult for a daughter to say no to her mother, no matter how uncomfortable she might be with the prospect of donating her eggs, or for a son to refuse to donate to his father. It is evident that there is an imbalance of power that exists between parent and child. The infertility counselor's responsibility is to address the inherent boundary violations in such arrangements that leave the family system or the relationships vulnerable and at risk.

The infertility counselor must also consider a son or daughter's relationship with the 'stepparent'. Are there any sexual overtones? Is there evidence of discomfort? When children donate to parents, the natural order of the relationships is transposed, whereby children are providing for their parents while these parents are still competent. However, when parents donate or gestate for their children, it is more often viewed as an indigenous extension of their caretaking responsibilities in which the 'natural order' is preserved. The question remains: Do children have the right to donate to parents if they so choose, and, if so, what are the responsibilities of the infertility counselor when confronted with these unique family-building scenarios? Can the child truly make an informed, not coerced, decision to donate or not to donate?

In other circumstances, intrafamilial donations might be fraught with less controversy, whereby participants—cousins, sisters, brothers—can enter these arrangements without the potential of inadvertently damaging, upsetting, or threatening the sanctity of the existing relationship or violating boundaries. That is not to say that all problems would necessarily be avoided. Sister-to-sister or brother-to-brother donation on many levels may appear to be ideal, but it is only as good as the health of the relationships between the two siblings and their respective spouses. Critical is their ability to come to a clear understanding of boundaries: who will be the parent and who will be aunt or uncle? Proximity alone might make this an even greater challenge as the donor or carrier watches the rearing of the child.

Careful considerations must be given to all forms of collaborative reproduction. The infertility counselor must help participants examine the potential pitfalls associated with all these arrangements, so the best possible resolution can be reached. Coercion must be avoided, and sometimes it is the counselor who needs to help one party say no to an uncomfortable request. To best accomplish the task of counseling in third-party arrangements, it is necessary to depart from the traditional therapeutic model whereby there is only one client. With prior consent (documented), all parties are first seen independently. If an ongoing relationship is an anticipated outcome, as would be the case in an intrafamilial donation or most surrogacy arrangements, then the participants would be seen together (see Chapters 18–21).

Motivations, concerns, expectations, wants, hopes, and fears are all part of the counseling agenda. The infertility coun-selor works through the issues involved in collaborative arrangements and makes appropriate recommendations to the participants.

Age Considerations

More recently, age minimums and max-imums in reproductive practice have been an area of dispute. Ethicists continue questioning how 'old' is too old and how 'young' is too young. Women in their 50s and 60s can successfully gestate and birth a baby created from sperm and a donated egg[36]. Donors are typically recruited on the basis of age, with younger donors being more coveted than older ones. Is there such a thing as a donor that is too young? What about encouraging older women to have children, challenging the natural aging process? How should age cutoffs be determined, and who should decide what these limits should be? Many programs look at the age of majority as a reasonable requirement for younger donors, but the ethical advisability of having an enforced maximum age remains in question.

Medical wisdom promotes the util-ization of young donors with minimum regard to psychological readiness, the maxim touted being 'the younger, the better'. Many egg donation programs and sperm banks recruit donors from colleges and universities. Consent revolves around medical risks and complications, with little regard given to the psychological com-plications potentially inherent in donation agreements. Infertility counselors involved in these procedures are obligated to review issues such as the donor's future fertility or infertility, as might be the unfortunate case; beliefs about genetic ties; and the ability to distinguish genetic, gestational, and rearing contributions. Donors need to understand and take responsibility for the emotional consequences of these donations that might emerge at a later time. They must be counseled about the procedure and the potential consequences of their donations, so that an informed decision can be reached, void of coercion factors or purely financial incentives.

A moral question that seems to resurface is whether or not a gamete donor who has never had a child can truly give psychological informed consent. Some practitioners liken gamete donation to bone marrow or kidney donation, despite the differences in risks, and believe that having had a child is irrelevant to the donation process. Others believe that it is ethically imprudent to use as donors women who have never had children. While many practitioners seem to be throwing caution to the winds concerning the use of young donors, there is the ecstasy voiced by reproductive practitioners on the success of impregnating senior women with younger women's fertilized eggs. Others argue that the medical and psychological risks for these older recipients and the children that they are hoping to bear outweigh the benefits[11].

Historically, there has been disparity on the issue of men and women having children later in life. Men who sire children in their later years are heralded and applauded, while women who want to have children later in life are looked on with disdain and a critical eye. Addressing the age issue is no easy task and, again, is more often coming under the auspices of infertility counselors as a result of an outcry disclaiming the rationality of these procedures. Infertility counselors can contribute by helping recipients think through the consequences of their decision with adequate information and counseling. Recognizing how egg donation challenges nature's original plan and therefore taking responsibility for the consequences of such disruption are sound ethical practice (see Chapter 15).

Terminating Treatment: Enough is Enough

The quintessential question that haunts medical and psychological practitioners is the dispute over when 'enough is enough'. Some patients are enticed into trying procedure after procedure, with medical innovations offering yet another chance and more hope. How many IVFs or intrauterine inseminations (IUIs) constitute a reasonable course of medical treatment?

Infertility counselors see patients in awe of other patients who finally achieved success after 21 or so IVF attempts or perhaps after 5 or 15 years of grueling treatment protocols, with intracytoplasmic sperm injection (ICSI) being offered as the new treatment of choice. These patients are viewed as Goliaths in the perseverance of their goal. They are held up as heroes by other patients experiencing a similar struggle. Less often does one see patients looking with a critical eye toward the negative side of an unrelenting pursuit of fertility.

What has happened to patients' lives in the midst of their fertility quest? Not enough mind has been paid to the emotional costs of such perseverance. It is on this issue that infertility counselors should focus. It is inevitable that patients, in time, become emotionally wounded by the repeated failures and draining experiences that the treatment process invites. It is not necessarily in every patient's best interest to continue treatment indefinitely, and knowing when to stop is a key ingredient in healthy as opposed to desperate decision-making.

What is the right path for one patient is not necessarily the right one for another. There are many contributing factors to consider in the choice of a particular treatment option. Infertility counselors can make sure that clients/patients have all the relevant information by encouraging them to ask prudent questions. Too often, one will see a 47-year-old woman repeatedly wanting to do 'just one more' IUI, believing that she will be the one to beat the odds and have that coveted biological child. Her physician just does not have the heart to say no, despite the dismal odds and increased risk of miscarriage and chromosomal anomalies should she actually beat the odds and conceive.

Although it is not an infertility counselor's job to tell patients when to terminate treatment, it is their professional responsibility to make sure that patients are armed with accurate information in an effort to increase the probability of wise decision-making. Patients need to be made aware when their own behavior interferes with their ability to act in their own best interest. It is not enough to just gather medical facts. Patients need to assess what the emotional costs of their fertility quest have been. Addressing quality-of-life issues is usually a helpful avenue to pursue with patients.

Nevertheless, it is very difficult for patients to give up on a life's dream and consider an alternate lifeplan, such as to use gamete donation, to adopt, or to be child-free. Yet if equipped with all the facts and given a supportive environment, most individuals will tend to find the resources to take better care of themselves and know when enough is enough.

Best Interests: His, Hers, Whose?

One of the most perplexing concerns for those immersed in the current reproduction hurricane concerns the concept of 'best interest'. Often, courts will rely on the 'best interest of the child' paradigm in an effort to make just and prudent decisions regarding custody and parental rights. This paradigm has been borrowed by critics of current reproductive medical practice, claiming that the best interest of the

potential offspring is in no way being served by those providers focused simply on creating pregnancies.

Practitioners of assisted reproductive technologies are further accused of abusing medical know-how for self-serving purposes. This is at the expense of their patient's well-being by underestimation of the implications of their technological successes. Even the more tolerant of these censors charge that because the technology is moving forward so quickly, due consideration has not been given to the social, physical, and psychological consequences of these medical advances.

It is evident that there are diverse perspectives held by different sectors of society when it comes to noncoital conception and having babies in today's world. The emerging issues stimulated by the advances in reproductive medicine lend themselves to the best-interest model, providing a context within which to examine some of the more pertinent dilemmas. However, reliance on the best-interest model alone cannot meet the needs of this challenge. Agreement on the best interests of a child is destined to be challenged by the immediate needs of the clients themselves. Only time and experience will bring even a semblance of clarity to these mind-boggling dilemmas. A number of burning ethical issues are currently being debated and scrutinized by both advocates and critics of reproductive medicine.

Anonymity or Nonanonymity: An Issue Unresolved

An increasingly common obstacle that patients face is the question of whether or not to participate in an open or closed third-party arrangement. (Open programs are nonanonymous arrangements in which the identity and information about the other is freely given. Closed or anonymous arrangements involves participants who have no identifying information about the other). Currently, many medical programs are based on what is now being challenged as an antiquated policy of anonymity. Until fairly recently, patients had little choice about whether or not they would have access to information about their third-party helper. Closed programs prevailed and were accepted as an appropriate path by which to pursue motherhood. Programs went to great lengths to protect the anonymity of participants, believing that this was in everyone's best interests. Participants did not have access to one another and were discouraged from asking for information about their donor or recipient.

Anonymity, however, is no longer the only option touted by professionals. More and more, one hears about the advantages of an open policy whereby information is provided to all participants. The level of openness might vary from program to program, but what seems clear is that there is an emerging trend toward more openness as opposed to strictly anonymous participation. The prudence of such programs is being debated among professionals, with mental health professionals becoming increasingly more uncomfortable with the typical anonymous policies that most collaborative programs advocate[37,38].

Infertility counselors are obligated to examine with their clients the pros and cons of such a policy, using the best-interest model, in an effort to make an informed choice. Unfortunately, because most programs are anonymous, patients do not really have the choice to select freely. Until clinics begin offering the option of non-anonymity or until a central donor registry is mandated in the USA as in other countries, patients may not independently select a 'known' donor.

Disclosure/Nondisclosure

Somewhat related to the concept of anonymity is the issue of disclosure: disclosure to the child, family, or friends concerning genetic origins and gestational ties. The traditional dictate was a non-disclosure policy whereby no one needed to know that the family came to be through nontraditional means. It was believed that there was no benefit in informing children about their genetic origins and that children did not have an inherent right to know about their genetic/ gestational beginnings. Over time, the judiciousness of this advice has come into question as professionals ponder the psychological issue of genealogical bewilderment[39] and the negative impact that secrecy[40-42] has on family dynamics (see Chapter 25).

How does an infertility counselor counsel patients vis-à-vis the issue of one's inalienable right to know one's genetic origins and the parents' right to privacy? How does the best-interest perspective stay in focus when the best interests of the parents seemingly conflict with the child's right to know?

In infertility counselors' probing of the reasons for not telling, shame emerges as a theme more often than not, and often is what fuels a nondisclosure stance. There exists the illusion that if they do not tell, they are all shielded from the sadness of not having a family by traditional means; therefore, they do not have to face the humiliation of that reality. A poignant question arises about the wisdom of allowing individuals to create children through a process that they see as shameful. If collaborative reproduction is indeed a loving act, then why taint it with lies and deception?

Families who protect secrets develop a complicated system of interpersonal relationships and positions of power that is different from that of families that hold no big secrets. There is the risk that the child picks up on subtle cues that tell something is not quite right. This undercurrent can impact the family in a profound and insidious way. It can inadvertently promote family estrangement and create unhealthy alliances between those who know and those who do not know[39].

A secret of such magnitude can undermine the trust that is vital to a health parent-child relationship. Parents often live in fear of the unanticipated revelation of the secret. Over time, lies are built on lies, and more and more energy must be exerted to protect the secret. The threat of betrayal lurks in the shadows of the family's existence; if the truth ever became known, it would inevitably break the bond of trust that children have with their parents[43].

The opposing views of whether or not a child has the right to know about his or her genetic origins are compelling and offer infertility counselors a rich abundance of material to ponder and examine with their clients. Infertility counselors are respons-ible for providing a forum for patients to safely explore their feelings, using the best-interest model. The goal is for them to understand why they made a particular choice and feel comfortable with that choice, whether it is to disclose or not to disclose.

Sex Selection

Although the option of choosing the sex of one's child is more widely practiced among the fertile than the infertile, it does come up often enough in the practice of reproductive medicine to warrant giving it some discussion. Specialists will discourage the use of sex selection if it at all compromises the success of the procedure. These recommendations are based on medical prudence (e.g., sex-linked genetic disorders) rather than on moral grounds.

It is one thing to yearn for a child and want to procreate in the way that most people do. It is another to choose the sex of the desired child through technological manipulation. Sex selection is believed by many to push beyond what is seen as a decadent playground where eugenics is the name of the game. Nevertheless, if the sex selection is not for medical reasons but represents clear cultural differences and prejudices favoring one sex over another, counseling for those clients requires a culturally specific approach. It is under these circumstances that infertility coun-selors need to be well versed in the biases of the particular culture in order for useful and relevant counseling to occur. If this is not possible, counselors should reveal their lack of knowledge to clients and refer them to appropriate resources, if at all possible.

An alternative plan is that clients could educate the infertility counselor on their culture's specific values and beliefs and work accordingly. Sex selection in the United States seems to be viewed with more distaste than would perhaps be evident elsewhere. Counseling considerations must address the reasons why one sex is preferred over the other, the psychological aftermath of the disappointment if the process fails, and the meaning to the family if they were to have a child of the nonselected sex. If the sex selection is for genetic reasons, issues of prenatal testing and termination of an affected but wanted child must be addressed. In these cases, culture bias and stigma may be even greater due to lack of understanding of the genetic reasons for sex selection and/or termina-tion. Again, it is prudent for infertility counselors to work from the best-interest perspective when tackling this sensitive issue.

Fetal Reduction and Disposition of Extra Embryos

Reproductive specialists have inadvertently paved the way for an increased need for patients to consider yet another tech-nological intervention, selective reduction. Fetal reduction is a technological tool often used to make good on what is retro-spectively an ill-conceived medical decision, that is, the transfer of too many embryos or proceeding with a superovul-ation cycle in which there is potential for excessive oocytes to be fertilized. In determining the optimal number of embryos to transfer, physicians struggle with finding the right balance between increasing the likelihood of success and minimizing the risk of a multiple gestation. Of course, this 'choice' is government-mandated in some countries (e.g., Great Britain, Canada).

Unfortunately, selective reduction is too often viewed as a quick fix to an unpalatable situation, with little fore-thought given to the psychological impli-cations for those involved. The parents have to live with their decision to eliminate one or more fetuses, and the child(ren) that are born could conceivable harbor un-resolved feelings of guilt from being the fetus(es) to survive. Infertility counselors, after the fact, often carry the burden of helping bereft patients make peace with a difficult and heartfelt decision. These patients, in the midst of their plight, are all too often ignorant of the fact that a multiple gestation is a feasible outcome. Their long struggle with infertility usually blinds them to this possibility, and often preprocedure counseling is not suggested or required by the medical clinic, highlighting why such care is imperative (see Chapters 12 and 24).

In other situations, infertility counselors may be called upon to assist in resolving a dispute regarding the disposition of jointly conceived embryos. Best-interest issues in these situations are difficult even under ideal circumstances. When couples have conflicting interests regarding their embryos, infertility counselors are chall-enged to help them reach an equitable resolution in an arena that has no precedent.

Bringing more havoc to the arena of technological reproduction is the dis-position of unused or 'extra' embryos. With increased successes, clinics have been forced to stockpile extra or abandoned cryopreserved embryos created by those patients successful in their initial attempts to conceive. The moral question crossing the minds of many involved in this field is what to do with this growing abundance of embryos. This is a moral question for which there are no simple answers. Most medical clinics have provisions for the disposition of extra embryos that usually include three options: donation, destruction, or research. Each option has moral implications and can weigh heavily on patients trying to make a decision where none of the choices feel quite right.

The question reemerges: What is the status of an embryo? Is an embryo a human being, or is an embryo property and to be treated as such? A related point of contention is: When does life begin, at conception or at birth. Although the philosophical discourse con-tinues, a middle-of-the-road position holds that embryos be given special status in regard to the potential to become a human being[14]. There are no pat solutions to these morally complex dilemmas. Infertility counselors can help patients find some peace in the choices that they make by acknowledging the difficulties surrounding these issues and, whenever possible, by ensuring or encourag-ing clear couple agreement about treatment.

Posthumous Conception

Posthumous conception has become increasingly available as technology im-proves and public awareness grows. The freezing of gametes for men and women about to undergo medical treatment that would compromise or harm their fertility has been accepted and utilized as a means to preserve genetic continuity. The intent is to reproduce a child after treatment ceases.

In some cases, his or her illness leads to death, and the surviving spouse may choose to use the gametes to have a child. The goal is not to parent posthumously, but ultimately to parent children with whom there is a genetic tie to the deceased. These medical applications are generally considered ethical and appropriate response to a potential life-altering illness.

However, as with many scientific advances, there is the potential of abusing the technology and going too far. Infertility counselors have been called on to help in the decision-making regarding extracting a deceased man's sperm for the purpose of having a child, whether it be with his wife, fiancee, or girlfriend, or to help parents become grandparents by using a deceased child's gametes for fertilization with a donor and/or surrogate. All too often, infertility counselors are not called on when such plans are set in motion, but after the fact, to 'mop up' deteriorating situations.

Clinicians must ask: What is the moral obligation to the child? What about the bereft individual wanting to use the embryos or sperm? This is an area that leaves almost everyone associated with these unusual situations uncomfortable and somewhat bewildered as to how to proceed. The counseling issues are multifaceted and complex and require careful consideration and exploration with the patient as to the implications of proceeding.

The focus in such cases should be on what would be in the *child's* best interest relative to the circumstances of his or her birth. Is it better to have never been born, or is it better to have been created and inherit a most challenging and controversial birthright? Infertility counselors are being asked to participate in such reproductive plans as a way to ease this questionable process for both clients who seek these services and medical providers who can make it happen. There are no immediate solutions to these ethically troubling issues.

FUTURE IMPLICATIONS

No consensus can be expected from the legal, psychological, medical, or religious communities on the ethical nature or legal status of the new reproductive technologies. The cliché that, in the world of reproductive medicine, choices are no longer black and white but all shades of gray is truly an understatement when it comes to the vast possibilities reproductive medicine holds up to vulnerable, desperate and pained individuals trying to do what most people can do so easily, naturally, and with so little forethought: conceive and grow a child.

Once seen as a shameful secret, infertility is emerging as a huge frontier of medicine with implications for the future that we can only begin to imagine. More and more, infertility counselors will encounter these issues and will be called upon to help patients and medical practitioners find their way. At a bare minimum, infertility counselors must be prepared and educated on the basic concepts. The controversies inherent to this highly specialized area only add to the growing list of contradictions and professional challenges.

The primary responsibilities of infertility counselors is to try to save clients from making careless or ill-advised decisions due to their own desperate state. They must listen, integrate, listen, and reintegrate the multifaceted concerns and issues that crowd the world of reproductive decision-making. Infertility counselors must examine and explore with clients the broad range of issues and perspectives that are relevant to each particular case. It is the infertility counselors' primary responsibility to demand (in a therapeutic sense) that clients look at as many ramifications of their decision-making as possible, to produce the best result for all concerned.

The longer mental health professionals work in the area of reproductive medicine, the more loaded the issues become. With scientists having now successfully cloned a sheep and monkey, praise, fear, and dread are emerging from various circles as we begin our descent of the slippery slope toward cloning a human being. Care must be taken to separate the cloning issue from reproductive medicine to protect ourselves and clients from a backlash that would put unreasonable constraints on the reproductive technologies currently available. Only time and experience will bring even a semblance of clarity to these mind-boggling dilemmas.

The jurisdiction of responsibility for infertility counselors is limitless, with vague parameters regarding guidance for patients. While addressing the needs of patients, infertility counselors must still respect the common good. Some of the ethical challenges are bound by legal jurisdiction, others by medical priorities and goals, and still others by religious perspectives, none of which is wholly adequate and many of which are contradictory. Infertility counselors are obligated to adjust the boundaries of traditional practice to meet the needs of this growing and changing field, while following their profession's dictates. As their client's advocate—whether the infertile, the surrogate, the gestational carrier, or the gamete donor—all mental health professionals must remain loyal to their professional ethics and personal legal liability, while protecting themselves from being drowned in waters that are getting as muddy as they are deep.

SUMMARY

- A practitioner must have and maintain expertise as an infertility counselor to avoid malpractice suits based on negligence.
- Infertility counselors should have all parties sign waivers of confidentiality, precluding suits based on breach of confidentiality and providing clarification of their role and duties.
- Infertility counselors are duty-bound to keep accurate records of all tests and interactions with clients and make sure that they are stored and/or disposed of properly.
- If an infertility counselor screens potential participants out of a program, it should be based on recognized psychological assessments and criteria.
- Financial separation from the medical team protects practitioners from claims of bias based on personal financial gain.
- Conflicts about release of records to potential offspring and recipients should be resolved before the parties begin participation.
- Clear and detailed psychological consent documents should be obtained and signed by all parties.
- Consent to release any psychological information or test results must be obtained prior to initiation of the assessment process.
- Third-party reproduction is an unsettled area of the law. Due to the absence of legislation, reproductive contracts may be ruled to be unenforceable.
- It is an infertility counselor's responsibility to inform all participants as to the role that (s)he will serve at the outset.
- Infertility counselors must be respectful of their clients' religious and cultural biases with regard to reproductive decision-making.
- Persons rejected from participation should be informed what the reason for the rejection is and whether there is any action that might change that decision.
- Infertility counselors should remove themselves from working on any cases in which their moral or personal

attitudes may interfere with their professional judgment.

• Indications of coercion or pathology in

collaborative arrangements are grounds for nonacceptance.

REFERENCES

1. American Psychological Association. *Ethical Principles of Psychologists and Code of Ethics*. Washington, DC: American Psychological Association, 1992
2. American Psychological Association. Ethical principles of psychologists and code of conduct. *Am Psychol* 1992
3. American Psychiatric Association. *Principles of Medical Ethics with Annotation. Especially Applicable to Psychiatry*. Washington, DC: American Psychiatric Association, 1994
4. National Association of Social Workers. *Code of Ethics of the National Association of Social Workers*. Washington, DC: National Association of Social Workers, 1993
5. California Association of Marriage and Family Therapists. *Ethical Standards for Marriage and Family Therapists*. San Diego, CA: California Association of Marriage & Family Therapists, 1992
6. Gelis J. *History of Childbirth*. Boston, MA: Northeastern University Press, 1991
7. Asbell B. *The Pill*. New York: Random House, 1995
8. Pope Paul VI. *Humanae Vitae*. Vatican, 1968
9. *Roe v Wade*, 410 US 113 (1973)
10. Constitution. Beijing: Chinese National People's Congress, 1982
11. Cohen C. *New Ways of Making Babies*. Bloomington, IN: Indiana University Press, 1996:156
12. In the matter of Baby M, 537 A2nd 1227 (NJ 1988)
13. *Johnson v Calvert*, 822 P2d 1317 (1992)
14. Hall C. Lover wins custody of dead man's sperm. *Los Angeles Times*, Feb. 23, 1997
15. Maugh II T. Scientists report cloning adult. *Los Angeles Times*, Feb. 25, 1997
16. Robertson JA. *Children of Choice*. Princeton, NJ: Princeton University Press, 1994
17. Alpern K. *Ethics of Reproductive Technology*. New York: Oxford University Press, 1992
18. Francoeur RT. *Biomedical Ethics: A Guide to Decision Making*. New York: John Wiley &.

Sons, 1983:36
19. Beauchamp TL, Childress JF. *Principles in Biomedical Ethics*, 4th edn. London: Oxford University Press, 1996
20. Engelhardt HT Jr. *The Foundations of Bioethics*, 2nd edn. London: Oxford University Press, 1996
21. Griswold v Connecticut, 381 US 479 (1965)
22. *Eisenstadt v Baird*, 405 US 438 (1972)
23. *Casey v Planned Parenthood*, 112 SCt 2791 (1992)
24. *California Senate Bill* 1555
25. Mental Health Professional Group of the American Society for Reproductive Medicine. *Qualification guidelines for mental health professionals in reproductive medicine*. Birmingham, AL: American Society for Reproductive Medicine, 1995
26. *Bruni v Tatsumi*, 346 NE2nd 673 (1976)
27. The Standard Evidence Code of the State of California, 1992: Secs. 1010–27
28. *Skinner v Oklahoma*, 316 US 535 (1942)
29. Ethics Committee of the American Society for Reproductive Medicine. *Ethical Considerations of Assisted Reproductive Technologies*. Birmingham, AL: American Society for Reproductive Medicine, 1994;62(suppl):s1
30. Ornstein P. Looking for a donor to call Dad. *New York Times Magazine*. June 18, 1995
31. *Salgo v Leland Stanford Jr University Board of Trustees*, 317 P2nd 170 (1957)
32. *Natanson v Kline*, 186 Kan 393 (1960)
33. Breckenridge Jr PG. *California Jury Instructions Civil, Book of Approved Jury Instruction* Vol. 1, 8th edn. St Paul, MN: West Publishing, 1994:198(6.11)
34. American Law Institute. *Restatement of the Law, Torts*. St. Paul, MN: American Law Institute Publishers 1991:240–2
35. Oocyte donation: Recommendation of the National Advisory Board on Ethics in Reproduction. *NABER Rep.* 1995;1:2

36. Freda MC. Childbearing, reproductive control, aging women and healthcare: The projected ethical debates. *J Obstet Gynecol Neonatal Nurs* 1994;23:144–51

37. Cooper SL, Glazer ES. *Beyond Infertility: The New Paths to Parenthood.* New York: Lexington Books, 1994

38. Imber-Black E. *Secrets in Families and Family Therapy.* New York: Norton, 1993

39. Brodzinsky D, Schechter DE, Henig RM. *Being Adopted: The Lifelong Search for Self.* New York: Doubleday, 1992

40. Mahlstedt PP, Greenfeld DA. Assisted reproductive technology with donor gametes: The need for patient preparation. *Fertil Steril* 1989;52:908–14

41. Baran A, Pannor R. *Lethal Secrets: The Psychology of Donor Insemination: Problems and Solutions.* New York: Warner, 1989

42. Noble E. *Having Your Baby by Donor Insemination: A Complete Resource Guide.* Boston, MA: Houghton Mifflin, 1987

43. Kirk HD. *Shared Fate: A Theory and Method of Adoptive Relationships.* Port Angeles, WA: Ben-Simon Publications

28

Physicians and Nurses: Counseling the Infertile Patient

Diane N. Clapp, BSN, RN, and G. David Adamson, MD

Healing depends on listening with the inner ear—
stopping the incessant blather, and listening.

Marion Woodman

HISTORICAL OVERVIEW

For many years, most physicians and many nurses were not aware of the significant psychological sequelae associated with infertility. Indeed, it was commonly believed that psychological problems caused infertility rather than being the result of them. It is true that disruption of the hypothalamic-pituitary-ovarian axis secondary to psychological stress can cause infertility. Theoretically, stress could also cause immune dysfunction affecting implantation or abnormal catecholamine release affecting tubal function. However, these are very uncommon causes of infertility. What we do know is that psychological stress almost always accompanies infertility and that serious dysfunction is not unusual.

Much of the credit for this awareness belongs to Barbara Eck Menning[1], who in 1980 described couples' response to the infertility experience based on the Kübler-Ross grief reaction. This seminal article, appearing in a highly regarded scientific journal, for the first time made many physicians and nurses aware of the psychological aspects of infertility. Since then significant efforts by National RESOLVE, the Nurses Professional Group, and the Mental Health Professional Group of the American Society for Reproductive Medicine have dramatically increased our understanding of and attention to this aspect of infertility care. Today, these organizations provide excellent educational and scientific support to the lay, nursing, mental health, and medical communities.

The purpose of this chapter is to further improve physician and nursing counseling of the infertile patients. It will address:

- a theoretical framework for identifying the important role physicians and nurses play in infertility counseling
- the focus of their counseling roles especially as it pertains to identifying appropriated referral sources, making a referral for counseling, and teamwork with infertility counselors
- strategies for helping couples identify their need for counseling and ways to cope with infertility.

REVIEW OF THE LITERATURE

Research in this area has been limited primarily because it has been difficult to perform well-designed trials in this area of medicine. We are not aware of any prospective randomized studies that reported outcomes assessment of physician and nurse office counseling. Yet our understanding of the clinical approach to infertile couples has become reasonably sophisticated through retrospective studies. The major obstacle is not so much knowing what to do as it is the education of health professionals and routine implementation of effective counseling in the daily care of infertile couples.

THEORETICAL FRAMEWORK

Infertility is described by Greil[2] as, 'Not really a pathological condition, rather it is the absence of a desired condition'. Mahlstedt[3] characterized the infertility experience as a series of losses: loss of a dream, loss of self-esteem, loss of security, and loss of fantasy. Later models described the infertility experience as a developmental challenge necessitating new coping mechanisms. Infertility has many of the characteristics of chronic illness. It often goes on for a prolonged period of time, outcome is uncertain, and the emotional effect can be significant. Like those suffering from chronic illness, the infertile couple usually feels that the quality of their life is adversely affected. Infertility begins to engulf their lives. Work schedules, vacations, sex life, and the ability to socialize with friends and family are all impacted. Clearly, infertility is not just a medical challenge, but one necessitating that a couple mobilize together to negotiate through the work-up, treatments, decision-making, and eventually resolution.

Recognizing the differences in how women and men perceive and respond to infertility is important. Generally, women perceive infertility as a direct threat to their personal, social, and cultural identity. Women often describe the feelings associated with infertility as a failure to live up to a lifelong expectation and as the loss of a dream. They express a sense of being out of control of their lifeplan and of their bodies. Statements such as 'feeling defective' are not uncommon. For men, the primary threat appears to be to their marital relationship. Men become preoccupied with the impact of infertility on their wife's quality of life. Men often are less in touch initially with the loss aspect of infertility and more concerned about how to help their partner cope with this experience. Men often discount their feelings as 'not worth dwelling on' and quickly refer to how difficult the experience has been for their partner[4]. Men and women tend to shield their partner from their individual distress, disappointment, and humiliation. Women take the emotional pain on themselves. Men sympathize and search for solutions. To the physician or nurse, the couple may appear as a 'united front' ready to comply with whatever is required. This may both mask the level of distress experienced by each partner and give the false impression that, 'As a couple, they are doing well'.

It has been suggested that there are four psychological tasks that infertile couples must complete in order to deal effectively with their infertility[5]:

- verbalization of their feelings
- grieving
- evaluation of the reasons why they want a child
- decision-making.

Both nurses and physicians must determine which tasks the couple is most involved with, so that an appropriate approach to meet their needs can be developed.

Davis and Dearman[6] identified six strategies for coping with infertility. These are:

- *Increasing space between themselves and reminders of infertility.* Physicians and nurses can assist patients by helping to identify activities and life work not associated with infertility. Some women find talking to others about their infertility helpful, while others do not. It is important to respect this difference and not make patients feel guilty about finding their own ways to create space for themselves away from infertility.

- *Regaining control of their lives,* which may mean providing information to patients and identifying sources of support, as well as helping them develop plans with time frames for dealing with their infertility. It is also helpful for physicians and nurses to help couples maintain a positive attitude about their ability to cope with their infertility and develop positive coping strategies.

- *Providing written treatment plans, long-range treatment goals, or decision trees, or assuring patients that they will be told if/when success appears unlikely.* This might involve optimizing their weight and appearance, discontinuing habits such as smoking, or being more creative sexually. Physicians and nurses should encourage their patients to identify areas in their lives in which they can excel or take control to help restore self-esteem and pursue activities that they enjoy.

- *Finding hidden meaning in infertility.* This may involve religion, faith, or spirituality, as defined by the patient, but it also involves stepping back and assessing positive aspects, for example, more information about etiology of infertility from a failed in vitro fertilization (IVF) cycle or better communication with their partner.

- *Giving in to feelings.* Physicians and nurses can help by validating the feelings and responses such as crying, avoiding unpleasant tasks (e.g., housekeeping) or being self-indulgent.

- *Sharing the burden,* perhaps with husband, family, friends, physicians, nurses, the infertility counselor and/or support groups.

It has also been found that physicians, nurses, and patients have different perceptions of the infertility experience[7]. Overall, nurses perceived the emotional and physical stress on infertile patients to be higher than the patients themselves perceived it to be, and physicians rated the stress on patients as lower than nurses or patients did. Physicians, nurses, and patients all rated the emotional difficulty of routines and events as being greater than the physical. All agreed that the most emotionally difficult ratings of infertility distress were associated with failed attempts at conception (e.g., interrupted IVF cycle, negative pregnancy test, onset of menses, ectopic pregnancy, or miscarriage). Next in degree of stress were specific procedures (e.g. gamete intrafallopian transfer, egg retrieval, laparotomy). Older physicians and nurses perceived patients to experience less stress than younger physicians and nurses. However, as the amount of professional experience with infertility increased, nurses perceived patients to have more stress, while physicians perceived less. There was no difference between male and female physicians. Interestingly, patients viewed the decision to begin adoption proceedings as less stressful than did their physicians and nurses.

Overall, nurses gave higher ratings of physical and emotional difficulty than physicians on all factors except medications. The presence of expanding technologies in reproductive medicine may put increasing demands on technical expertise and medical procedures for physicians and make it harder to focus on psychological aspects. This may create greater role separation between physicians, nurses, and mental health professionals. It is clear that a teamwork approach among physicians, nurses, and mental health workers, is necessary to optimize psychological care of infertile couples.

Berg and Wilson[8] showed that psychological issues change during the course of infertility treatment. Couples experienced more emotional stress in the first year, less in the second, and more again in the third. Bonding within the marriage and sexual fulfillment remained satisfactory in the first 2 years, but problems often developed in the third year. Areas of focus were sexual functioning, marital adjustment, and psychological distress. They concluded that psychological treatment should focus on communication issues at first, then feelings of low self-esteem, and then the sense of loss. Obviously, these stages can overlap and are not invariable. Physicians and nurses need to be aware of these stages in order to adapt their treatments and appropriately respond to patients.

Imparting knowledge can be difficult because of the complexity of the clinical situation[9]. Many factors affect how individuals process information, and couples routinely forget much of what they are told. Significantly, they are just as likely to forget critical information as the less meaningful information.

Importantly, several studies which have been reviewed by Reading and Kerrin[9] indicated that psychometric testing of infertile women showed them to be essentially normal. Therefore, psychological counseling is usually focused on communication issues, marital or sexual issues, or facilitation of decision-making—all issues directly resulting from infertility. Physicians and nurses must remember that not all couples are self-aware of the psychodynamics of their situation or the causes of their distress or depression. Additionally, while many couples say that psychological services are desired, most feel that they are more needed by others, and do not recognize how they may personally be helped by them. Careful questioning

and gentle recommendations for counseling are necessary in these situations. Suggestions for how to make referrals are found later in the chapter.

CLINICAL ISSUES AND THERAPEUTIC INTERVENTIONS

Physicians

Physicians and nurses have both similar and differing roles and responsibilities in counseling infertile patients. Physicians are responsible for consultation, medical decision-making, and provision of sophisticated technical, laboratory, and operative interventions. They must be able to provide these services, however, within the context of the psychological status of the patient and his/her partner. Therefore, they must be able to recognize and appreciate this context and be able to utilize additional nursing and mental health resources when necessary.

Part of the physician's role in counseling is to provide accurate and comprehensive facts to the couple to help them decide how to manage their infertility. Interventions that are generally worth considering include[10]:

- an accurate assessment of prognosis
- description of benefits (value and probabilities of success) and costs (financial, time, physical and emotional)
- discussion of loss of control and ways to increase control
- activities to decrease stress
- alternative forms of affection and sexual communication
- facilitation of access to information and emotional support.

Couples should be able to proceed at their own pace, within medically appropriate guidelines. Physicians should freely offer second opinions if patients appear to desire one or are excessively questioning or concerned about the treatment plan. Physicians should counsel patients that they may have problems coping with some aspects of their investigation and treatment because of the physical discomfort or emotional stress[11]. They need to counsel couples about problems associated with success, that is, the increased rate of pregnancy loss and other obstetrical and neonatal complications associated with infertile patients. Couples also need to be informed about the dramatic changes in lifestyle which occur with parenting and the need not to have unrealistic expectations for themselves or their child. Sometimes, the physician just needs to be 'there', to listen, to comfort, and 'to take on sadness from time to time', to become frustrated and tired, but not to lose patience[12].

It is important to have the best possible office ambience, including adequate facilities, congenial surroundings, an efficient and pleasant staff, and an ability to avoid stress-promoting situations. This requires the ability to see the man and woman separately or together, to provide adequate time for consultation, and to have special areas for infertile patients away from obstetrical patients. The whole team should be involved in the support effort, but it is the physician's responsibility to set the tone.

Easily recognizable signs that may alert physicians to patients having problems dealing with the psychological issues of infertility include:

- difficulty or delay in making decisions
- not following directed care
- obvious emotional distress at visits
- differences of opinion with spouse
- expressed difficulties at work
- financial problems associated with treatment
- sexual problems
- multiple phone calls
- missed appointments
- inappropriate behavior to office staff.

Overall, physicians need to provide counseling within the context of the primary focus of medical care. They must recognize the high degree of dependence patients have on them and their general reluctance to injure or threaten that relationship. They need to be especially sensitive to signs of difficulty, be able to provide timely, appropriate, and compassionate support and information, and refer patients to nursing staff or mental health professionals for specific situations as necessary. Most physicians do not have the time or expertise to provide sophisticated counseling services to infertile patients in serious need of help. It is important for physicians to help patients understand that they are not being pushed away but are being referred so that excellent care can be provided by health care personnel.

Nurses

Nurses are not only medical providers but also teachers and counselors, and have a pivotal role in patient care. Often, nurses will have a better 'feel' for the psychological status of the couple because they spend more time with them and have a different focus in their interactions. The couple may be more comfortable with nurses and unwilling to jeopardize their relationship with the physician. Nurses (as well as physicians) need to recognize the degree of distress, depression, and anxiety experienced by couples, and, in a limited period of time, identify the most critical areas on which to focus. These include:

- education
- assessment and support
- referral
- teamwork

Education

Education is a critical part of the nurse's counseling role. Patients need to know the specifics of procedures and tests. Knowing how long a test will take, how it is going to feel, when results will be returned, and what the treatment plan is can help patients feel some sense of control. Patients need to have specific instruction about injections, side effects of drugs, and procedures.

In the role as educator, nurses should recognize that the patient's high anxiety levels often preclude easy absorption of factual knowledge. Studies have shown that patients usually fail to remember as much as 50% of information presented to them in a consultation. For that reason, it is important to repeat instructions and have instructions in writing. Educational materials in handout form, as well as giving one-on-one instruction, reduces levels of anxiety and increases the patients' sense of control. Because of the significant isolation that patients experience, educational sessions run by the clinic as group instruction can be beneficial. Participants can benefit from others' questions as well as recognizing that they are not alone. Feeling less isolated can reduce anxiety and increase the ability to cope.

Part of the educational role of nurses is to normalize the typical emotional reaction to the infertility crisis. It is important to acknowledge studies which have shown that women experiencing infertility have the same depression and anxiety levels as women experiencing life-threatening diseases like cancer and heart disease[13]. This validates a couple's experience and demonstrates that the nurse is aware of how intensely infertility is causing distress and threatening their sense of well-being. In addition, the loss of innocence that couples experience when they confront the infertility experience can impact on how they navigate their course of treatment.

Anticipatory guidance is a form of education and counseling that can be well implemented by nurses. It is essential to explain to couples that rarely are couples 'in synch'. Men and women do not respond to infertility in the same way or necessarily at the same time. Mentioning that couples often experience tension as they navigate infertility and that infertility treatment can impact on sexuality and intimacy can be reassuring to couples. Discussing the fairly common problems of impotency during postcoital tests or difficulty in collecting a semen specimen for analysis can make couples feel more 'normal', as well as providing opportunities for them to think of solutions for themselves.

Explaining to couples that infertility treatment is elective, that they can stop any time and that the medical team recognizes the need for couples to take a break is important. It is helpful to ask the couple about how much money they anticipate spending on infertility treatment. In many states treatment is not well covered by insurance and this can deplete financial resources, causing an additional burden and stress. Helping couples set realistic financial and time limits can empower them when facing difficult decisions, which is not to say these cannot later be reevaluated.

Another aspect of education is discussion with couples of the availability of infertility counselors. Referencing this *before* a couple is in crisis can take away any stigma they may associate with 'going into therapy'. Information about support/discussion groups within the practice or through a local RESOLVE chapter or providing the phone number of a therapist can be invaluable. Isolation and loneliness are common feelings that infertile patients describe. Loneliness is inversely related to social support. Studies have shown how social support and spousal support can help patients adjust to distressing events. This is particularly true for those experiencing infertility.

Table 1 Would a support group be helpful for you?

You may be hesitant to join a support group because of some assumptions about what happens at the group:

Myth	Fact
Being in a RESOLVE support group is like going to therapy	No, a support group is not designed to offer professional counseling or psychological therapy. It is, however, therapeutic to talk with others about the intense experience of infertility
I'll have to bare my soul and talk about the most private areas of my life	It is up to you to decide how much information and emotion to share with the group. You remain in control
A support group will go on for months	RESOLVE support groups are limited to 10–12 sessions
Joining a support group of infertile women or couples will just make me feel worse	You will receive support for your pain and disappointment and will also learn new methods of coping that can help you move forward

If any of the following statements apply to you, you may want to consider joining a RESOLVE support group:

I'm feeling lonely and isolated.

I have very few people to talk with about my infertility. No one understands!

Everyone I know is pregnant or has children.

My husband/wife is the only one I have who provides emotional support.

Infertility is affecting my work and career.

I feel that my life plan is out of control.

I'm having trouble navigating through my medical treatment options.

I can't decide when 'enough is enough'.

Holidays and coping with family and friends are becoming more and more difficult.

An example of a tool that can help nurses identify couples who may be helped by support groups and counseling is shown in Table 1. Questionnaire tools may be helpful in measuring the specific effects of infertility on self-esteem, blame/guilt, and sexuality. Such educational tools can help the couple understand the impact of infertility on their lives and also provide physicians and nurses with information to help with management, counseling, and/or referral. Management plans need to be individualized[14].

Giving written materials about resources enables couples to save them for future use and not have to ask for them when they are in crisis. If the time comes for a nurse to refer a couple to a mental health professional, she can refer to the material provided at an earlier appointment.

If a gynecology or reproductive endocrinology clinic has a mental health professional who is part of the team, it is helpful to have a flyer sent to new patients introducing the mental health services, indicating the office location, office hours, fees, and types of services provided. If the office or clinic has a newsletter or publication for patients, having the mental health professional write an article about coping can be helpful. Including the mental health provider in staff meetings can enhance the team building approach to comprehensive care. Referrals to a mental health provider are made more easily when the patients feel that the mental health provider was recommended and held in high esteem by the physician and the nurse.

Assessment

Throughout the diagnostic and treatment phase, nurses should assess an individual's and couple's psychological status. There are verbal and non-verbal clues to be alert to. Three specific characteristics that influence infertile patients' behavior in the clinical setting result from infertility being an un-anticipated life crisis, a narcissistic injury, and a process which requires mourning and grieving before resolution. In terms of unanticipated life crisis and narcissistic injury, couples' behavior indicates that they feel confused and out of control with their bodies. Giving couples a sense of control whenever possible is important. Allowing them to determine how much of a diagnostic work-up they want to do, and when, and ensuring that they are informed consumers before making treatment choices helps them regain a sense of control. Patients frequently tell their nurses that they feel 'crazy' or 'disorganized'. At this stage they need reassurance and written information which can be filtered through their high anxiety levels. Infertility patients inevitably feel guilt about their infertility. They are plagued by the 'why me?' questions. Being aware of the potential for self-blame and reassuring patients that infertility is a disease, not something they caused by 'bad' behavior, is essential. Nurses should avoid using medical terminology such as 'hostile cervical mucus' and 'multiple aborter'; terminology that may increase patients' self-blame.

Some infertility patients may experience denial. Frequently, husbands and wives have different levels of denial. Husbands may feel hopeful and wives may feel despair. Often, at this stage, nurses and physicians witness the anger and bargaining behavior frequently resorted to by infertility patients. Bargaining behavior results from patients' efforts to hold at bay the grief that they sense may be ahead. An important role of nurses is to help patients do a reality test. Both physicians and nurses must be aware of how results and summaries of particular treatment cycles are presented to patients and keep in mind that for every statistical statement, there is a positive and negative interpretation[9]. If there is a 20% success rate, there is also an 80% failure rate. Nurses need to be aware of what patients' perceptions are of the success and failure rates.

Patients gradually begin to come to terms with the losses involved in infertility—the losses of their life-plans, and not being in synch with their peers in society. Often at this stage, the question of who and what to tell arises. Couples become isolated and find that holidays such as Christmas and Hanukkah, Thanksgiving, and even Halloween, are painful reminders of what is not happening in their lives.

How couples respond to the infertility life crisis depends on their individual resiliency in the face of life crises, their marital adjustment to this experience, and their history of coping with crisis as a couple. Long-term infertility can result in chronic grief. Each unsuccessful cycle can feel like a death to couples. There are no endings. The appointments and new therapies represent new hope but also are reminders of what has not worked. Some patients doggedly pursue treatment. They appear to be afraid of ending treatment for several different reasons. The couple may not agree about which options to consider in the future. This is particularly true if one partner wants to consider adoption or child-free living and the other does not. This difference may keep them in

Table 2 Questions that nurses can use to help individuals or couples address their feelings regarding unsuccessful treatment and to assess their coping skills

---

Have you and your partner talked about a time frame for continuing or ending treatment?

Are you aware that the monthly disappointments of not being pregnant result in feelings ranging from jealousy of pregnant women to grief and mourning? (It is important to validate this experience and, if appropriate, mention the various components such as disbelief, anger, guilt, and sorrow.)

What is the hardest part of having the treatment not work?

For you, is the greatest loss not experiencing a pregnancy or not being a parent?

Do you have any regrets or 'if onlys' that are troubling you?

Who is your source of emotional support and comfort?

Who, if anyone, would you be disappointing if treatment continues to be unsuccessful or you decide to stop treatment?

Are you beginning to gather information on other treatment options or family-building alternatives?

---

treatment, often in the face of dismal odds. The other reason that some patients persist in following medical options, often beyond what is 'reasonable', is that they do not feel strong enough to address the grief that stopping treatment would trigger. Table 2 identifies tools to help patients address when 'enough is enough'.

Referrals

Nurses and physicians should be alert to signs of distress which warrant referral to a mental health provider[15]:

- change in eating habits
- disturbed sleep patterns
- social isolation
- difficulty at work
- inability to concentrate
- increasing sense of hopelessness
- loss of interest in activities that used to give enjoyment
- problems with relationships
- expressions of suicidal thoughts
- primary sexual dysfunction (e.g., erectile dysfunction)

- obsessive-compulsive behaviors
- diffuse anxiety
- diminished ability to accomplish tasks
- decreased ability to focus
- change in appetite or weight
- increased use of drugs or alcohol or evidence of drug-seeking behaviors

Certain situations that are commonly part of the infertility experience can be helped by brief, focused counseling. These include[15]:

- decisions about assisted reproductive technologies, using donor gametes, stopping treatment, alternative treatments, or multifetal reduction
- couple distress as a result of the infertility experience
- intense or prolonged feelings of loss and grief
- symptoms of menopause
- single parenting
- previous elective abortion or multiple pregnancy losses
- prior adoption placement
- older parenting

Table 3 Questions that nurses can urge patients to ask in selecting a mental health professional

Where did the therapist attend college and what degree does he or she have?

What was the length and specific area of concentration of the professional's clinical training?

When was his/her practice established?

Which professional organizations is he or she a member of?

Does the counselor have experience with infertility issues and treatments including assisted reproductive technologies? Does the therapist have experience with pregnancy loss, adoption, surrogacy, donor gametes, or child-free issues?

What is the professional's approach? Is medication used? Are special techniques or 'homework' utilized? Is hypnotherapy used?

How often would the sessions be? How long are they?

What is the fee for the initial interview? What is the per-session fee? Is there a sliding scale or payment plan? Is insurance accepted?

Would the therapist like to talk with the medical personnel who have been involved with your care?

- critical health histories (e.g., cancer, sexual abuse)
- mourning after a pregnancy loss or selective fetal reduction
- need to explore other family-building options.

Helping patients recognize the need for a counseling referral and empowering them to follow through with the referral are the responsibility of nurses and physicians. A referral can be supported by statements such as, 'You deserve to have someone to talk to about these issues' or 'Many of our patients have benefited from talking with a counselor'. In addition, asking patients whether they would like the nurse or physician to speak to the therapist can reduce some of the anxiety that they may have about the referral. Nurses and physicians can help patients carefully evaluate the mental health professionals providing referral services (Table 3).

It is the physician's and nurse's responsibility to help set a sensitive environment for patients. It is essential to

have an atmosphere that supports couples dealing with infertility. This can extend to the type of artwork on the walls and the literature that is in the waiting room, as well as the quality of the staff and their sensitivity to the crisis that infertility patients may be experiencing. Nurses can be key in making sure that the team is sensitive and protective of couples, for example, by stressing the importance of privacy, such as not giving lab results over the phone when a whole waiting room can also hear. These small things can cause an emotional eruption in a patient who is already feeling fragile and vulnerable.

Deciding to end treatment is difficult not only for patients but also for nurses and physicians. At some point, couples have to move on to resolution and, in doing so, they may feel that they are disappointing the medical team. Feelings of loss as they terminate their relationship with the medical team that they may have known for months or years can be intense. It is helpful for physicians and/or nurses to do a follow-up letter, either personalized or generic, indicating that the practice is wishing the couple well and hopes to hear about what alternatives or options they decide upon. Having materials on alternatives in the waiting room, such as books on child-free living, adoption, donor insemination, donor egg, surrogacy, or newsletters from relevant organizations that discuss these alternatives, is essential. Follow-up calls to couples who have had a pregnancy loss also are part of the nurse's job as counselor. Grief following a pregnancy loss is intense and the nurse's reaching out is an important counseling tool.

Dealing with infertility and its resolution requires courage. Couples have to face deep pain as they grieve their physical and symbolic losses. Infertility forces them to make decisions that they did not want to make and to live a life that they would not have chosen. Nurses and physicians walk along the path with patients offering courage, hope, and counseling as needed. The goal of nurses working with infertility patients is to help couples to achieve not only live birth but also, in some cases, survive a life crisis and be able to look at options and make decisions that will lead to a full life after the exhausting experience of infertility.

Teamwork Among Physicians, Nurses, and Infertility Counselors

Physicians are responsible for overall patient care and are focused on the physical health of the patient and medical aspects of infertility treatment. They are trained to be able to diagnose and treat psychological problems and should be able to provide preliminary counseling for all patients. However, most physicians are limited by their interest, expertise, and time in providing sophisticated counseling services.

Many infertility nurses are very knowledgeable about the clinical issues of infertility. They have both a medical background and training in patient evaluation and counseling. Since they often spend more time with patients than physicians do, they are frequently able to provide excellent evaluation and counseling for infertile couples. However, many nurses are limited by training, experience, expertise, and/or time in dealing with the more serious or complex psychological issues of infertility, especially if these are compounded by other underlying pre-existing psychological issues.

Mental health professionals have training and experience in dealing with complex psychological issues and can provide the time and focus needed for management of these issues. However, they generally have more limited medical knowledge and may not be as aware of the subtleties of patients' medical care. The Mental Health Professional Group of the American Society for Reproductive Medicine has developed qualification guidelines for infertility counselors (see Appendix 1). These guidelines can be most helpful in evaluating the qualifications of a specific mental health professional.

It is clear that the optimal approach requires involvement of physicians, nurses, and mental health professionals. Most physicians will have a nurse or nurse practitioner working with them. It is physicians' responsibility to ensure that nurses are well trained in managing psychological issues. In large practices, it may be possible to have a nurse specializing in infertility counseling, but this is uncommon. In very large practices, it may be feasible to have an infertility counselor on staff to whom all patients are referred either before or after undergoing counseling with the nurse or as part of specific treatment plans (e.g., prior to IVF or donor insemination). The most critical aspect of this situation is to ensure that the roles of the physician, nurse, and mental health professional are clearly defined so that high quality, appropriate psychological support and care are provided.

Each infertility practice should establish guidelines for managing psychological issues. These might include providing all patients with educational materials regarding psychological issues they may experience, as well as the availability of support from the physician, nurse, RESOLVE and other support groups, and infertility counselors. This information should be reviewed briefly by the physician, and in more detail by the nurse.

In many practices, it is not possible to have a mental health professional on staff. It is important in these situations to identify at least one, and preferably more, infertility counselors skilled and interested in managing infertile patients. In these cases the mental health professionals should familiarize themselves with the practice, and the physician and/or nurse should ensure that the infertility counselor is aware of the expectations of the practice when patients are referred. In addition, it is important to have an agreement about how and what communications are desired and what the expectations of all the individuals involved are. In larger metropolitan areas, it may be possible to identify several infertility counselors, each of whom specializes in different areas of infertility (e.g., perinatal loss, third-party reproduction). This has the advantage of providing highly skilled counseling to patients who have different needs. However, it is imperative that effective communication be maintained between the practice and mental health professional to ensure consistency and realization of expectations.

Arguments can be made for both the employment of mental health professionals within an infertility clinic setting as well as their independent consulting outside of the clinic. The advantages of having infertility counselors on staff are that they are more familiar with the clinic protocols and issues,

have a better understanding of the expectations of the physicians and nurses, and can provide more specific and continuous input. They are also more available for crisis intervention and possibly more likely to be utilized. Advantages of external mental health consultants are that they are more independent of the clinics and are, theoretically, more objective in their management of couples because they have less conflict of interest. They may also be able to see patients from more than one practice and therefore have a more balanced view of different treatment approaches. In addition, some patients may need or want a different physical setting for discussing their feelings (see Chapter 26).

Since most infertile couples are dealing with a situational crisis alone, initial counseling may well consist of referral to RESOLVE and possibly a RESOLVE support group. Often, the education and support provided by RESOLVE are sufficient to help couples deal with their infertility. Such couples need to be willing and able to function in a support group setting.

Patients should have the choice of being referred for counseling or other support at any time. It is important that physicians and nurses be aware of resources in their practice and geographic area so that the best possible referrals can be made. Referrals may be to a nurse, a nurse specializing in infertility counseling, RESOLVE, or a mental health professional, depending on their evaluation of the problem in conjunction with the team.

Physicians or nurses may also suggest a referral based on their evaluation of the patient. Mandatory referral may be appropriate in selected situations, such as patients with a prior history of psychological problems, obvious unresolved psychological or marital distress, current psychological crisis (e.g., physical or sexual abuse, evidence of alcohol/drug abuse, or extreme psychiatric symptoms), or those considering the use of donor gametes or surrogacy.

FUTURE IMPLICATIONS

Assessment of the psychological needs of infertile couples is one important role of physicians and nurses in the psychological care of patients. Physicians and nurses need to be compassionate and empathetic and provide an environment conducive to discussion of psychological issues. Both physicians and nurses should be able to evaluate coping mechanics, and provide information on support groups, organizations, and infertility counselors.

Menning[1] has outlined the most important activities for physicians and nurses.

- treat infertility as a couple problem
- develop a plan of investigation and treatment
- offer emotional support and education, including giving permission to discontinue treatment
- respect the level of their expertise
- be accessible
- be aware of RESOLVE and other support group services.

Physicians and nurses also need to continue their efforts to educate medical professionals and the public about the psychological stresses of infertility. The benefits to a practice of providing good emotional support to their patients include[15]:

- more satisfied patients
- patients who take responsibility for their treatment choices
- patients who are happier and easier to treat
- patients who do not blame others
- patients who participate in treatment decisions
- emotionally healthy patients
- support for the medical staff
- resource for the medical staff.

SUMMARY POINTS

- Infertility is a life crisis resulting in a variety of responses from both involved partners.
- Physicians, nurses, and patients have different perspectives on the stresses involved.
- Understanding the male/female responses to infertility will assist the physician and nurse in counseling couples.
- Physicians and nurses have a responsibility to be aware of psychological issues affecting all patients and play a vital role in the team managing these issues.
- Physicians and nurses have a role in identifying and referring patients with unresolved psychological issues.
- Physicians and nurses have three roles: medical provider, patient educator, and counselor.
- Physicians and nurses need to provide anticipatory guidance regarding emotional stages that individuals usually experience throughout treatment.
- Physicians and nurses have an important role in assessing patients for signs of depression and other psychological problems and making correct referrals.
- Physicians and nurses have a role helping patients assess 'when enough is enough'.
- Sensitivity to the emotional state of infertility patients can be reflected in waiting room material, artwork, and in sensitizing support staff.
- Team work among physicians, nurses, and mental health professionals will ensure optimal patient outcomes.
- Different models for providing psychological support are appropriate in different clinical situations.
- Further education of physicians, nurses, patients, and the lay public is needed to improve the quality of counseling services for infertile patients.

REFERENCES

1. Menning BE. The emotional needs of infertile couples. *Fertil Steril* 1980;34:313–9
2. Greil AL. *Not Yet Pregnant.* NJ: Rutgers University Press, 1991
3. Mahlstedt P. The psychological component of infertility. *Fertil Steril* 1985;43:335–46
4. Cudmore L. Fertility counseling: A couple approach. *J Fertil Couns* 1996;2:13–16
5. Sawatzky M. Tasks of infertile couples. *J Obstet Gynecol Neonatal Nurs* 1981;10:132–3
6. Davis DC, Dearman CN. Coping strategies of infertile women. *J Obstet Gynecol Neonatal Nurs* 1991;20:221–8
7. Kopitzke EJ, Berg BJ, Wilson JF, Owens D. Physical and emotional stress associated with components of the infertility investigation: Perspectives of professionals and patients. *Fertil Steril* 1991;55:1137–43
8. Berg BJ, Wilson JF. Psychological functioning across stages of treatment for infertility. *J Behav Med* 1991;14:11–26
9. Reading AE, Kerrin J. Psychologic aspects of providing infertility services. *J Reprod Med* 1989;34:861–71
10. Sherrod RA. Coping with infertility: A personal perspective turned professional. *MCN* 1988;13:191–4
11. Harrison RF. Aims and objectives in the infertility clinic: The practical issues. *Int J Fertil* 1991;36:204–11
12. Bradney N. A piece of my mind. But not alone. *JAMA* 1986;255:41
13. Domar A, Zuttermeister B, Freidman R. The psychological impact of infertility: A comparison with patients with other medical conditions. *J Psychosom Obstet Gynaecol* 1993;14:45–52
14. Bernstein J, Mattox JH. An overview of infertility. *J Obstet Gynecol Neonatal Nurs* 1982;11:309–14
15. Mental Health Professional Group, American Society for Reproductive Medicine. *Physician's Guide For Referral to a Mental Health Practitioner.* Birmingham, AL: American Society for Reproductive Medicine, 1996

X. APPENDICES

Appendix 1

Qualification Guidelines for Mental Health Professionals in Reproductive Medicine

These guidelines were developed by the Mental Health Professional Group of the American Society for Reproductive Medicine to help determine the qualifications and training for mental health professionals working in reproductive medicine. Mental health professionals are playing an increasingly important role in reproductive medicine due to technological advances and recognition of the complex psychosocial issues faced by infertility patients. As a result, there is a growing need for the skills and services of trained infertility counselors to assist patients and staff. Infertility counseling includes psychological assessment, psychotherapeutic intervention, and psychoeducational support of individuals and couples who are experiencing fertility problems. A qualified infertility counselor should be able to provide the following services:

- psychological assessment and screening
- diagnosis and treatment of mental disorders
- psychometric testing (psychologist)
- decision-making counseling
- couple and family therapy
- grief counseling
- supportive counseling
- education/information counseling
- support group counseling
- referral/resource counseling
- staff consultation
- crisis intervention

- sexual counseling
- psychotherapy

The following guidelines suggest minimum qualifications and training of mental health professionals providing infertility counseling and psychological services. The mental health professional should have:

1. Graduate Degree in a Mental Health Profession

A master's or doctorate degree from an accredited program in the field of psychiatry, psychology, social work, psychiatric nursing, or marriage and family therapy. Curriculum and training should include psychopathology; personality theory; life cycle and family development; family systems theory; bereavement and loss theory; crisis intervention; psychotherapeutic interventions; individual, marital, and group therapy; and a supervised clinical practicum or internship in counseling.

2. License to Practice

A license (or registration/certification, where applicable) to practice in the mental health field in which the professional holds a graduate degree and as required by the state in which the individual practices.

3. Training in the Medical and Psychological Aspects of Infertility

Training in the medical aspects of infertility indicating knowledge of:

1. basic reproductive physiology
2. testing, diagnosis, and treatment of reproductive problems
3. etiology of male and female infertility
4. assisted reproductive technologies.

Training in the psychology of infertility indicating knowledge of:

1. marital and family issues associated with infertility, and the impact on sexual functioning
2. approaches to the psychology of infertility including psychological assessment, bereavement/loss, crisis intervention, post-traumatic stress, and typical/atypical responses
3. family-building alternatives including adoption, third-party reproduction, child-free lifestyle
4. psychological and couple treatments
5. the legal and ethical issues of infertility treatments

4. Clinical Experience

The mental health professional should have a minimum of one year clinical experience providing infertility counseling, preferably under the supervision of or in consultation with a qualified and experienced infertility counselor.

5. Continuing Education

Continuing education helps ensure continued growth in knowledge and skills. Regular attendance at course offered by the American Society for Reproductive Medicine or other professional organizations and educational institutions is recommended to provide continuing education in both the medical and psychological issues in reproductive health care.

Prepared by the Committee on Infertility Counseling Guidelines:

Sharon N. Covington, MSW, Chair
Linda D. Applegarth, EdD, Vice-Chair
Linda Hammer Burns, PhD, Vice-Chair
Suzan A Aydinel, PhD
Paul R Feldman, MD
Judith Parkes, MSW, RN
Deidra T Rausch, MSN, RNC

September 1995

Appendix 2

Comprehensive Psychosocial History for Infertility (CPHI)

This is not a psychometric test. Instead, it is a comprehensive psychological and social history of infertility designed to be used by a mental health or medical professional. It should provide the clinician with a global impression of the patient's history, stressors, functioning, and current psychosocial status relevant to infertility. Although the history provides guidelines for potentially disruptive responses, there are some areas that are red flags and indications for referral for more complete psychological evaluation and intervention. They include: (1) use or consideration of a donor/surrogate program, (2) prior psychiatric illness, (3) change in current mental status and/or exacerbation of prior psychiatric symptoms, (4) history of pregnancy loss, (5) history of cancer, (6) history of rape, (7) ambisexual patterns, and (8) current problems with substance abuse.

I. Reproductive History

A. Infertility
1. Current infertility: primary or secondary
2. History of past infertility

B. Pregnancy
1. Living children (stepchildren, adopted, donor offspring, placed for adoption)
2. Therapeutic abortion(s)
3. Spontaneous abortion(s)
4. Other perinatal loss: SIDS, death of child
5. High-risk pregnancy

C. History of genetic/chromosomal abnormalities
1. Cancer of the reproductive tract and/or chemotherapy
2. DES exposure
3. Congenital abnormalities of the reproductive tract
4. Family history of genetic disorders

II. Mental Status

A. Psychiatric history
1. Hospitalization for psychiatric illness
2. Psychiatric treatment
3. Treatment with psychotropic medication
4. Substance abuse

B. Current mental status
1. Symptoms of depression
2. Symptoms of anxiety/panic attacks
3. Symptoms of obsession
4. Current use of psychotropic medications
5. Current problem with substance abuse/addiction

C. Change in mental status

D. Exacerbation of prior psychiatric symptoms

III. Sexual History

A. Frequency and response

B. Function/dysfunction

C. Religious or cultural influence on sexual patterns or procreation beliefs

D. Sexual history
1. Function/dysfunction
2. Sexually transmitted disease
3. Prior sperm donor/surrogate

mother/consideration of use of donor gametes
4. Homosexual or ambisexual patterns
5. History of rape or incest

E. Changes in any sexual patterns secondary to infertility or medical treatment.

IV. Relationship Status

A. Marital
1. History of marriages/divorces
2. History of marital discord/therapy
3. Extramarital relationships
4. Current satisfaction/dissatisfaction

5. Ambivalence about medical treatment and reproductive technologies

B. Familial
1. History of dysfunctional family of origin
2. Recent deaths or births in family
3. History of numerous familial losses

C. Social
1. Available support system
2. Career disruptions or pressures
3. History of or current legal problems
4. Criminal conduct

(Reproduced from Burns LH, Greenfeld DA, for the Mental Health Professional Group. *CPHI: Comprehensive Psychosocial History for Infertility*. Birmingham, AL: American Society for Reproductive Medicine, 1990.)

Appendix 3
Personality Types and Infertility

Personality structure	Reaction to infertility
Obsessive: orderly, systematic, perfectionist, inflexible	Infertility is seen as punishment for letting things get out of control
Narcissistic: self-involved, angry, independent, perfectionist	Infertility is seen as an attack on autonomy and perfection of self
Borderline: demanding, impulsive, unstable	Infertility is seen as a threat of abandonment
Dependent: long suffering, depressed, submissive	Infertility is seen as expected punishment for worthlessness
Avoidant: remote, unsociable, uninvolved	Infertility and its procedures are seen as a dangerous invasion of privacy
Paranoid: wary, suspicious, blaming, hypersensitive	Infertility is seen as annihilating assault coming from everywhere outside of self

(Reproduced from Goldfarb JM, Rosenthal MB, Utian WH. Impact of psychological factors in the care of the infertile couple. *Semin Reprod Endocrinol* 1985;3:97; with permission.)

Appendix 4
Antepartum Questionnaire (APQ)

Directions: For questions 1–23 check the one answer that most closely applies to you.

1. Marital information:

0 ( ) married and living with husband

4 ( ) other (for example: single, separated, divorced)

2. I was separated from my mother when I was child or teenager:

4 ( ) yes

0 ( ) no

3. When I was growing up, my relationship with my mother was:

1 ( ) very close

2 ( ) close

3 ( ) fairly close

4 ( ) sometimes distant

5 ( ) distant

4. I believe that when I was growing up, my mother:

1 ( ) was very happy about being a mother

2 ( ) was satisfied with being a mother

3 ( ) accepted her role as a mother

4 ( ) was disappointed and frustrated in her role as a mother

5 ( ) was very unhappy in her role as a mother

5. When I was growing up, if I needed help or advice, I knew that I could count on my father:

1 ( ) almost always

2 ( ) usually

3 ( ) sometimes

4 ( ) hardly ever

5 ( ) never

6. When I was growing up, I felt that I was a worthwhile and important member of my family:

1 ( ) almost always

2 ( ) often

3 ( ) sometimes

4 ( ) hardly ever

5 ( ) never

7. When I am NOT pregnant, I feel that my general emotional state is:

1 ( ) excellent

2 ( ) good

3 ( ) fair

4 ( ) poor

5 ( ) very poor

8. When I am NOT pregnant, I generally feel sad:

5 ( ) almost always

4 ( ) often

3 ( ) sometimes

2 ( ) hardly ever

1 ( ) never

9. At the present time, I feel good about myself as a person:

1 ( ) almost all of the time

2 ( ) most of the time

3 ( ) some of the time

4 ( ) hardly ever

5 ( ) none of the time

534

10. Before pregnancy, when I menstruated, most of the time:

1 ( ) I felt comfortable enough to go about my normal routine

2 ( ) I may have had to take a few hours off for one day

3 ( ) I may have had to take a day off

4 ( ) I may have had to take two or more days off

5 ( ) I may have had to take off for my entire period

11. After the birth of one or more of my children, I:

5 ( ) was very depressed and had to have medical attention

4 ( ) was very depressed but did not have medical attention

3 ( ) was moderately depressed for more than a week

2 ( ) was not depressed

4 ( ) this is my first child

12. So far in this pregnancy, I have had nausea or vomiting:

2 ( ) almost all the time

1 ( ) often

0 ( ) sometimes

1 ( ) hardly ever

2 ( ) not at all

13. During this pregnancy I felt nervous and anxious:

5 ( ) almost all of the time

4 ( ) often

3 ( ) sometimes

2 ( ) hardly ever

1 ( ) not at all

14. During this pregnancy I have generally felt sad:

5 ( ) almost all of the time

4 ( ) often

3 ( ) sometimes

2 ( ) hardly ever

1 ( ) not at all

15. At the present time, I am satisfied with the amount of education I have had:

1 ( ) almost always

2 ( ) usually

3 ( ) sometimes

4 ( ) hardly ever

5 ( ) never

16. I feel that I can manage on my present income:

1 ( ) almost always

2 ( ) usually

3 ( ) sometimes

4 ( ) hardly ever

5 ( ) never

17. At the present time, my relationship with my mother is:

1 ( ) very close

2 ( ) close

3 ( ) fairly close

4 ( ) sometimes distant

5 ( ) distant

3 ( ) my mother is not living

18. My mother criticizes me:

2 ( ) almost all the time

1 ( ) too often

0 ( ) sometimes

1 ( ) hardly ever

2 ( ) never

3 ( ) my mother is not living

19. At the present time, when I really need help, I know that I can count on my father:

1 ( ) almost always

2 ( ) usually

3 ( ) sometimes

4 ( ) hardly ever

5 ( ) never

6 ( ) my father is not living

20. At the present time, my relationship with my father is:

1 ( ) very close

2 ( ) close

3 ( ) fairly close

4 ( ) sometimes distant

5 ( ) distant

6 ( ) my father is not living

21. At the present time, my relationship with my husband or boyfriend is usually:

1 ( ) excellent

2 ( ) good

3 ( ) fair

4 ( ) poor

5 ( ) very poor

22. If I need help or advice, I know that I can count on my husband or boyfriend:

1 ( ) almost always

2 ( ) usually

3 ( ) sometimes

4 ( ) hardly ever

5 ( ) never

1 ( ) almost all the time

2 ( ) most of the time

3 ( ) some of the time

4 ( ) hardly ever

5 ( ) none of the time

23. At the present time, I feel good about my life:

1 ( ) almost all the time

2 ( ) most of the time

3 ( ) some of the time

4 ( ) hardly ever

5 ( ) none of the time

24. At the present time, if I need help or advice, I can count on the following people: (check all that apply)

-1 ( ) my mother

-1 ( ) my father

-1 ( ) my husband or boyfriend

-1 ( ) a sister, brother or relative

-1 ( ) another person

0 ( ) no one

Directions for scoring:

1. Add algebraically the numerical value of the responses checked for all 24 questions.
2. A score of 46 or more suggests clinical potential for the development of postpartum depressive symptoms (PPDS).

This Questionnaire was developed by N.A. Posner, MD; R.R. Unterman, MA, MSW; K.N. Williams, PhD; and G.H. Williams, PhD; Department of Obstetrics and Gynecology, Albany Medical Center, 47 New Scotland Avenue, Albany, NY 12208.

Appendix 5

Clinical Protocols for Perinatal Loss

Maternal Cases

I. *Background:* age; marital status; race; ethnic membership; occupation; religion

II. *Circumstances of loss*
- A. *Nature of loss:* time elapsed since occurrence; whether planned pregnancy; kind of loss; how far along in pregnancy; medical complication; causality; suddenness or anticipation of loss; visible abnormalities; viability of fetus; concurrent stressors
- B. *Prior history:* infertility problems; fate of all other conceptions; months attempting this conception; family history of pregnancy losses and related difficulties; medical history (especially obstetric-gynecological problems)
- C. *Involvement with the baby:* knowledge of sex; contact (whether saw, touched, held); whether named; memorabilia (e.g., photographs, finger- or footprints); funeral or memorial service; fate of body
- D. *Future planning:* likelihood of recurrence; impact on future fertility; plans for future pregnancy (if felt as urgent); interval until next pregnancy

III. *Interpersonal reactions*
- A. *Medical:* reported quality and sensitivity of medical care; grieving suppressed or encouraged; information and advice provided; hospital procedures; any follow-up after discharge; change in relationship to medical caretakers
- B. *Spouse:* background information (age,

occupation, and so on); how involved with wife and unborn child during pregnancy; meaning of loss; course of grief; general personality and dynamics; availability to wife after loss; empathy with wife's grief; impact of loss on communication; closeness and sexual relations in marriage; prior and subsequent marital problems
- C. *Family* (children, parents, siblings): tolerance of maternal grief; quality of prior relationship; ability of parents to facilitate resolution of other children's grief (i.e., provide information, answer questions, support mourning, and empathize with feelings); expression of unresolved grief with children (e.g., overprotective, scapegoating, replacement dynamics); change in valuing of parental role and children
- D. *Friends:* tolerance of maternal grief; quality of prior relationship; impact of loss on relationship; change in empathy with others facing losses and hardship
- E. *Community:* availability of and participation in support groups; knowledge and sensitivity about perinatal loss on part of ministers and teachers; any change in religious identification; any change in job

IV. *Intrapsychic responses*
- A. *History:* prior deaths and unresolved losses; individual and family history of traumas; prior psychotherapy; relevant developmental history (person, parental, sexual)

B. *Psychodynamics*: symptoms; central dynamic issues and conflicts; character structure (with favored defenses); extent and tolerance of depression; gender identification; narcissistic deficits (stability of self-esteem and ego ideal); susceptibility to regression or decompensation; superego functioning; pregnancy dynamics (nature of prenatal attachment, conscious and unconscious wishes, conflicts over baby and motherhood, nature of infantile and maternal identifications)

C. *Reactions to loss*: nature of loss (narcissistic versus object); patterning of grief; defenses against mourning; meanings of loss

V. *Psychotherapy*

A. Treatment particulars: referral source; contract (length and frequency of recommended and actual plans); orientation of treatment; source of payment

B. Course of therapy: presenting problems (manifest description and latent association with loss); anniversary effects; focus of therapeutic work (facilitating mourning, providing insight, restoring narcissistic equilibrium); role of therapist; importance of transference; reactions to separations and interruptions in treatment; memorable material (sessions, dreams, and fantasies); termination (planned or abrupt, any acting-out, intensity of feelings over ending, interpretation and resolution of termination issues)

C. *Role of perinatal loss*: source of new disturbance: revival of earlier problems; stimulus to adaptation or growth

D. *Outcome*: resolution of perinatal loss and unrelated issues; comparison with preloss functioning; comparison with functioning upon entering treatment; unresolved disturbance and symptoms.

(Reproduced from Leon IG. *When a Baby Dies: Psychotherapy for Pregnancy and Newborn Loss*. New Haven, CT: Yale University Press, 1990;197–8; with permission.)

Appendix 6

Present Thoughts and Feelings about Your Loss (Short Form)

Each of the items is a statement of thoughts and feelings which some people have concerning a loss such as yours. There are no right or wrong responses to these statements. For each item, circle the number which best indicates the extent to which you agree or disagree with it at the present time. If you are not certain, use the 'neither' category. Please try to use this category only when you truly have no opinion.

	Strongly agree	Agree	Neither agree nor disagree	Disagree	Strongly disagree
1.(2.) I feel depressed.	1	2	3	4	5
2.(3.) I find it hard to get along with certain people.	1	2	3	4	5
3.(6.) I feel empty inside.	1	2	3	4	5
4.(10.) I can't keep up with my normal activities.	1	2	3	4	5
5.(11.) I feel a need to talk about the baby.	1	2	3	4	5
6.(14.) I am grieving for the baby.	1	2	3	4	5
7.(15.) I am frightened.	1	2	3	4	5
8.(19.) I have considered suicide since the loss.	1	2	3	4	5
9.(23.) I take medicine for my nerves.	1	2	3	4	5
10.(24.) I very much miss the baby.	1	2	3	4	5
11.(25.) I feel I have adjusted well to the loss.	1	2	3	4	5
12.(32.) It is painful to recall memories of the loss.	1	2	3	4	5

	Strongly agree	Agree	Neither agree nor disagree	Disagree	Strongly disagree
13.(35.) I get upset when I think about the baby.	1	2	3	4	5
14.(36.) I cry when I think about him/her.	1	2	3	4	5
15.(41.) I feel guilty when I think about the baby.	1	2	3	4	5
16.(43.) I feel physically ill when I think about the baby.	1	2	3	4	5
17(47.) I feel unprotected in a dangerous world since he/she died.	1	2	3	4	5
18.(50.) I try to laugh, but nothing seems funny anymore.	1	2	3	4	5
19.(51.) Time passes so slowly since the baby died.	1	2	3	4	5
20.(53.) The best part of me died with the baby.	1	2	3	4	5
21.(54.) I have let people down since the baby died.	1	2	3	4	5
22.(55.) I feel worthless since he/she died.	1	2	3	4	5
23.(58.) I blame myself for the baby's death.	1	2	3	4	5
24.(60.) I get cross at my friends and relatives more than I should.	1	2	3	4	5
25.(61.) Sometimes I feel like I need a professional counselor to help me get my life back together again.	1	2	3	4	5
26.(63.) I feel as though I'm just existing and not really living since he/she died.	1	2	3	4	5
27.(66.) I feel so lonely since he/she died.	1	2	3	4	5

	Strongly agree	Agree	Neither agree nor disagree	Disagree	Strongly disagree
28.(67.) I feel somewhat apart and remote, even among friends.	1	2	3	4	5
29.(68.) It's safer not to love.	1	2	3	4	5
30.(72.) I find it difficult to make decisions since the baby died.	1	2	3	4	5
31.(73.) I worry about what my future will be like.	1	2	3	4	5
32.(78.) Being a bereaved parent means being a 'second-class citizen.'	1	2	3	4	5
33.(79.) It feels great to be alive.	1	2	3	4	5

33-ITEM PERINATAL GRIEF SCALE

The following three subscales comprise the grief total for the 33-item scale. Each column lists the subscale number and name and the item numbers from the 84-item questionnaire that make up that subscale. Items marked (R) must be reversed in scoring.

Subscale 1	Subscale 2	Subscale 3
Active grief	**Difficulty coping**	**Despair**
2	3	23
6	10	41
11	19	43
14	25 (R)	47
15	54	50
24	60	53
32	61	55
35	63	58
36	67	68
51	72	73
66	79 (R)	78

NOTE: Reversing the items indicated is easiest but produces a scale wherein low scores are associated with higher grief. We do a second reversal on the scale so that high scores mean higher grief.

(Reproduced from: Pafvin L, Lasker J, Toedter L. Measuring grief. A short version of the perinatal grief scale. *J Psychopathol Behav Assess* 1989;11:29–45; with permission.)

Appendix 7

Recommended Guidelines for the Screening and Counseling of Oocyte Donors

Anonymous Oocyte Donor

I. Clinical interview: psychosocial history based on a semi-structured interview

A. Comprehensive Psychosocial History for Infertility (CPHI) (see Appendix 2)

B. If the CPHI is not used, then target these essential elements:
1. Family history (with or without genogram)—investigate history through grandparents and offspring.
2. Assessment of stability (e.g., job history, relationships)
3. Motivation to donate
4. Current life stressors and coping skills
5. Difficult or traumatic reproductive history
6. Interpersonal relationships
7. Sexual history (including sexual abuse)
8. History of major psychiatric disorders, including personality disorders
9. Alcohol, drug use, and/or dependence in donor and family of origin (current and past)
10. Legal history (lawsuits, misdemeanors, felonies)
11. History of abuse or neglect (sexual, physical)
12. Educational background

C. Determination of motivation to participate (psychological, financial, physical)

D. Ability to comprehend and assimilate information provided

E. Education about treatment for donor and recipient (and respective partners, if applicable)
1. Purpose
2. Description of procedures
3. Success and failure rates
4. Potential health risks and complications
5. Reasons why treatment would be discontinued
6. Financial issues
7. Time commitment
8. Potential psychological risks

F. Counseling: pre- and post-treatment and during treatment
1. Potential impact on relationships (e.g., marital, sexual, work, social, family)
2. Potential impact on relationship between donor and recipient (known donors)
3. Implications
   a. What if treatment is not successful
   b. What if pregnancy is not successful
   c. What if pregnancy is terminated or selectively reduced
   d. What if donor changes her mind
   e. What if the child has a physical problem

G. Counseling on recipient specific issues

1. Impact of the failure of treatment
   a. Emotional issues associated with infertility, including feeling out of control or failure
   b. Terminating treatment
   c. Grieving process
   d. Developing alternatives (e.g., child-free living or adoption)
2. Impact of success of treatment
   a. Feelings during pregnancy
   b. Transition to parenthood
   c. Privacy vs. openness with the child
   d. Potential impact of multiple pregnancy
   e. Parenting at an older age (if applicable)
   f. Family relationships

H. Information and consents
   1. Provide a reasonable time interval between giving of information, assessment, and consent
   2. Specifically state risks involved
   3. Specifically state who has parental rights and responsibilities
   4. State and designate financial responsibilities
   5. Require maintenance of medical records of all participants and applicable state law
   6. Delineate specific responsibilities of each participant
   7. Provide for anonymity of all parties to the best of the clinician's ability

II. Psychological testing

A. Structured personality tests (examples listed below)
   1. Minnesota Multiphasic Personality Inventory 2
   2. California Personality Inventory
   3. Personality Assessment Inventory
B. Self-report measures (examples listed below)
   1. Marital Satisfaction Inventory
   2. Dyadic Adjustment Scale
   3. Life Events Checklist
   4. Beck Depression or Anxiety Inventory
   5. Sentence Completion
   6. Pennsylvania Reproductive Associate Infertility Survey (PRAIS)
   7. Brief Symptom Inventory

III. Known oocyte donors

For known donors, the protocol of the interview and psychological testing is the same, although psychological testing is optional in some known-donor programs. The clinical interview should include the recipient and her husband/partner and the donor and her husband/partner. The interview should also include a group meeting in which all parties come together for discussion, summary, and recommendations. The interview should include the following elements that are not included in the anonymous donor interview.

A. Additional content areas for known donor interview
   1. Assessment for the presence of coercion (financial or emotional)
   2. Information from both the donor and recipient regarding their interpersonal relationship
   3. In sister-to-sister donation: parents' role
   4. Issues of disclosure or privacy
   5. Interactions among all three or four parties
   6. Dysfunctional family history
   7. Plans for future relationships
   8. Information regarding intentions of all four parties regarding custody arrangements in the event of the death of the recipients
   9. Issues regarding cryopreservation and future disposition of the frozen embryos

10. Prenatal testing and selective reduction
11. Donor's role and relationship with future child(ren)
12. Impact on donor if treatment is unsuccessful
13. Estimation of number of cycles in which donor is willing to participate

IV. Criteria for acceptance or rejection of oocyte donors

The following indicators can be used to decide on a case-by-case basis who is suitable as an oocyte donor. While the following list is not exhaustive and each program may over time add to or delete from this list, it is offered as a preliminary guide. The caveat is to err on the side of caution to protect all parties.

A. Positive indicators
1. Absence of significant psychopathology
2. Absence of unusual life stressors
3. Use of adaptive coping skills
4. Ability to provide informed consent
5. Supportive and stable interpersonal and/or marital relationships
6. Economic stability
7. Psychological testing within normal limits
8. Employment stability

B. Negative indicators
1. Significant DSM IV axis I or II disorder (including psychological standardized testing which is two standard deviations above the mean)
2. Positive family history for heritable psychiatric disorder (e.g., schizophrenia, bipolar disorders)
3. Two or more first degree relatives with substance dependence
4. Current use of psychoactive medications
5. Family history of sexual or physical abuse with no professional treatment for the donor
6. Chaotic lifestyle
7. Significant current stress
8. Marital instability
9. Impaired cognitive functioning or mental incompetence
10. History of legal difficulties

If the potential donor is in a crisis, appropriate psychological help should be provided. Objection to donation by the husband or partner of the donor should be grounds at least for a deferment of treatment.

(Developed by the Mental Health Professional Group Ovum Donor Task Force of the American Society for Reproductive Medicine, 1994.)

Appendix 8

Psychological Guidelines for Embryo Donation

These recommendations should be understood as general guidelines for addressing the many complex moral, ethical, and psychosocial issues which embryo donors, recipients, and potential offspring may confront as we move forward with this family-building option. Providing thorough information and adequate time for decision-making will increase the likelihood for establishing well-adjusted families.

I. Donors

1. Prior to signing an informed consent document, all potential donor couples should be educated about all aspects of their medical treatments and the relevant psychological and ethical issues inherent in donating embryos. These issues should be addressed during the clinical interview and are included in recommendations for the interview.

2. It is recommended that there should be a discussion of embryo disposition options at the time of cryopreservation. After couples have concluded their own reproductive attempts, they should again be apprised of embryo-disposition options, including donation.

3. Psychological assessment is strongly recommended to ascertain appropriateness of potential donors, including determining psychopathology. This assessment should include a clinical interview and psychological testing. The timing of this assessment should occur after couples have concluded their own reproductive attempts and have clearly indicated their desire to donate embryos (including signing informed consent),

and their embryos are medically appropriate for donation.

4. The clinical interview should include a psychosocial history of both partners which addresses: educational background, current life stressors, difficult or traumatic reproductive history, interpersonal relationships, sexual history, history of major psychiatric and personality disorders, legal problems, history of abuse or neglect, substance abuse, and family history (at least first-degree relatives) of major psychiatric and personality disorders, substance abuse, physical or sexual abuse, and legal problems.

5. The clinical interview should also address the unknown potential psychological impact and/or risks, assessment for presence of coercion (financial and/or emotional), emotional attachment to embryos, disclosure or non-disclosure of the donors' involvement, amount and type of information to be exchanged, if any, between donors and recipients.

6. Psychological testing is recommended to document and validate in a standardized, objective manner the information gathered from the clinical interview and should include an objective personality test and other self-report measures to assess potential instability or psychopathology.

7. Positive indicators for embryo donors include: absence of significant psychopathology, absence of current or significant history of substance abuse/ addiction, absence of unusual life

546

stressors, use of adaptive coping skills, ability to provide true informed consent, supportive and stable 'marital' relationship, economic stability, employment stability, lack of coercion, and psychological testing within normal limits.

8. Negative indicators for embryo donors include: presence of significant psychopathology, positive family history for heritable genetic and psychiatric disorders, substance abuse/addiction, two or more first-degree relatives with substance abuse, family history of sexual or physical abuse with no professional treatment, chaotic lifestyle, significant current life stress, 'marital' instability, impaired cognitive functioning or mental incompetence, history of legal difficulties, high-risk sexual practices, and objection by either partner.

9. A minimum 3-month waiting period is recommended between the time a couple signs the consent form to donate embryos and the actual donation to a recipient couple.

10. Employees of the infertility program or physician should be excluded from embryo donation within their own program.

11. Donors should not be compensated for their donated embryos.

12. Donors should be a least 21 years of age.

II. Recipients

1. Recipients of donor embryos should receive counseling about the potential psychosocial implications of this parenting option prior to signing an informed consent document.

2. Counseling should address the impact of success of treatment, such as the feelings during pregnancy, positive and negative aspects of disclosure and non-disclosure with offspring, potential impact of multiple pregnancy, transition to parenthood (if applicable), parenting at an older age (if applicable), and nongenetic parenting issues.

3. The impact of treatment failure should also be addressed, including treatment termination, the grieving process, and developing alternatives for the future.

4. Related issues such as the potential impact of the relationship between known donors and recipients and potential offspring should be addressed when relevant.

5. Psychological assessment is strongly recommended to assess appropriateness of potential recipients (not to assess parenting abilities). This assessment would attempt to rule out significant psychiatric illness, current substance abuse/addiction, and ability to cope with the stress of assisted reproductive technologies.

(Developed by the Mental Health Professional Group of the American Society for Reproductive Medicine Task Force on Embryo Donation, 1996.)

Appendix 9

Example of Informed Psychological Consent

Disclaimer: This is only an example.

Anonymous Oocyte (Egg) Donor

It is impossible to state with any degree of certainty or specificity the psychological implications of your participation as an oocyte donor in the egg donor program.

You have undergone a psychological evaluation, which included the MMPI-2, generally acknowledged to be accurate in the assessment of potential personality difficulties and pathology that would make you an inappropriate egg donor candidate. We have discussed feelings and thoughts related to egg donation so that you can make a responsible and informed decision.

A number of areas of potential difficulty were discussed, including (1) curiosity regarding the potential child or children, (2) break in the connectedness and continuity traditionally experienced in a genetic parent–child relationship, and (3) possible feelings and questions that may arise in the future.

By signing this document, you acknowledge that you have been informed of the potential psychological risks involved with your participation in an egg donor program to the best of our ability at this time. You acknowledge that you are a willing participant as an egg donor and that neither (*therapist's name*) nor anyone else in the program has acted in a coercive manner or pressured you to participate in any way.

Egg donor/Date
Egg donor's husband/Date
Witness/Date

Appendix 10

Example of Informed Psychological Consent

Disclaimer: This is only an example.

Recipients: Anonymous Egg Donation

It is impossible to state with any degree of certainty or specificity the psychological implications of your participation in the egg donor program as recipients of anonymously donated oocytes (eggs).

You have had a consultation with a mental health professional during which the psychosocial issues surrounding egg donation and the possible implications for your family were discussed. We have discussed your feelings and thoughts regarding building your family by egg donation so that you can make an informed and responsible choice.

The areas of potential difficulty that were discussed included: (1) possible curiosity in the child regarding his/her genetic heritage, (2) discontinuity of traditional biological connectedness in the parent–child relationship, and (3) questions and feelings that might arise in the future either within the child, you, or your partner. As with any child, temperament, personality, intelligence, and physical characteristics cannot always be known or accurately predicted.

By signing this document, you acknowledge that you have been informed of the potential psychological risks of your participation in the egg donor program to the best of our ability at this time. You acknowledge that you are a willing participant in the egg donor program and that neither (*therapist's name*) nor anyone else has acted in a coercive or pressuring manner toward you in any way.

Donated oocyte recipient/Date
Recipient's spouse or partner/Date

Appendix 11

Example of Consent for Release of Information

Disclaimer: This is only an example.

I,   , hereby authorize and request (*therapist's name, address*) to exchange all pertinent clinical information pertaining to me with:

I understand that I have no obligation whatsoever to disclose the requested information and that I may revoke this consent at any time by informing the above-named individuals in writing. I further understand that this authorization is valid only for the period of one year from the date of my signature below.
pregnancy

Signature/Date

Appendix 12

Example of Consent and Waiver Regarding Conflict of Interest

Disclaimer: This is only an example.

Egg Donation

We, the undersigned, acknowledge that (*therapist's name*) has assisted in the psychological screening, testing, and counseling of some or all of the parties to this agreement, pursuant to their involvement in the egg donation procedure.

Furthermore, we recognize that although (*therapist's name*) may receive her fees from the recipient or recipient couple, it is understood that the donor and her husband (if any) are the therapist's patients and, as such, her professional responsibility lies in her privileged relationship with them.

While it is the intention of the parties and (*therapist's name*) to assist in the successful completion of an egg donation cycle, the parties understand and agree that the therapist may ethically and legally advise the egg donor (and/or her husband) to act in a manner contrary to the interests and desires of the recipient and/or her partner.

If acting in the best interest of her patient, (*therapist's name*) advises actions that may constitute a breach of the egg donor contract, the recipient or recipient couple expressly release and hold harmless (*therapist's name*), her agents, and/or employees (if any) from all liability. In addition, this consent recognizes that her actions are based on her reasonable professional advice. Nothing contained in this consent and waiver is intended to release (*therapist's name*) from actions constituting malpractice or negligence.

Recipient /Date

Recipient's partner/Date

Egg donor/Date

Egg donor's partner/Date

Witness/Date

Appendix 13

Points to Consider for a Counselors' Retainer Agreement

Disclaimer: This is only an example.

WHEREAS, Intended Parents acknowledge that the Surrogate is the client of the Counselor, and the Counselor shall act as consultant to Intended Parents, that Intended Parents have retained the Counselor, and that this Retainer Agreement is intended to explain the nature of the services and charges that Intended Parents shall incur in connection with their surrogate parenting endeavors.

NOW, THEREFORE, for and in consideration of the foregoing premises and the mutual covenants between the parties, Intended Parents and the Counselor hereby enter into an agreement whereby the Counselor will provide psychological consultation services under the following terms and conditions, and intending to be legally bound:

Intended Parents acknowledge that:

A. The Counselor does not guarantee or warrant that the Surrogate and/or her husband, if any, will comply with the surrogate agreement and/or the advice of professionals involved. After Intended Parents and the Surrogate, and her Husband, if any, have met and agreed to work together, Intended Parents' independent legal counsel will provide Intended Parents and Surrogate and her Husband, if any, with legal contracts covering their relationship (hereinafter refereed to as 'Surrogate Agreement').

B. The Counselor is not trained in the field of medicine and is not acting in a medical capacity and cannot be held liable for medical decisions made by physicians.

C. The Counselor does not guarantee or warrant that the Surrogate will in fact conceive a child, nor does the Counselor guarantee that a child, if conceived, will be a healthy child free of congenital or birth defects or abnormalities.

D. Intended Parents acknowledge that third-party reproduction or surrogacy is a very expensive procedure and has unknown complications. This Retainer Agreement is intended to cover reasonable and customary psychological counseling services rendered to the Surrogate and Intended Parents during the course of a customary surrogate mother arrangement as defined and experienced by the Center.

Intended Parents shall meet with and have the final decision as to the selection of any potential Surrogate and her Husband, if any.

Intended Parents acknowledge that surrogate parenting and the resulting interpersonal relationship are new and unclear and that while the Counselor shall use her best professional skills and exert maximum effort, the results are not completely foreseeable. By signing this document, Intended Parents acknowledge that there are potential psychological risks involved in surrogacy.

While it is the intention of the Counselor herein to aid in the successful culmination of this Retainer Agreement, the Parties understand that the Counselor may ethically and legally have to advise or counsel the Surrogate and her husband, if any, to conduct themselves or act in a manner contrary to the interests of Intended Parents. Intended Parents are hereby advised that the Counselor has no obligation to relate certain information she learns from Surrogate, or any other person(s), to Intended Parents, if the Counselor believes that such information is not pertinent to this surrogacy relationship, or Surrogate requests this information is not relayed to Intended Parents and the Counselor agrees, or the Counselor decides that in her professional opinion, such information will not benefit Intended Parents with regards to this surrogacy relationship. Additionally, the Counselor has no obligation to advise Center or physician or attorneys involved in this relationship of information (regarding Surrogate and/or Intended Parents), which in her opinion is not pertinent to this surrogacy arrangement or which she feels is confidential information.

In the event that, in her professional opinion (so long as such an opinion is in the best interest of the party so advised), the Counselor advises either party to act in a manner contrary to the intentions of the Retainer Agreement, the non-breaching party, their employees, agents, heirs, assigns, and representatives shall release from liability the above-mentioned professional for any action taken by Intended Parents, the Surrogate and/or her husband, if any, their families, heirs, assigns, or representatives against said professionals, based on the reasonable professional advice of the Counselor. Any such professional advice shall not constitute a breach of any duty owed to Intended Parents or Surrogate and her husband, if any, or Center or physician or attorney involved in this relationship. This document is not intended to, nor does it, release any professional involved herein from professional malpractice or negligence.

Intended Parents, either together or individually, shall submit to psychological evaluation or counseling as deemed reasonably necessary by the Counselor.

Intended Parents further agree to install an answering machine/voice mail in their home and ensure that it is operational throughout the duration of their agreement with the Counselor.

Intended Parents further agree that they will release the Counselor from any and all liability associated with the surrogate mother procedure contemplated herein relating to claims for child support or maintenance, medical costs, loss of earnings, pain, suffering, emotional distress, and/or similar claims of the child, Surrogate, their respective families, heirs, or representatives.

Intended Parents further agree that they will release the Counselor from any and all liabilities associated with the surrogate procedure, except as a result of negligence of the Counselor. This paragraph is not an attempt to waive psychological malpractice as to any party.

Intended Parents acknowledge that the Counselor reserves the right to terminate this Agreement if the relationship with Intended Parents becomes no longer tenable, and/or if it is disclosed that Intended Parents have intentionally misrepresented themselves.

The Counselor recommends that Intended Parents consult with independent legal counsel prior to signing this Retainer Agreement.

Appendix 14

Acknowledgment, Waiver, and Consent Re: Conflict of Interest of Psychological Professionals

Disclaimer: This is only an example.

The undersigned acknowledges that while the Counselor involved in the surrogate parenting procedure contemplated herein, pursuant to the terms of this Retainer Agreement, may be paid by Intended Parents. The Surrogate and her husband, if any, as well as Intended Parents, are the clients of the Counselor. The Counselor must place the health and well-being of her clients above all else.

While it is the intention of Intended Parents and the Counselor herein to aid in the successful culmination of this Retainer Agreement, the parties understand that the Counselor may ethically and legally have to advise or counsel the surrogate and her husband, if any, to conduct themselves or act in a manner contrary to the interests of the Intended Parents.

In the event that, in her professional opinion, (so long as such an opinion is in the best interest of the party so advised), Counselor advises either party to act in a manner contrary to the intentions of the Retainer Agreement, the non-breaching party, their employees, agents, heirs, assigns, and representatives shall release from liability the above- mentioned professional for any action taken by Intended Parents, the Surrogate and/or her husband, if any, their families, heirs, assigns, or representatives against said professional based on the reasonable professional advice of the Counselor.

Any such professional advice shall not constitute a breach of any duty owed to Intended Parents or Surrogate and her husband, if any.

This document is not intended to, nor does it, release any professional involved herein from professional malpractice or negligence.

Appendix 15
Daily Record Keeping Sheet

INSTRUCTIONS FOR DAILY RECORD KEEPING SHEET

Fill in the personal code number, date and whether this is treatment week 1, 2, 3, 4, 5 or 6 of your IVF cycle in the space provided at the top right corner of the sheet.

Part 1

Day of treatment: *The first day of the IVF cycle (at the top of the chart) is calculated as the day you go for the first day scan.*

Date: *Record the dates of the month which correspond with the days of your IVF cycle.*

Treatment code: *In the box labeled "Treatment code" are the names of events or medical interventions occurring during treatment. Use these codes to indicate on the Treatment code line the events you experienced that day. For example, on the day you do a Pergonal injection you would put a 'PL' and on the day you have the egg retrieval you would put 'OR'. If you have more than one intervention, for example a Pergonal injection and an ultrasound scan, put the two codes, as in 'PL/U'. Be sure to indicate all the interventions you received that day.*

Medical feedback. *Use this space to indicate the days you received feedback about the progress of treatment from medical staff (doctors, nurses). Place a '+' sign for positive feedback (good news) and a '–' sign for negative feedback (bad news). If you cannot decide whether the feedback was good or bad, then place both signs (+/–). If you did not receive any feedback for that day, leave the corresponding box blank.*

Part 2

Symptoms: *A list of various emotional (Part 2) and physical symptoms (Part 3) possibly experienced during treatment are listed in the main chart. On a daily basis you are to rate the extent to which you experienced each one of these symptoms. You should fill in the chart at the same time each day, before you go to sleep, and reflect on the past 24 hours in terms of whether and to what extent the symptom occurred. These symptoms are graded as follows:*

Rating Scale

NONE	MILD	MODERATE	SEVERE
	1	2	3

None - Leave the box blank it the symptom is not present.
Mild - Place a '1' in the box if the symptom is present but does not interfere with daily activities.
Moderate - Place a '2' in the box if the symptom is present and interferes to some degree with daily activities.
Severe - Place a '3' in the box it the efficiency of performing some daily tasks is markedly reduced.

Part 4

Items: *A list of different ways of handling IVF are listed in the last section. On a daily basis indicate the extent to which you used each method by placing a '1' (used a little), '2' (used somewhat) or '3' (used a lot) in the corresponding box. It you did not use a method, leave the corresponding box blank.*

NB *The Record Keeping sheet is to be filled out on a daily basis from the first day scan until the third day after the IVF pregnancy test results. You have been provided with six charts, with each chart corresponding to 7 days (7 columns) of record keeping. At the end of each seven day period mail the form back in the pre-addressed, stamped envelope provided. It is very important to mail these sheets back on a weekly basis. In order to ensure that your responses remain confidential, use only your personal code number on this form.*

Daily Record Keeping Sheet

Date						
Treatment week	1	2	3	4	5	6
PART 1						
Day of treatment						
Date						
Treatment code						
Medical feedback +, − or +/−						
PART 2						
Nervous						
Anxious						
Hesitant						
Touchy/sensitive						
Peaceful						
Cautious						
Moody						
Pessimistic						
Doubtful						
Happy						
Unsure						
Angry						
Frustated						
Sad						
Content						
Tense						
Irritable						
Hassled						
Worried						
Fulfilled						
Optimistic: pregnancy						
PART 3						
Hot flushes/sweats						
Dizziness						
Fatigue/tired						
Breast tenderness						
Abdominal discomfort						
Ovarian pain						
Constipation						
Decreased appetite						
Headaches						

TREATMENT CODES

S	=	Spotting
SP	=	Suprefact, Nafarelin
PL	=	Pergonal, Metrodin, Humegon, Normagon
BD	=	Blood test
U	=	Ultrasound/Scan
PR	=	Profasi, Pregnyl
OR	=	Egg retrieval
ET	=	Embryo transfer
G	=	Gestone

RATING SCALE (use for Part 2, 3 and 4)

NONE	MILD	MODERATE	SEVERE
	1	2	3

PART 4						
I turned my attention away from treatment by thinking about other things or doing some activity						
I tried to see treatment in a different light that made it seem more bearable						
I thought about ways to make treatment more likely to work or did things to make a pregnancy more likely						
I expressed my feelings about treatment to reduce tension, anxiety or frustration						
I accept that there was nothing that I could do						
I sought or found emotional support from loved ones, friends or professionals						
I did something with the implicit intention of relaxing						
I sought or found spiritual comfort or support						

XI. RESOURCES

SECTION I: OVERVIEW OF INFERTILITY

Books

Barker GH, Bronson RA. *Your Search for Fertility*. New York: Morrow, 1981

Bellina JH, Wilson J. *You Can Have a Baby: Everything You Need to Know About Fertility*. New York: Crown Publishers, 1985

Berger GS, Goldstein M, Fuerst M. *The Couple's Guide to Fertility*. New York: Doubleday, 1989

Bridwell D. *The Ache for a Child*. Wheaton, IL: Victor Books, 1994

Chase ME. *Waiting for Baby: One Couple's Journey Through Infertility to Adoption*. New York: McGraw-Hill, 1990

Corson SL. *Conquering Infertility*. East Norwalk, CT: Appleton-Century-Crofts, 1983

Decker A, Lobel S. *Why Can't We Have a Baby? An Authority Looks at the Causes and Curses of Childlessness*. New York: Dial Press, 1978

Flemming B. *Motherhood Deferred: A Woman's Journey*. New York: G.P. Putnam Sons, 1994

Frank D, Vogel M. *The Baby Makers*. New York: Carroll and Graf Publishers, 1988

Frisch MJ, Rapoport G. *Getting Pregnant*. Tucson, AZ: The Body Press, 1987

Glazer E, Cooper S. *Without Child: Experiencing Resolving Infertility*. Lexington, MA: Lexington Books, 1988

Harkness C. *The Infertility Book: A Comprehensive Medical and Emotional Guide*. San Francisco, CA: Volcano Press, 1987

Houghton D, Houghton P. *Coping with Childlessness*. London: Allen and Unwin, 1984

Johnston PI. *Understanding: A Guide to Impaired Fertility for Family and Friends*. Fort Wayne, IN: Perspectives Press, 1987

Johnston PI. *Taking Charge of Infertility*. Indianapolis, IN: Perspectives Press, 1994

Lasker JN, Borg S. *In Search of Parenthood: Coping with Infertility and High-Tech Conception*. Boston: Beacon Press, 1987

Liebmann-Smith J. *In Pursuit of Pregnancy*. New York: New Market Press, 1987

Marrs R, Bloch LF, Silverman KK. *Dr Richard Marr's Fertility Book*. New York: Dell, 1998

Mason MC. *Male Infertility: Men Talking*. London: Routledge, 1993

McGuirk J, McGuirk ME. *For Want of a Child: A Psychologist and His Wife Explore the Emotional Effects and Challenges of Infertility*. New York: Continuum, 1991

Menning BE. *Infertility: A Guide for the Childless Couple*, 2nd edn. New York: Prentice-Hall, 1988

Mullens A. *Missed Conception*. Toronto: McGraw-Hill Ryerson, 1990

Nachtigall R, Mehren E. *Overcoming Infertility: A Practical Strategy for Navigating the Emotional, Medical, and Financial Minefields of Trying to Have a Baby*. New York: Doubleday, 1991

Payne NB, Richardson BL. *The Language of Fertility: A Revolutionary Mind/Body Program for Conscious Conception*. New York: Harmony Books, 1997

Perloe M, Christie LG. *Miracle Babies and Other Happy Endings*. New York: Rawson Associates, 1986

Pfeffer N, Woollett A. *The Experience of Infertility*. London: Virago Press, 1983

Pfeffer RA, Whitlock K. *Fertility Awareness*. Englewood Cliffs, NJ: Prentice-Hall, 1984

Rosenberg HS, Epstein YM. *Getting Pregnant—When You Thought You Couldn't*. New York: Warner Books, 1993

Silber S. *How to Get Pregnant*. New York: Warner Books, 1980

Stangel JJ. *Fertility and Conception: An Essential Guide for Childless Couples*. New York: Paddington Press, 1979

Stanway A. *Infertility: A Common Sense Guide for the Childless*. Rochester, VT: Thorsons Publishers House, 1985

Stout M. *Without Child: A Compassionate Look at Infertility*. Grand Rapids, MI: Zondervan Publishing House, 1985

Van Regenmorter J, Sylvia JS, McIlhaney JS. *Dear God, Why Can't We Have a Baby?* Grand Rapids, MI: Baker Book House, 1986

Vercollone C, Moss R, Moss H. *Helping the Stork: The Choices and Challenges of Donor Insemination*. New York: Macmillan, 1997

Wiscot A, Meldrum D. *New Options for Fertility*. New York: Pharos Books, 1990

Zoldbrod A. *Getting Around the Boulder in the Road: Using Imagery to Cope with Infertility Problems*. Lexington, MA: Center for Reproductive Problems, 1990

Zoldbrod A. *Men, Women and Infertility*. New York: Lexington Books, 1992

Videos

Meeting the Challenges of Infertility. Produced by the Ferre Institute, Inc., 258 Genesee Street, Suite 302, Utica, NY 13502. (315) 724-4348 Fax (315) 724-1360

To Have a Child: Seeking Treatment for Infertility. Produced by American Society for Reproductive Medicine, Distributed by Milner-Fenwick, Inc., 2125 Greenspring Drive, Timonium, MD 21093 Fax (410) 252-6136

Organizations

Access
Australia's National Infertility Network
PO Box 959, Parramatta NSW 2124
Australia
(61) 2-670-2380

American College of Obstetricians and Gynecologists
Resource Center
409 12 Street, NW
Washington, DC 20024
(202) 638-5577

American Society for Reproductive Medicine (formerly the American Fertility Society)
1209 Montgomery Highway
Birmingham, AL 35216-2809
205-978-5000
e-mail asrm@asrm.com

Centering Corporation
PO Box 3367
Omaha, NE 68103-0367

Ferre Institute, Inc
258 Genesee Street, Suite 302
Utica, NY 13502
(315) 724-4348 Fax (315) 724-1360

Infertility Awareness Association of Canada
206-2378 Holly Lane
Ottawa, Ontario K1V 7P1
Canada

International Federation of Infertility Patients Associations
Box 959
Parramatta NSW 2124
Australia

International Society of Nurses in Genetics
c/o Shirley L. Jones, MS
Genetics and IVF Institute
3020 Javier Road
Fairfax, VA 22031
(703) 698-3870

Issue (The National Fertility Association)
509 Aldridge Road
Great Barr
Birmingham B44 8NA
United Kingdom
(44) 1922 722 888

National Society of Genetic Counselors
233 Canterbury Drive
Wallingford, PA 19086
(215) 872-7608

National Women's Health Resource Center
2440 M Street NW, Suite 325
Washington, DC 20037

Perspectives Press
PO Box 90318
Indianapolis, IN 46290

RESOLVE, Inc
1310 Broadway
Somerville, MA 02144-1731
623-1156 (business office); (617) 623-0744
(helpline)

Tapestry Books
PO Box 359
Ringoes, NJ 08551
(800) 765-2367

SECTION II: ASSESSMENT

Counseling

Berger MM, ed. *Women Beyond Freud: New Concepts of Feminine Psychology*. New York: Brunner/Mazel, 1994

Bruckner-Gordon F, Gangi B, Wallman G. *Making Therapy Work*. New York: Harper & Row, 1988

Butcher JN, Williams CL. *Essentials of MMPI-2 and MMPI—A Interpretation*. Minneapolis, MN: University of Minnesota Press, 1993

Gerald A. *A Guide to Psychotherapy*. Lanham, MD: University Press of America, 1983

Greene RL. *The MMPI-2/MMPI: An Interpretative Manual*. Boston: Allyn and Bacon, 1991

Groth-Marnat G. *Handbook of Psychological Assessment*, 3rd edn. New York: Wiley, 1997

Hales D, Hales RE. *Caring for the Mind: The Comprehensive Guide to Mental Health*. New York: Bantam Books, 1995

Meth RL, Pasick RS. *Men in Therapy: The Challenge of Change*. New York: Guilford Press, 1990

Philpot CL, Brooks GR, Luterman D, Nutt RL. *Bridging Separate Gender Worlds*. Washington DC: American Psychological Association, 1997

Raphael B. *The Anatomy of Bereavement*. New York: Basic Books, 1983

Staudacher C. *Men and Grief*. Oakland, CA: New Harbinger Publications, 1991

Mental Health

Books

Casper RC, ed. *Women's Health: Hormones, Emotions and Behavior*. Cambridge University Press, 1997

Demers LM, McGuire JL, Phillips A, Rubinow DR, eds. *Premenstrual, Postpartum, and Menopausal Mood Disorders*. Baltimore: Urban & Schwarzenberg, 1989

Gallant SJ, Keita GP, Royak-Schaler R, eds. *Health Care for Women: Psychological, Social, and Behavioral Influences.* Washington, DC: American Psychological Press, 1997

Goodwin FK, Jamison KR. *Manic-Depressive Illness.* New York: Oxford University Press, 1990

Hales RE, Yudofsky S, Talbott J, eds. *American Psychiatric Press Textbook of Psychiatry*, 2nd edn. Washington, DC: American Psychiatric Press, 1994

Hollander E. *Obsessive-Compulsive Related Disorders.* Washington, DC: American Psychiatric Press, 1993

Jensvold MF, Halbreich U, Hamilton JA, eds. *Psychopharmacology and Women: Sex, Gender, and Hormones.* Washington DC: American Psychiatric Press, 1996

Kaplan HI, Sadock BJ. *Comprehensive Textbook of Psychiatry*, 5th edn., vol. 2. Baltimore: Williams & Wilkins, 1989

Linehan MM. *Cognitive-Behavioral Treatment of Borderline Personality Disorder.* New York: Guilford Press, 1993

Lion JR, ed. *Personality Disorders: Diagnosis and Management*, 2nd edn. Baltimore: Williams & Wilkins, 1981

Meyer RG, Deitsch SE, eds. *The Clinician's Handbook*, 4th edn. Boston: Allyn and Bacon, 1996

Nicholi AM, ed. *The New Harvard Guide to Psychiatry.* Cambridge, MA: Belknap Press, 1988

Schatzberg AF, Cole JO. *Manual of Clinical Psychopharmacology.* Washington, DC: American Psychiatric Press, 1991

Stanton AL, Gallant SJ. *The Psychology of Women's Health.* Washington, DC: American Psychological Press, 1995

Stewart DE, Stotland NL, eds. *Psychological Aspects of Women's Health Care.* Washington, DC: American Psychiatric Press, 1993

Stotland NL. *Social Change and Women's Reproductive Health Care: A Guide for Physicians and Their Patients.* New York: Praeger, 1988

Stoudemire A, ed. *Clinical Psychiatry for Medical Students.* Philadelphia: JB Lippincott, 1990

Organizations

American Anorexia/Bulimia Association, Inc
418 East 76th Street
New York, NY 10021
(212) 734-1114

Anxiety Disorders Association of America
6000 Executive Blvd., Suite 513
Rockville, MD 20852
(301) 231-8368

Depression Awareness, Recognition and Treatment—DART Program
National Institute of Mental Health
5600 Fishers Lane, Room 15C-05
Rockville, MD 20857
(301) 443-4513

Depression and Related Affective Disorders Association
600 N. Wolfe Street
Meyer 3-181
Baltimore, MD 21287-7381
(410) 955-4647

National Alliance for the Mentally Ill (NAMI)
2101 Wilson Blvd., #302
Arlington, VA 22201
(703) 524-7600

National Depression and Manic Depression
Association
730 N. Franklin Street, #501
Chicago, IL 60610
(800) 326-3632

National Foundation for Depressive Illness
2 Pennsylvania Plaza
New York, NY 10121
(800) 248-4344

National Mental Health Association
1021 Prince Street
Alexandria, VA 22314-2971
(800) 969-6642

Obsessive Compulsive Disorder Foundation
PO Box 9573
New Haven, CT 06535
(203) 772-0565

SECTION III: TREATMENT MODALITIES

Individual Counseling

Berson AR. Quality of life issues of reproductive endocrinology. *Clin Consult Obstet Gynecol* 1994;6

Greenfeld DA, ed. Psychological issues in infertility. *Infertil Reprod Med Clin North Am* 1993;4:517–31

Infertility Counselling Guidelines for Practice. London: British Infertility Counselling Association, 1991, 1996

Jennings SE, ed. *Infertility Counselling.* London: Blackwell Press, 1995

King's Fund Centre Report. *Counselling for Regulated Infertility Treatments: The Report of the Counselling Committee.* London: King's Fund Centre, 1991

Leiblum SR, ed. *Infertility: Psychological Issues and Counseling Strategies.* New York: Wiley, 1997

Shapiro C. *When Part of the Self is Lost: Helping Clients Heal After Sexual and Reproductive Losses.* San Francisco, CA: Jossey-Bass, 1993

Valentine D, ed. *Infertility and Adoption: A Guide for Social Work Practice.* New York: Haworth Press, 1987

Couples Counseling

Becker, G. *Healing the Infertile Family: Strengthening Your Relationship in the Search for Parenthood.* New York: Bantam Books, 1990

McDaniel S, Hepworth J, Doherty W. *Medical Family Therapy.* New York: Basic Books, 1992

Mikesell RH, Lusterman D, McDaniel SH, eds. *Integrating Family Therapy: Handbook of Family Psychology and Systems Theory.* Washington, DC: American Psychological Press, 1995

O'Hanlon-Hudson P, Hudson-O'Hanlon W. *Rewriting Love Stories: Brief Marital Therapy.* New York: Norton, 1991

Philpot CL, Brooks GR, Lusterman D, Nutt RL. *Bridging Separate Gender Worlds.* Washington, DC: American Psychological Press, 1997

Salzer L. *Infertility: How Couples Can Cope.* Boston: GK Hall, 1986

Group Counseling

Mazor MD, Simons HF, eds. *Infertility: Medical, Emotional, and Social Considerations.* New York: Human Sciences Press, 1984

Shapiro C. *Infertility and Pregnancy Loss: A Guide for the Helping Professionals.* San Francisco, CA: Jossey-Bass, 1988

Behavioral Medicine

Bellina JH, Wilson J. *The Stress of Infertility: The Complete Fertility Book.* New York: Crown Publishers, 1985

Blechman E, Brownell K, eds. *Behavioral Medicine for Women.* New York: Pergamon Press, 1987

Craighead LW, Craighead WE, Kazdin AE, Mahoney MJ. *Cognitive and Behavioral Interventions: An Empirical Approach to Mental Health Problems.* Boston: Allyn and Bacon, 1994

Domar AD, Dreher H. *Healing Mind, Healthy Woman.* New York: Henry Holt, 1996

Goldberger L, Breznitz S, eds. *Handbook of Stress: Theoretical and Clinical Aspects*, 2nd edn. New York: Free Press, 1993

Hafen BQ, Karren KJ, Frandsen KJ, Smith NL, eds. *Mind/Body Health: The Effects of Attitudes, Emotions, and Relationships.* Boston: Allyn and Bacon, 1996

Rosenthall D, ed. *Family Stress.* Rockville, MD: Aspen Publishers, 1987

Salzer L. *Surviving Infertility: A Compassionate Guide Through the Emotional Crisis of Infertility.* New York: Harper Perennial, 1991

Stanton AL, Dunkel-Schetter C, eds. *Infertility: Perspectives from Stress and Coping Research.* New York: Plenum, 1991

Tunks E, Bellissimo A. *Behavioral Medicine: Concepts and Procedures.* New York: Pergamon Press, 1991

Woolfolk RL, Lehrer PM, eds. *Principles and Practices of Stress Management.* New York: Guilford Press, 1984

Sexual Counseling

Books

Baker R. *Sperm Wars: The Science of Sex.* New York: Basic Books, 1996

Barbach L. *For Yourself: The Fulfilment of Female Sexuality.* New York: Doubleday, 1975

Barbach L. *For Each Other: Sharing Sexual Intimacy.* New York: Doubleday, 1982

Barbach L. *Pleasures: Women Write Erotica.* New York: Harper & Row, 1985

Barbach L, Geisinger DL. *Going the Distance: Finding and Keeping Lifelong Love.* New York: New American Library/Dutton, 1993

Barbach L, Levine L. *Shared Intimacies: Women's Sexual Experiences.* New York: Doubleday, 1980

Heiman J, LoPiccolo J. *Becoming Orgasmic: A Personal and Sexual Growth Program for Women.* Englewood Cllffs, NJ: Prentice-Hall, 1988

Kaplan H. *How to Overcome Premature Ejaculation.* New York: Brunner/Mazel, 1989

Keesling B. *Sexual Healing: A Self-Help Program to Enhance Your Sexuality and Overcome Common Sexual Problems.* Claremont, CA: Hunter House, 1990

Levine L, Barbach L. *The Intimate Male: Candid Discussions About Women, Sex, and Relationships.* New York: New American Library/Dutton, 1985

Masters WH, Johnson VE, Kolodny RC. *Human Sexuality*, 4th edn. New York: Harper College, 1991

Money J. *Gay, Straight and In-Between: The Sexology of Erotic Orientation*. London: Oxford University Press, 1988

Valins L. *When a Woman's Body Says No to Sex: Understanding and Overcoming Vaginismus*. New York: Penguin Books, 1988, 1992

Zilbergeld B. *Male Sexuality*. New York: Bantam Books, 1978

Videos

Becoming Orgasmic. Sinclair Institute, PO Box 8865, Chapel Hill, NC 27515. (919) 929 3797 Fax (919) 942-0792

Treating Vaginismus; Treating Erectile Problems. Focus International, 14 Oregon Drive, Huntington Station, New York 1746. (800) 843-0305

Organizations

American Association of Sex Educators, Counselors and Therapists (AASECT)
435 North Michigan Avenue, Suite 1717
Chicago, IL 60611-4067
(312) 644-0828

Impotence Information Center
PO Box 9
Minneapolis, MN 55440
(800) 843-4315; (612) 933-4666 (in Minnesota)

Kinsey Institute for Research in Sex, Gender, and Reproduction
313 Morrison Hall
Indiana University
Bloomington, IN 47405
(812) 855-7686

SEICUS Report
Sex Information and Education Council of the United States
130 West 42nd Street, Suite 2500
New York, NY 10036
(212) 819-9770

SECTION IV: MEDICAL COUNSELING ISSUES

Medical Conditions

Ambiguous Genitalia
428 E. Elm Street, #4/D
Lodi, CA 95240
(209) 369-0414

American Cancer Society
1599 Clifton Road
NE Atlanta, GA 30329
(800) ACS-2345 (patient information)
(Pamphlets available: Sexuality and Cancer: For the Man Who Has Cancer, and His Partner; Sexuality and Cancer: For the Woman Who Has Cancer, and Her Partner)

American Society for Reproductive Medicine
1209 Montgomery Highway, Birmingham, AL 35216-2809
(205) 978-5000
(Pamphlets available: Endometriosis: A Guide for Patients; Fertility After Cancer Treatment: A Guide for Patients)

Cystic Fibrosis Foundation (CFF)
6931 Arlington Road
Bethseda, MD 20814
(800) 322-4823

DES Action
1615 Broadway, Suite 510
Oakland, CA 9461
(800) DES-9288; (510) 465-4011

Endometriosis Association
8585 N. 76th Place
Milwaukee, WI 53223
(800) 992-ENDO (3636) (recorded message); (414) 355-2200 (office)

FRAXA Research Foundation
PO Box 935
Westbury, MA 01985-0935
(508) 462-1990

Hysterectomy Educational Resources and Services
501 Woodbrook Lane
Philadelphia, PA 19119
(215) 247-6232

Hysterectomy Support Group
The Venture
Green Lane, Upton
Huntington PE 17 5YE
United Kingdom
(44) 181-690-5987

Klinefelter Syndrome and Association (KS)
PO Box 119
Roseville, CA 95678-0119
(916) 773-1449

Klinefelter's Syndrome Association
Route 1, Box 93
Pine River, WI 54965
(414) 987-5782

March of Dimes Birth Defects Foundation
1275 Mamaroneck Avenue
White Plains, NY 10526
(914) 428-7100

National Cancer Institute
Building 31, Room 10A16
9000 Rockville Pike
Bethseda, MD 20982

National Down's Syndrome
666 Broadway
New York, NY 10012-2317
(800) 221-4602

National Endometriosis Society
35 Belgrave Square
London SW1X 8QB
United Kingdom
(44) 171-235-4137

National Fragile X Foundation
1411 York Street, Suite 303
Denver, CO 80265
(800) 688-8765

Parent Assistance Committee on Down's Syndrome
208 Lafayette Avenue
Peerskill, NY 10566
(914) 739-4085

RESOLVE, Inc
1310 Broadway
Somerville, MA 02144
(617) 623-0744 (national helpline)
(Fact sheets available: Cancer and Infertility; Endometriosis; Three Doctors Look at Endometriosis)

Support and Education for Klinefelter's Syndrome
SEEK'S, Inc
1417 25th Avenue Drive W
Bradenton, FL 34205-6449
(813) 750-8044

Turner's Syndrome Society of USA
15500 Wayzata Blvd., #811
Twelve Oaks Center
Wayzata, MN 55391
(800) 365-9944

Genetic Conditions

Books

Bartels DM, LeRoy BS, Caplan A, eds. *Prescribing Our Future: Ethical Challenges in Genetic Counseling*. New York: Aldine de Gruyter, 1993

Beyond Prenatal Choice. Omaha, NE: Centering Corporation, 1990

Blatt R. *Prenatal Tests: What They Are, Their Benefits and Risks, and How to Decide Whether to Have Them or Not*. New York: Vintage Books, 1988

Crespigny L, Dredge R. *Which Tests for My Unborn Baby?: Ultrasound and Other Prenatal Tests*. Melbourne, Australia: Oxford University Press, 1991, 1996

Difficult Decisions. Omaha, NE: Centering Corporation, 1990

Fine BA, Gettig EL, Greendale K, et al., eds. *Strategies in Genetic Counseling: Reproductive Genetics and New Technologies*. White Plains, NY: March of Dimes Defects Foundation, 1990

Isle S. *Precious Lives, Painful Choices: A Prenatal Decision-Making Guide*. Maple Plain, MN: Wintergreen Press, 1990

Jackson JF. *Genetics and You*. Totowa NJ: Humana Press, 1996

Kolata G. *The Baby Doctors: Probing the Limits of Fetal Medicine*. New York: Delacorte Press, 1990

Minnick MA, Delp KJ, eds. *A Time to Decide, A Time to Heal*, 2nd edn. Mullett Lake, MI: Pineapple Press, 1991

Romero R, Pilu P, Jeanty A, et al. *Prenatal Diagnosis of Congenital Abnormalities*. East Norwalk, CT: Appleton & Lange, 1988

Rothenberg KH, Thomson EJ, eds. *Women and Prenatal Testing: Facing the Challenges of Genetic Technology*. Columbus: Ohio State University Press, 1994

Rothman BK. *The Tentative Pregnancy: How Amniocentesis Changes the Experience of Motherhood*. New York: Norton, 1986, 1993

Schild S, Black RB. *Social Work and Genetics: A Guide for Practice*. New York: Haworth Press, 1984

Organizations

Alliance of Genetic Support Groups
PO Box 8738
Reno, NV 89507-8738
(702) 826-7332

A Heartbreaking Choice
35 Wisconsin Circle, Suite 440
Chevy Chase, MD 20815
(301) 652-5553; (800) 336-4363

Support for Prenatal Decision
PO Box 1161
San Bernardino, CA 92402
(714) 794-5196; (714) 792-2113; (714) 361-0407

Pregnancy Loss

Books

Allen M, Marks S. Miscarriage. *Women Sharing from the Heart*. New York: Wiley, 1993

Covington S. *Silent Birth: If Your Baby Dies*. 1996. (Booklet available in English and Spanish for purchase: 9707 Medical Center Drive, #230, Rockville, Maryland 20850)

DeFrain J. *Stillborn: The Invisible Death*. New York: Lexington Books, 1986

Friedman R, Gradstein B. *Surviving Pregnancy Loss: A Complete Source Book for Women and Their Families*. Boston–Toronto: Little Brown, 1982.

Ilse S, Burns LH. *Miscarriage: A Shattered Dream*. Long Lake, MN: Wintergreen Press, 1985

Jacobs S. *Pathologic Grief: Maladaptation to Loss*. Washington, DC: American Psychiatric Press, 1993

Kohn I, Moffitt P. *A Silent Sorrow: Pregnancy Loss: Guidance and Support for You and Your Family*. New York: Delacorte Press, 1992

Leon IG. *When a Baby Dies: Psychotherapy for Pregnancy and Newborn Loss*. New Haven. CT: Yale University Press, 1990

Mehren E. *Born Too Soon*. New York: Doubleday, 1991

Minnik M, Delp K. *A Time to Decide, A Time to Heal*, 2nd edn. Mullett Lake, MI: Pineapple Press, 1991

Peppers LG, Knapp RJ. *Motherhood and Mourning: Perinatal Death*. New York: Praeger, 1980

Pizer H, O'Brien C. *Coping With a Miscarriage*. New York: New American Library, 1981

Shapiro CH. *Infertility and Pregnancy Loss*. San Francisco: Jossey-Bass, 1988

Worden JW. *Grief Counseling and Grief Therapy: A Handbook for the Mental Health Practitioner*. New York: Springer, 1983

Woods R, Esposito J, eds. *Pregnancy Loss: Medical Therapeutics and Practical Considerations*. Baltimore: Williams & Wilkins, 1987

Videos

At a Loss for Words (For Family and Caregivers); *Footprints on our Hearts* (for Parents). Paraclete Press, PO Box 1568, Orleans, MA 02653. (800) 451 5006

Organizations

Alliance of Genetic Support Groups
35 Wisconsin Circle, Suite 440
Chevy Chase MD 20815
(301) 652-5553; (800) 336-4363

Compassionate Friends, Inc
PO Box 3696
Oakbrook, IL 60522
(708) 990-0010

Miscarriage Association
Clayton Hospital
Northgate
Wakefield
West Yorkshire WF1 3JS
United Kingdom
(44) 1924-200-799

Pregnancy and Infant Loss Center
1421 E. Wayzata Blvd., Suite 30
Wayzata, MN 55391
(612) 473-9372

Resolve Thru Sharing
Gunderson Lutheran Hospital
1910 South Avenue
Lacrosse, WI 54601
(608) 785-0530 (ext. 4747)

SHARE, Inc
St. Joseph Health Center
300 First Capitol Drive
St Charles, MO 63301
(314) 947-6164; (800) 821-6819
www.nationalshareoffice.com

Stillbirth and Neonatal Death Society
28 Portland Place
London W1N 4DE
United Kingdom
(44) 171-436-5881

Sudden Infant Death Syndrome Alliance
1314 Bedford Avenue, Suite 210
Baltimore, MD 21208
(800) 221-7437

SECTION V: SPECIAL POPULATIONS

Cross-Cultural Counseling

Anderson AK. *Taste of Tears, Touch of God.* Nashville, TN: Oliver-Nelson Books, 1984

Berry JW, Toortnga Y, Segall MH, Dasen PR. *Cross-Cultural Psychology: Research and Application.* Cambridge, UK: Cambridge University Press, 1992

Boyd-Franklin N. *Black Families in Therapy: A Multisystems Approach.* New York: Guilford Press, 1989

Comas-Diaz L, Griffith EEH, eds. *Clinical Guidelines in Cross-Cultural Mental Health.* New York: Wiley, 1988

Gaw AC, ed. *Culture, Ethnicity, and Mental Illness.* Washington, DC: American Psychiatric Press, 1993

Grazi R. *Be Fruitful and Multiply: Fertility Therapy and the Jewish Tradition.* Spring Valley, NY: Feldheim Publishers, 1995

Greil AL. *Not Pregnant Yet: Infertile Couples in Contemporary America.* New Brunswick and New Jersey: Rutgers University Press, 1991

Marsh M, Ronner W. *The Empty Cradle: Infertility in America from Colonial Times to the Present.* Baltimore: Johns Hopkins University Press, 1996

Martin E. *The Woman in the Body: A Cultural Analysis of Reproduction.* Boston: Beacon Press, 1987

May ET. *Barren in the Promised Land: Childless Americans and the Pursuit of Happiness.* New York: Basic Books, 1995

McGoldrick M. *Ethnicity and Family Therapy: An Overview.* New York: Guilford Press, 1982

Ramierez M. *Psychotherapy and Counseling with Minorities.* New York: Pergamon Press, 1991

Sha JL. *Mothers of Thyme: Customs and Rituals of Infertility and Miscarriage.* Ann Arbor MI: Lida Rose Press, 1990

Stigger JA. *Coping with Infertility.* Minneapolis, MN: Augsburg, 1983

Sue DW, Sue D. *Counseling the Culturally Different: Theory and Practice,* 2nd edn. New York: Wiley, 1990

Tseng W, Hsu J. *Culture and Family: Problems and Therapy.* New York: Haworth Press, 1991

Tseng W, McDermott JF. *Culture, Mind, and Therapy.* New York: Brunner/Mazel, 1981

Tyler EM. *Barren in the Promised Land.* New York: Basic Books, 1995

Single and Lesbian Mothers

Books

Boston Lesbian Psychologies Collective, eds. *Lesbian Psychologies: Explorations and Challenges.* Urbana, IL: University of Illinois Press, 1987

Bowers K. *Single Pregnancy, Single Parenting.* Pleasant Hill, CA: Park Alexander Press, 1996

Braude M, ed. *Women, Power and Therapy: Issues for Women.* New York: Haworth Press, 1988

Chambers D. *Solo Parenting: Raising Strong and Happy Families.* Minneapolis, MN: Fairview Press, 1997

Clunis DM, Green GD. *The Lesbian Parenting Book.* Seattle, WA: Seal Press, 1995

Melina LR. *Making Sense of Adoption: A Parent's Guide*. New York: Harper & Row, 1989

Miller N. *Single Parents by Choice: A Growing Trend in Family Life*. New York: Plenum, 1992

Pies C. *Considering Parenthood: A Workbook for Lesbians*. San Francisco, CA: Spinsters/Aunt Lute, 1985

Bozett, F, ed. *Gay and Lesbian Parents*. New York: Praegar, 1987; 165–74

Bozett FW, Sussman MB, eds. *Homosexuality and Family Relations*. New York: Haworth Press, 1990;137–54

Vida G, ed. *Our Right to Make Love: A Lesbian Resource Book*. Englewood Cliffs, NJ: Prentice-Hall, 1978

For Children

Elwin R, Paulse M. *Asha's Mums*. Toronto: Women's Press, 1990

Jenness A. *Families: A Celebration of Diversity, Commitment and Love*. Boston: Houghton Mifflin, 1990

Newman L. *Heather Has Two Mommies*. Boston: Alyson Wonderland, 1989

Organizations

Committee for Single Adoptive Parents
PO Box 15084
Chevy Chase, MD 20815

DI Network
PO Box 265
Sheffield S3 7YX
United Kingdom

Donors' Offspring
PO Box 33
Sarcoxie, MO 64862

Gay and Lesbian Parents' Coalition
International
PO Box 50360
Washington, DC 20091

National Organization of Single Mothers
PO Box 6
Midland, NC 28107-006

Parents Without Partners
8807 Colesville Road
Silver Springs, MD 20910
(301) 588-9354

Single Mothers by Choice, Inc
200 East 84th Street
New York, NY 10028

Older Infertile Patients

Books

Carnoy M, Carnoy D. *Fathers of a Certain Age: The Joys and Problems of Middle-Age Fatherhood*. Minneapolis, MN: Fairview Press, 1995

Daniels P, Weingarten KI. *Sooner or Later: The Timing of Parenthood in Adult Lives*. New York: Norton, 1982

Morris M. *Last-Chance Children: Growing Up with Older Parents*. New York: Columbia University Press, 1988

Price J. *You're Not Too Old to Have a Baby*. New York: Farrar, Strauss, and Giroux, 1977

Yarrow A. *Latecomers*. New York: Free Press, 1991

Pregnancy and the Older Mother

Curtis GB. *Your Pregnancy after 30*. Tucson, AZ: Fisher Books, 1996

Kitzinger S. *Birth Over Thirty-Five*. New York: Penguin Books, 1982, 1994 .

McCauley C. *Pregnancy After 35*. New York: Dutton, 1976

Organizations

Parenthood After Thirty
451 Vermont
Berkeley, CA 94707
(415) 524-6635

Remarriage and Stepfamilies

Books

Berman C. *Making It as a Stepparent: New Roles, New Rules*. New York: Harper & Row, 1986

Clark LF, Burns C. *Stepmotherhood: How to Survive Without Feeling Frustrated, Left Out, or Wicked*. New York: Times Books, 1985

Hetherington EM, Arastek J, eds. *The Impact of Divorce, Single-Parenting and Step Parenting on Children*. Hillsdale, NJ: Lawrence Erlbaum, 1988

Martin D, Martin M. *Stepfamilies in Therapy*. San Francisco: Jossey-Bass, 1992

Papernow PL. *Becoming a Stepfamily*. San Francisco: Jossey-Bass, 1993

Pasley K, Inhinger-Tallman M, eds. *Remarriage and Step Parenting Today: Current Research and Theory*. New York: Guilford Press, 1987

Pickhardt CE. *Keys to Successful Step-fathering*. Hauppauge, NY: Barron's Education Series, 1997

Visher EB, Visher JS. *Step Families: A Guide to Working with Stepfamilies and Stepchildren*. New York: Bruner/Mazel, 1979

Visher EB, Visher JS. *Old Loyalties, New Ties: Therapeutic Strategies with Step Families*. New York: Brunner/Mazel, 1988

Visher EB, Visher JS. *How to Win as a Step-Family*, 2nd edn. New York: Brunnel/Mazel, 1991

Sager CJ, Brown HS, Crohn H, et al., eds. *Treating the Remarried Family*. New York: Brunnel/Mazel, 1983

Organizations

Stepfamily Association of American, Inc
National Headquarters
602 E. Joppa Road
Baltimore, MD 21204
(301) 823-7570

Step Family Association of America
212 Lincoln Center
215 S. Centennial Mall
Lincoln, NE 68508-1834
(800) 735-0329

The Step Family Foundation
333 West End Avenue
New York, NY 10023

Secondary Infertility

Simons HF. *Wanting Another Child: Coping with Secondary Infertility*. New York: Lexington Books, 1995

Hawke S, Know D. *One Child by Choice*. Englewood Cliffs, NY: Prentice-Hall, 1977

Kappelman M. *Raising the Only Child*. New York: New American Library, 1977

Newman S. *Parenting an Only Child*. New York: Doubleday, 1990

Sifford D. *Only Child: Being One, Loving One, Understanding One, Raising One*. New York: Harper & Row, 1989

SECTION VI: THIRD-PARTY REPRODUCTION

Books

Andrews L. *Between Strangers: Surrogate Mothers, Expectant Fathers, and Brave New Babies*. New York: Harper & Row, 1990

Baran A, Pannor R. *The Shocking Consequences and Unsolved Problems of Artificial Insemination*. New York: Warner Books, 1989

Baran A, Pannor R. *Lethal Secrets: The Psychology of Donor Insemination—Problems and Solutions*. New York: Warner Books, 1993

Cohen CB. *New Ways of Making Babies: The Case of Egg Donation*. Bloomington, IN: Indiana University Press, 1996

Dutton G. *A Matter of Trust: Guide to Gestational Surrogacy*. Irvine, CA: Clouds Publications, 1997

Friedeman JS. *Building Your Family Through Egg Donation: What You Will Want to Know About the Emotional Aspects, Bonding, and Disclosure Issues*. Ft. Thomas, KY: Jolance Press, 1996

Glazer E, Cooper S. *Beyond Infertility: The New Paths to Parenthood*. New York: Lexington Books, 1994

Keane NP, Breo D. *The Surrogate Mother*. New York: Everest House, 1981

McWhinnie A. *Families Following Assisted Conception: What Do We Tell Our Child?* Dundee: University of Dundee, 1997. (Write to: Ann Wallace, Dept. of Social Work, University of Dundee, Frankland Bldg., Dundee DD1 5HN, United Kingdom)

Noble E. *Having Your Baby by Donor Insemination: A Complete Resource Guide*. Boston: Houghton Mifflin, 1987

Ragone H. *Surrogate Motherhood: Conceptions in the Heart*. San Francisco: Westview Press, 1994

Robinson S, Pizer HE. *Having a Baby Without a Man: The Woman's Guide To Alternative Insemination*. New York: Simon & Schuster, 1985

Schlaff WD, Vercollone CF. *Understanding Artificial Insemination*. Aurora, CO: Zetek Inc., 1987

Seibel MM, Crockin SL., eds. *Family Building Through Egg and Sperm Donation: Medical, Legal, and Ethical Issues*. Boston: Jones and Bartlett, 1996

Singer P, Wells D. *The Reproductive Revolution: New Ways of Making Babies*. Oxford, UK: Oxford University Press, 1984

Snowden R, Mitchell GD. *The Artificial Family: A Consideration of Artificial Insemination by Donor*. London: George Allen and Unwin, 1981

Books for Children

Gordon E. *Mommy, Did I Grow in Your Tummy? Where Some Babies Come From*. Santa Monica, CA: EM Greenburg Press, 1992

Hoberman M. *Fathers, Mothers, Sisters, Brothers: A Collection of Family Poems*. New York: Puffin Books, 1991

My Story. University Department of OB/GYN, Jessop Hospital for Women. Sheffield, England: Infertility Research Trust, 1991. (Order from Kris Probasco, LSCSW, 144 Westwood Dr., Liberty, MO 64068; $14.95)

New South Wales Infertility Social Workers Group, Paul J, ed. *How I Began: The Story of Donor Insemination*. Carleton, Victoria, Australia: The Fertility Society of Australia, 1988. [Order: C/-ACTS, GPO Box 2200, Canberra ACT 2601, Australia; phone (61) 6-257-3299]

Pellegrini N. *Families Are Different*. New York: Holiday House, 1991

Schaffer P. *How Babies and Families Are Made (There is More Than One Way!)*. Berkeley, CA: Tabor Sarah Books, 1988

Schnitter J. *Let Me Explain: A Story About Donor Insemination*. Indianapolis, IN: Perspectives Press, 1995

Simon N. *All Kinds of Families*. Niles, IL: Albert Whitman & Co., 1976

Simon N. *Why Am I Different?* Morton Grove, IL: Albert Whitman & Co., 1976

Snyder GS. *Test-Tube Life*. Englewood Cliffs, NJ: Prentice Hall, 1982

Organizations

Childlessness Overcome Through Surrogacy (COTS)
C/o Gena Dodd, Secretary
Loandu Cottage
Gruids, Lairg
Sutherland IV27 4EF
United Kingdom
www.surrogacy.com

Di Network
Po Box 265
Sheffield S3 7YX
United Kingdom

Donor Conception Support Group
Po Box 53
Georges Hall
New South Wales 2198
Australia

Donors' Offspring
Po Box 33
Sarcoxie, MO 64862

New Reproductive Alternatives Society
641 Cadogan Street
Nanaimo, British Columbia V9S 1T6
Canada

Organization of Parents through Surrogacy
National Headquarters
Shirley Zaeger
PO Box 213
Wheeling, IL 60090
(805) 482-1566 (California, main number); (708) 394-4116 (Illinois); (201) 384-9409 (New Jersey); (617) 740-1783 (Massachusetts)
www.opts.com

SECTION VII: ALTERNATIVE FAMILY-BUILDING

Adoption

Books

Adamac CA. *There ARE Babies to Adopt*. New York: Pinnacle, 1991

Alexander-Roberts C. *The Essential Adoption Handbook*. Dallas, TX: Taylor Publishing, 1993

Beauvais-Godwin L, Godwin R. *The Independent Adoption Manual*. Lakewood, NJ: The Advocate Press, 1993

Benet MK. *The Politics of Adoption*. New York: Free Press, 1976

Bolles EB. *The Penguin Adoption Handbook*. New York: Penguin Books, 1984

Brodzinsky D, Schechter M, eds. *The Psychology of Adoption*. New York: Oxford University Press, 1990

Brodzinsky D, Schechter DE, Henig RM. *Being Adopted: The Lifelong Search for Self*. New York: Doubleday, 1992

Glazer ES. *The Long-Awaited Stork: A Guide to Parenting after Infertility*. New York: Lexington Press, 1990

Gilman L. *The Adoption Resource Book*. New York: HarperCollins, 1992

Johnston P. *Adopting After Infertility*. Indianapolis, IN: Perspectives Press, 1992

Kirk HD. *Shared Fate: A Theory and Method of Adoptive Relationships*. Port Angeles, WA: Ben-Simon Publications, 1984

Lindsay J. *Open Adoption: A Caring Option*. Buena Park, CA: Morning Glory Press, 1987

Lindsay J, Monserrat C. *Adoption Awareness: A Guide for Teachers, Counselors, Nurses and Caring Others*. Buena Park, CA: Morning Glory Press, 1989

Melina LR. *Raising Adopted Children*. New York: Harper and Row, 1986

Melina LR. *Making Sense of Adoption: A Parent's Guide*. New York: HarperCollins, 1990

Melina LR, Roszia SK. *The Open Adoption Experience*. New York: HarperCollins, 1993

Michaelman S, Schneider M. *The Private Adoption Handbook: A Step-by-Step Guide to Independently Adopting a Baby*. New York: Dell, 1988

Pulmez JH. *Successful Adoption*. New York: Harmony Books, 1987

Reitz M, Watson KW. *Adoption and the Family System*. New York: Guilford Press, 1992

Rosenberg EB. *The Adoption Life Cycle*. New York: Free Press, 1992

Schaffer J, Lindstrom C. *How to Raise an Adopted Child*. New York: Crown Publishers, 1989

Smith J, Miroff F. *You're Our Child: The Adoption Experience*. Lanham, MD: Madison Books, 1987

Winkler RC, Brown DW, van Keppel M, Blanchard A. *Clinical Practice in Adoption*. New York: Pergamon Press, 1988

Organizations

Adoptive Families of America, Inc. (AFA)
3333 Highway 100 North
Minneapolis, MN 55422
(612) 537-0316

American Academy of Adoption Attorneys
PO Box 33053
Washington, DC 20033

American Adoption Congress (AAC)
PO Box 44040
L'Enfant Plaza Station
Washington, DC 20026

Child Welfare League of America
440 First Avenue, NW
Washington, DC 20001
(202) 638-2952

Committee for Single Adoptive Parents
PO Box 15084
Chevy Chase, MD 20815

International Concerns Committee for
Children
911 Cypress Drive
Boulder, CO 80303

Latin American Adoptive Families (LAAF)
40 Upland Road
Duxbury, MA 02332

National Adoption Information
Clearinghouse (NAIC)
11426 Rockville Pike, Suite 410
Rockville, MD 20852
(301) 231-6512

National Council for Adoption
1930 17th Street, NW
Washington, DC 20009
(202) 328-1200

North American Council on Adoptable
Children (NACAC)
970 Raymond Avenue, Suite 106
St. Paul, MN 55114
(612) 644-3036

Child-free Living

Books

Anton HL. *Never to Be a Mother: A Guide for All Women Who Didn't—or Couldn't—Have Children*. San Francisco: HarperCollins, 1992

Bartlett J. *Will You Be Mother? Women Who Choose to Say No*. New York: University Press, 1994

Bombardieri M. *The Baby Decision: How to Make the Most Important Choice of Your Life*. New York: Rawson Wade, 1981

Burgwyn D. *Marriage Without Children*. New York: Harper & Row, 1982

Campbell E. *The Childless Marriage: An Exploratory Study of Couples Who Do Not Want Children*. New York: Tavistock Publications, 1985

Carter J, Carter M. *Sweet Grapes: How to Stop Being Infertile and Start Living Again*. Indianapolis, IN: Perspectives Press, 1989

Lafayette L. *Why Don't You Have Kids? Living a Full Life Without Parenthood*. New York: Kensington Publishing, 1995

Lang SS. *Women Without Children: The Reasons, the Rewards, the Regrets*. New York: Pharos Books, 1991

Lindsay K. *Friends as Family*. Boston: Beacon Press, 1981

Safer J. *Beyond Motherhood: Choosing a Life Without Children*. New York: Simon & Schuster, 1996

Stout M. *Without Child: A Compassionate Look at Infertility*. Grand Rapids, MI: Zondervan Publishing House, 1985

Whelan EM. *A Baby? Maybe*. Indianapolis, IN: Bobbs-Merrill, 1975

Wilk CA. *Career Women and Childbearing: A Psychological Analysis of the Decision Process*. New York: Van Nostrand Reinhold, 1986

Organizations

Childfree Network
7777 Sunrise Blvd
Citrus Heights, CA 95610
(916) 773-7178 Fax (916) 786-0513

National Organization of Single Mothers
PO Box 6
Midland, NC 28107-006

Parents Without Partners
8807 Colesville Road
Silver Spring, MD 20910
(301) 588-9354

SECTION VIII: POSTINFERTILITY COUNSELING ISSUES

Pregnancy After Infertility

Books

Cherry SH. *Understanding Pregnancy and Childbirth*, 3rd edn. New York: Collier Books, 1992

Colman LL, Colman A. *Pregnancy: The Psychological Experiences*. New York: Noonday Press/Farrar, Straus, and Giroux, 1991

Diamond K. *Motherhood after Miscarriage*. Holbrook, MA: Bob Adams Publications, 1991

Eisenberg A, Murkoff HE, Hathway SE. *What to Expect When You're Expecting*. New York: Workman Publishing, 1996

Kitzinger S. *The Complete Book of Pregnancy and Childbirth*. New York: Knopf, 1980

Leonhardt-Lupa M. *A Mother Is Born: Preparing for Motherhood During Pregnancy*. Westport, CT: Bergin & Garvey, 1995

Mathews AM. *Excited, Exhausted, Expecting: The Emotional Life of Mothers-to-Be*. New York: Perigee Book 1995

Raphael-Leff J. *Pregnancy: The Inside Story*. London: Jason Aronson, 1993

Complicated Pregnancies

Freeman RK, Pescar SC. *Safe Delivery: Protecting Your Baby During High Risk Pregnancy*. New York: Facts on File, 1982

Gregg R. *Pregnancy in a High-Tech Age: Paradoxes of Choice*. New York: New York University Press, 1995

Hales D, Creasy RK. *New Hope for Problem Pregnancies: Helping Babies BEFORE They're Born*. New York: Harper & Row, 1982

Hales D, Johnson TRB. *Intensive-Caring: New Hope for High-Risk Pregnancy*. New York: Crown Publishers, 1990

Johnson SH, Kraut DA. *Pregnancy Bedrest: A Guide for the Pregnant Woman and her Family*. New York: Henry Holt, 1990

Katz M, Gill P, Turiel J. *Preventing Preterm Birth: A Parent's Guide*. Health Publishing, 1988

Nance S. *Premature Babies: A Handbook for Parents*. New York: Arbor House, 1982

Rakusen J, Davidson N. *Out of Our Hands: What Technology Does to Pregnancy*. London: Pan Books, 1982

Rick L. *When Pregnancy Isn't Perfect: A Layperson's Guide to Complications in Pregnancy*. New York: Dutton, 1991

Robertson PA, Berlin PH. *The Premature Labor Handbook: Successfully Sustaining Your High-Risk Pregnancy*. New York: Doubleday, 1986

Semchyshyn S, Colman C. *How to Prevent Miscarriage and Other Crises of Pregnancy*. New York: Collier Books, 1989

Pregnancy with Multiples

Bryan E. *Twins, Triplets and More: From Pre-Birth Through High School—What Every Parent Needs to Know When Raising Two or More*. New York: St. Martin's Press, 1992

Noble E. *Having Twins*. New York: Houghton Mifflin, 1980, 1991

Rothbart B. *Multiple Blessings: From Pregnancy Through Childhood: A Guide for Parents of Twins, Triplets, and More*. New York: Hearst, 1994

Pregnancy and Sexuality
Bing E, Colman L. *Making Love During Pregnancy*. New York: Farrar, Straus, and Giroux, 1977

Video
After Loss: Journey of the Next Pregnancy. c/o Abbott Northwestern Hospital, Pregnancy After Loss Program, 28th at Chicago, Minneapolis, MN 55407-1320

Organizations
Birthways
127 Telegraph Avenue
Oakland, CA 94609
(415) 653-7300

Center for Loss in Multiple Birth (CLIMB)
PO Box 1064
Palmer, AK 99645
(907) 746-6123

Intensive Caring Unlimited (ICU)
910 Bent Lane
Philadelphia, PA 19118
(215) 233-4723

Parent Care
University of Utah Medical Center
50 North Drive, Room 2A210
Salt Lake City, UT 84132
(801) 581-5323

Parents of Prematures
c/o Houston Organization for Parent Education, Inc
2990 Richmond, Suite 204
Houston, TX 77098
(713) 524-3089

Parenthood After Infertility
Books
Anthony EJ, Benedek T, eds. *Parenthood: Its Psychology and Psychopathology*. Boston: Little, Brown, 1970

Belsky J, Kelly J. *The Transition to Parenthood: How a First Child Changes a Marriage*. London: Vermilion, 1994

Cohen RS, Cohler BJ, Weissman SH, eds. *Parenthood: A Psychodynamic Perspective*. New York: Guilford Press, 1984

Curran D. *Traits of a Healthy Family*. New York: Ballentine Books, 1983

Curran D. *Stress and the Healthy Family*. New York: Harper & Row, 1985

Doherty WJ. *The Intentional Family*. Reading, MA: Addison-Wesley, 1997

Friedland R, Kent C, eds. *The Mother's Book*. Boston: Houghton Mifflin, 1981

Genevive L, Magolis E. *The Motherhood Report: How Women Feel About Being Mother*. New York: Macmillan, 1987

Glazer E. *The Long Awaited Stork: A Guide to Parenting After Infertility*. Boston: Lexington Books, 1990

Hass A. *The Gift of Fatherhood*. New York: Fireside Press, 1994

LaRossa R. *The Modernization of Fatherhood*. Chicago: University of Chicago Press, 1997

McBride AB. *The Growth and Development of Mothers*. New York: Harper & Row, 1981

Niven CA. *Psychological Care for Families: Before, During, and After Birth*. Oxford: Butterworth-Heinemann, 1992

Rich A. *Of Woman Born: Motherhood as an Experience and Institution*. London: Virago, 1984

Williams LH, Berman HS, Rose L. *The Too-Precious Child*. New York: Warner Books, 1987

Postpartum Mental Health

Dalton K, Holton W. *Depression After Childbirth: How to Recognize, Treat, and Prevent Postnatal Depression*. Oxford: Oxford University Press, 1996

Dix C. *The New Mother Syndrome*. New York: Pocket Books, 1985

Dunnewold A. *Evaluation and Treatment of Postpartum Emotional Disorders*. Sarosta, FL: Professional Resource Exchange, 1997

Hamilton JA, Harberger PN. *Postpartum Psychiatric Illness: A Picture Puzzle*. Philadelphia: University of Pennsylvania Press, 1992

Kleiman K, Raskin V. *This Isn't What I Expected*. New York: Bantam Books, 1994

Placksin S. *Mothering the New Mother*. New York: Newmarket Press, 1994

For Children

Bernstein A. *The Flight of the Stork: What Children Think (and When) about Sex and Family Building*, rev ed. Indianapolis, IN: Perspectives Press, 1994

Magazines

Twins Magazine
5350 S. Roslyn Street, Suite 400
Englewood, CO 80011

Organizations

Depression After Delivery
PO Box 1282
Morrisville, PA 19067
(800) 944-4773

International Twins Association
6898 Channel Road, NE
Minneapolis, MN 55432
(612) 571-3022

The Marce Society
c/o Michael O'Hara, PhD
Department of Psychology
University of Iowa
Iowa City, IA 52242
(319) 335-2405

Multiple Birth Foundation
Institute of Obstetrics and Gynaecology
Queen Charlotte's Hospital
Goldhawk Road
London W6 OXG
United Kingdom
(44) 181-740-3519

National Organization of Mothers of Twins Clubs (NOMOTC)
12404 Princess Jeanne, NE
Albuquerque, NM 87112
(505) 275-0955

Only Child Association
9810 Magnolia Avenue
Riverside, CA 92503

Parents of Only Children
4719 Reed Road, Suite 121
Columbus, OH 43220
(614) 442-0873

PASS-CAN
PO Box 7282
Oakville, Ontario L6J 6L6
Canada
(905) 844-9009

Postpartum Support International
927 Kellogg Avenue
Santa Barbara, CA 93111
(805) 967-7636

Society for Reproductive and Infant
Psychology
c/o Dieter Wolke
Psychology Division
University of Hertfordshire

Hatfield
Herts AL 10 9AB
United Kingdom
www.dur.ac.uk~dps0rfd/srip.htm

SECTION IX: INFERTILITY COUNSELING IN PRACTICE

Integrating Counseling

American Association for Marriage and
Family Therapy (AAMFT)
1717 K Street, NW, Suite 407
Washington, DC 20006
(202) 452-0109; (800) 374-2638

American Association of Pastoral
Counselors
9508A Lee Highway
Fairfax, VA 22031
(703) 385-6967

American Psychiatric Association
1400 K Street, NW
Washington, DC 20005
(202) 682-6000

American Psychological Association
750 1st Street, NW
Washington, DC 20002
(202) 336-5500

Australian and New Zealand Infertility
Counsellors Association (ANZICA)
c/o Kay Oke
RBU Royal Women's Hospital
Melbourne, Australia
(64) 9-523 3007 (New Zealand); (61) 2-438
7580 (New South Wales); (61) 7-832 4262
(Queensland); (61) 8-243 6782 (South
Australia); (61) 3-344 2143 (Victoria); (61)
9-386 2088 (Western Australia)

British Infertility Counsellors Association
69 Division Street
Sheffield S1 4G
United Kingdom

British Psychological Society
St. Andrews House
48 Princess Road East
Leicester LE1 7DR
United Kingdom

International Society of Psychosomatic
Obstetrics and Gynecology
c/o Eylard V. Van Hall
Department of Gynaecology
University Hospital
PO Box 9600
2300 RC Leiden
The Netherlands

Mental Health Professional Group
American Society for Reproductive
Medicine (formerly American Fertility
Society)
1209 Montgomery Highway
Birmingham, AL 35216-2809
(205) 978-5000

National Association of Perinatal Social
Workers
11 Wintergreen Hall
Danbury, CT 06812
(304) 589-4869

National Association of Social Workers
750 1st Street, NE, Suite 700
Washington, DC 20002
(202) 408-8600

North American Society of Psychosocial
Obstetrics and Gynecology (NASPOG)
409 12th Street, SW
Washington, DC 20024-2188
(202) 863-1645

Southern Ontario Network of Infertility
Counselors (SONIC)
c/o Sherry Franz, MSW, CSW
790 Bay Street, 8th Floor
Toronto, Ontario
Canada
M5G 1N9
(416) 410-8904

Working Group on Training for Infertility
Counselling
Dr Jim Monach
BICA Executive Committee
Department of Psychiatry
SCHARR
University of Sheffield
Regent Court
30 Regent Street
Sheffield S1 4DA
United Kingdom
(44) 114-222-0775 Fax (44) 114-272-4095
e-mail j.h.monach@sheffield.ac.uk

Internet

Infertility counseling discussion group:
infertility-counselling@sheffield.ac.uk

Ethical and Legal Issues

Books/Journals

Adler N, Keyes S, Robertson P, eds. *Women
and New Reproductive Technologies:
Medical, Psychological, Legal, and Ethical
Dilemmas.* Hillsdale, NJ: Lawrence
Erlbaum, 1991

Alpern KD, ed. *The Ethics of Reproductive
Technology.* New York: Oxford University
Press. 1992

Arditti R, Klein RD, Minden S, eds. *Test-
Tube Women: What Future for Motherhood?*
London: Pandora Press, 1984

Bartholet E. *Family Bonds.* Boston:
Houghton Mifflin, 1993

Baruch D *et al.* eds. *Embryos, Ethics and
Women's Rights: Exploring the New
Reproductive Technologies.* New York:
Harrington Park Press, 1988

Beauchamp TL, Childress JF. *Principles of
Biomedical Ethics*, 4th edn. London:
Oxford University Press, 1994

Bromham DR, Daltom ME, Jacson JC, eds.
*Philosophical Ethics in Reproductive
Medicine.* Manchester, UK: Manchester
University Press, 1990

Canter MB, Bennett BE, Jones SE, Nagy
TF. *Ethics for Psychologists: A Commentary
on the APA Ethics Code.* Washington, DC:
American Psychological Association,
1994

Corea G. *The Mother Machine: Reproductive
Technologies from Artificial Insemination to
Artificial Wombs.* New York: Harper &
Row, 1985

Daly M. *Gynecology: The Metaethics of Radical
Feminism.* Boston: Beacon Press, 1978

Engelhardt HT Jr. *The Foundations of
Bioethics*, 2nd edn. London: Oxford
University Press, 1996

Ethics Committee of the American Fertility
Society. *Ethical Considerations of Assisted
Reproductive Technologies.* Birmingham,
AL: The American Fertility Society, 1994

Ethics Committee of American Society for
Reproductive Medicine. Ethical
considerations of assisted reproductive
technologies. *Fertil Steril* 1994;62 (suppl
1):5

Klein R, ed. *The Exploitation of Infertility:
Women and Reproductive Technologies.*
London: The Women's Press, 1989

The National Advisory Board on Ethics in
Reproduction. *NABER Report* 1995;1(2)

National Bio-ethics Consultative Committee. *Reproductive Technology Counselling: Final Report for the Australian Health Ministers Conference, Commonwealth of Australia*, 1991

O'Brien M. *The Politics of Reproduction*. Boston: Routledge & Kegan Paul, 1981

Peters T. *For the Love of Children: Genetic Technology and the Future of the Family*. Chicago: University of Chicago Press, 1997

Ratcliff KS, Ferree MM, Mellow GO, eds. *Healing Technologies: Feminist Perspectives*. Ann Arbor, MI: University of Michigan Press, 1989

Raymond JG. *Women as Wombs: Reproductive Technologies and the Battle Over Women's Freedom*. San Francisco: Harper San Francisco, 1993

Reidy M, ed. *Ethical Issues in Reproductive Medicine*. Dublin: Gill & Macmillan, 1982

Robertson JA. *Children of Choice: Freedom and the Next Reproductive Technologies*. Princeton, NJ: Princeton University Press, 1994

Royal Commission on New Reproductive Technologies. *Proceed with Care: Final Report of the Commission on New Reproductive Technologies*. Ottawa, Ontario, Canada, 1993

Spallone P. *Beyond Conception: The New Politics of Reproduction*. Granby, MA: Bergin & Garvey Publishers, 1989

Spallone P, Steinberg DL, eds. *Made to Order: The Myth of Reproductive and Genetic Progress*. Oxford: Pergamon Press, 1987

Yeh J, Yeh MV. *Legal Aspects of Infertility*. Boston: Blackwell Scientific, 1992

Organizations

American Bar Association
Family Law Section
Laws of Reproduction and Genetics
Technology Committee
750 N. Lakeshore Drive
Chicago, IL 60611
(312) 988-5000

Human Fertilisation and Embryology
Authority
Paxton House
30 Artillery Lane
London E1 7LS
United Kingdom
(44) 171-600 3272

Physicians and Nurses
Books

Braverman AM, ed. Role of the nurse in infertility. *Infertil Reprod Med Clin North Am* 1996;7

Garner C. *Principles of Infertility Nursing*. Boco Raton, Florida: CRC Press, 1991

Organizations

American College of Obstetricians and Gynecologists (ACOG)
600 Maryland Avenue, SW, Suite 300 East
Washington, DC 20024

American Nurses Association
2420 Pershing Road
Kansas City, MO 64108
(816) 474-5720

American Society of Andrology
309 W Clark Street
Champaign, IL 61820
(217) 356-3182

American Urological Association, Inc
1120 North Charles Street
Baltimore, MD 21201
(301) 727-1100

Australian Fertility Society
Unit 4 24-26 Mort Street
Braddon-GPO Box 2200
Canberra ACT 2601
Australia

British Fertility Society
Room 2/62, 2nd Floor
Birmingham Maternity Hospital
Edgbaston
Birmingham B15 2TG
United Kingdom

Canadian Fertility and Andrology Society
2065 Alexander de Seve, Suite 409
Montreal, Quebec H2L 2W5
Canada
(514) 524-9009

Nurses Professional Group
American Society for Reproductive
Medicine (formerly American Fertility
Society)
1209 Montgomery Highway
Birmingham, AL 35216-2809
(315) 724-4348

European Society of Human Reproduction
and Embryology (ESHRE)
Central Office
A. Van Aken Straat 41
B-1850 Grimbergen
Belgium
(32) 2 269 5600

XII. GLOSSARY

Glossary

Abruptio placentae. During pregnancy, the placenta separates from the lining of the uterus causing bleeding and pain.

Acquired immune deficiency syndrome (AIDS). A disease caused by the human immunodeficiency virus that impairs the body's immune system and leads to severe infections and eventually death.

Acrosome. An enzyme-filled membrane on the sperm head that releases enzymes necessary to penetrate the egg's outer covering (zona pellucida).

Adhesions (scar tissue). Bands of fibrous scar tissue that may bind the pelvic organs and/or loops of bowel together. Adhesions can result from previous infections, endometriosis, or surgeries.

Adoptive parents. Parents who have children by adoption.

Agency adoption. An adoption that takes place through an established institution, either public or private, that exists for the purpose of facilitating adoptions.

Agenesis. An imperfect development of organ or other part.

Amenorrhea. Complete absence or suppression of menstrual periods.

American Society for Reproductive Medicine (ASRM). A professional medical organization of more than 10,000 health care specialists interested in reproductive medicine.

Amniocentesis. A procedure in which a small amount of amniotic fluid is removed through a needle from the fetal sac at about 16 weeks of pregnancy. The fluid is studied for chromosomal abnormalities that may affect fetal development.

Androgens. In men, androgens are the 'male' hormones produced by the testes that are responsible for encouraging masculine characteristics. In women, androgens are produced in small amounts by both the adrenal glands and ovaries. In women, excess amounts of androgens can lead to irregular menstrual periods, obesity, excessive growth of body hair (hirsutism), and infertility.

Andrologist. Laboratory scientist who studies and works with male hormones and sperm.

Anovulation. Absent ovulation; failure of the ovary to ovulate regularly.

Antibody. Protein produced by the body to attack and destroy foreign substances, such as bacteria and viruses. Antibodies are an important part of the body's immune system.

Anticardiolipin antibody. Type of a group of antiphospholipid antibodies that may be associated with miscarriage.

Antisperm antibody. Immune or protective proteins (immunoglobulins) that attack and destroy the sperm because they recognize it as a foreign substance. Antisperm antibodies may be present in men in blood or sperm or in women in blood or cervical mucus.

ART (assisted reproductive technologies). Procedures performed in a laboratory or physician office that facilitate pregnancy. Examples of ART include in vitro fertilization (IVF) and gamete intrafallopian transfer (GIFT).

Assay. A medical term meaning *test*.

Assisted reproductive technology (ART). All treatments that include laboratory handling of eggs, sperm, and/or embryos. Some examples of ART are in vitro fertilization (IVF), gamete intrafallopian transfer (GIFT), pronuclear stage tubal transfer (PROST), tubal embryo transfer (TET), and zygote intrafallopian transfer (ZIFT).

Autoimmune. A condition in which the body's immune system attacks its own tissues, falsely recognizing them as foreign.

Azoospermia. Complete absence of sperm in the semen.

Basal body temperature (BBT). The body temperature at rest. The temperature is taken orally each morning immediately upon awakening. The readings help identify ovulation, which is indicated by a temperature rise of 0.4°F or more.

Bicornuate uterus. Birth defect in which the uterus appears to be heart-shaped with a central indentation. This condition may result in premature labor or abnormal positioning of the fetus in the uterus.

Biochemical pregnancy. Pregnancy detected by a rise of the pregnancy hormone (human chorionic gonadotropin [hCG]) in the blood, but no fetus is visible on ultrasound and the woman has a menstrual period.

Biofeedback. Techniques using equipment to help people gain control over involuntary body functions; often used to control pain or stress.

Biological child. Child produced by the union of the sperm and the egg of the birth parents.

Biological parents. Parents who supply the egg and the sperm that produce a child.

Biopsy. Removal of a small tissue sample for microscopic examination. The term also refers to the tissue removed during the procedure.

Carcinoma. The medical term for cancer.

CBAVD. See congential bilateral absence of vas deferens, cystic fibrosis.

Cerclage. Placement of a nonabsorbable suture around an incompetent (weak) cervical opening in an attempt to keep it closed and thus prevent miscarriage; also known as a cervical stitch.

Cervical agenesis. An undeveloped or absent cervix that obstructs the opening of the uterus.

Cervical mucus. Substance in the cervix through which sperm must swim in order to enter the uterus.

Cervix. Lower narrow end of the uterus that connects the uterine cavity to the vagina.

Chemical pregnancy. See Biochemical pregnancy.

Chemotherapy. Treatment of diseases with chemicals that may also be acutely harmful to the individual and have a toxic effect on the disease-causing process.

Chlamydia. Genus of sexually transmitted bacteria that cause pelvic infections and subsequent damage to the fallopian tubes.

Chorionic villus sampling (CVS). Procedure in which a small sample of cells is taken from the placenta early in a pregnancy for chromosomal testing. Also known as placental bipsy or placentocentesis.

Chromosome. Rod-shaped structure located in the nucleus (center) of a cell that contains hereditary (genetic) material. Humans have 23 pairs of chromosomes (46 total). Two of the 46 are the sex chromosomes, which are the X and Y chromosomes. Normally, women have two X chromosomes and men have one X and one Y chromosome.

Cleavage. Cell division of a fertilized egg.

Clinical pregnancy. A pregnancy confirmed by an increasing level of human chorionic gonadotropin (hCG) and the presence of a gestational sac detected by ultrasound.

Clomid. See Clomiphene citrate.

Clomiphene citrate. An oral antiestrogen drug used to induce ovulation in women. It is also sometimes used to increase testosterone levels in infertile men, which may in turn improve sperm production. Trade names are Clomid and Serophene.

Closed adoption. An adoption in which no information is exchanged between the birthparents and the adoptive parents.

Congenital. A physical abnormality that is present at birth. The defect(s) may be due to an inherited problem, such as abnormal chromosomes or genes, or to an influence occurring during pregnancy.

Congenital bilateral absence of vas deferens. Genetic disorder causing azoospermia, also known as genital cystic fibrosis, as men with the disorder are either carriers or affected by cystic fibrosis (although it may be a mild form in which men are asymptomatic and unaware of disorder before diagnosis of azoospermia).

Contraindication. A medical situation that suggests that a particular medication or treatment should not be used because of possible risks and/or side effects.

Controlled superovulation. Administration of hormone medications (ovulation drugs) that stimulate the ovaries to produce multiple eggs; sometimes called enhanced follicular recruitment or controlled ovarian hyperstimulation.

Cordocentesis. Removal of a sample of fetal blood by inserting a needle, under ultrasound guidance, through the abdominal wall of a pregnant woman into the umbilical vein. The fetal blood is used for chromosome analysis.

Corpus luteum. Tissue formed in the ovary from a mature follicle that has released its egg at ovulation. The corpus luteum secretes progesterone and estrogen during the second half of a normal menstrual cycle. The secreted progesterone prepares the lining of the uterus (endometrium) to support a pregnancy.

Crohn's disease. Inflammatory bowel disease that causes painful ulcers to form within the bowel.

Cryopreservation. Freezing at a very low temperature, such as in liquid nitrogen (−196°C), to keep embryos viable so as to store them for future transfer into a uterus or to keep sperm viable for future insemination or assisted reproductive technology procedures. At present, eggs and ovary tissue have limited success being cryopreserved.

Cystic fibrosis (fibrocystic disease of pancreas, mucoviscidosis). Hereditary disease affecting the exocorin gland, resulting in the production of thick mucus that obstructs intestinal glands, pancreas, and bronchi.

Danazol. Androgen-like drug, used to treat endometriosis, that blocks ovulation and suppresses estrogen levels. The trade name is Danocrine.

DES. See Diethylstilbestrol.

Diabetes mellitus. Condition due to abnormal production of insulin, resulting in abnormally elevated blood glucose (sugar) levels.

Diagnostic hysteroscopy. Insertion of a long, thin, lighted telescope-like instrument, called a hysteroscope, through the vagina and cervix, and into the uterus in order to look inside the uterine cavity.

Diagnostic laparoscopy. Insertion of a long, thin, lighted telescope-like instrument, called a laparoscope, through the navel into the abdomen in order to look at the internal pelvic organs, such as the uterus, ovaries, and fallopian tubes.

Didelphic uterus. Complete double uterus and double cervix. It is often also associated with a partial or complete double vagina.

Diethylstilbestrol (DES). Synthetic hormone given from 1938–1971 in part during pregnancy to prevent miscarriage. Children from treated pregnancies can have abnormalities of the reproductive system, including an increased risk of ectopic pregnancy, undescended testicles, and infertility.

Dilation and curettage (D & C). An outpatient surgical procedure during which the cervix is dilated and the lining of the uterus is scraped out. The tissue is often used for microscopic examination for the presence of abnormality or pregnancy tissue.

Dilator. Instrument(s) used to enlarge a small opening, such as the cervix and the vagina.

Disorders of fusion. Birth defects in the female reproductive system that result from the failure of the two müllerian ducts to join together. See Rokitansky-Küster-Hauser syndrome.

Distal tubal blockage. Blockage at the end of the fallopian tube farthest away (distal) from where it joins the uterus and near where it meets the ovary.

Domestic adoption. Adoption of a child from the same country of citizenship as the adoptive parents.

Donor. A woman who provides eggs, a man who provides sperm, or a couple who provide embryos for a recipient man, woman, or couple.

Donor egg. Egg taken from the ovaries of a fertile woman and donated to an infertile woman to be used in an assisted reproductive technology procedure, i.e., IVF or GIFT. See also Egg donation.

Donor embryo. Embryos produced from the sperm and the egg of one couple and donated to an infertile woman or couple.

Donor embryo transfer. Transfer of an embryo donated by a couple into the uterus of an infertile woman.

Donor insemination (DI). Process of placing sperm from a donor (a man who is not a woman's sexual partner) into a woman's reproductive tract for the purpose of producing a pregnancy. The resulting child will be biologically related to the woman but not to her partner.

Donor sperm. Sperm donated by a male donor to be used in a donor insemination procedure. See also Donor insemination.

Down syndrome. Genetic disorder caused by the presence of an extra chromosome (21) and characterized by mental retardation, abnormal facial features, and medical problems such as heart defects.

Dysfunctional uterine bleeding (DUB). Abnormal uterine bleeding with no evidence of mechanical or structural cause. The cause of DUB is deficient or excessive production of estrogen and/or progesterone.

Dyspareunia. Pain with intercourse; sometimes a symptom of endometriosis.

Early menopause. Cessation of menstrual periods due to failure of the ovaries before age 40. The average age of menopause in the United states is 52. See also Premature ovarian failure.

Ectopic (extrauterine) pregnancy. A pregnancy that implants outside of uterus, usually in the fallopian tube. The tube may rupture or bleed as the pregnancy grows becoming a serious medical situation.

Egg donation. Process of fertilizing eggs from a donor with the male partner's sperm in a laboratory dish and transferring the resulting embryos to the female partner's uterus. The female partner will not be biologically related to the child, although she will be the birth mother on record. The male partner will be biologically related to the child.

Egg retrieval (harvest). Procedure by which eggs (oocytes) are obtained by inserting a needle into the ovarian follicle and removing the fluid and the egg by suction; also called oocyte aspiration.

Egg. The female sex cell (ovum or oocyte) produced by the female's ovaries, which, when fertilized by a male's sperm, produces an embryo, the earliest form of human life.

Ejaculation. Expulsion of semen (sperm and glandular fluid) from the urethra at the time of male orgasm. Semen is also referred to as the *ejaculate*.

Embryo. The earliest stage of early human development arising after the union of the sperm and the egg (fertilization).

Embryo transfer. Placement of an embryo into the uterus through the vagina and cervix or, in the case of zygote intrafallopian transfer (ZIFT) or tubal embryo transfer (TET), into the fallopian tube.

Embryologist. A scientist who studies the growth and development of the embryo from fertilization until birth. The embryologist is an important member of the assisted reproduction team.

Empirical therapy. When medications or other treatments reportedly work for some patients but are unproven to work consistently in large research studies. Empirical therapy is tried without proven effects.

Endometrial biopsy. Removal of a small piece of tissue from the endometrium (lining of the uterus) for microscopic examination. The results may indicate whether or not the endometrium is at the appropriate stage for successful implantation of a fertilized egg (embryo) and/or whether it is inflamed or diseased.

Endometrioma. Blood-filled cyst that can occur when endometrial tissue develops in the ovary.

Endometriosis. Condition in which patches of endometrium-like tissue (the tissue that lines the uterus) develop outside of the uterine cavity in abnormal locations such as the ovaries, fallopian tubes, and abdominal cavity. Endometriosis can grow with hormonal stimulation, causing pelvic pain, inflammation, and scar tissue. It also may be associated with infertility.

Endometritis. Inflammation of the endometrial lining caused by bacterial invasion.

Endometrium. The lining of the uterus that is shed each month with the menstrual period. As the monthly cycle progresses, the endometrium thickens and thus provides a nourishing site for the implantation of a fertilized egg.

Epididymis. A tightly coiled system of tiny tubing where sperm collect after leaving the testes. Sperm continue to mature as they are pushed through the epididymis, which covers the top and back sides of each testis.

Estradiol. The predominant estrogen (hormone) produced by the follicular cells of the ovary.

Estrogen. The female sex hormones produced by the ovaries that are responsible for the development of female sex characteristics. Estrogens are largely responsible for stimulating the uterine lining to thicken during the first half of the menstrual cycle in preparation for ovulation and possible pregnancy. They are also important for healthy bones and overall health. These hormones are also produced in small amounts in men when testosterone is converted to estrogen.

Estrogen replacement therapy. Use of synthetic or natural estrogenic hormones to replace the hormones that are lost due to menopause; also known as hormone replacement therapy.

Fallopian tubes. A pair of hollow tubes attached one on each side of the uterus, through which the egg travels from the ovary to the uterus. Fertilization usually occurs in the fallopian tube. The fallopian tube is the most common site of ectopic pregnancy.

Fecundity. Probability of conception occurring in a given period of time, usually 1 month.

Fertility drugs. Drugs that stimulate the ovaries to produce and mature eggs so that they can be released at ovulation.

Fertilization. Fusion of the sperm and the egg.

Fetoscopy. Inspection of the fetus before birth by passing a special fiberoptic instrument (fetoscope) through the abdomen of a pregnant woman into her uterus, allowing visualization of the fetus for abnormalities.

Fetus. An unborn child.

Fibroid. Benign (noncancerous) tumor of the uterine muscle wall that can cause abnormal uterine bleeding; also known as leiomyoma or myoma.

Fimbriae. The flared end (fingers) of the fallopian tube that sweep over the surface of the ovary and help to direct the egg into the tube.

Follicle. Fluid-filled sac located just beneath the surface of the ovary, containing an egg (oocyte) and cells that produce hormones. The sac increases in size and volume during the first half of the menstrual cycle. At ovulation, the follicle matures and ruptures, releasing the egg. As the follicle matures, it can be visualized by ultrasound.

Follicle-stimulating hormone (FSH). In women, FSH is the pituitary hormone responsible for stimulating follicular cells in the ovary to grow, stimulating egg development and the production of the female hormone estrogen. In men, FSH is the pituitary hormone that travels through the bloodstream to the testes and helps stimulate the manufacture of sperm. FSH can also be given as a medication; brand names are Metrodin and Fertinex.

Follicular phase. First half of the menstrual cycle (beginning on day one of bleeding), during which the dominant follicle grows, matures, and secretes large amounts of estrogen.

Galactorrhea. A small amount of breast milk production by a woman who is not nursing, caused by elevated levels of the pituitary hormone prolactin.

Gamete intrafallopian transfer (GIFT). An assisted reproductive technology that involves surgically removing eggs from a woman's ovary, combining them with sperm, and immediately injecting the eggs/sperm mixture into the fallopian tube. Fertilization then hopefully takes place inside the fallopian tube, as it does in nature. One disadvantage of GIFT is the inability to know whether or not fertilization took place if the woman does not become pregnant.

Gamete. Any germ cell, whether ovum (oocyte) or sperm.

Genes. Structures located on chromosomes that contain 'blueprints' for inherited characteristics.

Genetic. Referring to inherited conditions, usually due to the genes located on the chromosomes.

Genetic testing. See Karyotyping.

Gestation. Pregnancy.

Gestational carrier. A woman who carries an embryo to delivery. The embryo is derived from the egg and the sperm of persons not related to the carrier; therefore the carrier has no genetic relationship with the resulting child.

Gestational sac. Fluid-filled sac surrounding an embryo that develops within the uterine cavity. Ultrasound can detect the sac in the uterus at a very early stage of pregnancy.

Gonadotropin-releasing hormone (Gn-RH). Natural hormone secreted by the hypothalamus that prompts the pituitary gland to release follicle-stimulating hormone (FSH) and luteinizing-hormone (LH) into the bloodstream. This in turn stimulates the ovaries to produce estrogen and progesterone and to ovulate. Factrel and Lutrepulse are trade names.

Gonadotropin-releasing hormone (Gn-RH) agonists. Synthetic hormones similar to natural Gn-RH secreted by the hypothalamus. When given in short pulses, Gn-RH agonists stimulate FSH and LH production by the pituitary gland. However, when given in more prolonged doses, they decrease FSH and LH production by the pituitary, which in turn decreases ovarian hormone production.

Gonadotropin-releasing hormone (Gn-RH) analog. A long-acting drug that blocks the release of hormones, stops ovulation, and decreases the body's production of estrogen. Prolonged use of Gn-RH analogs causes decreased hormone production and menopausal levels of estrogen. Some trade names include Lupron, Depo Lupron, Synarel, and Zolodex.

Gonadotropin. Follicle-stimulating hormone (FSH) and luteinizing hormone (LH). FSH and LH may be purified or synthetically produced to be used as ovulatory drugs. Pergonal, Humegon, and Metrodin are trade names.

Gonorrhea. A sexually transmitted disease caused by the gonococcus bacterium that can cause pelvic infections, scar tissue, and tubal damage in women. In men, gonorrhea can cause obstructions in the ducts that transport sperm.

Hamster egg penetration test. See Sperm penetration assay.

Heparin. A blood-thinning medication given by injection, sometimes used in treating disorders causing repeat miscarriages (e.g., antiphospholipid antibodies).

Hirsutism. The growth of long, coarse hair on the face, chest, upper arms, and upper legs of women in a pattern similar to that of men.

Home study. Part of the adoptive process, either public or private, in which an adoption worker examines the home environment where the adoptive child will be placed.

Hormones. Substances secreted from organs of the body, such as the pituitary gland, adrenal gland, or ovaries, that are carried by a bodily fluid, such as blood, to other organs or tissues where the substances exert a specific action.

Hormone replacement therapy. Use of synthetic hormonal medications (estrogen sometimes with progesterone) to substitute for the natural hormones that are lost due to menopause.

Huhner test. See postcoital test.

Human chorionic gonadotropin (hCG). A hormone that increases early in pregnancy; it is produced by the placental tissue. Its detection is the basis of pregnancy tests. It can also be used as an luteinizing hormone (LH) substitute to trigger ovulation in conjunction with clomiphene or gonadotropin therapy.

Human immunodeficiency virus (HIV). A retrovirus that causes acquired immune deficiency syndrome (AIDS), a disease that destroys the body's ability to protect itself from infection and disease. It is transmitted by the exchange of bodily fluids or blood transfusions.

Human menopausal gonadotropins (hMG). Fertility drug containing follicle-stimulating hormone (FSH) and luteinizing hormone (LH). It is derived from the urine of postmenopausal women. Trade names are Pergonal, Humegon, and Metrodin.

Humegon. See Gonadotropins and Human menopausal gonadotropins (hMG).

Husband insemination (HI). Procedure in which sperm from a woman's partner is placed into her reproductive tract for the purpose of increasing the chance of pregnancy. Also known as artificial insemination from husband (AIH).

Hydramnios. Presence of abnormally large amount of amniotic fluid surrounding the fetus after about the fifth month of pregnancy.

Hyperemesis gravidarum. Severe vomiting during pregnancy.

Hyperstimulation syndrome. A constellation of signs and symptoms which indicate excessive stimulation of the ovaries with effects ranging from mild discomfort to severe complications.

Hysterectomy. Surgical removal of the uterus. It may be performed through an abdominal incision (laparotomy), through the vagina (vaginal hysterectomy), or through laparoscopy-assisted vaginal hysterectomy (LAVH). Sometimes, the ovaries and fallopian tubes are also removed.

Hysterosalpingography. An x-ray procedure in which a special iodine-containing solution is injected through the cervix into the uterine cavity to illustrate the inner shape of the uterus and degree of openness (patency) of the fallopian tubes.

Hysteroscopy. Insertion of a long, thin, lighted telescope-like instrument, called a hysteroscope, through the cervix and into the uterus to examine the inside of the uterus. Hysteroscopy can be used to both diagnose and surgically treat uterine conditions.

Identified adoption. An adoption in which the prospective adoptive parents locate a child or birth parents and utilize the services of an agency to assist with and finalize the adoption; also known as agency-assisted adoption.

Idiopathic. Unexplained.

Immunologic factors. Antibodies or allergic responses that may cause certain types of infertility.

Implantation. Process whereby an embryo embeds in the uterine lining in order to obtain nutrition and oxygen. Sometimes, an embryo will implant in areas other than the uterus, such as in a fallopian tube. This is known as an ectopic pregnancy.

Impotence. Inability of a male to achieve or maintain an erection.

In vitro fertilization (IVF). A method of assisted reproduction that involves combining an egg with sperm in a laboratory dish. If the egg fertilizes and begins cell division, the resulting embryo is transferred into the woman's uterus, where it can implant in the uterine lining and further develop. IVF is generally performed in conjunction with medications that stimulate the ovaries to produce multiple eggs in order to increase the chances of successful fertilization and implantation. IVF bypasses the fallopian tubes and is often the treatment choice for women who have badly damaged or absent tubes.

Incompetent cervix. A cervix (the narrow, lower end of the uterus) that is incapable of staying closed and holding a pregnancy without surgical correction.

Independent or private adoption. An adoption that takes place outside an agency. It is usually facilitated by a lawyer, minister, and/or physician who serves as an intermediary between the birth parents and the adoptive parents.

Infertility. Infertility is the result of a disease of the male or female reproductive tract that prevents the conception of a child or the ability to carry a pregnancy to delivery. The duration of unprotected intercourse with failure to conceive should be about 12 months or more before an investigation is undertaken, unless medical history, age, and physical findings dictate earlier evaluation and treatment.

Infertility work-up. Series of tests performed to determine the cause(s) of infertility.

Insemination. Placement of sperm via a syringe into a woman's uterus or cervix for the purpose of producing a pregnancy.

International adoption. Adoption of a child from a country other than that of the adoptive parents.

Interracial adoption. Adoption of a child of a race other than that of the adoptive parents.

Intracervical insemination (ICI). Placement of semen via a syringe directly into the cervical canal.

Intracytoplasmic sperm injection (ICSI). A micromanipulation technique that involves injecting a sperm directly into an egg in order to facilitate fertilization.

Intramural fibroid. Fibroid located in the muscular wall of the uterus.

Intrauterine device (IUD). Contraceptive device placed within the uterus; also sometimes used to prevent scar tissue formation following uterine surgery.

Intrauterine insemination (IUI). Process whereby a sperm preparation is injected directly into the uterine cavity in order to bypass the cervix and place the sperm closer to the egg. The sperm are usually washed first to remove chemicals that can irritate the uterine lining and to increase sperm motility and concentration.

Intrauterine pregnancy. An embryo that has implanted appropriately on the wall of the uterus.

Irritable bowel syndrome (IBS). Bowel condition associated with alternating diarrhea and constipation and bowel discomfort. IBS may be aggravated by stress and may improve with changes in the diet.

Karyotyping. A blood or tissue test that analyzes a person's chromosomes.

Klinefelter's syndrome. Chromosomal anomaly (47,XXY), congenital endocrine condition of primary testicular failure, usually not evident prior to puberty. Testes small and firm, gynecomastia, abnormally long legs, and subnormal intelligence usually present. Occurs in 1 of 700 live male births.

Laparoscopy. Insertion of a long, thin, lighted, telescope-like instrument, called a laparoscope, into the abdomen through an incision, usually in the navel, to visually inspect the organs in the abdominal cavity. Other small incisions may also be made and additional instruments inserted to facilitate diagnosis and allow surgical correction of abnormalities. The surgeon can sometimes remove scar tissue and open closed fallopian tubes during this procedure. This is usually out-patient, same-day surgery.

Laparotomy. Major abdominal surgery through an incision in the abdominal wall.

Leiomyoma. See Fibroid and Myoma.

Lesion. A growth or abnormality of normal anatomy. Examples include scar tissue, polyps, and uterine fibroids.

LH surge. Rapid rise of luteinizing hormone (LH) released by the pituitary gland in the middle of the menstrual cycle to trigger ovulation.

Libido. Sexual drive and desire.

Lupron. Trade name of leuprolide acetate. See Gonadotropin-releasing hormone (Gn-RH) analog.

Luteal phase. Second half of the menstrual cycle after ovulation when the corpus luteum secretes large amounts of progesterone, important in preparing the endometrium to receive an embryo for implantation.

Luteal phase defect. A shorter than normal luteal phase or one with a progesterone deficit; a condition present when the lining of the uterus (endometrium) does not mature or develop properly in response to progesterone secretion by the ovaries after ovulation. A luteal phase defect can result in early pregnancy loss.

Luteinizing hormone (LH). In women, the pituitary hormone that triggers ovulation and stimulates the corpus luteum of the ovary to secrete progesterone and other hormones during the second half of the menstrual cycle. In men, LH is the pituitary hormone that stimulates the testes to produce the male hormone testosterone.

Macrosomia. A fetus of abnormally large size usually associated with diabetes.

Male factor. A problem in the male reproductive tract that may result in infertility; for example, inability to ejaculate or insufficient number of sperm (low sperm count).

Mammogram. An x-ray examination of the breasts.

Marriage and family therapist. Mental health professional who has earned a graduate degree (masters (MA) or doctorate (PhD)) in marriage and family therapy.

Maternal serum AFP. Noninvasive prenatal testing involving blood testing AFP (alphafetoprotein, chorionic gonadotropin (hCG), and estriol (Ue3/Ue4)).

Menarche. Age at which an adolescent female experiences her first menstrual period. The average age of menarche is approximately 12.8 years in the United States.

Menometrorrhagia. Heavy or irregular bleeding during and between menstrual periods.

Menopause. Natural cessation of ovarian function and menstruation. It can occur between ages 42 and 56 but usually occurs around age 51, when the ovaries stop producing eggs and estrogen levels decline.

Menorrhagia. Regular but heavy menstrual bleeding that is excessive in either amount (greater than 80 cc—approximately five tablespoons) or duration (greater than 7 days).

Mental Health Professional Group (MHPG). Society affiliated with the American Society of Reproductive Medicine (ASRM) comprised of mental health professionals working in the field of reproductive medicine. Formerly known as the Psychological Special Interest Group (PSIG) and Psychological Aspects of Infertility Special Interest Group (PAISIG).

Methotrexate. Medication that hastens reabsorption of tissue in a woman with an ectopic pregnancy.

Metrodin. Trade name of an ovulation-induction drug containing follicle-stimulating hormone (FSH). See also FSH.

Metrorrhagia. Irregular bleeding from the uterus between normal menstrual periods.

Microdeletion. When part of a chromosome is missing.

Microinsemination. The IVF laboratory process whereby a small number of sperm are concentrated and placed close to the eggs to maximize the chance of fertilization.

Micromanipulation. Manipulation of eggs, sperm, and embryos with the aid of a microscope. Micromanipulation techniques to facilitate fertilization include injection of a single sperm into an egg (intracytoplasmic sperm injection [ICSI]), injection of sperm under the membrane surrounding the egg (subzonal injection [SUZI]), and drilling a small hole in the membrane to allow the sperm easier access to the egg (partial zonal dissection [PZD]). Embryos may be micromanipulated before embryo transfer. The two most common embryo micromanipulation procedures are assisted hatching and embryo biopsy. Assisted hatching is a procedure in which the zona pellucida (outer covering) of the embryo is partially disrupted, usually by injection of acid, to facilitate embryo implantation and pregnancy. Embryo biopsy is a procedure in which one or more cells are removed from the embryo

596

for the purposes of preimplantation genetic diagnosis.

Microsurgery. Type of surgery that uses magnification, meticulous technique, and fine suture material to get precise surgical results. Microsurgery is important for certain types of tubal surgery in women, as well as for vasectomy reversal in men.

Microsurgical epididymal sperm aspiration (MESA). Surgical removal of sperm directly from the epididymis thereby bypassing the vas deferens and/or need for ejaculation.

Miscarriage. The naturally occurring expulsion of a nonviable fetus and placenta from the uterus; also known as spontaneous abortion or pregnancy loss.

Mittelschmerz. A pain in the lower abdomen that is associated with ovulation.

Morphology. The form, structure, and shape of sperm.

Mosaicism. Condition in which the cells of an individual do not all contain identical chromosomes. In affected individuals, the chromosome defect is usually not fully exposed.

Motility. Percentage of all moving sperm in a semen sample. Normally, 50% or more are moving rapidly.

Müllerian anomalies. Congenital abnormalities (birth defects) of the female reproductive organs that are derived from the müllerian ducts.

Müllerian duct system. A pair of ducts parallel to the vertebrae in embryonic life. They develop into the female reproductive tract (fallopian tubes, uterus, cervix, and upper vagina).

Müllerian dysgenesis. Birth defect in which the internal female reproductive organs do not develop completely, generally leading to the absence (agenesis) of the uterus, cervix, and upper part of the vagina; also known as Rokitansky-Küster-Hauser syndrome or Rokitansky syndrome.

Multifetal pregnancy reduction (MPR) or selective reduction. Procedure to reduce the number of fetuses in the uterus that may be considered for women who are pregnant with multiple fetuses. As the risk of extreme premature delivery, miscarriage (spontaneous abortion), and other problems increases with the number of fetuses present, this procedure may be performed in an attempt to prevent the entire pregnancy from aborting or severe health problems in the mother.

Myoma. Benign (noncancerous) tumor of the uterine muscle wall that can cause abnormal uterine bleeding and miscarriage. See also Fibroid.

Neural tube defect. Incomplete closure of the spine during fetal development that may involve an opening of the spine and protrusion of spinal cord contents, also known as spina bifida and anencephaly

Neurotransmitter. Chemical substance released from nerve endings that transmits impulses between the nerves and the muscles or glands that they supply.

Neurotropic. Affecting neural tissue, usually viruses, chemicals, or toxins.

Oligo-ovulatory. Infrequent ovulation.

Oligomenorrhea. Light or infrequent uterine bleeding occurring at intervals of greater than 35 days.

Oocyte. Egg; also called ovum.

Oophorectomy. Surgical removal of an ovary.

Open adoption. Adoption in which information is exchanged between birth parents and adoptive parents.

Operative hysteroscopy. Surgery, such as removal of adhesions or tumors, performed inside the uterus using a hysteroscope.

Operative laparoscopy. Surgery, such as removal of adhesions or endometriosis, performed inside the abdomen with a laparoscope and other long, slender instruments. The surgeon can sometimes cut and remove scar tissue and open closed fallopian tubes during this procedure.

Oral contraceptive (birth control pills). Pills containing a mixture of synthetic estrogen and progestin. Proper usage prevents pregnancy by suppressing ovulation and decreasing the ovarian secretion of hormones, including androgens.

Ova (plural of ovum). Eggs.

Ovarian cyst. Fluid-filled cyst on the ovaries.

Ovarian hyperstimulation syndrome (OHS). Condition that may result from ovulation induction, characterized by enlargement of the ovaries, fluid retention, and weight gain.

Ovaries. The paired female sex glands in the pelvis, located one on each side of the uterus. They produce eggs and hormones including estrogen, progesterone, and androgens.

Ovulation. Release of a mature egg from its developing follicle in the outer layer of the ovary. This usually occurs approximately 14 days preceding the next menstrual period (the 14th day of a 28-day cycle). This is triggered by the patient's own LH surge or by an injection of human chorionic gonadotropin (hCG).

Ovulation detection kit. Commercially available kits using paper dipsticks that show changes in the levels of luteinizing hormone (LH) in the urine. Once the LH surge has occurred, ovulation usually takes place within 12–44 hours. Urine testing usually begins 2 days prior to the expected day of ovulation.

Ovulation induction. Administration of hormone medications (ovulation drugs) to stimulate the ovaries to ovulate.

Partial salpingectomy. Operation in which the section of a fallopian tube containing an ectopic pregnancy is removed. This procedure attempts to preserve most of the tube for subsequent reattachment using microsurgery in order to maintain future fertility.

PCOS. See Polycystic ovarian syndrome.

Pelvic inflammatory disease (PID). Infection in the uterus, fallopian tubes, and ovary that may cause pain and scar tissue formation (adhesions).

Pergonal. See Gonadotropins and Human menopausal gonadotropins (hMG).

Perimenopausal transition. The end of a woman's reproductive years, when the ovaries lose their ability to secrete estrogen and progesterone in a regular fashion.

Perimenopause. The years that immediately precede cessation of menstrual periods (menopause); usually about 5 years before menopause.

Perinatologist. A maternal–fetal medicine specialist.

Peritoneum. The smooth transparent membrane that lines the abdominal and pelvic cavities.

Pituitary adenoma. Benign (noncancerous) tumor of the pituitary gland often associated with excessive prolactin production.

Pituitary gland. A small hormone-producing gland just beneath the hypothalamus in the brain, which controls the ovaries, thyroid, and adrenal glands. Ovarian function is controlled through the secretion of follicle-stimulating hormone (FSH) and luteinizing hormone (LH). Disorders of this gland may lead to irregular or absent ovulation in women and abnormal or absent sperm production in men.

Placenta. Disk-shaped vascular organ attached to the wall of the uterus and to the fetus by the umbilical cord. It provides nourishment to the fetus.

Placenta previa. During pregnancy, the placenta rests in the lower part of the uterus, typically near the cervix, potentially causing bleeding and hemorrhaging.

Polycystic ovarian disease (PCOD). See Polycystic ovarian syndrome.

Polycystic ovarian syndrome (PCOS). Condition in which the ovaries contain many cystic follicles that are associated with chronic anovulation and overproduction of androgens (male hormones). The cystic follicles exist presumably because the eggs are not expelled at the time of ovulation. Symptoms may include irregular menstrual periods, obesity, excessive growth of central body hair (hirsutism), and infertility. It can also be associated with heart disease, hypertension, or diabetes; also called Stein-Leventhal syndrome.

Polymenorrhea. Uterine bleeding occurring at regular intervals of fewer than 21 days.

Polyp. General term describing any mass of tissue that bulges or projects outward or upward from the normal surface level.

Postcoital test (PCT). Microscopic analysis of a sample of cervical mucus, usually collected within 18 hours after intercourse, for the purpose of determining the quality of cervical mucus, the number of sperm, and the ability of sperm to enter and penetrate the mucus; also called the Huhner test.

Postmenopausal. Term used to refer to the time after menopause.

Preimplantation genetic diagnosis (PGD). Screening of embryos for genetic disorders before implantation involving IVF, embryo biopsy, and molecular genetic testing.

Premature ovarian failure (POF). Cessation of menstrual periods due to failure of the ovaries before age 40; also known as early menopause.

Primary dysmenorrhea. Lower abdominal pain associated with menstrual periods that decreases with age.

Private adoption. Adoption that takes place outside an agency. It is usually facilitated by a lawyer, minister, or physician who serves as an intermediary between the potential birth parents and the adoptive parents.

Progestational agent. Any medication that mimics the effect of progesterone.

Progesterone. Female hormone normally secreted by the corpus luteum after ovulation during the second half of the menstrual cycle (luteal phase). It prepares the lining of the uterus (endometrium) for implantation of a fertilized egg and also allows complete shedding of the endometrium at the time of menstruation. In the event of pregnancy, the progesterone level remains stable beginning a week or so after conception.

Progestin. Synthetic hormone that has an action similar to progesterone; synonymous with progestational hormones.

Prolactin. Hormone secreted by the pituitary gland into the bloodstream for the purpose of maintaining milk production during lactation. When secreted in excessive amounts, it may lead to irregular or absent menstrual periods and may produce a milk-like discharge from the breasts. See galactorrhea

Pronuclear stage. Early stage of fertilization when the sperm has penetrated the egg but before cell division has begun: The nucleus of the sperm and the nucleus of the egg (pronuclei) are visible under a microscope. The pronuclei contain the genetic material. The egg and sperm pronuclei later fuse to establish the correct number of chromosomes for a human.

Pronuclear stage transfer (PROST). See Zygote intrafallopian transfer (ZIFT).

Prostaglandin. Any of a class of acids found throughout the body, especially in semen, that stimulate smooth muscle and affect blood pressure, metabolism, body temperature, and other body processes. In women, prostaglandins are hormone-like chemicals produced in large amounts by endometrial cells. They stimulate the uterine muscles to contract and are largely responsible for menstrual cramps.

Prostate gland. Gland located below the bladder in men where the ejaculatory ducts and the urethra join. It also contributes fluid to the ejaculate.

Proximal tubal blockage. Tubal blockage that occurs near where the fallopian tubes join the uterus.

Pseudomenopause. Hormonal state created by taking medication that mimics the symptoms of menopause and characterized by low estrogen levels similar to those found at menopause.

Psychiatric nurse. Mental health professional who has a nursing degree and has completed additional graduate level training in psychiatric nursing.

Psychiatrist. Mental health professional who completed medical school and a residency (special training) in psychiatry. Psychiatrists as physicians are the only mental health professionals typically able to prescribe medications.

Psychologist. Mental health professional who has earned a graduate degree (typically a doctorate (PhD)) in a field of psychology. Psychologists are the only mental health professionals qualified to perform psychological testing.

Pubis. The bony region at the base of the abdomen.

Radiation therapy. Treatment with high-energy rays to kill or damage cancer cells. External radiation therapy uses a machine to aim high-energy rays at the cancer growth. Internal radiation therapy is the placement of radioactive material inside the body as close as possible to the cancer.

Recipient. A woman/couple that receives donated eggs, sperm, or embryos.

Recurrent miscarriage. Consecutive pregnancy loss (two or three) before 20 weeks gestation. The fetus usually weighs less than 1 pound.

Retrograde ejaculation. Condition that causes the ejaculate to be released backward into the bladder at male climax.

Reversible menopause. Temporary hormonal state, created by taking Gn-RH analogs, in which estrogen levels fall to menopause levels, ovulation does not occur, endometrium does not grow, and menstruation does not occur.

Rh factor. Condition determined by heredity and present in red blood cells. It may cause adverse reactions during pregnancy if a woman without an Rh factor (Rh negative) has become sensitized to the Rh factor and the fetus is Rh positive.

Rheumatoid arthritis. Chronic autoimmune disease of the joints characterized by inflammation, discomfort, and deterioration of the bones.

Rokitansky-Küster-Hauser syndrome. See Müllerian dysgenesis, also known as Rokitansky syndrome. Congenital endocrine syndrome affecting 1 in 4000 to 5000, causing amenorrhea as a result of absences of the uterus, cervix, and/or upper portion of the vagina.

Salpingectomy. Operation in which one or both of the fallopian tubes are removed.

Salpingo-oophorectomy. Removal of the fallopian tube and ovary together.

SART Registry. Ongoing collection of results from participating assisted reproductive technology clinics in the United States developed and maintained by the Society for Assisted Reproductive Technology (SART), a society affiliated with the American Society for Reproductive Medicine (ASRM).

Scrotum. Pouch of skin and other tissues that contain the testes in males.

Secondary dysmenorrhea. Lower abdominal pain associated with menstrual periods that begins later in a woman's reproductive life span. It may be due to an abnormal condition such as endometriosis or infection.

Semen. Sperm and fluid that come out of the urethra when a man ejaculates.

Semen analysis. Microscopic examination of semen to determine the number of sperm (sperm count), their shapes (morphology), and their ability to move (motility).

Semen viscosity. Thickness of semen. Semen is ejaculated as a liquid, becomes jelly-like, and then turns to liquid again.

Semen volume. Amount of semen. The normal amount of semen per ejaculate is 2–5 milliliters (approximately one teaspoon).

Seminal plasma. Fluid in which the sperm is ejaculated. Seminal plasma makes up most of the fluid volume of semen.

Seminal vesicles. Two oblong glands located behind the bladder that join each vas deferens and empty into the urethra. They contribute about 90% of the fluid volume of semen.

Septate uterus. Congenital abnormality (birth defect) in which the uterus has a normal-appearing outer surface but has a central wall of fibrous tissue (septum) within the uterine cavity.

Serophene. See Clomiphene citrate.

Sexually transmitted diseases (STDs). Infections, such as chlamydiosis or gonorrhea, that are transmitted by sexual activity. In women, some STDs can cause pelvic infections and lead to infertility by damaging the fallopian tubes and increasing the risk of ectopic pregnancy. In men, STDs can cause blockage of the ductal system that transports sperm.

Social worker. Mental health professional who has earned a graduate degree (masters (MA) or doctorate (PhD)) in social work.

Society for Assisted Reproductive Technology (SART). A society affiliated with the American Society for Reproductive Medicine (ASRM) and comprising representatives from assisted reproductive technology programs that have demonstrated their ability to perform IVF and other assisted reproductive technologies.

Sonogram. Image produced by ultrasound, using high-frequency sound waves to form a picture of internal organs on a monitor screen.

Sonohysterography. Technique involving injection of fluid into the uterus and fallopian tubes and using ultrasound to observe the image of these structures on a monitor screen.

Special-needs adoption. Adoption of a child who has special health or emotional needs.

Sperm. The male reproductive cells that fertilize a woman's egg. The sperm head carries genetic material (chromosomes), the midpiece produces energy for movement, and the long, thin tail wiggles to propel the sperm.

Sperm antibody test. Test in which blood, semen, or cervical mucus is examined to detect antibodies to sperm. Antibodies can contribute to infertility in men or women.

Sperm autoimmunity. Allergy to sperm that may be present in a man against his own sperm. This can lead to abnormalities of sperm function and infertility.

Sperm capacitation. Laboratory process for increasing the ability of sperm to penetrate and fertilize an egg.

Sperm count. Number of sperm per milliliter of semen. A normal count is usually 20 million or more per milliliter.

Sperm morphology. The shape of individual sperm as seen under a microscope. At least 50% of the sperm in a routine semen analysis should have oval heads and slightly curving tails.

Sperm motility. Percentage of all moving sperm in a semen sample. Normally, 50% or more are moving rapidly.

Sperm penetration assay. Test to help evaluate the fertilizing ability of a man's sperm. A semen sample is incubated with specially treated hamster eggs to determine whether or not the sperm can penetrate them.

Sperm washing. Procedure for removing seminal fluid from sperm cells before intrauterine insemination (IUI) or other assisted reproductive technologies.

Spermatogenesis. Process whereby mature spermatozoa are produced in the testes.

Spina bifida. See neural tube defects.

Stein-Leventhal syndrome. See polycystic ovarian syndrome.

Superovulation with timed intrauterine insemination. Procedure for facilitating fertilization whereby a woman is given ovulation-inducing drugs that cause her ovaries to produce multiple eggs. When the eggs are ready to be released, the woman is inseminated with her partner's sperm or donated sperm.

Surrogacy/surrogate. In traditional surrogacy, a woman (surrogate) is inseminated with the sperm of a man who is not her partner in order to conceive and carry a child to be reared by the biologic (genetic) father and his partner. In this procedure, the surrogate is genetically related to the child. The biologic father and his partner must usually adopt the child after its birth. Another type of surrogate is a gestational carrier, a woman who is implanted with the fertilized egg (embryo) of another couple in order to carry the pregnancy. The gestator is not genetically related to the child in this case.

Tay-Sachs disease. A fatal heredity disorder characterized by mental retardation and paralysis. This condition is most common in offspring from Jewish couples.

Testes. The two male reproductive glands located in the scrotum that produce testosterone and sperm.

Testicular sperm extraction (TESE). Also known as testicular sperm aspiration (TSA). Surgical removal of sperm directly from the testes thereby bypassing the vas deferens and/or need for ejaculation.

Testosterone. In men, the primary male hormone produced by the testes; it is responsible for the development of sperm, male physical characteristics, and sex drive. It is also produced in small quantities by the ovaries in women.

Tocolytics. Medications used to prevent preterm labor.

Traditional surrogate. See Surrogacy/surrogate.

Transcervical balloon tuboplasty. A method of treatment for fallopian tube obstruction which utilizes the hysteroscope or the fluoroscope.

Transvaginal ultrasound. Imaging technique using a smooth cylindrical probe placed in the vagina and sound waves to view organs on a monitor screen.

Transvaginal ultrasound aspiration. Ultrasound-guided technique for egg retrieval. A long, thin needle is passed through the vagina into the ovarian follicle, and suction is applied to retrieve the egg; also known as ultrasound-guided egg aspiration and transvaginal egg retrieval.

Tubal (ectopic) pregnancy. A fertilized egg that implants within the fallopian tube rather than the uterine cavity. Under these conditions, the tube can rupture and bleed. Tubal pregnancies can be fatal if they are not identified and treated early.

Tubal embryo transfer (TET). Process whereby a fertilized and dividing egg (early cleavage stage embryo) is transferred to the fallopian tube.

Tubal ligation. Surgical procedure in which the fallopian tubes are clamped, clipped, or cut to prevent pregnancy.

Tubal reanastomosis. Reconnection of the fallopian tubes, usually after tubal ligation, often utilizing microsurgical techniques.

Turner's syndrome. Condition in which the female has only one X chromosome instead of two. It is associated with short stature, failure to undergo normal sexual development, and other physical abnormalities.

Ultrasound. Imaging technique in which a picture of internal organs is produced by high-frequency sound waves and viewed on a video screen; it is used to monitor growth of ovarian follicles or a fetus and to retrieve eggs. It can be performed either abdominally or vaginally. Also known as sonogram.

Ultrasound-guided egg aspiration (retrieval). Technique in which an ultrasound-guided needle is passed into the ovary and an egg is removed by suction. Usually, the needle is passed through the vagina; also known as transvaginal ultrasound aspiration.

Unicornuate uterus. Congenital abnormality (birth defect) in which only one-half of the uterus is formed from only one-half of the müllerian duct system. See Rokitansky syndrome.

Ureter. Tube connecting each kidney to the bladder, often abnormal in women with müllerian duct defects or men with an absent vas deferens.

Urethra. In men, the tube leading from the bladder that carries urine and semen out of the body. In women, the tube leading from the bladder that carries urine out of the body.

Uterine fibroid. Abnormal mass of smooth muscle tissue (noncancerous tumor) that grows within the uterine wall; also called fibroid, myoma, or leiomyoma.

Uterus (womb). The hollow, muscular female reproductive organ in the pelvis where an embryo implants and grows during pregnancy. The lining of the uterus, called the endometrium, produces the monthly menstrual blood flow when there is no pregnancy.

Vagina. The canal in the female that leads to the cervix, which leads to the uterus.

Vaginal hysterectomy. Removal of the uterus through the vagina.

Vaginal suppository. A soluble cone of medicated material inserted into the vagina.

Vaginoplasty. Surgical creation of a vagina.

Varicocele. A varicose or dilated vein within the scrotum that can cause infertility in some men.

Vas deferens. The two muscular tubes that carry sperm from the epididymis to the urethra.

Vasectomy. Surgical procedure to sever the vas deferens (tubes leading from the testes to the urethra), usually for the purposes of sterilization. Although vasovasotomy can be performed to reconnect the severed ends, sperm antibodies may have developed in the interim causing infertility.

Vasoepididymostomy. Surgical procedure to connect the vas deferens to the epididymis in order to bypass an obstruction in the epididymis, sometimes used for vasectomy reversal.

Vasovasostomy. Surgical procedure to reconnect the severed ends of the vas deferens; often called vasectomy reversal.

Viable intrauterine pregnancy. An embryo that has implanted appropriately in the wall of the uterus and appears to be growing well.

Vulva. Outer lips of the vagina.

Zona pellucida. The egg's tough outer layer that functions somewhat like a shell. Sperm must penetrate this 'shell' in order to fertilize the egg.

Zygote. A fertilized egg before cell division (cleavage) begins.

Zygote intrafallopian transfer (ZIFT). An assisted reproductive technology procedure in which eggs are collected and combined in a laboratory dish with sperm, and the resulting zygote is then transferred to the fallopian tube at the pronuclear stage.

(Used with permission of the American Society of Reproductive Medicine. Birmingham, AL, 1997)

Subject Index

Author Index